Handbook of Renal Biopsy Pathology

Handbook of Renal Biopsy Pathology

Edited by Ricardo Clinton

hayle medical

New York

Hayle Medical,
750 Third Avenue, 9th Floor,
New York, NY 10017, USA

Visit us on the World Wide Web at:
www.haylemedical.com

ISBN: 978-1-63241-659-9

The publisher's policy is to use permanent paper from mills that operate a sustainable forestry policy. Furthermore, the publisher ensures that the text paper and cover boards used have met acceptable environmental accreditation standards.

Printed in China.

Cataloging-in-Publication Data

Handbook of renal biopsy pathology / edited by Ricardo Clinton.
p. cm.
Includes bibliographical references and index.
ISBN 978-1-63241-659-9
1. Kidneys--Biopsy. 2. Kidneys--Diseases. 3. Nephrology. 4. Pathology. I. Clinton, Ricardo.
RC903.9 .H36 2019
616.61--dc23

Table of Contents

Preface

Renal biopsy is a form of medical procedure in which a small piece of kidney is extracted from the body for examination. The examination is usually done under a microscope. It helps in the diagnosis, monitoring and the treatment of kidney problems. Renal biopsy is commonly used in those cases where other less invasive tests are insufficient. Haematuria, proteinuria, kidney failure or kidney tumor are some of the common cases in which a renal biopsy is performed. An ultrasound is usually performed before the biopsy to assess the current structure, position and condition of the kidneys. A nephrologist or interventional radiologist is the one who supervises and performs a renal biopsy. This book contains some path-breaking studies in the field of renal biopsy. It will also provide interesting topics for research which interested readers can take up. Those in search of information to further their knowledge will be greatly assisted by this book.

All of the data presented henceforth, was collaborated in the wake of recent advancements in the field. The aim of this book is to present the diversified developments from across the globe in a comprehensible manner. The opinions expressed in each chapter belong solely to the contributing authors. Their interpretations of the topics are the integral part of this book, which I have carefully compiled for a better understanding of the readers.

At the end, I would like to thank all those who dedicated their time and efforts for the successful completion of this book. I also wish to convey my gratitude towards my friends and family who supported me at every step.

Editor

1

Urinary and Plasma Levels of Vasohibin-1 Can Predict Renal Functional Deterioration in Patients with Renal Disorders

Norikazu Hinamoto[1], Yohei Maeshima[1,2]*, Daisuke Saito[1], Hiroko Yamasaki[1], Katsuyuki Tanabe[1], Tatsuyo Nasu[1], Hiroyuki Watatani[1], Haruyo Ujike[1], Masaru Kinomura[1], Hitoshi Sugiyama[1,3], Hikaru Sonoda[4], Yasufumi Sato[5], Hirofumi Makino[1]

1 Department of Medicine and Clinical Science, Okayama University Graduate School of Medicine, Dentistry and Pharmaceutical Sciences, Okayama, Japan, **2** Department of Chronic Kidney Disease and cardiovascular disease, Okayama University Graduate School of Medicine, Dentistry and Pharmaceutical Sciences, Okayama, Japan, **3** Center for Chronic Kidney Disease and Peritoneal Dialysis, Okayama University Graduate School of Medicine, Dentistry and Pharmaceutical Sciences, Okayama, Japan, **4** Discovery Research Laboratories, Shionogi, Osaka, Japan, **5** Department of Vascular Biology, Institute of Development, Aging, and Cancer, Tohoku University, Sendai, Japan

Abstract

Vasohibin-1 (VASH-1) is a negative feedback regulator of angiogenesis, and a small vasohibin-binding protein (SVBP) serves as its secretory chaperone and contributes to its antiangiogenic effects. In the present study, we aimed to define the clinical significance of VASH-1 and SVBP in patients with chronic kidney disease (CKD). We recruited 67 Japanese hospitalized patients with renal disorders with (n = 45) or without (n = 22) renal biopsy samples and 10 Japanese healthy controls. We evaluated the correlations between the plasma and urinary levels of VASH-1/VASH-1-SVBP complex/SVBP and the clinicopathological parameters. The plasma levels of VASH-1 were inversely correlated with age and systolic and diastolic blood pressure and positively correlated with crescent formation. Increased plasma and urinary levels of VASH-1 and VASH-1-SVBP complex were significantly correlated with worse renal outcomes. These results demonstrate an association between elevated urinary and plasma levels of VASH-1 and progressive decline of the renal function, thus suggesting a potential role for VASH-1 in predicting a worse renal prognosis in patients with renal disease, including CKD.

Editor: Valquiria Bueno, UNIFESP Federal University of São Paulo, Brazil

Funding: A portion of this study was supported by JSPS KAKENHI Grant Number (20590958, 23591193, YM) and the Cooperative Research Project Program of Joint Usage/Research Center at the Institute of Development, Aging and Cancer, Tohoku University (2010–2013, YM). The funders had no role in study design, data collection and analysis, decision to publish, or preparation of the manuscript.

* E-mail: ymaeshim@md.okayama-u.ac.jp

Introduction

Chronic kidney disease (CKD) is associated with an increased risk of end-stage renal disease (ESRD) and cardiovascular morbidity and mortality. Since the number of patients with ESRD is increasing worldwide, establishing biomarkers to predict renal functional deterioration and prevent the progression of CKD by initiating early medical intervention is required.

Glomerulosclerosis and tubulointerstitial alterations are the most common characteristic histological alterations observed in patients with renal disorders. In general, deterioration of the renal function correlates better with the degree of tubulointerstitial injury than do glomerular alterations [1]. Experimental and biopsy studies have shown that the loss of podocytes [2,3,4,5] and renal capillaries [6] is closely linked with the progression of CKD and renal scarring.

Vasohibin-1 (VASH-1), an endogenous angiogenesis inhibitor, was originally identified in a microarray analysis assessing genes up-regulated by vascular endothelial growth factor (VEGF)-A, a major pro-angiogenic factor [7], in endothelial cells [8]. The human VASH-1 protein is composed of 365 amino acid residues [8] and regulates the proliferation and migration of endothelial cells in an autocrine manner and thus is considered to be a negative feedback regulator of angiogenesis [8]. More recently, the critical role of VASH-1 in the maintenance of endothelial cells against cellular stressors and the regulatory mechanisms of its synthesis via posttranscriptional regulation mediated by the binding of HuR proteins to AU-rich elements in the 3′ untranslated region of VASH-1 mRNAs have been reported [9]. VASH-1 does not contain a classic signal sequence; rather, a small vasohibin-binding protein (SVBP) serves as its secretory chaperon and contributes to its antiangiogenic effects [10]. To date, no cell surface receptors for VASH-1 have been identified. The therapeutic efficacy of VASH-1 in experimental models of tumors, atherosclerosis, proliferative retinopathy [8,11,12] and diabetic nephropathy [13,14] has been reported. However, the circulating and urinary levels of VASH-1 in patients with renal disorders have not been examined to date.

In the present study, we aimed to elucidate the clinical significance of VASH-1 in patients with renal disorders. We determined the plasma, urinary levels of VASH-1 and evaluated the correlations between these parameters and clinical as well as histological variables. This is the first study to examine the clinical significance of VASH-1 in patients with renal disorders, indicating the potential of VASH-1 as a predictive biomarker for progressive renal functional deterioration.

Results

Characteristics of the study groups

The mean age of the patients was 50±18 years, the mean estimated glomerular filtration rate (eGFR) was 60.3±34.7 mL/min/1.73 m^2 and the mean daily level of proteinuria was 2.1±2.9 g/day. The prevalence of hypertension, diabetes mellitus and dyslipidemia was 44%, 22% and 57%, respectively (Table 1). Only the age (51±5 years, 1 unknown), gender (Male 5/Female 4, 1 unknown), and VASH-1-related data were available for the healthy control subjects. The baseline clinical data of healthy controls and classified according to the renal disorder diagnosed by renal biopsies are shown in Table 2. No significant differences were observed among any of the groups. Due to the small number of patients in membranous nephropathy, minimal change, crescentic glomerulonephritis, lupus nephritis, diabetic nephropathy and nephrosclerosis, it was difficult to show the statistical significances among those disorders.

Correlations between the plasma and urinary levels of VASH-1 and various clinical/histological parameters

The plasma levels of VASH-1 detected using enzyme-linked immunosorbent assay (ELISA) were found to be inversely correlated with age and systolic/diastolic blood pressure (SBP/DBP) (Figure 1, panels A, C and E) but not with eGFR or daily proteinuria (Figure 1, panels G and I). The ratio of the urinary level of VASH-1 to creatinine (urinary levels of VASH-1) were not significantly correlated with age, SBP, DBP, eGFR or daily proteinuria (Figure 1, panels B, D, F, H and J). There were no significant correlations between the plasma and urinary levels of VASH-1 (data not shown). There were also no significant correlations between the plasma/urinary levels of VASH-1 and other clinical parameters (gender, body mass index, hemoglobin, HbA1c, fasting plasma glucose, total cholesterol, low-density lipoprotein cholesterol, high-density lipoprotein cholesterol and triglycerides) (data not shown).

The plasma levels of VASH-1 were positively correlated with the presence of crescent formation (Table 3). There were no significant differences in the plasma/urinary levels of VASH-1 among the patients with various renal disorders (Figure 2).

Correlations between the plasma/urinary levels of the VASH-1-SVBP complex and SVBP and various clinical/histological parameters

The plasma levels of the VASH-1-SVBP complex were positively correlated with the plasma levels of VASH-1. The urinary levels of the VASH-1-SVBP complex were positively correlated with the presence of mesangial hypercellularity and crescent formation and the urinary levels of VASH-1. The plasma and urinary levels of SVBP were inversely correlated with age (Table 4).

Correlation between VASH-1 and renal outcomes

The plasma and urinary levels of VASH-1 and the plasma levels of the VASH-1-SVBP complex were inversely correlated with the annual change rates in eGFR, with statistical significance (Table 5). The annual change rates were evaluated as follows: the annual change in eGFR was divided by the eGFR at baseline. We next performed a Kaplan-Meier analysis to evaluate the potential clinical usefulness of the plasma and urinary levels of VASH-1 and the plasma levels of the VASH-1-SVBP complex in predicting poor renal outcomes. The patients were stratified into two or three groups for the Kaplan-Meier analysis. The cutoff values (median)

Table 1. Clinical parameters of the patients with renal disorders ($n = 67$).

Age	50±18	(17–82)
Gender (male/female)	28/39	
BMI (kg/m^2)	23.6±3.7	(16.6–33.8)
SBP (mmHg)	130±20	(82–168)
DBP (mmHg)	77±13	(48–107)
Hemoglobin (g/dL)	12.5±2.1	(8.3–16.6)
HbA1c (NGSP) (%)	6.0±1.0	(4.8–9.8)
FPG (mg/dL)	111.8±39.0	(74–331)
T-cho (mg/dL)	227.8±80.7	(106–590)
LDL-C (mg/dL)	132.2±59.1	(29–417)
HDL-C (mg/dL)	60.1±24.5	(27–170)
TG (mg/dL)	149.4±87.5	(42–476)
eGFR (mL/min/1.73 m^2)	60.3±34.7	(6.1–132.4)
Daily proteinuria (g/day)	2.1±2.9	(0.0–13.1)
Hypertension (%)	43.9	
Diabetes mellitus (%)	22.2	
Dyslipidemia (%)	56.5	

Abbreviations: BMI, body mass index; DBP, diastolic blood pressure; eGFR, estimated glomerular filtration rate; FPG, fasting plasma glucose; HDL-C, high-density lipoprotein cholesterol; LDL-C, low-density lipoprotein cholesterol; NGSP, national glycohemoglobin standardization program; SBP, systolic blood pressure; T-cho, total cholesterol; TG: triglycerides. The values are presented as the means ± SD. The values in the parenthesis are minimum to maximum.

Table 2. Characteristics of the patients with renal biopsy and the control subjects (at baseline).

	n	Age (years)	sCr (mg/dL)	eGFR (mL/min/1.73 m^2)	Proteinuria (g/day)	SBP (mmHg)	DBP (mmHg)
Control	10	51±5	-	-	-	-	-
MN	3	66±11	1.2±0.4	57.1±22.2	4.9±3.4	145±10	92±2
MC	3	39±18	0.7±0.2	86.1±34.2	6.0±3.2	111±10	72±2
Crescentic GN	5	64±10	1.2±0.4	53.4±22.4	0.5±0.5	126±11	75±11
IgA N	15	40±16	0.8±0.4	79.0±24.1	0.6±0.6	127±19	81±12
Lupus N	3	43±10	1.0±0.4	55.9±21.1	1.1±0.3	140±20	82±13
Diabetic N	2	65±1	1.0±0.2	59.8±14.3	3.1±1.0	147±9	68±10
Nephrosclerosis	3	65±2	0.6±0.1	88.2±25.8	0.1±0.0	144±5	76±20
Others	11	34±14	0.8±0.3	87.4±29.0	2.3±3.8	113±22	71±16

Abbreviations: DBP, diastolic blood pressure; eGFR, estimated glomerular filtration rate; GN, glomerulonephritis; MC, minimal change; MN, membranous nephropathy; N, nephropathy; SBP, systolic blood pressure; sCr, serum creat nine. The values are expressed as the means ± SD.

for the plasma and urinary levels of VASH-1 were set at 609 fmol/mL and 21 fmol/mg, respectively, and three groups (<316, 316 to 408 and >408 fmol/mL) were used for the Kaplan-Meier analysis of the plasma levels of the VASH-1-SVBP complex, as shown in Figure 3. We defined a composite renal event as an eGFR decline of greater than 30% from baseline, the initiation of renal replacement therapy or kidney disease-related death. The patients with elevated plasma levels of VASH-1 exhibited a significantly higher incidence of composite renal events and odds ratio than the patients with lower plasma levels of VASH-1 (Figure 3, panel A; Table 6). The patients with elevated urinary levels of VASH-1 also tended to experience a higher incidence of renal events and tended to show a lower odds ratio than the patients with lower urinary levels of VASH-1 (Figure 3, panel B; Table 6). The patients with the highest plasma levels of the VASH-1-SVBP complex exhibited a significantly higher incidence of composite renal events and odds ratio than the patients with the intermediate or the lowest plasma levels of the VASH-1-SVBP complex (Figure 3, panel C; Table 6). The changes in the eGFR and the number of the events in the overall patients and patients with classified renal disorders (diagnosed by renal biopsy) during the three-year follow-up are shown in Table 7. The clinical data for the overall patients and patients with classified renal disorders (diagnosed by renal biopsy) at the final follow-up (after three years) are shown in Tables S1 and S2 in File S1.

The characteristics of the patients classified by the plasma and urinary levels of VASH-1 and the plasma levels of the VASH-1-SVBP complex at baseline and at the final follow-up (after three years) are shown in Tables S3 and S4 in File S1. The follow-up data regarding the changes in the eGFR and the number of the events during the three years of follow-up in the patients classified by the plasma and urinary levels of VASH-1 and the plasma levels of the VASH-1-SVBP complex are shown in Table S5 in File S1. At baseline, the SBP was significantly lower in the group with elevated plasma levels of VASH-1 compared with the group with lower plasma levels of VASH-1 (Table S3 in File S1). Similarly, the SBP was significantly lower in the group with elevated plasma levels of VASH-1-SVBP complex compared with lower plasma levels (Table S3 in File S1). The group with elevated urinary levels of VASH-1 was older and exhibited lower renal function compared with the group with lower levels at both baseline and at all of the follow-up examinations (Tables S3, S4 and S5 in File S1).

The renal function was worse at every time point examined, and the number of composite renal events was greater in patients without a renal biopsy compared with patients who underwent a renal biopsy (Table 7). Most of the patients without renal biopsies were at CKD stage G3b to G5 at baseline. On the other hand, most of the patients who underwent renal biopsies were at CKD stage G1 to G3a at baseline (Table S6 in File S1). The characteristics of the patients with or without renal biopsies classified by the plasma levels of VASH-1 at baseline and at the final follow-up are shown in Table 8 and Table S7 in File S1, respectively. In the patients who underwent a renal biopsy, the group with elevated plasma levels of VASH-1 exhibited preserved renal function, a younger age and lower SBP at the baseline examination (Table 8) and a lower SBP after three years (Table S7 in File S1) compared with the group with lower levels. In patients who did not undergo a renal biopsy, the group with elevated plasma levels of VASH-1 exhibited lower renal function and an older age compared with the group with lower levels after three years (Table S7 in File S1). In the patients without a renal biopsy, the group with elevated plasma levels of VASH-1 exhibited a

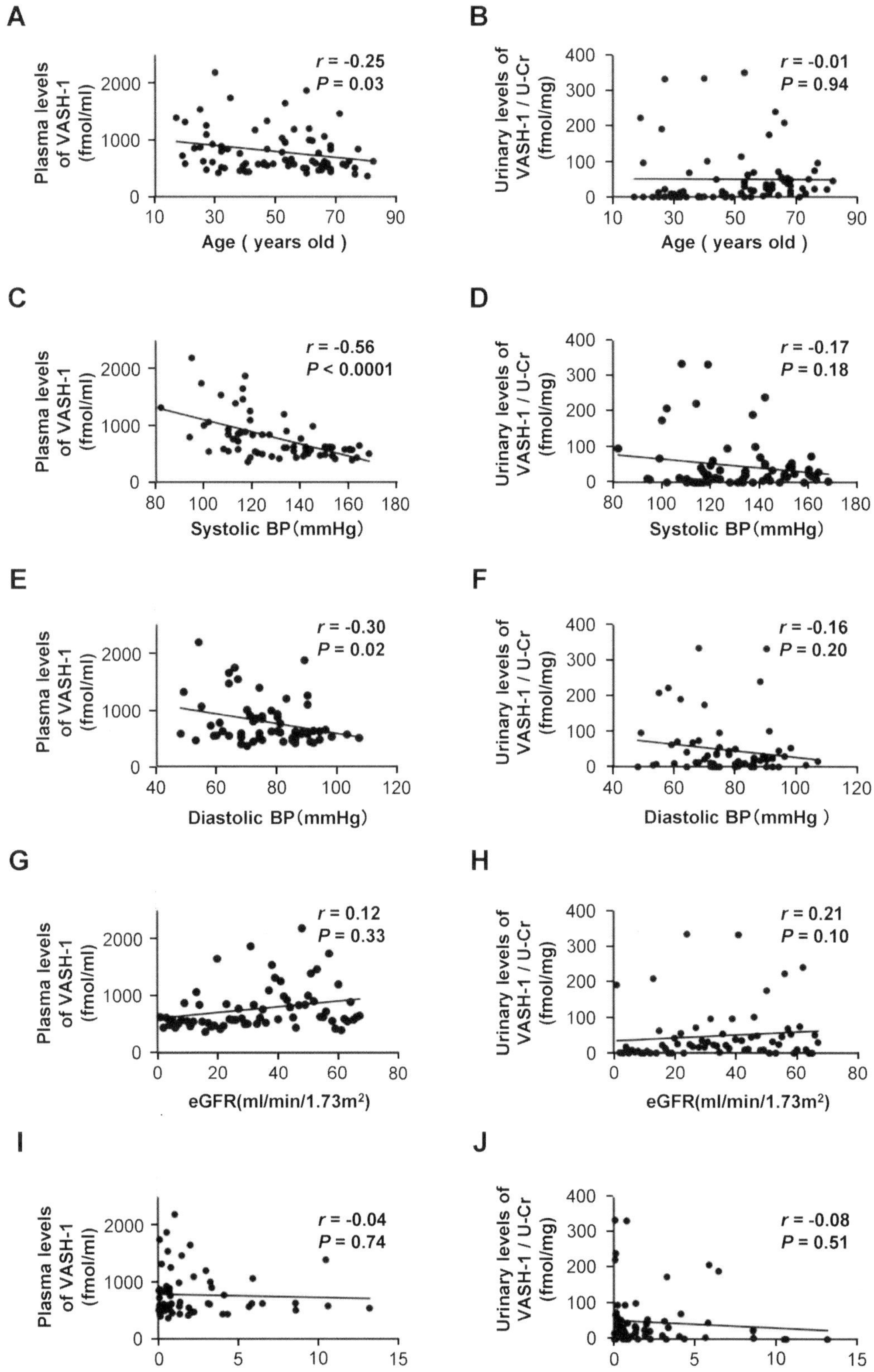

Figure 1. Correlations between the plasma/urinary levels of vasohibin-1 and the clinical parameters. (A) Correlations between the plasma/urinary levels of VASH-1 and age. (B) Correlation between the urinary VASH-1/Cr ratio and age. (C) Correlation between the plasma level of VASH-1 and systolic blood pressure. (D) Correlation between the urinary VASH-1/Cr ratio and systolic blood pressure. (E) Correlation between the plasma level of VASH-1 and diastolic blood pressure. (F) Correlation between the urinary VASH-1/Cr ratio and diastolic blood pressure. (G) Correlation between the plasma level of VASH-1 and eGFR. (H) Correlation between the urinary VASH-1/Cr ratio and eGFR. (I) Correlation between the plasma level of VASH-1 and proteinuria. (J) Correlation between the urinary VASH-1/Cr ratio and proteinuria. Abbreviations: BP, blood pressure; eGFR, estimated glomerular filtration rate; U-Cr, urinary level of creatinine; VASH-1, vasohibin-1.

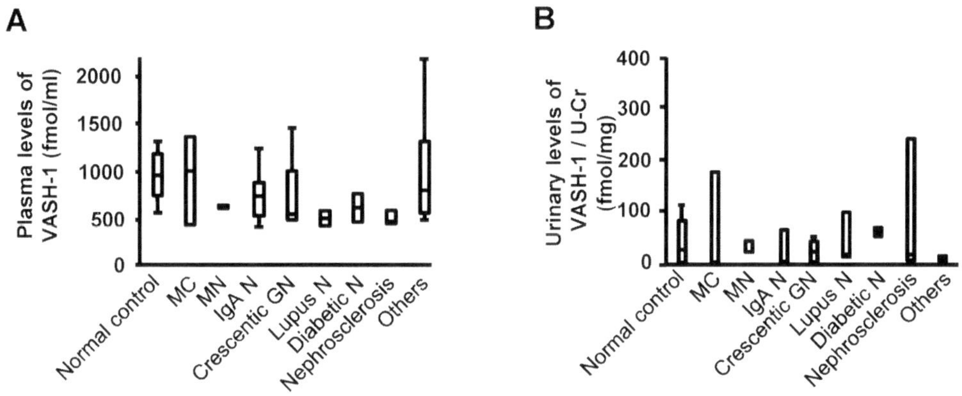

Figure 2. Plasma/urinary levels of vasohibin-1 in patients with various renal disorders. (A) The plasma levels of VASH-1 in patients with various renal disorders. (B) The urinary VASH-1/Cr ratios in patients with various renal disorders. Abbreviations: GN, glomerulonephritis; MC, minimal change; MN, membranous nephropathy; N, nephropathy; U-Cr, urinary level of creatinine; VASH-1, vasohibin-1.

significantly higher incidence of composite renal events during three years compared with the group with lower levels (Table 9).

In patients with or without renal biopsies, the groups with elevated urinary levels of VASH-1 were significantly older compared with the groups with lower VASH-1 levels at baseline (Table S8 in File S1). In patients without renal biopsies, the group with elevated urinary levels of VASH-1 exhibited significantly lower levels of proteinuria compared with the group with lower VASH-1 levels at baseline (Table S8 in File S1). The changes in the eGFR and the number of events in the patients with or without renal biopsies classified by the urinary levels of VASH-1 are shown in Table S9 in File S1, but no statistically significant differences were observed among the groups.

Discussion

Angiogenesis is involved in physiological processes as well as pathological disorders [15]. Angiogenesis-associated factors are involved in the development of the kidneys [16,17,18]. Experimental studies have demonstrated the involvement of an imbalance in angiogenesis-related factors in the progression of CKD [19,20,21,22,23,24,25] and the potential therapeutic effects on CKD achieved by modulating these factors [6,26,27,28,29,30,31,32,33].

The clinical usefulness of angiogenesis-associated factors, such as VEGF-A, sVEGFR-1/2 and Angiopoietin-1/2, in CKD patients has recently been demonstrated [34,35,36,37,38,39]. There are as yet no reports investigating the clinical role of VASH-1 in CKD patients.

In general, VASH-1 is primarily synthesized and secreted by vascular endothelial cells. An inverse correlation between the plasma levels of VASH-1 and age/blood pressure has been observed in CKD patients. At baseline, the SBP was significantly lower in the groups with elevated plasma levels of VASH-1 or VASH-1-SVBP complex compared with the groups with lower levels. However, the differences in the SBP at baseline were not observed when patients were categorized based on the urinary levels of VASH-1. These results suggest that the production of VASH-1 by vascular endothelial cells might be reduced in elderly and hypertensive patients due to systemic arteriosclerotic alterations accompanied by endothelial cell dysfunction, consistent with recent findings suggesting VASH-1 to be a critical factor for the maintenance of endothelial cells [9].

On the other hand, the plasma and urinary levels of VASH-1 and the plasma levels of the VASH-1-SVBP complex at baseline were inversely correlated with the annual rate of changes in the eGFR. The Kaplan-Meier analysis further indicated that elevated plasma levels of VASH-1 and the VASH-1-SVBP complex at

Table 3. Correlations between the plasma and urinary levels of vasohibin-1, and the histological parameters.

	Plasma levels of VASH-1 (fmol/mL)		Urinary levels of VASH-1/U-Cr (fmol/mg)	
	r	*P*	*r*	*P*
Mesangial hypercellularity	−0.01	0.92	0.02	0.93
Mesangial sclerosis	−0.08	0.60	0.03	0.87
Crescent formation	0.38	0.01[a]	−0.01	0.96
Global sclerosis	−0.15	0.31	−0.08	0.66
Interstitial cell infiltration	−0.02	0.92	0.04	0.81
Interstitial fibrosis	−0.17	0.28	0.00	0.98
Tubular atrophy	−0.23	0.13	0.02	0.90
Arteriosclerosis	0.15	0.33	0.10	0.58

Abbreviations: U-Cr, urinary level of creatinine; VASH-1, Vasohibin-1.
[a] $P<0.05$.

Table 4. Correlations between the plasma and urinary levels of vasohibin-1-small vasohibin-binding protein complex and small vasohibin-binding protein, and the clinical/histological parameters and the plasma/urinary levels of vasohibin-1.

	Plasma levels of VASH-1-SVBP complex (fmol/mL)		Urinary levels of VASH-1-SVBP complex (fmol/mg)		Plasma levels of SVBP (fmol/mL)		Urinary levels of SVBP (fmol/mg)	
	r	*P*	*r*	*P*	*r*	*P*	*r*	*P*
Age	−0.11	0.34	−0.12	0.31	−0.25	0.03[a]	−0.32	0.004[b]
Hemoglobin	−0.02	0.87	0.09	0.46	0.13	0.28	0.08	0.54
eGFR	0.01	0.93	0.16	0.20	0.06	0.62	0.14	0.26
Mesangial hypercellularity	−0.15	0.32	0.60	<0.0001[b]	−0.05	0.74	0.17	0.28
Mesangial sclerosis	−0.15	0.33	0.10	0.53	−0.08	0.62	−0.03	0.83
Crescent formation	0.17	0.25	0.32	0.03[a]	−0.04	0.81	0.14	0.35
Global sclerosis	−0.02	0.88	−0.16	0.30	−0.02	0.90	−0.16	0.30
Interstitial cell infiltration	0.05	0.74	0.14	0.37	0.14	0.35	0.21	0.17
Interstitial Fibrosis	−0.09	0.54	0.07	0.65	−0.02	0.90	−0.01	0.94
Tubular atrophy	−0.16	0.30	0.11	0.49	0.03	0.84	−0.03	0.82
Arteriosclerosis	0.19	0.22	−0.16	0.30	0.11	0.46	−0.06	0.70
Plasma levels of VASH-1 (fmol/mL)	0.54	<0.0001[b]	−0.02	0.88	0.16	0.16	−0.10	0.37
Urinary levels of VASH-1/U-Cr (fmol/mg)	−0.004	0.97	0.33	0.003[b]	0.16	0.16	0.11	0.34

Abbreviations: eGFR, estimated glomerular filtration rate; SVBP, small vasohibin-binding protein; U-Cr, urinary level of creatinine; VASH-1, vasohibin-1.
[a]$P<0.05$.
[b]$P<0.01$.

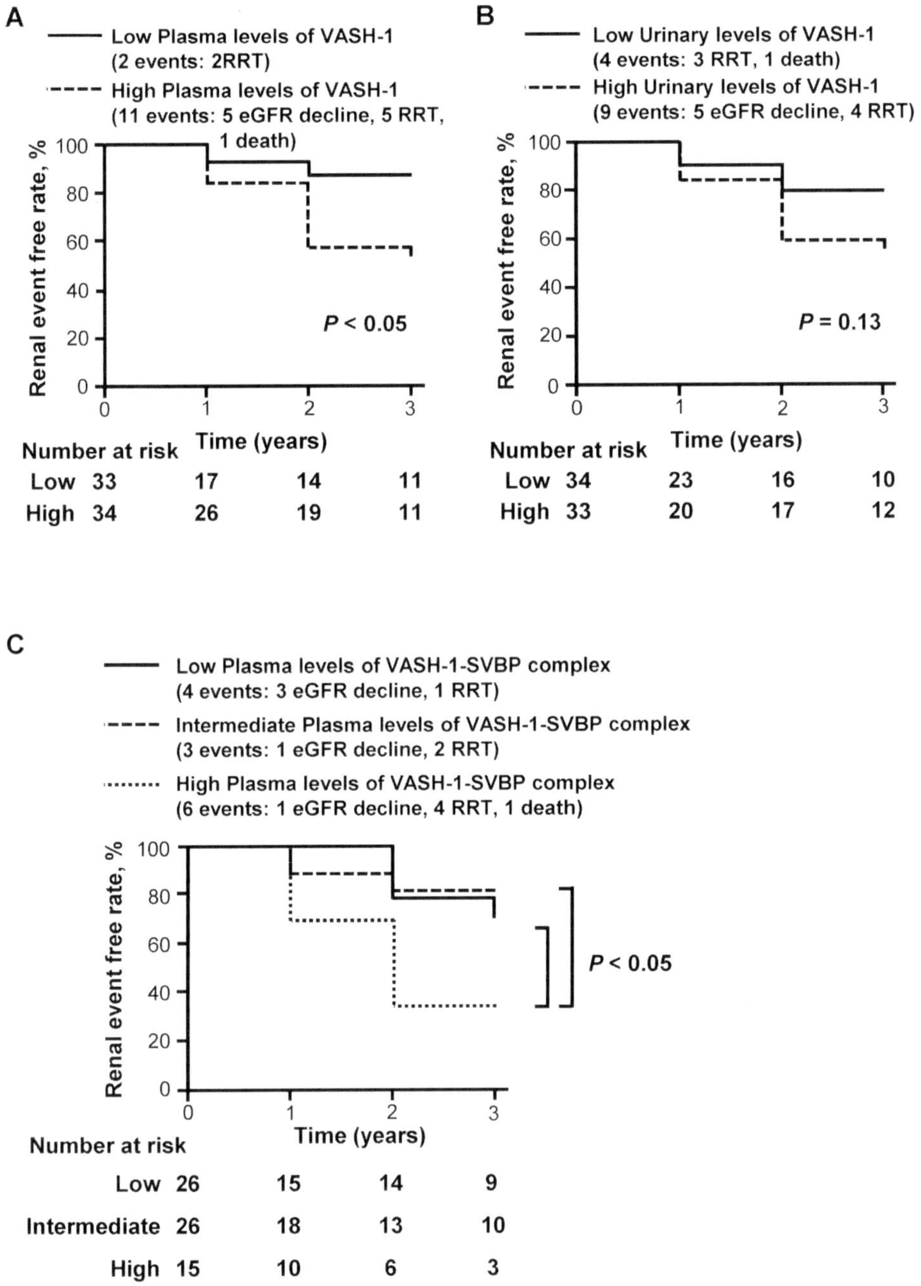

Figure 3. The results of the Kaplan-Meier analysis of the composite renal endpoint. A composite renal event was defined as a decline in the eGFR of more than 30% of the baseline value, initiation of renal replacement therapy or death associated with a renal disorder. In order to perform a Kaplan-Meier analysis of the plasma and urinary levels of VASH-1, the patients were stratified into two groups using the median (609 fmol/mL for the plasma level and 21 fmol/mg for the urinary level of VASH-1) as the cutoff point. The log-rank test was used to compare differences between the two groups. (A and B) Increased plasma levels of VASH-1 were significantly correlated and the urinary levels of VASH-1 tended to be correlated with worse renal outcomes. (C) In order to perform a Kaplan-Meier analysis of the plasma levels of the VASH-1-SVBP complex, the patients were stratified into three groups (<316, 316 to 408 and >408 fmol/mL). The group with the highest plasma levels of the VASH-1-SVBP complex exhibited significantly worse renal outcomes than the groups with moderate or low plasma levels. Abbreviations: eGFR, estimated glomerular filtration rate; RRT, renal replacement therapy, SVBP, small vasohibin-binding protein; VASH-1, vasohibin-1.

baseline successfully predicted a poor renal outcome. In addition, elevated plasma levels of VASH-1 and the VASH-1-SVBP complex at baseline were the significant determinants of a poor renal outcome in the multivariate analysis.

We next classified the patients into groups based on whether they had undergone a renal biopsy. Most of the patients who had not undergone renal biopsies were at CKD stage G3b-G5 (eGFR<45 mL/min/1.73 m^2). Among them, the eGFR of the patients with elevated plasma levels of VASH-1 consistently tended to be lower throughout the observational period compared with the group with lower levels of VASH-1. With regard to the composite renal endpoint, a significantly higher incidence was noted in the patients with elevated plasma levels of VASH-1 compared with the group with lower levels of VASH-1.

Table 5. Correlations between the plasma and urinary levels of vasohibin-1, the vasohibin-1-small vasohibin-binding protein complex and small vasohibin-binding protein, and the annual change rates in the estimated glomerular filtration rate.

	Plasma levels of VASH-1 (fmol/mL)		Urinary levels of VASH-1/U-Cr (fmol/mg)		Plasma levels of VASH-1-SVBP complex (fmol/mL)		Urinary levels of VASH-1-SVBP complex (fmol/mg)		Plasma levels of SVBP (fmol/mL)		Urinary levels of SVBP (fmol/mg)	
	r	*P*	*r*	*P*	*r*	*P*	*r*	*P*	*r*	*P*	*r*	*P*
Annual change rates in eGFR	−0.33	0.04[a]	−0.46	0.02[a]	−0.36	0.03[a]	0.05	0.77	−0.04	0.80	0.19	0.27

Abbreviations: eGFR, estimated glomerular filtration rate; SVBP, small vasohibin-binding protein; U-Cr, urinary level of creatinine; VASH-1, vasohibin-1. The annual change rates in eGFR were evaluated as follows: the annual change in eGFR was divided by the eGFR at baseline.
[a]$P<0.05$.

In the patients who underwent renal biopsies, most of the patients were at CKD stage G1-G3a (eGFR 45 mL/min/1.73 m^2 or higher). Among them, the group with elevated plasma levels of VASH-1 at baseline was younger and exhibited significantly a higher eGFR compared with the group with lower plasma levels of VASH-1. However, the group with elevated plasma levels of VASH-1 tended to experience an increased number of occurrences of the renal endpoint during the three-year observational period. To further investigate these findings, we classified the patients into groups based on whether they had renal disorders diagnosed by renal biopsy. Since the sample size was not large enough to make comparisons among the various renal disorders, the significance of VASH-1 for each particular renal disorder requires further study.

Similar to the present findings, previous reports had demonstrated that an elevated expression of VASH-1 predicted a worse clinical outcome in patients with cancer [40,41,42,43,44,45]. In various experimental disease models, including those of cancer and diabetic nephropathy, the administration of adenoviral vectors encoding VASH-1 results in therapeutic effects [8,12,13,14,46,47,48,49]. More recent findings have demonstrated the role of VASH-1 in enhancing the stress resistance of endothelial cells [9]. Therefore, we suppose that endogenous VASH-1 is upregulated in a compensatory manner in response to increased disease activities and endothelial cell stress in patients with CKD.

Previous reports have demonstrated the expression of VASH-1 in various organs, with a predominant expression observed in the brain and placenta and, to a lesser extent, in the heart and kidneys [8]. In general, the urinary, rather than the plasma, levels of certain factors are supposed to reflect the renal expression. Determining the origin of VASH-1 in the plasma of CKD patients, i.e., the kidney or other distant organs, requires further investigation.

In this study, the plasma and urinary levels of VASH-1 did not exhibit any statistically significant correlations with the renal function or proteinuria. Considering the relatively large molecular size of VASH-1 (42 kDa), it does not easily pass through the glomerular filtration barrier; thus, the urinary levels of VASH-1 are not directly influenced by the amount of VASH-1 in the plasma. Although podocytes may synthesize VASH-1, the lack of a correlation between proteinuria and the urinary VASH-1 level does not support podocytes as the primary source of the urinary VASH-1. On the other hand, VASH-1 may originate from the endothelial cells of the peritubular capillaries in the interstitium, and diffuse into the tubular lumens, thus influencing the urinary levels of VASH-1. Altered tubular reabsorption of VASH-1 due to tubulointerstitial injury may be the alternative factor influencing the urinary levels of VASH-1. However, these speculations require confirmation in further investigations.

In this study, the plasma and urinary levels of SVBP, a secretory chaperone for VASH-1 [10], were inversely correlated with age but not SBP or DBP (data not shown). To date, there is no information available regarding the link between SVBP and clinical parameters, and the causal relationship between SVBP and age may require further investigation. In addition, the urinary levels of the VASH-1-SVBP complex, but not VASH-1, were significantly correlated with the presence of mesangial hypercellularity and crescent formation. In association with these findings, previous reports demonstrated the anti-inflammatory action of VASH-1 and suppressive effects of VASH-1 on mesangial matrix expansion in experimental diabetic nephropathy models [13,14]. The present results suggest that the urinary levels of the VASH-1-

Table 6. Results of the multivariate logistic analysis of the risk of composite renal events.

Plasma levels of VASH-1 (fmol/mL)	OR (95% CI)	*P*-value
Model 1		
<609	1 (referent)	
≥609	9.6 (1.5, 104)	0.02
Model 2		
<609	1 (referent)	
≥609	7.9 (1.1, 95)	0.04
Urinary levels of VASH-1/U-Cr (fmol/mg)		
Model 1		
<21	1 (referent)	
≥21	0.39 (0.03, 3.4)	0.41
Model 2		
<21	1 (referent)	
≥21	0.23 (0.01, 2.7)	0.26
Plasma levels of VASH-1-SVBP complex (fmol/mL)	OR (95% CI)	*P*-value
Model 1		
<316	0.02 (0.0, 0.3)	0.003
316 to 408	0.01 (0.0, 0.2)	0.001
>408	1 (referent)	
Model 2		
<316	0.02 (0.0, 0.4)	0.01
316 to 408	0.01 (0.0, 0.2)	0.002
>408	1 (referent)	

Abbreviations: CI, confidence interval; eGFR, estimated glomerular filtration rate; OR, odds ratio; SVBP, small vasohibin-binding protein; U-Cr, urinary level of creatinine; VASH-1, vasohibin-1. A composite renal event was defined as a decline in the eGFR of more than 30% of the baseline value, initiation of renal replacement therapy or death associated with a renal disorder. In order to perform a multivariate logistic analysis of the plasma and urinary levels of VASH-1, the patients were stratified into two groups using the median value as the cutoff point, and the plasma levels of the VASH-1-SVBP complex, the patients were stratified into three groups.
Model 1: adjusted for age and gender.
Model 2: adjusted for age, gender and systolic blood pressure.

SVBP complex reflect the disease activity in the relatively acute phase of renal disorders.

There are several limitations in the present study. The sample size was not adequate for making comparisons between the patients with various renal disorders. With regard to the healthy control subjects, information other than the age, gender and VASH-1-related measurements were not available. In addition, the precise mechanisms underlying the relationships between the plasma/urinary levels of VASH-1 and the renal outcomes were not fully clarified. To further elucidate these precise mechanisms, basic research on VASH-1 *in vitro* and *in vivo*, including animal models of renal disorders, is required.

In conclusion, our present results demonstrated for the first time the potential role of the plasma/urinary level of VASH-1 and the plasma level of the VASH-1-SVBP complex in predicting future renal functional deterioration in patients with renal disorders.

Materials and Methods

Study population

We studied 67 Japanese hospitalized CKD patients with (n = 45) or without (n = 22) renal biopsy samples and 10 healthy control subjects only assented to the disclosure of their age and gender.

All patients attended the Department of Nephrology at Okayama University Hospital (Okayama, Japan) between the years 2007 and 2009. The histological evaluations of the biopsies were performed by two renal pathologists. To measure the eGFR, the modified MDRD equation for Japanese individuals [50] was used. The medical records from the day of the renal biopsy were evaluated. The protocol of the current study was approved by the Institutional Ethical Review Board of Okayama University Hospital (No. 471, Oct. 23, 2007), and written informed consent was obtained from all subjects.

The patients were followed up annually for three years. We defined a composite renal event as an eGFR decline of greater than 30% from baseline, initiation of renal replacement therapy or kidney disease-related death. GFR categories in CKD were defined by KDIGO 2012 Clinical Practice Guideline for the Evaluation and Management of Chronic Kidney Disease.

ELISA for VASH-1, SVBP and the VASH-1-SVBP complex

The plasma and urinary concentrations of VASH-1, SVBP and the VASH-1-SVBP complex were determined using sandwich ELISA, as previously described [10], utilizing monoclonal antibodies raised against human VASH-1 (VR1 12E7) for capture and horseradish peroxidase-conjugated anti-human VASH-1 antibodies (VC 12F6) for detection. ELISA of the VASH-1-SVBP complex was performed as previously described [10]. All samples were examined in duplicate, and the mean values of the individual samples were utilized for the statistical analysis.

Table 7. The changes in the estimated glomerular filtration rate and the number of events in the overall patients and patients with classified renal disorders.

	Baseline		One year		Two years		Three years		Number of events	
	n	eGFR	*n*	eGFR	*n*	eGFR	*n*	eGFR	Total	RRT or Death
All patients	67	60±35	37	58±31	30	56±30	25	57±30	13	8
Patients without RB	22	28±23[a]	13	31±23[a]	11	31±23[a]	10	38±28[a]	10[a]	7[a]
Patients with RB	45	75±29	24	74±24	19	71±21	15	71±21	3	1
MN	3	57±22	2	35±24	1	50	1	44	1	0
MC	3	86±34	3	80±21	2	85±27	1	64	0	0
Crescentic GN	5	53±22	3	62±30	3	51±24	1	65	1	1
IgA N	15	79±24	8	81±16	6	75±6	4	74±9	0	0
Lupus N	3	56±21	2	59±42	2	60±39	2	57±50	0	0
Diabetic N	2	60±14	1	59	1	51	1	43	1	0
Nephrosclerosis	3	88±26	1	94	1	94	1	89	0	0
Others	11	87±29	4	86±18	3	86±18	4	90±18	0	0

Abbreviations: eGFR, estimated glomerular filtration rate (mL/min/1.73 m^2); GN, glomerulonephritis; MC, minimal change; MN, membranous nephropathy; N, nephropathy; RB, renal biopsy; RRT, renal replacement therapy. A composite renal event was defined as a decline in the eGFR of more than 30% of the baseline value, initiation of RRT or death associated with a renal disorder. The values are expressed as the means ± SD.

[a]$P<0.01$ versus patients with RB.

Table 8. The baseline characteristics of the patients with or without renal biopsy, classified by the plasma levels of vasohibin-1.

	n	VASH-1 (fmol/mL)	Age (years)	sCr (mg/dL)	eGFR (mL/min/1.73 m^2)	Proteinuria (g/day)	SBP (mmHg)
The plasma levels of VASH-1 in patients with RB							
Low (<609 fmol/mL)	23	516±55	52±15	1.0±0.4	67±28	1.4±2.8	137±17
High (≥609 fmol/mL)	22	1036±417[b]	40±19[b]	0.8±0.3	84±27[a]	2.2±3.0	117±19[b]
The plasma levels of VASH-1 in patients without RB							
Low (<609 fmol/mL)	10	500±89	56±19	2.1±1.3	36±26	3.5±3.7	144±21
High (≥609 fmol/mL)	12	1014±396[b]	60±14	3.6±2.3	20±18	2.0±1.7	129±17

Abbreviations: eGFR, estimated glomerular filtration rate; RB, renal biopsy; SBP, systolic blood pressure; sCr, serum creatinine; VASH-1, vasohibin-1. The values are expressed as the means ± SD.
[a]$P<0.05$ versus the Low group.
[b]$P<0.01$ versus the Low group.

Table 9. The changes in the estimated glomerular filtration rate and the number of events in the patients with or without renal biopsy, classified by the plasma levels of vasohibin-1.

	Baseline		One year		Two years		Three years		Number of events	
	n	eGFR	*n*	eGFR	*n*	eGFR	*n*	eGFR	Total	RRT or Death
The plasma levels of VASH-1 in patients with RB										
Low (<609 fmol/mL)	23	67±28	10	80±22	8	73±19	6	70±26	0	0
High (≥609 fmol/mL)	22	84±27[a]	14	69±25	11	70±24	9	73±22	3	1
The plasma levels of VASH-1 in patients without RB										
Low (<609 fmol/mL)	10	36±26	6	43±28	4	51±26	5	51±32	2	2
High (≥609 fmol/mL)	12	20±18	7	22±9	7	19±13	5	20±13	8[a]	5

Abbreviations: eGFR, estimated glomerular filtration rate (mL/min/1.73 m^2); RB, renal biopsy; RRT, renal replacement therapy; VASH-1, vasohibin-1. A composite renal event was defined as a decline in the eGFR of more than 30% of the baseline value, initiation of RRT or death associated with a renal disorder. The values are expressed as the means ± SD. The average eGFR did not include the values from the patients who received RRT or died.
[a]$P<0.05$ versus the Low group.

Histological analysis

Formalin-fixed, paraffin-embedded sections were stained with periodic acid-Schiff (PAS), periodic acid-methenamine-silver (PAM) or Masson's trichrome for light microscopic observation. Renal histological alterations were semiquantitatively evaluated by scoring. The mean percentage of glomeruli with crescent formation and global sclerosis was also determined. The histological evaluation was performed in a blinded fashion by two investigators, and the results were averaged.

Statistical analysis

All values are expressed as the mean ± standard deviation (SD). Pearson's correlation coefficients were used to evaluate the association between two continuous variables. The Mann-Whitney U-test was used to compare the levels of VASH-1 in the control subjects and patients with renal disorders. Statistical significance was defined as a *P*-value of <0.05. The composite renal event rates were estimated using the Kaplan–Meier method and compared using the log-rank test. A multivariate logistic analysis was performed to examine the correlations between the plasma and urinary levels of VASH-1 and the plasma levels of the VASH-1-SVBP complex according to variables such as age, gender and systolic blood pressure. All statistical tests were performed using the JMP version 9 software package (SAS Institute Inc. Cary, NC, USA).

Supporting Information

File S1 Tables S1–S9. Table S1. The clinical parameters of the study groups after three years ($n = 25$). Table S2. The final (after three years) characteristics of the patients with renal biopsy ($n = 15$). Table S3. The baseline characteristics of the patients classified by the plasma and urinary levels of vasohibin-1 and the plasma levels of the vasohibin-1-small vasohibin-binding protein complex. At baseline, the SBP was significantly lower in the group with elevated plasma levels of VASH-1 compared with the group with lower plasma levels of VASH-1. Similarly, the SBP was significantly lower in the group with elevated plasma levels of VASH-1-SVBP complex compared with lower plasma levels. The group with elevated urinary levels of VASH-1 was older and exhibited lower renal function compared with the group with lower levels at baseline. Table S4. The final (after three years) characteristics of the patients classified by the plasma and urinary levels of vasohibin-1 and the plasma levels of the vasohibin-1-small vasohibin-binding protein complex ($n = 25$). The group with elevated urinary levels of VASH-1 was older and exhibited lower renal function compared with the group with lower levels at the final follow-up (after three years). Table S5. The changes in the estimated glomerular filtration rate and the number of events in the patients classified by the plasma and urinary levels of vasohibin-1 and the plasma levels of the vasohibin-1-small vasohibin-binding protein complex. The group with elevated urinary levels of VASH-1 exhibited lower renal function compared with the group with lower levels at all of the follow-up examinations. Table S6. The CKD stage of the patients with or without renal biopsy. Most of the patients without renal biopsies were at CKD stage G3b to G5 at baseline. On the other hand, most of the patients who underwent renal biopsies were at CKD stage G1 to G3a at baseline. Table S7. The final (after three years) characteristics of the patients with or without renal biopsy, classified by the plasma levels of vasohibin-1 ($n = 25$). In the patients who underwent a renal biopsy, the group with elevated plasma levels of VASH-1 exhibited a lower SBP compared with the group with lower levels after three years. In patients who did not undergo a renal biopsy, the group with elevated plasma levels of VASH-1 exhibited lower renal function and an older age compared with the group with lower levels after three years. Table S8. The baseline characteristics of the patients with or without renal biopsy, classified by the urinary levels of vasohibin-1. In patients with or without renal biopsies, the groups with elevated urinary levels of VASH-1 were significantly older compared with the groups with lower VASH-1 levels at baseline. In patients without renal biopsies, the group with elevated urinary levels of VASH-1 exhibited significantly lower levels of proteinuria compared with the group with lower VASH-1 levels at baseline. Table S9. The changes in the estimated glomerular filtration rate and the number of events in patients with or without renal biopsy, classified by the urinary levels of vasohibin-1. No statistically significant differences were observed among the groups.

Acknowledgments

A portion of this study was presented in abstract form at the annual meeting of the American Society of Nephrology, San Diego, CA, Nov. 1–4, 2012.

Author Contributions

Conceived and designed the experiments: YM HM. Performed the experiments: NH DS HY KT TN HW HU MK H. Sugiyama. Analyzed the data: NH. Contributed reagents/materials/analysis tools: H. Sonoda YS. Wrote the paper: NH YM.

References

1. Nasu T, Kinomura M, Tanabe K, Yamasaki H, Htay SL, et al. (2012) Sustained-release prostacyclin analog ONO-1301 ameliorates tubulointerstitial alterations in a mouse obstructive nephropathy model. Am J Physiol Renal Physiol 302: F1616–1629.
2. Thorner PS, Ho M, Eremina V, Sado Y, Quaggin S (2008) Podocytes contribute to the formation of glomerular crescents. J Am Soc Nephrol 19: 495–502.
3. Lemley KV, Lafayette RA, Safai M, Derby G, Blouch K, et al. (2002) Podocytopenia and disease severity in IgA nephropathy. Kidney Int 61: 1475–1485.
4. Macconi D, Bonomelli M, Benigni A, Plati T, Sangalli F, et al. (2006) Pathophysiologic implications of reduced podocyte number in a rat model of progressive glomerular injury. Am J Pathol 168: 42–54.
5. Wang G, Lai FM, Kwan BC, Lai KB, Chow KM, et al. (2009) Podocyte loss in human hypertensive nephrosclerosis. Am J Hypertens 22: 300–306.
6. Kang DH, Hughes J, Mazzali M, Schreiner GF, Johnson RJ (2001) Impaired angiogenesis in the remnant kidney model: II. Vascular endothelial growth factor administration reduces renal fibrosis and stabilizes renal function. J Am Soc Nephrol 12: 1448–1457.
7. Ferrara N, Carver-Moore K, Chen H, Dowd M, Lu L, et al. (1996) Heterozygous embryonic lethality induced by targeted inactivation of the VEGF gene. Nature 380: 439–442.
8. Watanabe K, Hasegawa Y, Yamashita H, Shimizu K, Ding Y, et al. (2004) Vasohibin as an endothelium-derived negative feedback regulator of angiogenesis. J Clin Invest 114: 898–907.
9. Miyashita H, Watanabe T, Hayashi H, Suzuki Y, Nakamura T, et al. (2012) Angiogenesis inhibitor vasohibin-1 enhances stress resistance of endothelial cells via induction of SOD2 and SIRT1. PLoS One 7: e46459.
10. Suzuki Y, Kobayashi M, Miyashita H, Ohta H, Sonoda H, et al. (2010) Isolation of a small vasohibin-binding protein (SVBP) and its role in vasohibin secretion. J Cell Sci 123: 3094–3101.
11. Shen J, Yang X, Xiao WH, Hackett SF, Sato Y, et al. (2006) Vasohibin is up-regulated by VEGF in the retina and suppresses VEGF receptor 2 and retinal neovascularization. Faseb J 20: 723–725.
12. Yamashita H, Abe M, Watanabe K, Shimizu K, Moriya T, et al. (2006) Vasohibin prevents arterial neointimal formation through angiogenesis inhibition. Biochem Biophys Res Commun 345: 919–925.
13. Nasu T, Maeshima Y, Kinomura M, Hirokoshi-Kawahara K, Tanabe K, et al. (2009) Vasohibin-1, a negative feedback regulator of angiogenesis, ameliorates

renal alterations in a mouse model of diabetic nephropathy. Diabetes 58: 2365–2375.
14. Saito D, Maeshima Y, Nasu T, Yamasaki H, Tanabe K, et al. (2011) Amelioration of renal alterations in obese type 2 diabetic mice by vasohibin-1, a negative feedback regulator of angiogenesis. Am J Physiol Renal Physiol 300: F873–886.
15. Folkman J (1995) Angiogenesis in cancer, vascular, rheumatoid and other disease. Nat Med 1: 27–31.
16. Kitamoto Y, Tokunaga H, Tomita K (1997) Vascular endothelial growth factor is an essential molecule for mouse kidney development: glomerulogenesis and nephrogenesis. J Clin Invest 99: 2351–2357.
17. Tufro A, Norwood VF, Carey RM, Gomez RA (1999) Vascular endothelial growth factor induces nephrogenesis and vasculogenesis. J Am Soc Nephrol 10: 2125–2134.
18. Woolf AS, Yuan HT (2001) Angiopoietin growth factors and Tie receptor tyrosine kinases in renal vascular development. Pediatr Nephrol 16: 177–184.
19. Hara A, Wada T, Furuichi K, Sakai N, Kawachi H, et al. (2006) Blockade of VEGF accelerates proteinuria, via decrease in nephrin expression in rat crescentic glomerulonephritis. Kidney Int 69: 1986–1995.
20. Kang DH, Anderson S, Kim YG, Mazzalli M, Suga S, et al. (2001) Impaired angiogenesis in the aging kidney: vascular endothelial growth factor and thrombospondin-1 in renal disease. Am J Kidney Dis 37: 601–611.
21. Kang DH, Joly AH, Oh SW, Hugo C, Kerjaschki D, et al. (2001) Impaired angiogenesis in the remnant kidney model: I. Potential role of vascular endothelial growth factor and thrombospondin-1. J Am Soc Nephrol 12: 1434–1447.
22. Cooper ME, Vranes D, Youssef S, Stacker SA, Cox AJ, et al. (1999) Increased renal expression of vascular endothelial growth factor (VEGF) and its receptor VEGFR-2 in experimental diabetes. Diabetes 48: 2229–2239.
23. Long DA, Woolf AS, Suda T, Yuan HT (2001) Increased renal angiopoietin-1 expression in folic acid-induced nephrotoxicity in mice. J Am Soc Nephrol 12: 2721–2731.
24. Yuan HT, Tipping PG, Li XZ, Long DA, Woolf AS (2002) Angiopoietin correlates with glomerular capillary loss in anti-glomerular basement membrane glomerulonephritis. Kidney Int 61: 2078–2089.
25. Rizkalla B, Forbes JM, Cao Z, Boner G, Cooper ME (2005) Temporal renal expression of angiogenic growth factors and their receptors in experimental diabetes: role of the renin-angiotensin system. J Hypertens 23: 153–164.
26. Masuda Y, Shimizu A, Mori T, Ishiwata T, Kitamura H, et al. (2001) Vascular endothelial growth factor enhances glomerular capillary repair and accelerates resolution of experimentally induced glomerulonephritis. Am J Pathol 159: 599–608.
27. Shimizu A, Masuda Y, Mori T, Kitamura H, Ishizaki M, et al. (2004) Vascular endothelial growth factor165 resolves glomerular inflammation and accelerates glomerular capillary repair in rat anti-glomerular basement membrane glomerulonephritis. J Am Soc Nephrol 15: 2655–2665.
28. Ostendorf T, Kunter U, Eitner F, Loos A, Regele H, et al. (1999) VEGF(165) mediates glomerular endothelial repair. J Clin Invest 104: 913–923.
29. Kim YG, Suga SI, Kang DH, Jefferson JA, Mazzali M, et al. (2000) Vascular endothelial growth factor accelerates renal recovery in experimental thrombotic microangiopathy. Kidney Int 58: 2390–2399.
30. de Vriese AS, Tilton RG, Elger M, Stephan CC, Kriz W, et al. (2001) Antibodies against vascular endothelial growth factor improve early renal dysfunction in experimental diabetes. J Am Soc Nephrol 12: 993–1000.
31. Flyvbjerg A, Dagnaes-Hansen F, De Vriese AS, Schrijvers BF, Tilton RG, et al. (2002) Amelioration of long-term renal changes in obese type 2 diabetic mice by a neutralizing vascular endothelial growth factor antibody. Diabetes 51: 3090–3094.
32. Sung SH, Ziyadeh FN, Wang A, Pyagay PE, Kanwar YS, et al. (2006) Blockade of vascular endothelial growth factor signaling ameliorates diabetic albuminuria in mice. J Am Soc Nephrol 17: 3093–3104.
33. Kim W, Moon SO, Lee SY, Jang KY, Cho CH, et al. (2006) COMP-angiopoietin-1 ameliorates renal fibrosis in a unilateral ureteral obstruction model. J Am Soc Nephrol 17: 2474–2483.
34. Hirokoshi K, Maeshima Y, Kobayashi K, Matsuura E, Sugiyama H, et al. (2007) Elevated serum sFlt-1/Ang-2 ratio in women with preeclampsia. Nephron Clinical practice 106: c43–50.
35. Mallamaci F, Benedetto FA, Tripepi G, Cutrupi S, Pizzini P, et al. (2008) Vascular endothelial growth factor, left ventricular dysfunction and mortality in hemodialysis patients. J Hypertens 26: 1875–1882.
36. Guo Q, Carrero JJ, Yu X, Barany P, Qureshi AR, et al. (2009) Associations of VEGF and its receptors sVEGFR-1 and -2 with cardiovascular disease and survival in prevalent haemodialysis patients. Nephrol Dial Transplant 24: 3468–3473.
37. Futrakul N, Butthep P, Futrakul P (2008) Altered vascular homeostasis in chronic kidney disease. Clin Hemorheol Microcirc 38: 201–207.
38. Shulman K, Rosen S, Tognazzi K, Manseau EJ, Brown LF (1996) Expression of vascular permeability factor (VPF/VEGF) is altered in many glomerular diseases. J Am Soc Nephrol 7: 661–666.
39. Hohenstein B, Colin M, Foellmer C, Amann KU, Brekken RA, et al. (2010) Autocrine VEGF-VEGF-R loop on podocytes during glomerulonephritis in humans. Nephrol Dial Transplant 25: 3170–3180.
40. Miyazaki Y, Kosaka T, Mikami S, Kikuchi E, Tanaka N, et al. (2012) The prognostic significance of vasohibin-1 expression in patients with upper urinary tract urothelial carcinoma. Clin Cancer Res 18: 4145–4153.
41. Wang Q, Tian X, Zhang C (2012) Upregulation of vasohibin-1 expression with angiogenesis and poor prognosis of hepatocellular carcinoma after curative surgery. Med Oncol 29: 2727–2736.
42. Yoshinaga K, Ito K, Moriya T, Nagase S, Takano T, et al. (2008) Expression of vasohibin as a novel endothelium-derived angiogenesis inhibitor in endometrial cancer. Cancer Sci 99: 914–919.
43. Tamaki K, Moriya T, Sato Y, Ishida T, Maruo Y, et al. (2009) Vasohibin-1 in human breast carcinoma: a potential negative feedback regulator of angiogenesis. Cancer Sci 100: 88–94.
44. Tamaki K, Sasano H, Maruo Y, Takahashi Y, Miyashita M, et al. (2010) Vasohibin-1 as a potential predictor of aggressive behavior of ductal carcinoma in situ of the breast. Cancer Sci 101: 1051–1058.
45. Yoshinaga K, Ito K, Moriya T, Nagase S, Takano T, et al. (2011) Roles of intrinsic angiogenesis inhibitor, vasohibin, in cervical carcinomas. Cancer Sci 102: 446–451.
46. Hosaka T, Kimura H, Heishi T, Suzuki Y, Miyashita H, et al. (2009) Vasohibin-1 expression in endothelium of tumor blood vessels regulates angiogenesis. Am J Pathol 175: 430–439.
47. Li D, Zhou K, Wang S, Shi Z, Yang Z (2010) Recombinant adenovirus encoding vasohibin prevents tumor angiogenesis and inhibits tumor growth. Cancer Sci 101: 448–452.
48. Heishi T, Hosaka T, Suzuki Y, Miyashita H, Oike Y, et al. (2010) Endogenous angiogenesis inhibitor vasohibin1 exhibits broad-spectrum antilymphangiogenic activity and suppresses lymph node metastasis. Am J Pathol 176: 1950–1958.
49. Watanabe T, Okada Y, Hoshikawa Y, Eba S, Notsuda H, et al. (2012) A potent anti-angiogenic factor, vasohibin-1, ameliorates experimental bronchiolitis obliterans. Transplant Proc 44: 1155–1157.
50. Horio M, Imai E, Yasuda Y, Watanabe T, Matsuo S (2010) Modification of the CKD epidemiology collaboration (CKD-EPI) equation for Japanese: accuracy and use for population estimates. Am J Kidney Dis 56: 32–38.

Urinary Retinol Binding Protein Is a Marker of the Extent of Interstitial Kidney Fibrosis

Nicolas Pallet[1,2,3,6]*, Sophie Chauvet[3,6], Jean-François Chassé[1,6], Marc Vincent[1], Paul Avillach[5,6], Charlene Levi[3,6], Vannary Meas-Yedid[4], Jean-Christophe Olivo-Marin[4], Diane Nga-Matsogo[3], Philippe Beaune[1,2,6], Eric Thervet[3,6], Alexandre Karras[3]

1 INSERM U775, Centre Universitaire des Saints Pères, Paris, France, **2** Service de Biochimie, Hôpital Européen Georges Pompidou, Assistance Publique-Hôpitaux de Paris, Paris, France, **3** Service de Néphrologie, Hôpital Européen Georges Pompidou, Assistance Publique-Hôpitaux de Paris, Paris, France, **4** Unité d'Analyse d'image quantitative, Institut Pasteur, Paris, France, **5** Departement d'informatique médicale, Hôpital Européen Georges Pompidou, Assistance Publique-Hôpitaux de Paris, Paris, France, **6** Université Paris Descartes, Paris, France

Abstract

Currently, a non-invasive method to estimate the degree of interstitial fibrosis (IF) in chronic kidney disease is not available in routine. The aim of our study was to evaluate the diagnostic performance of the measurement of urinary low molecular weight (LMW) protein concentrations as a method to determine the extent of IF. The urines specimen from 162 consecutive patients who underwent renal biopsy were used in the analysis. Numerical quantification software based on the colorimetric analysis of fibrous areas was used to assess the percentage IF. Total proteinuria, albuminuria, and the urinary levels of retinol binding protein (RBP), alpha1-microglobulin (α1MG), beta 2-microglobulin (β2MG), transferrin, and IgG immunoglobulins were measured. There was a significant correlation between the degree of IF and the RBP/creatinine (creat) ratio ($R2$: 0.11, $p<0.0001$). IF was associated to a lesser extent with urinary β2MG and α1MG; however, there was no association with total proteinuria or high molecular weight (HMW) proteinuria. The correlation between IF and RBP/creat remained significant after adjustment to the estimated glomerular filtration rate, age, body mass index, α1MG, and β2MG. The specificity of the test for diagnosing a fibrosis score of >25% of the parenchyma was 95% when using a threshold of 20 mg/g creat. In conclusion, RBP appears to be a quantitative and non-invasive marker for the independent prediction of the extent of kidney IF. Because methods for the measurement of urinary RBP are available in most clinical chemistry departments, RBP measurement is appealing for implementation in the routine care of patients with chronic kidney disease.

Editor: Aristidis S. Charonis, Biomedical Research Foundation of the Academy of Athens, Greece

Funding: The authors have no support or funding to report.

* E-mail: npallet@yahoo.fr

Introduction

Kidney disease evolution invariably lead to interstitial fibrosis (IF), which is the main factor contributing to kidney structural deterioration and loss of function [1,2], and its extent is positively correlated with adverse outcomes [3,4,5,6]. Therefore, IF may be may be considered a surrogate marker and its evaluation is of important prognostic value

The development of non-invasive biomarkers of kidney status and outcome is challenging but can result in individualized therapies for patients with chronic kidney disease (CKD) [7,8]. Although experimental and clinical evidence has contributed greatly to our knowledge of the pathophysiological role of the various molecular components of proteinuria in the progression of chronic kidney injury, namely, inflammation, tubular atrophy (TA), and IF, none of the urinary markers used routinely in clinical chemistry has been investigated as a predictor of the extent of IF [9,10]. Regardless, current evidence indicates that low molecular weight (LMW) and/or high molecular weight (HMW) proteinuria could serve as a non-invasive marker of kidney histological damage and may predict kidney survival in specific patients, including kidney transplant recipients (KTRs) and CKD patients [11,12,13]

In this study, we have hypothesized that IF (independent of the cause) promotes a defect in the proximal reabsorption of LMW proteins and that the urinary concentration of these proteins is an indication of the extent of kidney fibrosis. To test this hypothesis, we measured the urinary concentration of LMW proteins (retinol-binding protein, RBP; β2-microglobulin, β2MG; and α1-microglobulin, α1MG), HMW proteins (albumin, Alb; transferrin, TRF; and immunoglobulins G, IgG), and total proteins in 189 consecutive patients who underwent a kidney biopsy. Next, we measured the strength of the association between these proteins and the percentage IF, measured using a color segmentation image analysis technique. Our data indicated that the urinary concentration of LMW proteins was positively correlated with the degree of IF, and urinary RBP was independently associated with the extent of IF in CKD patients.

Methods

Patient population

Between March 2012 and March 2013, 189 consecutive patients who were referred to the Nephrology Department at the Georges Pompidou European Hospital (Paris, France) for kidney biopsy were evaluated for potential inclusion in the study. Indications for biopsy were estimated GFR<60 ml/min and/or proteinuria>0.5 g/l. Kidney biopsies were not performed for the purpose of this non interventional study, but only for patient care. We excluded from the study all patients with acute kidney injury and KTRs. At the time of biopsy, urine and blood samples were collected for routine clinical chemistry analyses and stored at −80°C. Detailed information regarding the clinical, medical, demographic, biological, and histological status of the patients was collected using an information-based data warehouse [14]. Analysis were performed anonymously. Paris Descartes University ethics comity (Comité de Protection des Personnes/Patients Protection Comity, representative: Dr Marie-France Mamzer) approved this observational study. Research was not performed out of France. Participants provided written consents, and the ethic committee approved this consent procedure. There is no difference in the distribution of histological diagnoses compared with the previous year (2011–2012), which confirms that this study is observational. The prevalence of glomerular diseases was 55% in 2012–2013 compared with 51% in 2011–2012; the prevalence of tubular and interstitial diseases was 22% in 2012–2013 compared with 25% in 2011–2012; the prevalence of vascular diseases was 16% in 2012–2013 compared with 15% in 2011–2012.

Clinical chemistry analyses

The urine protein measurements were performed at the Clinical Chemistry Department of the European Georges Pompidou Hospital. The urinary total protein concentration was quantified by measuring pyrogallol red at 600/800 nm absorbance (urinary CSF protein assay, Beckman Coulter), and the Alb concentration was measured by immunoturbidimetry analysis (DIAgAM assay, Beckman Coulter) using a Beckman Coulter AU680 analyzer. The urinary levels of α1MG, β2MG, TRF, RBP, and IgG were measured using a Siemens BN II nephelometer Analyzer II and kits from Siemens. Values considered normal were as follows: α1MG<15 mg/L; β2MG<350 μg/L; RBP<0.5 mg/L; TRF<2.2 mg/L, IgG<3.6 g/L, and Alb<20 mg/L [15,16]. The urine samples were alkalinized prior to measuring the β2MG level. The urine protein concentrations were corrected for creatinine levels, which were measured using a colorimetric assay (modified kinetic Jaffe method) on a Beckman Coulter DXC analyzer (serum) or a Beckman Coulter AU680 analyzer (urine). The glomerular filtration rate (eGFR) was estimated using the modification of the diet in renal disease (MDRD) formula [17].

Automated measurement of interstitial fibrosis

Masson's trichrome-stained kidney sections were analyzed using color segmentation image analysis software for the quantification of IF [18]. An image of the cortical section of each kidney biopsy was captured using the Hamamatsu slide scanner, Nanozoomer with an objective 20×, NA = 0.75, and a Hamamatsu 3-CCD camera. The cortex areas of the biopsy were analyzed, whereas the medulla was excluded from analysis. The images were analyzed using color segmentation image analysis software that automatically extracts the green color areas characteristic of IF; the renal capsule, tubular basement membranes, glomeruli, and vessel were automatically excluded from the analysis. The method for fibrosis quantification has been developed in details elsewhere. Briefly, the protocol for quantification consists of two steps: (1) segmentation to extract green areas and the biopsy area; (2) postprocessing to compute the IF index. The postprocess to compute the IF index is based on the exclusion of non-fibrotic areas. In order to keep only the IF area, the following regions are automatically detected and excluded from analysis. The index of the IF surface is defined as the ratio between the IF surface area and the total surface of the cortex area in the biopsy. More technical details can be found in [18] and particularly in the supplemental part (http://links.lww.com/TP/A493).

Statistical analysis

The results were expressed as the frequencies and percentages for the categorical variables and as the mean ± SEM for the continuous variables. Associations between the clinical and biological features of the patients were tested using the Student T test, Mann-Whitney test or through the estimation of the Pearson correlation coefficient (Pearson coefficient $= \sqrt{R^2}$), where appropriate. The variables correlating with the extent of IF by univariate analysis were included in a multivariate linear regression model. The variables correlating with the extent of IF by univariate analysis were included in a multivariate linear regression model. To check that despite this overlap RBP can help improve the prediction of fibrosis, we fitted and compared two linear models, one including known predicting factors alone (α1MG, β2MG and DFG) and one including both these factors and RBP. The two models were compared based on a Likelihood ratio test, where the deviance follows a Chi-square distribution with number of degrees equal to the difference of included variables in the two nested models. A backward stepwise linear regression analysis was used to identify the clinical factors independently associated with the extent of the IF. Power calculation is not necessary, because our principal objective was not to compare two groups of patients towards an end point to test the null hypothesis, with an alpha and beta risk. Rather, we performed uni and multivariate linear regression analysis; and we evaluated the performance of a diagnostic biomarker. The statistical analyses were performed using the R framework (http://www.R-project.org/).

Results

Characteristics of CKD patients

Of the 189 patients who entered the study between March 2012 and March 2013, 27 were excluded because of the absence of an analyzable histological sample (less than 10 glomeruli). The demographic and medical characteristics of the remaining 162 patients are listed in **Table 1.** Importantly, approximately half of the patient population was not of Caucasian origin. The vast majority of the kidney disease etiologies were of glomerular origin, which may explain the high mean level of proteinuria (2.3 g/L). Advanced kidney disease was common; more than 50% of the patients exhibited an eGFR <30 ml/min (**Fig. 1A**). The patients with glomerular disease exhibited better renal function compared to those with tubulo-intertitial or vascular nephropathy (**Fig. 1B**).

LMW proteinuria but not HMW proteinuria is associated with low eGFR

We characterized the proteinuria expression patterns in the 162 CKD patients. The LMW proteins strongly correlated with each other but not with the HMW proteins and total proteinuria (**Fig. 2A and B, Table 2, Fig. S1A-C**). As expected, HMW proteinuria was significantly higher in patients with glomerular disease compared to patients with tubular and vascular diseases (**Fig. 2C, Fig. S1D**), whereas LMW proteinuria was higher in patients with tubular disease compared to patients with vascular and glomerular diseases (**Fig. 2D, Fig. S1E and F**). Although a higher IgG concentration was expected in patients with glomerular disease (**Fig. 2E**), IgG concentration surprisingly did not

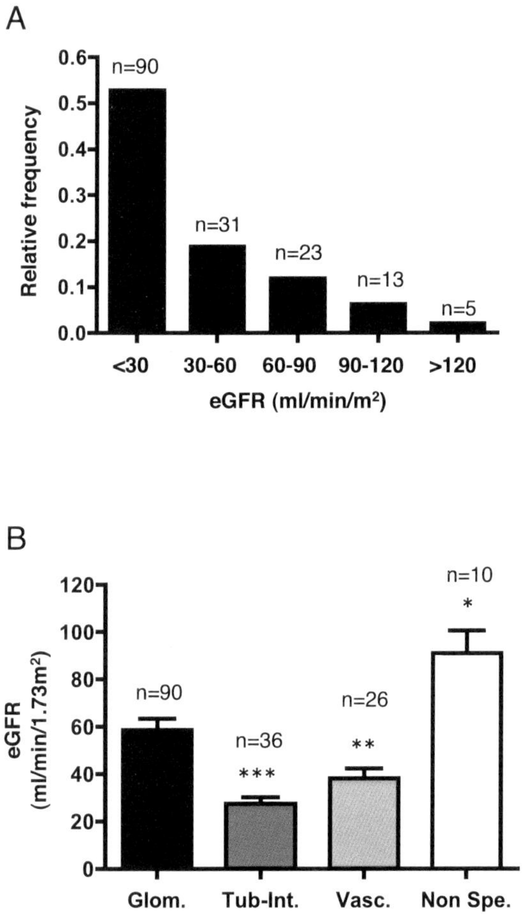

Figure 1. Distribution of estimated glomerular filtration rates. **A**. Histogram showing the distribution of the study population according to the eGFR level at inclusion. **B**. Histogram showing eGFR values according to the type of kidney disease. eGFR is expressed as the mean ± sem. *p<0.05, **p<0.01, ***p<0.001 compared to glomerular disease using Student's T test; the Mann-Whitney test was used for the glomerular vs. comparison with non-specific lesions. Glom: glomerular diseases; Tub-Int: tubular and/or interstitial diseases; Vasc: vascular diseases; Non-spe: non-specific.

Table 1. Baseline characteristics of the study cohort (n = 162).

Demographics	
Age (years)	52.6±18.2
Gender (male)	88 (54)
Caucasian patients	86 (53)
Body Mass Index (kg/m^2)	25.4±4.8
Hypertension	79 (48)
Hyperlipidemia*	37 (22)
Diabetes	17 (10)
Cancer**	25 (15)
Etiology of CKD	
FSGS/minimal changes disease	23 (14)
ANCA-mediated vasculitidis	15 (9)
IgA nephropathy	14 (8.5)
Primary Glomerulonephritis	14 (8.5)
Lupus	11 (6.5)
Diabetes	10 (6)
Tubule-interstitial nephropathy	10 (6)
Hypertensive nephropathy	10 (6)
Non specific***	10 (6)
Myeloma cast nephropathy	9 (5.5)
Other	36 (22)
Medications	
ACEI/ARB	69 (43)
Diuretics	27 (17)
Beta blockers	19 (12)
Calcium Channel Inhibitors	37 (23)
Others	7 (4)
Clinical Chemistry	
Serum creatinine (mg/dl)	2.08±1.45
eGFR (ml/min/1.73 m^2)	47.4±33.3
Proteinuria (g/l)	2.3±2.7
Albuminuria (g/l)	1.3±2.4

Continuous variables are expressed as the mean ± sem; categorical variables are expressed as n (%).
*Hyperlipidemia: total cholesterol >200 mg/dl and/orTriglycerides >200 mg/dl, and/or LDL cholesterol>130 mg/dl.
**Cancer: Multiple myemoma (= 13), Urogenital (= 7), Breast (= 2), Lung (= 1).
***Non specific: no diagnosis, moderate interstitial fibrosis and/or glomerulosclerosis.

discriminate a particular group of diseases. Total proteinuria was only weakly higher in the patients with glomerular disease than in patients with the other diseases (p = 0.046) (**Fig. S1G**).

The distribution of proteinuria according to the eGFR levels was analyzed. LMW proteinuria was significantly higher among the patients with a mean eGFR value <30 ml/min (**Fig. 3A, Fig. S2A and B**) compared to the patients with eGFR values >30 ml/min, whereas HMW and total proteinuria were not significantly different among the eGFR groups (**Fig. 3B and C, Fig. S2C and D**). These data indicated that LMW proteinuria but not total or HMW proteinuria was a characteristic of patients with low eGFR in this CKD population.

The extent of IF is correlated with a lower eGFR

We next analyzed the characteristic features of IF in the CKD patients. As proof of the deleterious effect of interstitial fibrosis in CKD, we determined that the extent of IF was negatively associated with the eGFR ($R^2 = 0.24$, $p<0.0001$) (**Fig. 4A, Table 2**), and that this correlation was highly significant for glomerular disease but not for tubular or vascular diseases (**Fig. 4B-D**). There was no difference in the IF percentages between the types of nephropathies even though, as expected, the IF percentage in the normal biopsies was significantly lower (**Fig. 4E**). These results indicated that in our population, the extent of IF was correlated significantly with a low eGFR, at least in patients with glomerular disease.

LMW proteinuria but not HMW proteinuria is correlated with higher IF

We next examined the association between LMW proteinuria and the extent of IF. The univariate analysis indicated that LMW proteinuria but not HMW or total proteinuria correlated significantly with the extent of IF; RBP ($R^2 = 0.11$, $p<0.0001$); α1MG ($R^2 = 0.08$, $p = 0.0004$); and β2MG ($R^2 = 0.03$, $p = 0.02$) (**Fig. 5, Table 2, Fig. S3**). This association was significant in

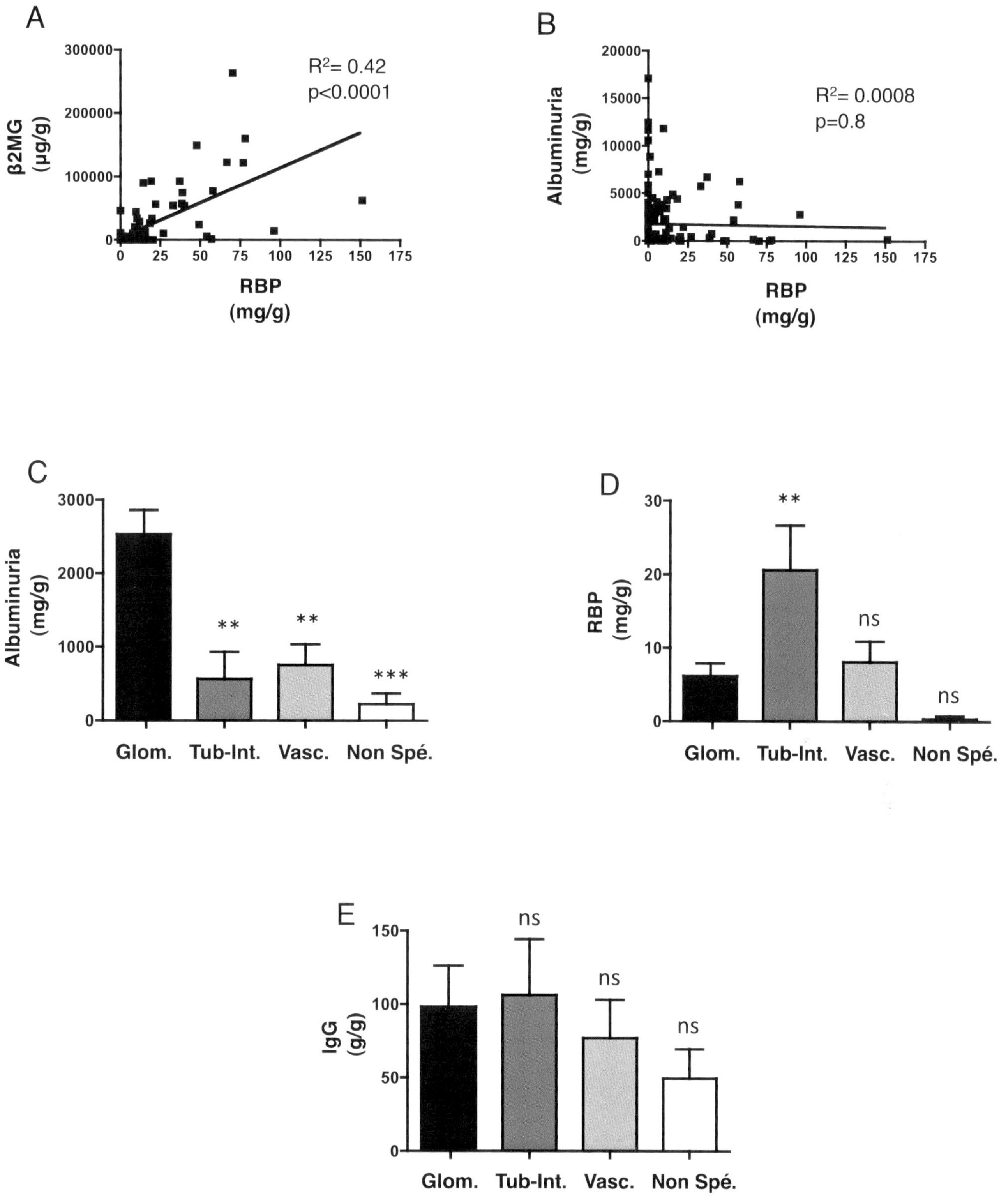

Figure 2. Expression patterns of proteinuria. A, B. Best-fit slope of the linear regression between RBP and β2MG (A) and RBP and Alb (B). **C, D, E.** Histogram showing Alb (A), RBP (B), and IgG (C) values according to the type of kidney disease. Protein concentrations are expressed as the mean ± sem. **p<0.01, ***p<0.001 compared to glomerular disease using Student's T test; the Mann-Whitney test was used for the glomerular vs. comparison with non-specific lesions. Glom: glomerular diseases; Tub-Int: tubular and/or interstitial diseases; Vasc: vascular diseases; Non-spe: non-specific.

Table 2. Summary of correlative data.

Covariate	R^2	p
Retinol Binding Protein		
β2MG	0.42	<0.0001
α1MG	0.66	<0.0001
Proteinuria	0.02	0.07
TRF	0.006	0.3
Albuminuria	0.0008	0.8
Fibrosis (glomerular diseases)	0.18	0.001
Fibrosis (tubule and interstitial diseases)	0.1	0.2
Fibrosis (vascular diseases)	0.008	0.5
eGFR		
Fibrosis (glomerular)	0.26	<0.0001
Fibrosis (vascular)	0.05	0.2
Fibrosis (tubule and interstitial diseases)	0.001	0.5
Fibrosis		
RBP	0.11	<0.0001
α1MG	0.08	0.0004
β2MG	0.03	0.03
TRF	0.01	0.2
Proteinuria	0.007	0.2
IgG	0.002	0.5
Albuminuria	0.0002	0.8

patients with glomerular disease ($R^2 = 0.11$, $p = 0.001$) but not in patients with tubule-interstitial disease ($R^2 = 0.10$, $p = 0.06$) or vascular disease ($R^2 = 0.08$, $p = 0.1$) despite a clear trend (**Fig. S4**).

Of the LMW proteins, RBP was the better predictor of IF; therefore, we performed a multivariate analysis to test whether this association was independent of other parameters. Given that α1MG, β2MG, and eGFR were correlated with the extent of IF, indicating that a portion of the information generated by RBP may also be provided by α1MG, β2MG, and eGFR, we fitted and compared two linear models, one including α1MG, β2MG, and eGFR and the other including these factors plus RBP. The two models were compared based on a likelihood ratio test in which the deviance follows a Chi-square distribution with the number of degrees equal to the difference of the variables included in the two nested models. The multiple linear regression analysis indicated that the model with RBP was significantly better than the model without RBP ($p = 0.03$), demonstrating that RBP was independently correlated with the extent of IF.

Finally, we analyzed the efficiency of testing urinary RBP levels for diagnosing the extent of IF. RBP/creat ratio has a high specificity in detecting cases with >25% fibrosis (the median value of fibrosis in our cohort, which also correlates with an altered prognosis in numerous settings, including chronic allograft nephropathy and chronic kidney diseases [4,5,6]; Recipient-Operating Characteristic curve (ROC curve area 0.7, $p = 0.0003$) indicates a high specificity in detecting cases with >25% fibrosis. For example, an RBP/creat ratio above 20 mg/g predicted a fibrosis score > 25% with a specificity of 95% but with a sensitivity of 20%. The likelihood ratio of this cutoff is 4, which indicates that a patients with a RBP ratio>20 mg/g is 4 times more likely to have >25% fibrosis. This observation indicated that a high concentration of urinary RBP was associated the extent of IF in non-selected CKD patients, with very few false positives; however, a normal or low value did not exclude the presence of IF.

Discussion

In this study, we demonstrated that the concentration of LMW proteins but not total or HMW proteins was positively associated with the degree of IF and altered renal function. The RBP/creat ratio was independently correlated with the extent of IF and could be useful for predicting renal fibrosis with a high specificity, especially in patients with glomerular diseases. To our knowledge, this study is the first to demonstrate a significant correlation between urinary RBP and kidney IF in a prospective and non-selected population of CKD patients. Given that the extent of fibrosis correlates with adverse outcomes, a non-invasive diagnosis of the extent of interstitial fibrosis is usefull tool for the management of CKD patients, both in terms of prognosis and therapeutic and nephroprotective strategies.

eGFR is a good predictor of fibrosis. The ROC curves of the two predictors are similar in terms of diagnostic performance, and the addition of RBP to eGFR does not increase the performance of the prediction (not shown). This raises the question of the prognostic value of RBP of the decline of renal function, which remains to be examined. Our results suggest that IF promotes loss of function and eGFR decline, and IF promotes tubular dysfunction and RBP loss. This point is supported but the results of the regression analysis indicating that RBP and GFR correlate with IF, and that RBP is independent of GFR.

The proposed rationale for the detection of increased LMW protein concentrations in the urine from patients with extended fibrosis of the kidneys is based on the hypothesis that IF is frequently associated with TA, leading to the defective proximal reabsorption of physiologically filtered LMW. Any increase in the urinary excretion of β2MG or RBP is highly specific for tubular disease, whereas the increased excretion of α1MG is observed in glomerular proteinuria [19,20]. This non-specific degenerative tubulopathy associated indirectly with LMW output and extended urinalysis (including glucosuria or aminoaciduria) could be used to confirm this hypothesis. There is indirect evidence to support this concept. For example, the reduction in the maximal reabsorption rate of filtered phosphates, which are reabsorbed mainly by the proximal tubules and are excreted in excess urine in cases of proximal tubulopathy, is proportional to the reduction in eGFR [21]. The concept that tubular dysfunction is related to IF is also supported by the recent demonstration of a strong correlation between RBP and Banff classification scores and TA in a series of KTRs; the protein measurements correlated with the interstitial Banff scores at the one-year biopsy [22]. However, for reasons that are unclear, the LMW and HMW protein levels observed in the study correlated strongly with each other and with graft function, histology, and survival; associations that were not observed in our study.

An advantage of our study is that the large panel of proteins tested in our center used validated methods used routinely in clinical chemistry laboratories, and the cost was relatively low (7 USD per RBP measurement). In comparison, the cost of a urinary electrophoretic profile is 10.5 USD and an albuminuria measurement is 3 USD. Importantly, the performance of these methods has been validated, including the interlaboratory reproducibility of the tests, and the practical outcome is that almost all clinicians can evaluate the extent of IF in CKD patients through measuring the RBP concentration [23,24]. To date, few non-invasive markers of the extent of kidney fibrosis have been tested, including polypeptide-like urinary procollagen III amino-

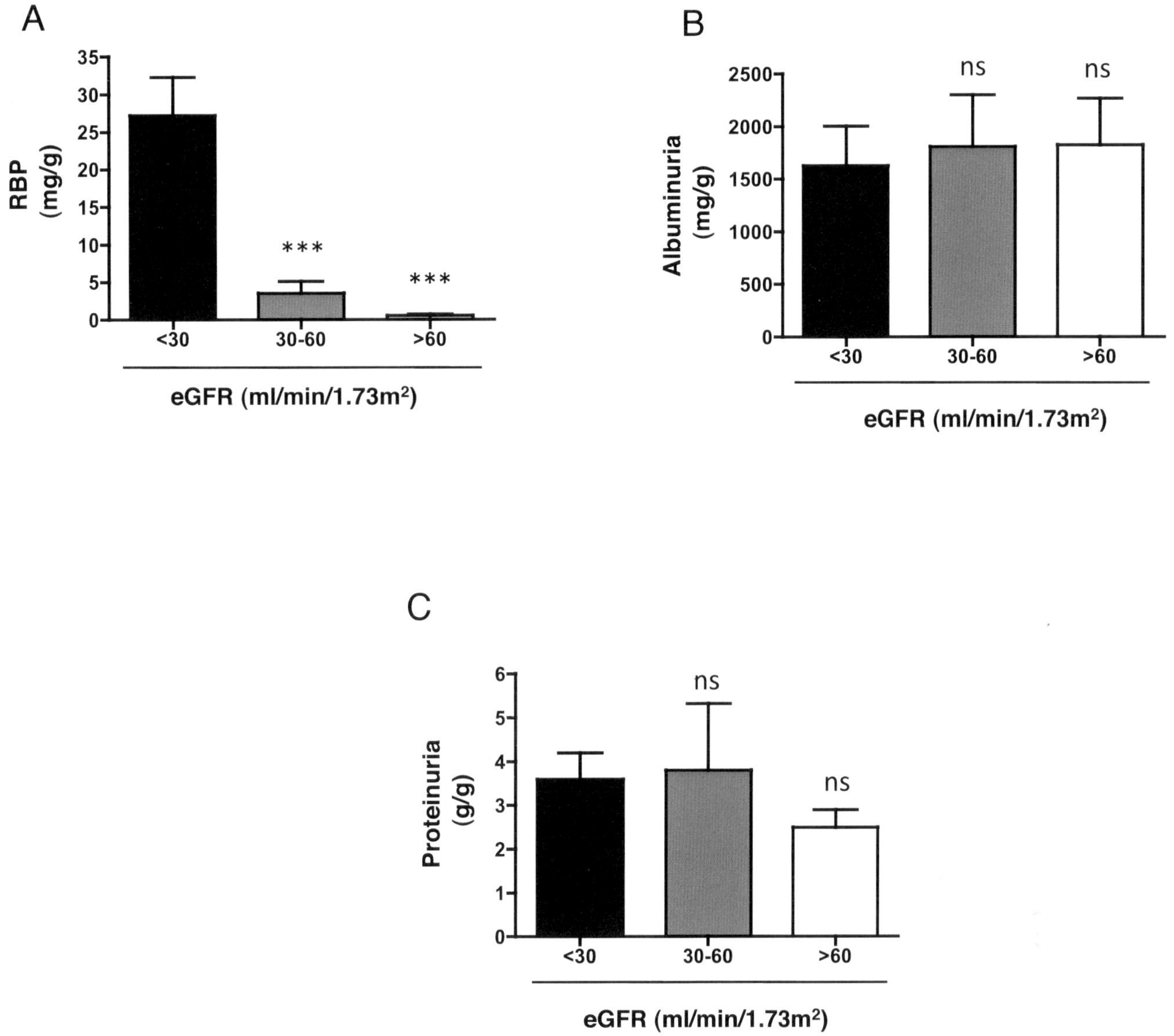

Figure 3. Distribution of proteinuria according to the estimated glomerular filtration rate. A, B, C. Histogram showing Alb (A), RBP (B), and total proteinuria (C) values according to the level of eGFR. Protein concentrations are expressed as the mean ± sem. **$p<0.01$, ***$p<0.001$ compared to eGFR <30 ml/min, using Student's T test.

terminal propetide (PIIINP) [10]. PIIINP levels have been correlated with the extent of kidney fibrosis; however, the association has not been tested using a multivariate analysis. Moreover, PIIINP analysis is not performed routinely, and the interlaboratory reproducibility of the test is unknown [10]. Regardless, together with our study, these studies demonstrated that non-invasive markers are associated with the extent of IF, which can be evaluated using the robust and reproducible method of color segmentation image analysis. This computerized method for IF quantification has been validated both in KTR [25] and CKD patients [10], and the results are predictive of renal prognosis.

We observed that RBP correlated with IF in sthe group of patients with glomerular disease but not in the patients with tubular or vascular disease. Despite this clear trend, the lack of a positive correlation in these two disease categories may be explained by the relatively low size of these subgroups of patients compared with the glomerular disease subgroup. Additionally, this finding may indicate that the tubule-interstitial injury induced by proteinuria secondary to glomerular disease impedes LMW reabsorption to a greater extent than in primitive tubulo-interstitial diseases. Recently, the effect of LMW proteinuria on the prognosis of glomerular disease was highlighted in a study of membranous nephropathy, demonstrating that LMW proteinuria is associated with the progression of kidney dysfunction[11].

Another intriguing finding was the pattern of urinary IgG expression, which, in contrast to previous studies in KTRs and membranous nephropathies [11,22], was not associated with any relevant variable in our study. More importantly, the mean concentration of IgG did not differ between etiologic groups, suggesting that despite the high MW of IgG (160 kD), the loss of glomerular permeability does not always result in IgG proteinuria. Our findings are corroborated by the normal IgG excretion rate demonstrated in a series of patients with membranous nephrop-

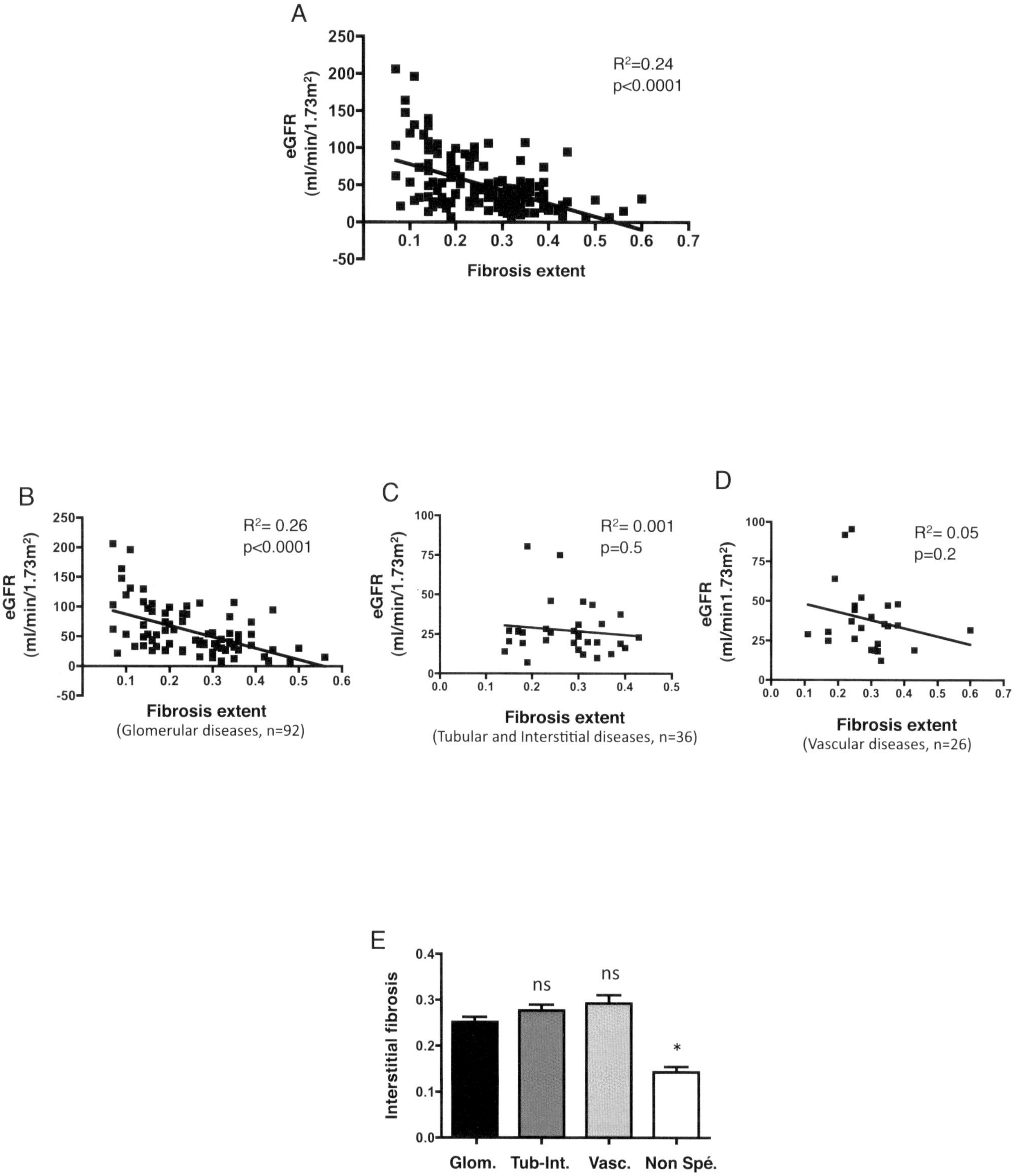

Figure 4. Correlation between the estimated glomerular filtration rate and extent of interstitial fibrosis. A. Best-fit slope of the linear regression between eGFR and extent of fibrosis. **B**, **C**, **D**. Best-fit slope of the linear regression between eGFR and extent of fibrosis in glomerular disease (B), tubular disease (C), and vascular disease (D). **E**. Histogram of the distribution of the extent of interstitial fibrosis according to the type of kidney disease. The percentages of interstitial fibrosis are expressed as the mean ± sem. *$p<0.05$ compared to glomerular disease, using Student's T test; the Mann-Whitney test was used for the glomerular vs. non specific lesions comparison. Glom: glomerular diseases; Tub-Int: tubular and/or interstitial diseases; Vasc: vascular diseases; Non-spe: non-specific.

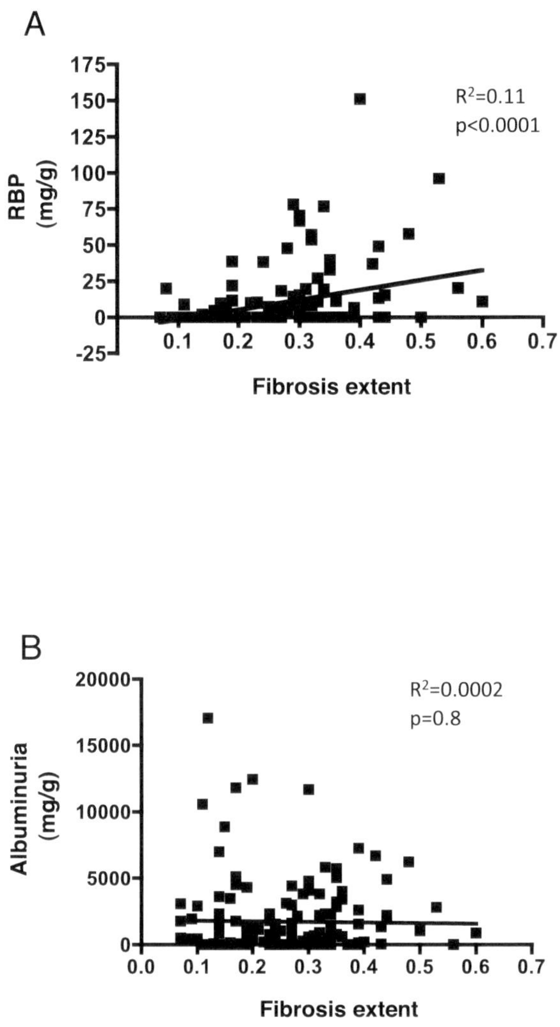

Figure 5. Correlation between proteinuria and the extent of interstitial fibrosis. A, B. Best-fit slope of the linear regression between RBP (A) and Alb (B) and extent of fibrosis extent.

athy [11]. The possibility of IgG or IgM being produced locally in the interstitium and secreted in the urine has been raised by a number of authors [22]; however, this phenomenon has not been demonstrated. Overall, our study challenged the usefulness of assaying urinary IgG levels in terms of characterizing the type of nephropathy and for purposes of identifying markers of tubulo-interstitial injury.

TA has not been evaluated in this study because to our knowledge, there is no validated automatized method for TA quantification in kidney tissue, and there is a need for tools providing continuous values of TA rather that semi-quantitative score. The only validated system of TA scoring is the Banff system, which is widely used, but with numerous limitations, and provides validated information in kidney transplant patients only. There is always a strong correlation between IF and TA scores in models in which they have be evaluated, mostly in kidney transplant recipients, which indicates the score of IF in somehow reveals the TA. The absence of TA measurement does not change the conclusion of our study regarding the performance of the measurement of the concentrations of RBP in urines in predicting the extent of IF.

In conclusion, we demonstrated that an increase in the excretion of LMW proteins, particularly RBP, is a non-invasive marker that can independently predict the extent of kidney IF. However, further studies are needed to validate our findings. Because the measurement of RBP is implemented routinely in clinical chemistry departments, RBP is an appealing marker to assess the severity of chronic kidney damage. Studies are ongoing to determine whether LMW protein levels independently predict CKD progression.

Supporting Information

Figure S1 Distribution of proteinuria in the 162 CKD patients. A,B,C. Best-fit slope of linear regression between α1MG and RBP (A), TRF and RBP (B), and proteinuria and RBP (C). D, E, F, G. Histograms showing TRF (D), α1MG (E), β2MG (F) and total proteinuria (G) values according to the type of kidney disease. Protein concentrations are expressed as mean±sem. *$p<0.05$, **$p<0.01$, ***$p<0.001$, compared to glomerular disease, Student T test, except Mann-Whitney test for Glomerular vs Non specific comparison and ANOVA for (G). Glom = glomerular disease; Tub-Int = tubular and interstitial diseases; Vasc = vascular diseases; Non-spe = non-specific lesions.

Figure S2 Distribution of proteinuria according to estimated glomerular filtration rates. Histograms showing α1MG (A), β2MG (B), IgG (C) and TRF (D) values according to the type of kidney disease. Protein concentrations expressed as mean±sem. *$p<0.05$, **$p<0.01$, ***$p<0.001$, as compared to eGFR<30 ml/min.

Figure S3 Correlation between proteinuria and the extent of interstitial fibrosis. Best-fit slopes of linear regression between α1MG (A), β2MG (B), TRF (C), IgG (D), and proteinuria (E) and the extent of interstitial fibrosis.

Figure S4 Correlation between proteinuria and the extent of interstitial fibrosis according to the type of nephropathy. Best-fit slope of linear regression between fibrosis extent and RBP according to the type of nephropathy: glomerular (A), tubular (B), and vascular (C).

Author Contributions

Conceived and designed the experiments: NP ET AK. Performed the experiments: SC JFC MV PA CL VMY JCOM DNM PB. Analyzed the data: NP AK. Contributed reagents/materials/analysis tools: SC JFC CL VMY JCOM DNM PB. Wrote the paper: NP.

References

1. Zeisberg M, Neilson EG (2010) Mechanisms of tubulointerstitial fibrosis. J Am Soc Nephrol 21: 1819–1834.
2. Liu Y (2011) Cellular and molecular mechanisms of renal fibrosis. Nat Rev Nephrol 7: 684–696.
3. Roberts IS, Cook HT, Troyanov S, Alpers CE, Amore A, et al. (2009) The Oxford classification of IgA nephropathy: pathology definitions, correlations, and reproducibility. Kidney Int 76: 546–556.
4. Cattran DC, Coppo R, Cook HT, Feehally J, Roberts IS, et al. (2009) The Oxford classification of IgA nephropathy: rationale, clinicopathological correlations, and classification. Kidney Int 76: 534–545.
5. Farris AB, Adams CD, Brousaides N, Della Pelle PA, Collins AB, et al. (2011) Morphometric and visual evaluation of fibrosis in renal biopsies. J Am Soc Nephrol 22: 176–186.

6. Hertig A, Anglicheau D, Verine J, Pallet N, Touzot M, et al. (2008) Early epithelial phenotypic changes predict graft fibrosis. J Am Soc Nephrol 19: 1584–1591.
7. Weiss RH, Kim K (2011) Metabolomics in the study of kidney diseases. Nat Rev Nephrol 8: 22–33.
8. Cravedi P, Ruggenenti P, Remuzzi G (2012) Proteinuria should be used as a surrogate in CKD. Nat Rev Nephrol 8: 301–306.
9. Mirkovic K, Doorenbos CR, Dam WA, Lambers Heerspink HJ, Slagman MC, et al. (2013) Urinary vitamin D binding protein: a potential novel marker of renal interstitial inflammation and fibrosis. PLoS One 8: e55887.
10. Ghoul BE, Squalli T, Servais A, Elie C, Meas-Yedid V, et al. (2010) Urinary procollagen III aminoterminal propeptide (PIIINP): a fibrotest for the nephrologist. Clin J Am Soc Nephrol 5: 205–210.
11. van den Brand JA, Hofstra JM, Wetzels JF (2011) Low-molecular-weight proteins as prognostic markers in idiopathic membranous nephropathy. Clin J Am Soc Nephrol 6: 2846–2853.
12. Halimi JM, Matthias B, Al-Najjar A, Laouad I, Chatelet V, et al. (2007) Respective predictive role of urinary albumin excretion and nonalbumin proteinuria on graft loss and death in renal transplant recipients. Am J Transplant 7: 2775–2781.
13. Amer H, Fidler ME, Myslak M, Morales P, Kremers WK, et al. (2007) Proteinuria after kidney transplantation, relationship to allograft histology and survival. Am J Transplant 7: 2748–2756.
14. Post AR, Kurc T, Cholleti S, Gao J, Lin X, et al. (2013) The Analytic Information Warehouse (AIW): A platform for analytics using electronic health record data. J Biomed Inform 46: 410–424.
15. Dati F, Schumann G, Thomas L, Aguzzi F, Baudner S, et al. (1996) Consensus of a group of professional societies and diagnostic companies on guidelines for interim reference ranges for 14 proteins in serum based on the standardization against the IFCC/BCR/CAP Reference Material (CRM 470). International Federation of Clinical Chemistry. Community Bureau of Reference of the Commission of the European Communities. College of American Pathologists. Eur J Clin Chem Clin Biochem 34: 517–520.
16. Gressner A, Thomas L (1995) Proteinstoffwechel; Greiling H, Gressner A, editors. Stuttgart; New York: Schattauer. 225 p.
17. Levey AS, Greene T, Beck GJ, Caggiula AW, Kusek JW, et al. (1999) Dietary protein restriction and the progression of chronic renal disease: what have all of the results of the MDRD study shown? Modification of Diet in Renal Disease Study group. J Am Soc Nephrol 10: 2426–2439.
18. Servais A, Meas-Yedid V, Buchler M, Morelon E, Olivo-Marin JC, et al. (2007) Quantification of interstitial fibrosis by image analysis on routine renal biopsy in patients receiving cyclosporine. Transplantation 84: 1595–1601.
19. Tomlinson PA (1992) Low molecular weight proteins in children with renal disease. Pediatr Nephrol 6: 565–571.
20. Kirsztajn GM, Nishida SK, Silva MS, Ajzen H, Moura LA, et al. (2002) Urinary retinol-binding protein as a prognostic marker in glomerulopathies. Nephron 90: 424–431.
21. Iwasawa H, Nakao T, Matsumoto H, Okada T, Nagaoka Y, et al. (2013) Phosphate handling by end-stage kidneys and benefits of residual renal function on phosphate removal in patients on haemodialysis. Nephrology (Carlton) 18: 285–291.
22. Amer H, Lieske JC, Rule AD, Kremers WK, Larson TS, et al. (2013) Urine high and low molecular weight proteins one-year post-kidney transplant: relationship to histology and graft survival. Am J Transplant 13: 676–684.
23. Twyman SJ, Overton J, Rowe DJ (2000) Measurement of urinary retinol binding protein by immunonephelometry. Clin Chim Acta 297: 155–161.
24. Parviainen MT, Ylitalo P (1983) Immunonephelometric determination of retinol-binding protein in serum and urine. Clin Chem 29: 853–856.
25. Meas-Yedid V, Servais A, Noel LH, Panterne C, Landais P, et al. (2011) New computerized color image analysis for the quantification of interstitial fibrosis in renal transplantation. Transplantation 92: 890–899.

3

Laser Capture Microdissection and Multiplex-Tandem PCR Analysis of Proximal Tubular Epithelial Cell Signaling in Human Kidney Disease

Ray Wilkinson[1,2,4,5]*, Xiangju Wang[1,2], Andrew J. Kassianos[1,2], Steven Zuryn[1,2], Kathrein E. Roper[1,2], Andrew Osborne[1,2], Sandeep Sampangi[1,2], Leo Francis[3], Vishwas Raghunath[2], Helen Healy[1,2]

1 Conjoint Kidney Research Laboratory, Pathology Queensland, Brisbane, Queensland, Australia, **2** Department of Renal Medicine, Royal Brisbane and Women's Hospital, Brisbane, Queensland, Australia, **3** Pathology Queensland, Brisbane, Queensland, Australia, **4** Institute of Health and Biomedical Innovation, Queensland University of Technology, Brisbane, Queensland, Australia, **5** Medical School, University of Queensland, Brisbane, Queensland, Australia

Abstract

Interstitial fibrosis, a histological process common to many kidney diseases, is the precursor state to end stage kidney disease, a devastating and costly outcome for the patient and the health system. Fibrosis is historically associated with chronic kidney disease (CKD) but emerging evidence is now linking many forms of acute kidney disease (AKD) with the development of CKD. Indeed, we and others have observed at least some degree of fibrosis in up to 50% of clinically defined cases of AKD. Epithelial cells of the proximal tubule (PTEC) are central in the development of kidney interstitial fibrosis. We combine the novel techniques of laser capture microdissection and multiplex-tandem PCR to identify and quantitate "real time" gene transcription profiles of purified PTEC isolated from human kidney biopsies that describe signaling pathways associated with this pathological fibrotic process. Our results: (i) confirm previous in-vitro and animal model studies; kidney injury molecule-1 is up-regulated in patients with acute tubular injury, inflammation, neutrophil infiltration and a range of chronic disease diagnoses, (ii) provide data to inform treatment; complement component 3 expression correlates with inflammation and acute tubular injury, (iii) identify potential new biomarkers; proline 4-hydroxylase transcription is down-regulated and vimentin is up-regulated across kidney diseases, (iv) describe previously unrecognized feedback mechanisms within PTEC; Smad-3 is down-regulated in many kidney diseases suggesting a possible negative feedback loop for TGF-β in the disease state, whilst tight junction protein-1 is up-regulated in many kidney diseases, suggesting feedback interactions with vimentin expression. These data demonstrate that the combined techniques of laser capture microdissection and multiplex-tandem PCR have the power to study molecular signaling within single cell populations derived from clinically sourced tissue.

Editor: Aristidis S. Charonis, Biomedical Research Foundation of the Academy of Athens, Greece

Funding: Funding provided by Chemical Pathology, Queensland Health; SERTF Trust Fund, Queensland Health; Private Practice Trust Fund, RBWH, Queensland. The funders had no role in study design, data collection and analysis, decision to publish, or preparation of the manuscript.

* E-mail: ray.wilkinson@qimr.edu.au

Introduction

It is widely acknowledged that the epithelial cells of the proximal tubule (PTEC) play a central role in interstitial fibrosis, following cellular insults such as excessive protein exposure and oxidative stress [1–5]. These insults lead to perturbation of the complex interactions of growth factors, cytokines and chemokines which maintain the homeostasis of these cells, leading to the over-expression of genes involved in inflammatory responses [6–8] and epithelial to mesenchymal transition (EMT) [9–12], both patho-biological processes resulting in a fibrotic phenotype. However, research implicating PTEC involvement in interstitial fibrosis comes predominantly from animal models or in-vitro studies using transformed cell lines or primary PTEC cultures. The relevance of translating PTEC knowledge derived from these models to human disease has not been established. Attempts to elucidate transcription profiles in human kidney disease tissue have generally taken a global approach, analyzing gene expression from whole kidney biopsies [13,14] or tissue sections with mixed cellular populations [15].

In this work we exploit the recent developments in microscopic dissection using Laser Capture Microdissection (LCM) to target the single cell PTEC population ex-vivo. The technology allows the visualisation of proximal tubules within renal biopsies from patients with kidney disease and the subsequent capture/isolation of PTEC from these tubules using laser catapult energy [16]. This technology has been recently used in human kidney research of gene expression in the glomerulus [17–19], to study one or two genes across different compartments of the kidney [20,21] or to analyse PTEC collected from proteinuric disease biopsies using gene microarray technology [22,23]. Gene microarray analysis studies provide vast amounts of transcriptional data but have a number of inherent difficulties including: (i) difficult and expensive to undertake, (ii) require duplicate samples to eliminate artifactual data, (iii) take weeks or months to analyse the large volumes of data and (iv) require large amounts of input RNA or, when not

Table 1. MT-PCR genes examined and the associated disease pathway.

	Gene Symbol	Official Name
House Keeping	GAPDH	glyceraldehyde-3-phosphate dehydrogenase
	BTF3	basic transcription factor 3
Fibrosis	TGFB1	transforming growth factor, beta 1
	SERPINE1	serpin peptidase inhibitor, clade E, member 1
	SMAD3	SMAD family member 3
	COL3A1	collagen, type III, alpha 1
	COL1A2	collagen, type I, alpha 2
	P4HA2	proline 4-hydroxylase, alpha polypeptide II
	SERPINH	serpin peptidase inhibitor, clade H (heat shock protein 47), member 1
	THBS1	thrombospondin 1
Inflammation	TNF	tumor necrosis factor (TNF superfamily, member 2)
	IL6	interleukin 6 (interferon, beta 2)
	IL8	interleukin 8
	NFKB1	nuclear factor of kappa light polypeptide gene enhancer in B-cells 1
	CCL2	chemokine (C-C motif) ligand 2/monocyte chemotactic protein 1
	C3	complement component 3
	BMP7	bone morphogenetic protein 7 (osteogenic protein 1)
	BMP6	morphogenetic protein 6
	Kim-1	kidney injury molecule-1/hepatitis A virus cellular receptor 1
	SPP1	secreted phosphoprotein 1 (osteopontin, early T-lymphocyte activation 1)
EMT	VIM	vimentin
	ACTA2	actin, alpha 2, smooth muscle, aorta
	TJP1	tight junction protein 1 (zona occludens 1)
	S100A4	S100 calcium binding protein A4
	TWIST1	twist homolog 1
	SNAI1	snail homolog 1
Apoptosis	BCL2	B-cell CLL/lymphoma 2
	BAD	BCL2-antagonist of cell death
	BAX	BCL2-associated X protein
	CASP3	caspase 3, apoptosis-related cysteine peptidase
	CASP8	caspase 8, apoptosis-related cysteine peptidase
	FAS	Fas (TNF receptor superfamily, member 6)

available as occurs in the clinical setting, non-specific pre-amplification of high quality RNA.

To remove bias, commonly encountered when non-specifically pre-amplifying the picogram quantities of RNA typically obtained from human biopsies using LCM, we utilised targeted gene transcription analysis using primer-specific nested amplification. This methodology, known as multiplex tandem-PCR (MT-PCR), has been reported to amplify cDNA from as little as 10 picograms of RNA and was designed to amplify degraded RNA recovered from formalin-fixed paraffin embedded tissue [24]. Here we use MT-PCR analysis of LCM-isolated PTEC from clinical human kidney biopsies to provide transcriptional data on the four major pathobiological pathways associated with kidney fibrosis: (i) inflammation, (ii) collagen deposition, (iii) EMT and (iv) apoptosis. We relate changes in the transcriptional profiles of the pathways to the clinical phenotype of the patients. These technologies are readily translatable to human diagnostics of the future where the prognostic power of PTEC may direct therapies to specific targets.

Methods

Patient and Tissue sample details

Control tissues were obtained from the healthy portions of malignant nephrectomies (n = 8) and were validated as normal at the macroscopic and microscopic level by the consulting renal pathologist. Diseased samples (n = 96) were collected from native kidney biopsy material that were surplus to diagnostic requirements. Biopsies were frozen in OCT within 20 minutes of collection and stored at −80°C prior to processing. When biopsies/patients were grouped according to the clinical diagnosis of acute or chronic disease, defined clinically prior to histopathological diagnosis, we had a total of 26 acute, 16 chronic, 51 acute-on-chronic and 3 undefined. Final disease diagnoses, of which there were three or more patients per disease group (n = 87), included IgA nephropathy (IgAN; n = 14), focal segmental glomerulosclerosis (FSGS; n = 11), pauci-immune glomerulonephritis (PI; n = 11), membranous nephropathy (MN; n = 9), interstitial nephritis (IN; n = 7), protein deposition disease (PDD;

n = 7), minimal change disease (MCD; n = 6), diabetic nephropathy (DN; n = 6), lupus nephritis (LN; n = 5), membranoproliferative glomerulonephritis (MPGN; n = 4), thrombotic microangiopathy (TMA; n = 4) and acute tubular necrosis (ATN; n = 3). The renal pathologist also scored the histological grading of the interstitium of all disease biopsies using a scale modified from the Banff system [25]. Briefly, overall cortical inflammation (OCI), unscarred cortical inflammation (UCI) and interstitial fibrosis/tubular atrophy (IF/TA) were each graded on a scale of 0–4 (0 = not present, 1 = up to 5%, 2 = 6–25%, 3 = 26–50% and 4 = greater than 50%) and yes/no for the presence of acute tubular injury (ATI), neutrophils and eosinophils. This grading was based upon the analysis of twenty individual 4 μm sections from each biopsy, which had been stained with haematoxylin and eosin or Masson's trichrome. Kidney function (estimated glomerular filtration rate (eGFR)) was calculated using the MDRD method by AUSLAB (Queensland Health) and proteinuria was described by urine protein to creatinine ratio (uPCR).

Ethics statement

All disease biopsy samples were used following written informed patient consent under human ethics approval from the Royal Brisbane and Women's Hospital (RBWH) (2002/011) and the Queensland Institute of Medical Research (QIMR) (P293).

LCM

10 μm thick cryosections were cut under RNase-free conditions and mounted on MembraneSlide 1.0 PEN slides (Carl Zeiss, Munich, Germany) treated with 20 min of UV exposure prior to use. Cryosections were stored at −80°C for a maximum of 48 hours or processed immediately for staining of endogenous alkaline phosphatase, exclusively expressed by PTEC in kidney cortex, by a one minute fixation in 70% ethanol followed by staining with SigmaFast BCIP/NBT (Sigma-Aldrich, St Louis, MO, USA) for 5 min. Cryosections were then dehydrated for 1 min each in 70%, 90% and 100% ethanol and PTEC were collected from these sections for a maximum time of 30 min, after which the process was repeated with additional sections until a total of one million μm^2 of tissue was collected. The PALM Microlaser System (PALM Microlaser Technologies, Zeiss, Jena, Germany) equipped with the PALM RoboSoftware controlled microscope stage and micromanipulator was used for LCM. PTEC were outlined at the basement membrane using the software and isolated from surrounding tissue by laser ablation prior to being catapulted into a Zeiss AdhesiveCap 500 Opaque collection cap (Zeiss) for subsequent RNA isolation. One cap per "section collection" was used and caps were replaced on their tube and stored on dry ice prior to RNA extraction using the Absolutely RNA Nanoprep kit (Stratagene, Santa Clara, CA, USA) with on-column DNase digestion. Confirming PTEC purity, initial quantitative RT-PCR optimization experiments failed to amplify non-PTEC expressed genes (aquaporin-2 and tamm-horsfall protein) from three million μm^2 LCM isolated PTEC (data not shown).

Table 2. The mean log relative gene expression (normalised to GAPDH) of nine genes able to differentiate disease from healthy control biopsies.

	Mean Control	Mean Disease	Disease-Control	p-value
Kim-1	0.24	2.17	1.93	<0.001
P4HA2	6.24	4.33	−1.91	0.002
C3	0.55	2.15	1.6	0.024
THBS1	8.37	6.45	−1.93	0.038
COL3A1	0.43	4.20	3.76	<0.001
ACTA2	5.88	3.83	−2.05	0.012
TJP1	2.40	3.86	1.46	0.033
VIM	0.22	4.34	4.12	<0.001
FAS	4.17	6.32	2.16	0.005

Kim-1, P4HA2 and C3 also demonstrated significant differences within disease groups based on histology (OCI, UCI, IF/TA, ATI and presence of neutrophils/eosinophils), kidney function (eGFR) or proteinuria (uPCR), compared to controls.

Multiplex Tandem-PCR

This methodology uses two-step MT-PCR gene-disc technology developed in commercial collaboration with AusDiagnostics Pty Ltd (Sydney, Australia). In the first step the RNA from a single one million μm^2 PTEC extraction was converted to cDNA and amplified in a multiplex single tube reaction for 25 cycles using AusDiagnostics gene-specific primers and master mix reagents. The product was then diluted 1/200 and dispensed into duplicate individual tubes containing specific nested primers for each gene of interest and amplified using real-time PCR for a further 45 cycles with a SYBR Green master mix in a Rotor-Gene Q thermal cycler (QIAGEN, Hilden, Germany). Genes were "called" by AusDiagnostics Software protocols that analyze products based upon melt temperature, purity and quantity values. All "called" results were manually verified during data analysis. Expression levels were normalised to the internal house-keeping genes GAPDH and BTF3 which were assigned an arbitrary value of 1000. Primer and product sequences are not reported due to commercial in-confidence agreements with AusDiagnostics Pty Ltd. We analyzed a total of 30 genes in duplicate for every sample. Genes are listed in Table 1.

Quantitative RT-PCR

Real-time PCR (RT-PCR) primers were designed and supplied by AusDiagnostics Pty Ltd. Three million μm^2 of PTEC were extracted by LCM from biopsies and total RNA was isolated from cells with the Absolutely RNA Nanoprep Kit (Stratagene) according to the manufacturer's instructions. Reverse transcription was performed using random hexamers (Invitrogen, Grand Island, NY, USA) and Superscript III Reverse Transcriptase (Invitrogen). RT-PCR reactions were performed using RT^2 SYBR Green qPCR master mix (QIAGEN). GAPDH was used for normalization of cDNA input, and RT-PCR reactions were performed using a Rotor-Gene Q thermal cycler (QIAGEN) according to the manufacturer's instructions: initial denaturation at 95°C for 10 min, followed by 45–50 cycles at 95°C for 15 sec and at 60°C for 60 sec. Data analysis was performed using Rotorgene software (QIAGEN) and the delta delta Ct (ΔΔCt) method.

Immunohistochemistry

6 μm cryosections were prepared and dried overnight prior to fixation in acetone/ethanol. Sections were blocked for 30 min in 4% milk and 15 min in 10% goat serum and incubated with primary Ab diluted in Tris-buffered saline (TBS) for 1 hour at room temperature. Primary Abs were mouse anti-human Kim-1 (Clone 219211; R&D Systems, Minneapolis, MN, USA), mouse anti-human Collagen III (Clone FH-7A; Abcam, Hong Kong) and mouse anti-human Vimentin (Clone V9; Dako, Glostrup, Denmark). Following three 5 min washes in TBS, sections were treated

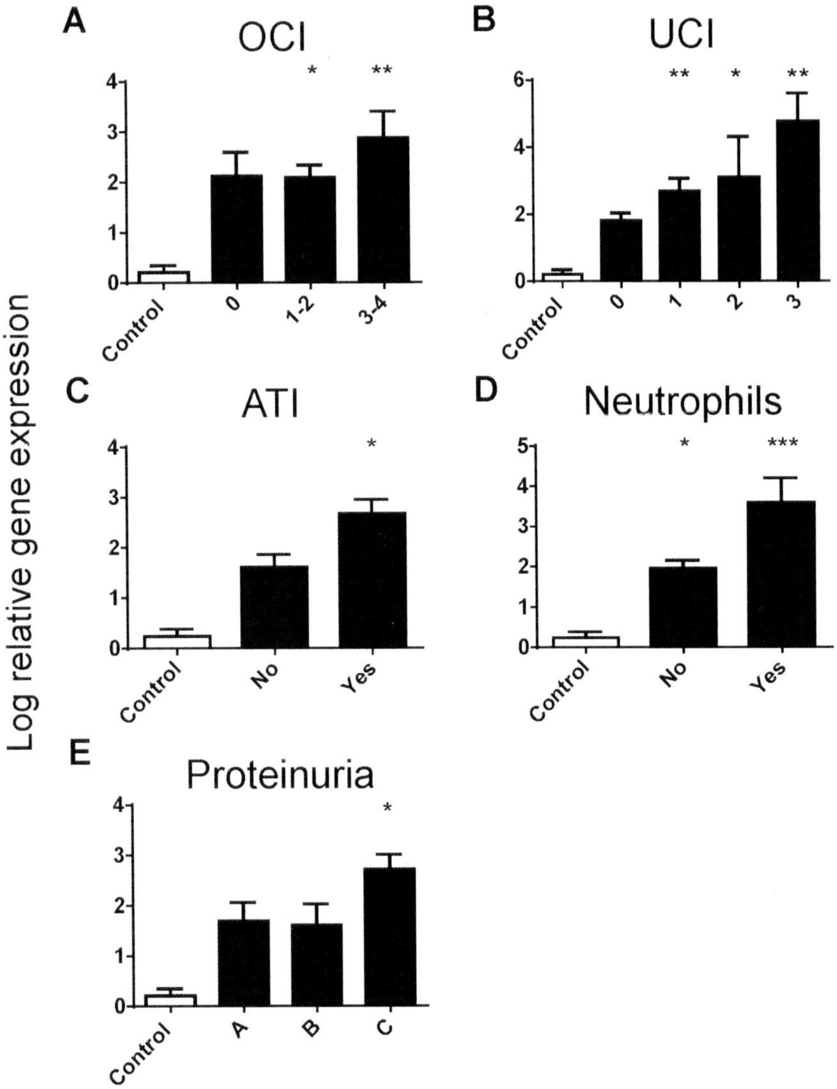

Figure 1. Kim-1 log relative gene expression (normalised to GAPDH) from normal biopsies (Control) and biopsies with (A) overall cortical inflammation (OCI, 0 = absent, 1–2 = 5–25%, 3–4 = 26–>50%), (B) unscarred cortical inflammation (UCI, 0 = absent, 1 = <5%, 2 = 6–25%, 3 = 26–50%), (C) the presence of acute tubular injury, (D) the presence of neutrophils and (E) proteinuria, defined using a urine protein to creatinine ratio (uPCR) (A = < 100 mg/mmol, B = 100–299 mg/mmol, C = ≥300 mg/mmol). Values are means ± SEM. *P<0.05, **P<0.01, ***P<0.001, one-way ANOVA with Dunnett's post-test.

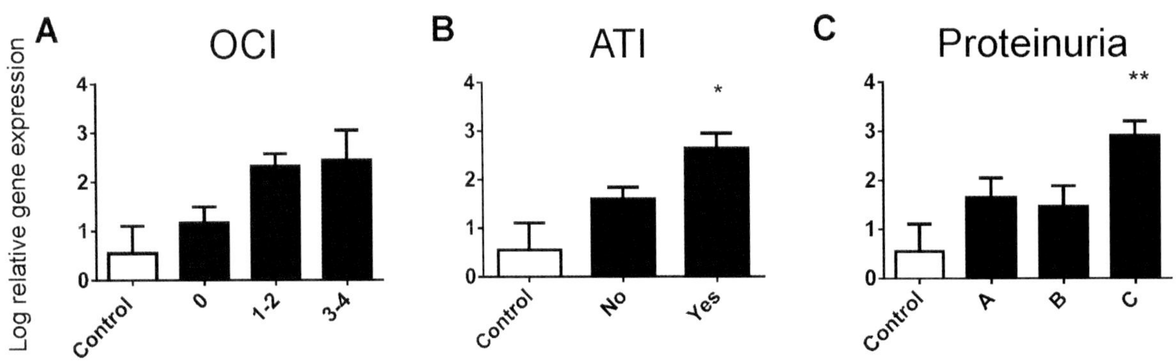

Figure 2. C3 log relative gene expression (normalised to GAPDH) from normal biopsies (Control) and biopsies with (A) overall cortical inflammation (OCI, 0 = absent, 1–2 = 5–25%, 3–4 = 26–>50%), (B) the presence of acute tubular injury and (C) proteinuria, defined using a urine protein to creatinine ratio (uPCR) (A = <100 mg/mmol, B = 100–299 mg/mmol, C = ≥300 mg/mmol). Values are means ± SEM. *P<0.05, **P<0.01, one-way ANOVA with Dunnett's post-test.

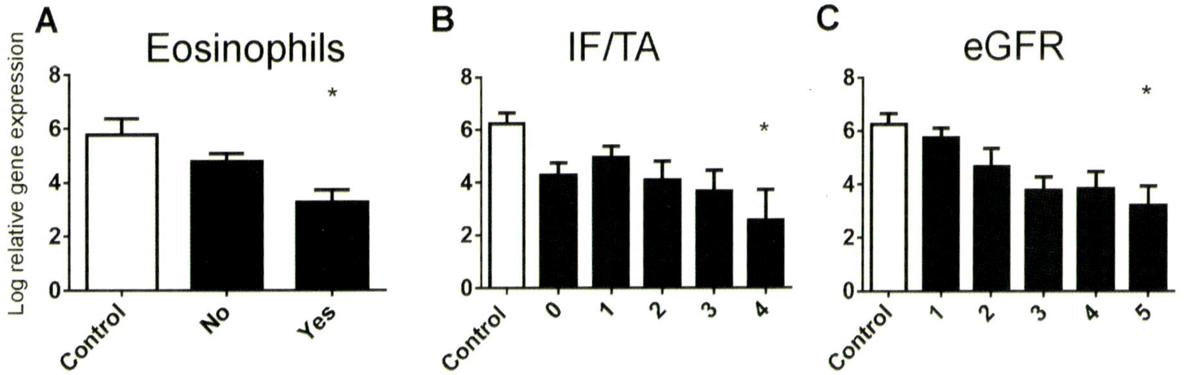

Figure 3. P4HA2 log relative gene expression (normalised to GAPDH) from normal biopsies (Control) and biopsies with (A) the presence of eosinophils, (B) interstitial fibrosis/tubular atrophy (IF/TA, 0 = absent, 1 = <5%, 2 = 6–25%, 3 = 26–50%, 4 = >50%) and (C) chronic kidney disease (CKD) defined by estimated glomerular filtration rate (eGFR, 1 = ≥90 ml/min/1.73 m^2, 2 = 60–89 ml/min/1.73 m^2, 3 = 30–59 ml/min/1.73 m^2, 4 = 15–29 ml/min/1.73 m^2, 5 = <15 ml/min/1.73 m^2). Values are means ± SEM. *P<0.05, one-way ANOVA with Dunnett's post-test.

with 1% H_2O_2 in TBS for 10 min to block endogenous peroxidase prior to 30 min incubation in goat anti-mouse horseradish peroxidase. Sections were then washed 3 times in TBS and developed with DAB for 5 min prior to light counterstaining with haematoxylin and eosin.

Statistical Analysis

Due to the skewed and wide distribution of the data, gene expression values were log transformed, which enabled the application of parametric statistics. As the log of zero is undefined, one was added to all measurements in order to preserve the zeros in the derived data set. Multiple comparisons of gene expression values for disease biopsies (stratified on histopathology, renal function, proteinuria and clinical diagnosis) against healthy controls were performed using a one-way ANOVA with Dunnett's post-test. Statistical tests were performed using Prism 5.0 analysis software (GraphPad Software, La Jolla, CA, USA). P values ≤0.05 were considered statistically significant.

Results

Multiplex Tandem-PCR – PTEC gene expression levels correlate with histology, renal function and proteinuria

We initially compared the means of the disease group to the control group for all 30 genes in the panel. A total of 9 genes discriminated disease samples from controls: Kim-1, C3, P4HA2, THBS1, COL3A1, ACTA2, TJP1, VIM and FAS (Table 2). For example, the expression of Kim-1 was, on average, 1.93 units higher in the disease group as compared to the control group and P4HA2 was, on average, 1.91 units lower in the disease group as compared to the control group.

We then stratified MT-PCR derived gene transcript data from diseased samples based on: (i) histological criteria (OCI, UCI, IF/TA, ATI and the presence of neutrophils or eosinophils), (ii) kidney function (eGFR) and (iii) degree of proteinuria (uPCR levels). Within these groupings, three genes, Kim-1, C3 and P4HA2 demonstrated significant differences compared to controls.

Levels of Kim-1 significantly correlated with increasing OCI (Fig 1a), and Kim-1 expression was significantly elevated in all disease groupings with UCI (Fig 1b). In line with the literature, Kim-1 expression was significantly higher in biopsies with ATI (Fig 1c) and infiltrating neutrophils (Fig 1d), histological markers of acute kidney disease. Biopsies from patients with the heaviest proteinuria, a marker for progression of uncontrolled kidney disease, also demonstrated significantly elevated levels of Kim-1 expression (Fig 1e). C3 expression levels correlated positively with OCI when compared to no inflammation and controls (Fig 2a). Furthermore, a significant increase in C3 expression was demonstrated in biopsies from patients with acute tubular injury (Fig 2b) and those with the heaviest proteinuria (Fig 2c). In contrast, P4HA2 expression was significantly lower in diseased biopsies with eosinophils (Fig 3a), whilst a trend for decreasing expression of P4HA2 with increasing levels of IF/TA (Fig 3b) and decreasing kidney function (eGFR) (Fig 3c) was observed.

Multiplex Tandem-PCR – PTEC gene expression levels correlate with clinical diagnosis

When we stratified gene results against clinical acute, chronic and acute-on-chronic groups, we found increased expression compared to controls of Kim-1, C3, COL3A1, VIM, SMAD3 and TJP1 across all clinical groupings and decreased expression of P4HA2 compared to controls across all clinical groupings (Fig 4). However there were no significant differences of gene expression patterns between groups for each individual gene.

When we compared gene results against biopsies grouped into disease diagnoses, Kim-1, P4HA2, COL3A1, VIM, SMAD3 and TJP1 were consistently expressed at different levels to control biopsies across a number of primary diagnoses (Fig 5). The mean expression of Kim-1 was higher than controls in biopsies from all disease groups except TMA, and significantly higher than controls in patients with IgAN, DN and PI (Fig 5a). The mean expression of P4HA2 was lower than controls in biopsies from all disease groups except MCD and significantly lower in patients with TMA and PDD (Fig 5b). The mean expression of COL3A1 was higher than controls in biopsies from all disease groups, and significantly higher than controls in patients with IgAN, MN, IN, DN, PI, ATN, PDD and FSGS (Fig 5c). The mean expression of VIM was higher than controls in biopsies from all disease groups and significantly higher than controls in all groups except MN (Fig 5d). The mean expression of SMAD3 was lower than controls in biopsies from all disease groups and significantly lower in biopsies from PDD patients (Fig 5e). The mean expression of TJP1 was higher than controls in biopsies from all disease groups except TMA and significantly higher than controls in patients with DN, LN and PI (Fig 5f).

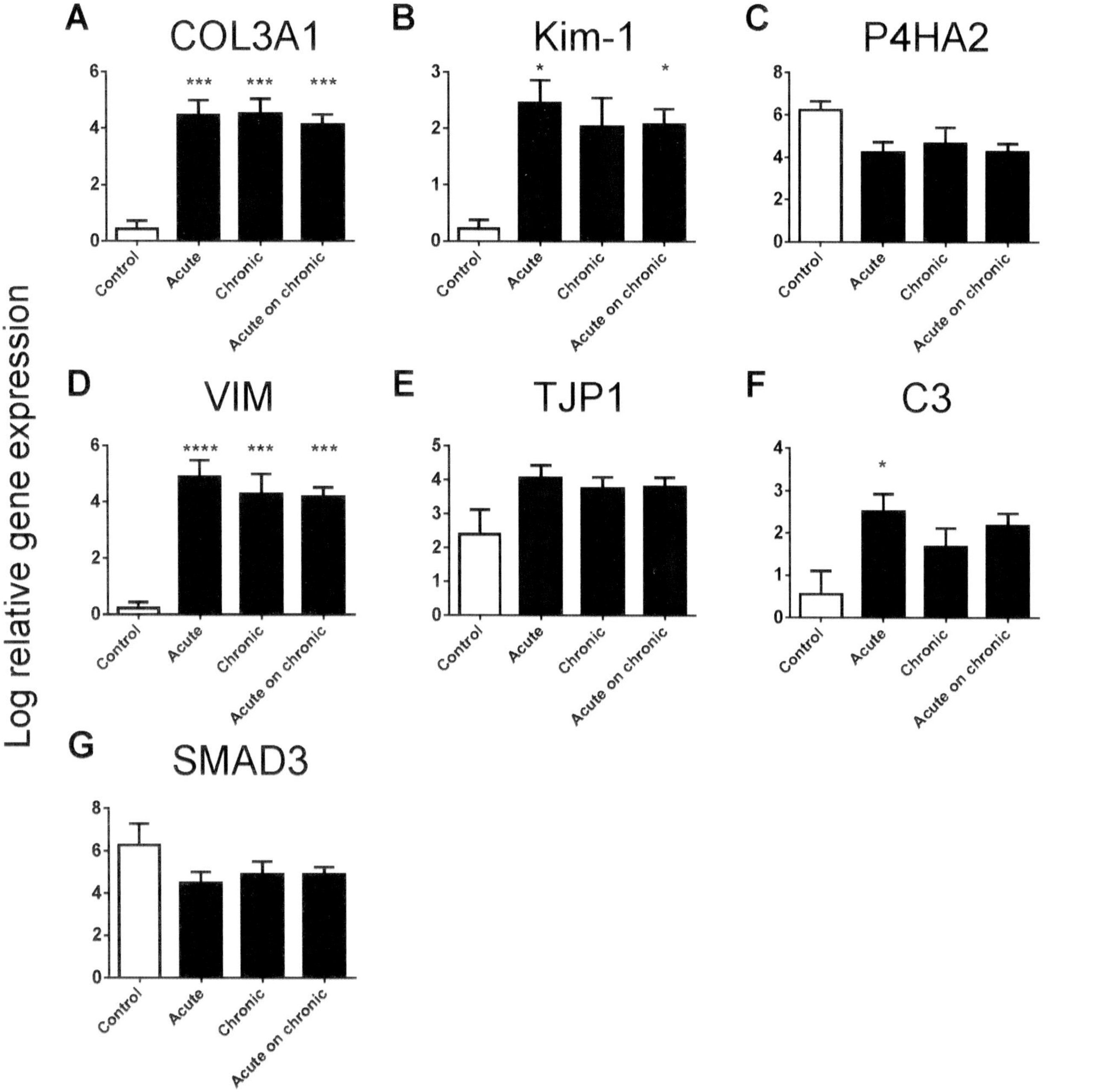

Figure 4. The log relative gene expression (normalised to GAPDH) of COL3A1, Kim-1, P4HA2, VIM, TJP1, C3 and SMAD3 across clinical acute, chronic and acute-on-chronic diagnoses. Values are means ± SEM. *P<0.05, ***P<0.001, ****P<0.0001, one-way ANOVA with Dunnett's post-test.

Confirmation of MT-PCR results at the molecular and protein level

To confirm our MT-PCR results at the molecular level, we undertook standard quantitative RT-PCR analysis of three candidate genes from our MT-PCR screening panel. We analyzed three different patient biopsies that had high expression of the relevant gene by MT-PCR and three different patient biopsies which had low/negative expression of the relevant gene by MT-PCR. We consistently detected greater levels of Kim-1, COL3A1 and VIM from biopsies with high expression of the respective genes compared to biopsies with no/low gene expression (Fig 6). We performed immununohistochemical analysis of these three gene products to correlate gene transcription levels to protein expression in tissue. We confirmed strong staining for Kim-1, COL3A1 and VIM in PTEC of biopsies that expressed high transcript levels by MT-PCR, with low or negative staining patterns in biopsies that had negative or very low transcript expression levels by MT-PCR (Fig 7). Extracellular staining of Kim-1 in the proteinacious material of the proximal tubule and of COL3A1 in the interstitium, adjacent to the basement membrane, was also noted.

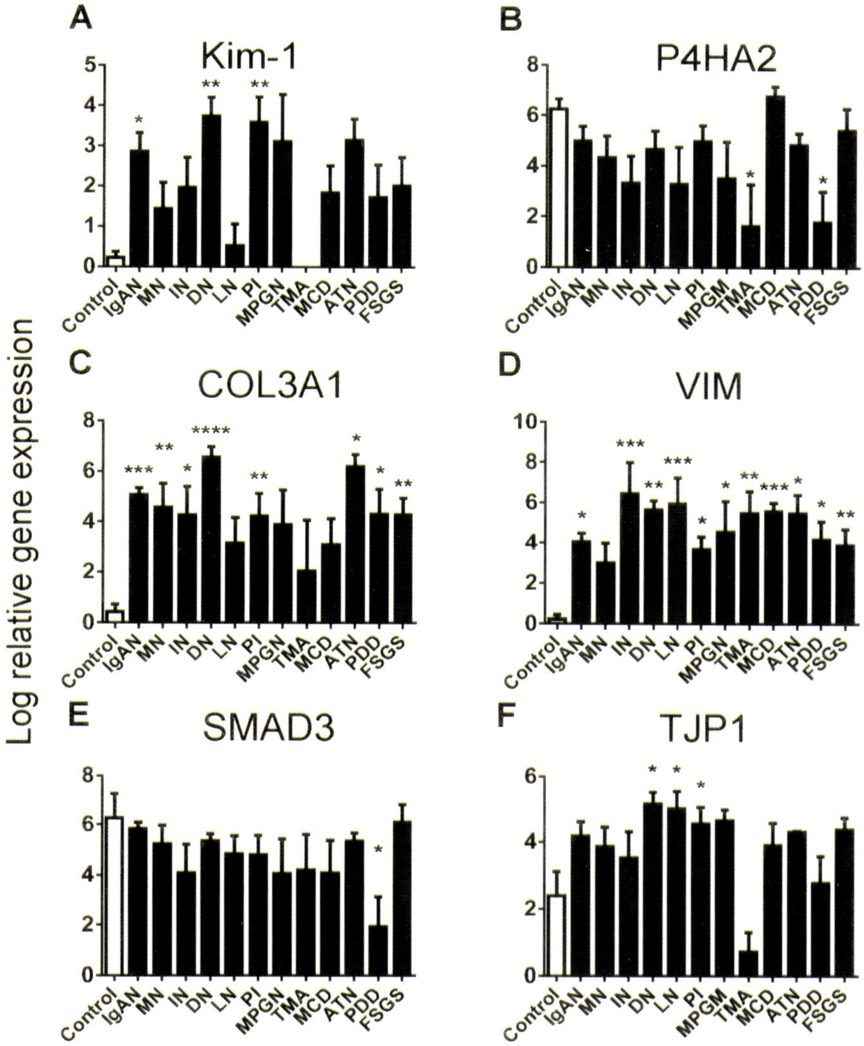

Figure 5. The log relative gene expression (normalised to GAPDH) of Kim-1, P4HA2, COL3A1, VIM, SMAD3 and TJP1 across disease diagnoses. Values are means ± SEM. *P<0.05, **P<0.01, ***P<0.001, ****P<0.0001, one-way ANOVA with Dunnett's post-test.

Discussion

PTEC are believed to play a central role in the progression of many different types of kidney disease, irrespective of whether the initiating aetiology occurs in the glomerulus or the interstitium. Various insults including increased protein, elevated glucose, AGE-modified proteins, oxidative stress, toxins, drugs and cytokines from infiltrating inflammatory cells can all impact on PTEC and perturb their normal physiology. The functional consequences of this perturbed function including aberrant chemokine secretion, EMT and cell death have primarily been studied in cell culture and animal model systems. Using the novel techniques of LCM and MT-PCR we have been able to demonstrate for the first time that PTEC purified from diseased human kidney demonstrate altered gene transcription profiles representing multiple pathobiological pathways that associate with markers of the clinical phenotypes of both acute and chronic kidney disease.

Kim-1 is a phosphatidylserine receptor that recognises stress and danger signals, like oxidized lipoproteins and apoptotic cells, and directs them to lysosomes [26]. Kim-1 gene expression appears quiescent under normal physiological conditions in the kidney but is rapidly up-regulated and transcribed into protein following injury. Kim-1 then localizes at very high levels on the apical membrane of PTEC where its extracellular domain is susceptible to metalloproteinase-mediated Kim-1 cleavage [26]. This soluble Kim-1, excreted in the urine, is a recognized acute kidney injury biomarker. Our findings that PTEC expression of Kim-1 is up-regulated in biopsies with acute tubular injury compared to both control and disease biopsies with no acute tubular injury is in line with the established literature. Not unexpectedly, high Kim-1 levels in PTEC are also associated with the presence of neutrophils, a cell of acute inflammation, in the interstitium.

Our findings also describe a relationship between Kim-1 expression in PTEC and the histological severity of kidney inflammation, renal function and amount of proteinuria. In addition, we report significantly elevated levels of Kim-1 in biopsies from patients diagnosed with IgA, DN and PI compared to controls. A review of the literature reveals elevated levels of Kim-1 in a number of kidney diseases. Kwon *et al* recently

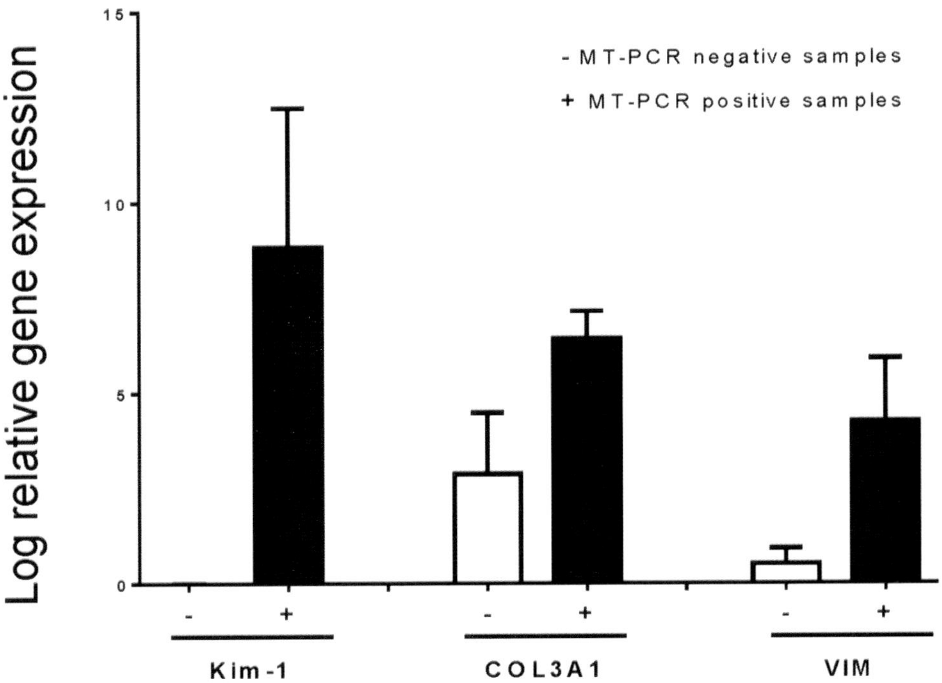

Figure 6. The log relative gene expression (normalised to GAPDH) of Kim-1, COL3A1 and VIM defined by real-time PCR from 3 biopsies with low/no MT-PCR expression (−) and 3 biopsies with medium/high MT-PCR expression (+) for that gene. Values are means ± SEM.

demonstrated that Kim-1 expression predicts renal outcomes in IgA nephropathy [27], whilst elevated Kim-1 levels have also been reported in DN [28] and decreasing levels associated with regression of microalbuminuria in type 1 diabetes, suggesting that tubular dysfunction is a critical component of the early course of DN [29]. This corroboration of our findings with the established literature is proof of concept of the validity of our LCM/MT-PCR approach to identifying PTEC specific genes involved in the pathobiology of kidney disease.

C3 is pivotal in the activation of the complement system and its processing by C3 convertase to C3a and C3b is the central reaction in both the classical and alternative complement pathways. C3 is a known inflammatory mediator, with C3a increasing vascular permeability and C3b promoting inflammatory cell interactions. PTEC production of C3 gene transcripts and protein has been reported in both in-vitro and in-vivo models [30,31] and Zoja *et al* [31] reported the co-localisation of interstitial inflammatory infiltrates with C3 expressing proximal tubules. Welsh *et al* also reported focal PTEC expression of C3 was always associated with localised interstitial infiltrate or focal tubular atrophy [32]. This is supported in our findings where there is a strong trend for increased C3 expression in disease biopsies with OCI and a significant positive relationship between expression of C3 and acute tubular injury. Our results support a therapeutic strategy akin to antibiotics; that is, time dependent therapeutic inhibitory targeting of C3 whilst the inflammatory process is active in the pathogenesis, possibly with proteinuria as a surrogate, and not during other pathological processes.

P4HA2 catalyses the post-translational formation of 4-hydroxyproline in -Xaa-Pro-Gly- sequences in collagens and other proteins and is essential to the proper three-dimensional folding of newly synthesized procollagen chains. To our knowledge, no other groups have studied P4HA2 transcription in human PTEC and only Rastaldi et al [33] have reported on the apparent up-regulation of its protein in diseased biopsies. The significance of decreased expressions levels of this gene in PTEC from biopsies with moderate to severe CKD and IF/TA is therefore counter-intuitive. However, prolyl hydroxylation via P4HA2 is part of the pathway by which hypoxia inducible factor-1 (HIF-1) is degraded. HIF-1 is known to regulate many important genes involved in angiogenesis, glucose utilization, proliferation and survival including erythropoietin, vascular endothelial growth factor and hemeoxygenase-1 [34]. It could be hypothesized that a decrease in PTEC expression of P4HA2 would promote the expression and activity of HIF-1, resulting in the expression of many genes required for survival within the compromised kidney environment of CKD. Therefore, our findings that decreased levels of P4HA2 correlate with reduced kidney function provide a new finding that warrants further investigation.

COL3A1 participates in the fibrotic process in the renal tubulo-interstitium, where the abnormal extracellular matrix (ECM) in fibrosis consists of an excess of normal components, such as collagen type IV, and an accumulation of proteins that are absent in the normal ECM, such as collagen type I and type III [35]. Although most collagen type III is reported to be produced by myofibroblasts in the kidney, it has also been demonstrated to be produced by PTEC cell lines *in vitro* [36] and by PTEC in diseased kidney biopsies [33]. The finding here that PTEC also produce COL3A1 *in vivo*, across a range of disease aetiologies, adds novel findings to the PTEC literature.

VIM is the characteristic cytoskeletal protein of mesenchymal cells and its expression in epithelial cells is a de-differentiation marker representing an early step in EMT. In their immunohistochemical studies on EMT in human biopsies, Rastaldi *et al* were unable to detect any vimentin positive tubules in healthy biopsies but reported vimentin positive PTEC from most disease biopsies

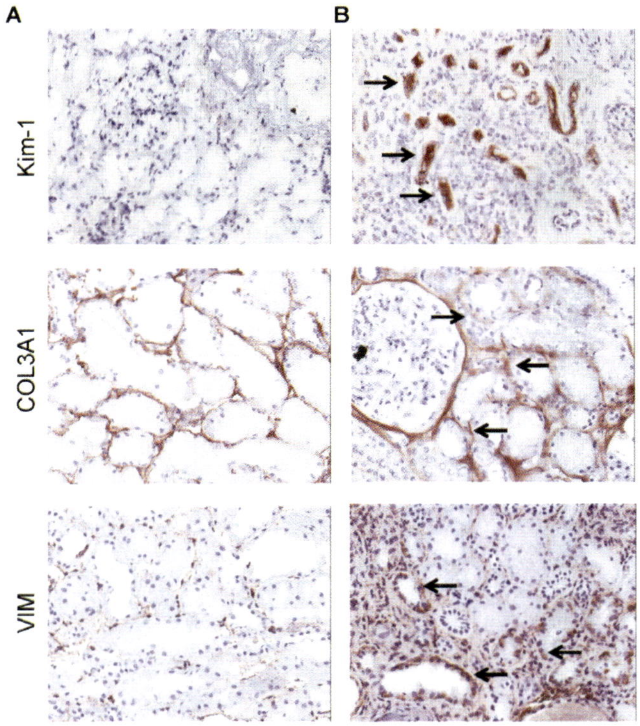

Figure 7. Immunohistological localization of Kim-1, COL3A1 and VIM in frozen kidney sections undertaken on (A) biopsy negative for that gene by MT-PCR and (B) biopsy positive for that gene by MT-PCR. Arrows indicate positive staining within PTEC. A representative result from three donor experiments are shown (mag ×100). There is evidence of Kim-1 staining from the protainaceous material within the lumen of some proximal tubules and COL3A1 staining is evident both within PTEC and in the interstitium, adjacent to the basement membrane.

studied [33]. We hypothesize that the increased PTEC expression of VIM transcripts in our disease biopsies reflects an early pathological response because we rarely detected increased ACTA2, a second, and later, marker of EMT, within PTEC. Galichon and Hertig came to a similar conclusion, reporting that vimentin is an early and reversible marker of EMT in kidney disease [37]. Thus, transcription of vimentin may have potential as a kidney disease biomarker at early and potentially reversible stages. Our observations that ACTA2 itself did not correlate with fibrosis scores or other markers of pathology was somewhat surprising to us as the product of this gene has been implicated in the fibrotic process, particularly in animal models [38]. However, others such as Rastaldi *et al* [33] have also reported minimal increases of smooth muscle actin in PTEC from human fibrotic biopsies.

SMAD3 is a member of the receptor-activated Smads (R-Smads) which are central mediators of TGF-β signaling. Induction and activation of the profibrotic cytokine TGF-β in the kidney, either alone or in combination with other cytokines such as epidermal growth factor, fibroblast growth factor-2 or angiotensin II, induces kidney damage through a range of pathobiological processes, including EMT, apoptosis and fibrosis (reviewed [39]). SMAD3 is also involved in other non-redundant signaling pathways and biological functions (reviewed [40]). We were quite surprised to note that all of our disease biopsies had lower SMAD3 levels than our control biopsies. However the literature reports that TGF-β can down-modulate SMAD3 gene expression in human glomerular mesangial cells over the short term (24 hours) and in renal tubular epithelial cells over the longer term (5–7 days) [41]. Therefore, our group hypothesize, for the first time, that the transcriptional inhibition of SMAD3 may form part of a biological control loop for TGF-β within human PTEC.

TJP1 or ZO-1 is a scaffolding protein that interacts with multiple other proteins to form and maintain tight junctions between cells. Levels of TJP1 are relatively low in proximal tubules compared to distal tubules (reviewed by [42]) reflecting their greater paracellular transport functions. As proximal tubule cells become fully differentiated they express more TJP1 [43]. This raises the intriguing possibility that our observed increases in TJP1 transcription in most disease states is a counter-regulatory response to the vimentin up-regulation induced early stages of PTEC EMT– counter acting forces in the de-differentiation:differentiation of PTEC homeostasis.

Collectively our study demonstrates that the technologies of LCM coupled with MT-PCR are feasible in the clinical setting where levels of PTEC RNA are available only in picogram amounts. Despite the incredible complexity of PTEC transcriptional profiles, their products and interactions, these technologies provide simultaneous experimental observations of multiple molecules of interest, informing better targeting of therapies and potential new renal biomarkers. However, our findings do not, at this stage, define a PTEC consensus chronic kidney disease transcript signature, aligning with the concept that chronic disease represents the cumulative dynamics of transient, repetitive or persistent acute insults varying over time.

Although we have used MT-PCR to examine genes involved in kidney pathobiology, the technique can be modified to examine any genes or gene pathways of interest. For instance, we have recently reported that human PTEC are able to modulate autologous immune responses [44,45] and we are currently modifying our protocols to examine the expression of immune mediator genes in PTEC derived from inflammatory disease biopsies.

In conclusion, using novel methods that give unprecedented access to real time human kidney tissue, we report alterations in PTEC gene and protein expression, representing multiple pathobiological pathways that associate with markers of the clinical phenotypes of both acute and chronic kidney disease. Where the amount of starting RNA is small, MT-PCR has the power to simultaneously observe multiple molecules representing several signaling pathways at the level of a single cell population. We found the diversity of pathways implicated in kidney disease include inflammatory, complement, collagen folding, fibrosis, cytoskeletal and cell scaffolding pathways, ascribing PTEC a pivotal role in regulatory networks of kidney homeostasis in health and disease.

Acknowledgments

The authors would like to thank the patients who donated tissue to this study, the renal and urology consultants of the RBWH, the pathologists and scientists of the Pathology Department, Queensland Health, for providing access to diagnostic biopsies, Dr Andrew Mallett and Dr Ross Francis of Queensland Health for clinical insight and constructive comments on the manuscript and Leesa Wockner of the QIMR statistics department for statistical analysis assistance.

Author Contributions

Conceived and designed the experiments: RW HH. Performed the experiments: RW XW AK SZ KR AO SS. Analyzed the data: RW XW AK SZ KR AO SS LF VR HH. Contributed reagents/materials/analysis tools: RW LF HH VR. Wrote the paper: RW AK HH. Provision of clinical disease interpretation: VR LF HH. Disease allocation: LF HH RW. Histopathological analysis: LF.

References

1. Eddy AA (1996) Molecular insights into renal interstitial fibrosis. J Am Soc Nephrol 7: 2495–2508.
2. Diwakar R, Pearson AL, Colville-Nash P, Brunskill NJ, Dockrell ME (2007) The role played by endocytosis in albumin-induced secretion of TGF-beta1 by proximal tubular epithelial cells. Am J Physiol Renal Physiol 292: F1464–1470.
3. Harris RC, Neilson EG (2006) Toward a unified theory of renal progression. Annu Rev Med 57: 365–380.
4. Shalamanova L, McArdle F, Amara AB, Jackson MJ, Rustom R (2007) Albumin overload induces adaptive responses in human proximal tubular cells through oxidative stress but not via angiotensin II type 1 receptor. Am J Physiol Renal Physiol 292: F1846–1857.
5. Wynn T (2008) Cellular and molecular mechanisms of fibrosis. J Pathol 214: 199–210.
6. Zheng G, Wang Y, Mahajan D, Qin X, Wang Y, et al. (2005) The role of tubulointerstitial inflammation. Kidney Int 67: S96–S100.
7. Sheerin NS, Risley P, Abe K, Tang Z, Wong W, et al. (2008) Synthesis of complement protein C3 in the kidney is an important mediator of local tissue injury. Faseb J 22: 1065–1072.
8. Takase O, Minto AW, Puri TS, Cunningham PN, Jacob A, et al. (2008) Inhibition of NF-kappaB-dependent Bcl-xL expression by clusterin promotes albumin-induced tubular cell apoptosis. Kidney Int.
9. Zhang C, Meng X, Zhu Z, Liu J, Deng A (2004) Connective tissue growth factor regulates the key events in tubular epithelial to myofibroblast transition in vitro. Cell Biol Int 28: 863–873.
10. Kida Y, Asahina K, Teraoka H, Gitelman I, Sato T (2007) Twist Relates to Tubular Epithelial-Mesenchymal Transition and Interstitial Fibrogenesis in the Obstructed Kidney. J Histochem Cytochem 55: 661–673.
11. Li Y, Dai C, Wu C, Liu Y (2007) PINCH-1 Promotes Tubular Epithelial-to-Mesenchymal Transition by Interacting with Integrin-Linked Kinase. J Am Soc Nephrol 18: 2534–2543.
12. Yoshino J, Monkawa T, Tsuji M, Inukai M, Itoh H, et al. (2007) Snail1 is involved in the renal epithelial-mesenchymal transition. Biochem Biophys Res Commun 362: 63–68.
13. Teteris SA, Menahem SA, Perry G, Maguire JA, Dowling JP, et al. (2007) Dysregulated growth factor gene expression is associated with tubulointerstitial apoptosis and renal dysfunction. Kidney Int 71: 1044–1053.
14. Yang XJ, Zhou M, Hes O, Shen S, Li R, et al. (2008) Tubulocystic carcinoma of the kidney: clinicopathologic and molecular characterization. Am J Surg Pathol 32: 177–187.
15. Langham RG, Kelly DJ, Gow RM, Zhang Y, Cox AJ, et al. (2008) Increased renal gene transcription of protein kinase C-beta in human diabetic nephropathy: relationship to long-term glycaemic control. Diabetologia 51: 668–674.
16. Blakey GL, Laszik ZG (2004) Laser-assisted microdissection of the kidney: fundamentals and applications. J Mol Histol 35: 581–587.
17. Schmid H, Henger A, Cohen CD, Frach K, Grone HJ, et al. (2003) Gene expression profiles of podocyte-associated molecules as diagnostic markers in acquired proteinuric diseases. J Am Soc Nephrol 14: 2958–2966.
18. Baelde HJ, Eikmans M, Lappin DW, Doran PP, Hohenadel D, et al. (2007) Reduction of VEGF-A and CTGF expression in diabetic nephropathy is associated with podocyte loss. Kidney Int 71: 637–645.
19. Bennett MR, Czech KA, Arend LJ, Witte DP, Devarajan P, et al. (2007) Laser capture microdissection-microarray analysis of focal segmental glomerulosclerosis glomeruli. Nephron Exp Nephrol 107: e30–40.
20. Reich HN, Oudit GY, Penninger JM, Scholey JW, Herzenberg AM (2008) Decreased glomerular and tubular expression of ACE2 in patients with type 2 diabetes and kidney disease. Kidney Int 74: 1610–1616.
21. Prabakaran T, Christensen EI, Nielsen R, Verroust PJ (2012) Cubilin is expressed in rat and human glomerular podocytes. Nephrology Dialysis Transplantation 27: 3156–3159.
22. Rudnicki M, Eder S, Perco P, Enrich J, Scheiber K, et al. (2007) Gene expression profiles of human proximal tubular epithelial cells in proteinuric nephropathies. Kidney Int 71: 325–335.
23. Rudnicki M, Perco P, Enrich J, Eder S, Heininger D, et al. (2009) Hypoxia response and VEGF-A expression in human proximal tubular epithelial cells in stable and progressive renal disease. Lab Invest 89: 337–346.
24. Stanley KK, Szewczuk E (2005) Multiplexed tandem PCR: gene profiling from small amounts of RNA using SYBR Green detection. Nucleic Acids Res 33: e180.
25. Racusen LC, Solez K, Colvin RB, Bonsib SM, Castro MC, et al. (1999) The Banff 97 working classification of renal allograft pathology. Kidney Int 55: 713–723.
26. Bonventre JV (2009) Kidney injury molecule-1 (KIM-1): a urinary biomarker and much more. Nephrology Dialysis Transplantation 24: 3265–3268.
27. Kwon SH, Park MY, Jeon JS, Noh H, Choi SJ, et al. (2012) KIM-1 expression predicts renal outcomes in IgA nephropathy. Clin Exp Nephrol 17: 359–364.
28. van Timmeren MM, van den Heuvel MC, Bailly V, Bakker SJL, van Goor H, et al. (2007) Tubular kidney injury molecule-1 (KIM-1) in human renal disease. The Journal of Pathology 212: 209–217.
29. Vaidya VS, Niewczas MA, Ficociello LH, Johnson AC, Collings FB, et al. (2011) Regression of microalbuminuria in type 1 diabetes is associated with lower levels of urinary tubular injury biomarkers, kidney injury molecule-1, and N-acetyl-beta-D-glucosaminidase. Kidney Int 79: 464–470.
30. Zhou W, Marsh JE, Sacks SH (2001) Intrarenal synthesis of complement. Kidney Int 59: 1227–1235.
31. Zoja C, Morigi M, Remuzzi G (2003) Proteinuria and Phenotypic Change of Proximal Tubular Cells. Journal of the American Society of Nephrology 14: S36–S41.
32. Welch TR, Beischel LS, Witte DP (1993) Differential expression of complement C3 and C4 in the human kidney. J Clin Invest 92: 1451–1458.
33. Rastaldi MP, Ferrario F, Giardino L, Dell'Antonio G, Grillo C, et al. (2002) Epithelial-mesenchymal transition of tubular epithelial cells in human renal biopsies. Kidney Int 62: 137–146.
34. Semenza GL (2001) Hypoxia-inducible factor 1: oxygen homeostasis and disease pathophysiology. Trends in Molecular Medicine 7: 345–350.
35. Fogo AB (1999) Mesangial Matrix Modulation and Glomerulosclerosis. Nephron Experimental Nephrology 7: 147–159.
36. Skill NJ, Johnson TS, Coutts IGC, Saint RE, Fisher M, et al. (2004) Inhibition of Transglutaminase Activity Reduces Extracellular Matrix Accumulation Induced by High Glucose Levels in Proximal Tubular Epithelial Cells. Journal of Biological Chemistry 279: 47754–47762.
37. Galichon P, Hertig A (2011) Epithelial to mesenchymal transition as a biomarker in renal fibrosis: are we ready for the bedside? Fibrogenesis Tissue Repair 4: 11.
38. Prakoura N, Politis PK, Ihara Y, Michalak M, Charonis AS (2013) Epithelial calreticulin up-regulation promotes profibrotic responses and tubulointerstitial fibrosis development. Am J Pathol 183: 1474–1487.
39. Garcia-Sanchez O, Lopez-Hernandez FJ, Lopez-Novoa JM (2010) An integrative view on the role of TGF-[beta] in the progressive tubular deletion associated with chronic kidney disease. Kidney Int 77: 950–955.
40. Massagué J, Seoane J, Wotton D (2005) Smad transcription factors. Genes & Development 19: 2783–2810.
41. Poncelet A-C, Schnaper HW, Tan R, Liu Y, Runyan CE (2007) Cell Phenotype-specific Down-regulation of Smad3 Involves Decreased Gene Activation as Well as Protein Degradation. Journal of Biological Chemistry 282: 15534–15540.
42. Denker BM, Sabath E (2011) The biology of epithelial cell tight junctions in the kidney. J Am Soc Nephrol 22: 622–625.
43. Lima WR, Parreira KS, Devuyst O, Caplanusi A, N'Kuli F, et al. (2010) ZONAB Promotes Proliferation and Represses Differentiation of Proximal Tubule Epithelial Cells. Journal of the American Society of Nephrology 21: 478–488.
44. Kassianos AJ, Sampangi S, Wang X, Roper KE, Beagley K, et al. (2013) Human proximal tubule epithelial cells modulate autologous dendritic cell function. Nephrol Dial Transplant 28: 303–312.
45. Wilkinson R, Wang X, Roper KE, Healy H (2011) Activated human renal tubular cells inhibit autologous immune responses. Nephrology Dialysis Transplantation 26: 1483–1492.

4

Angiotensin-Converting Enzyme Insertion/Deletion Polymorphism Contributes High Risk for Chronic Kidney Disease in Asian Male with Hypertension–A Meta-Regression Analysis of 98 Observational Studies

Chin Lin[1], Hsin-Yi Yang[2], Chia-Chao Wu[3], Herng-Sheng Lee[4], Yuh-Feng Lin[3,5], Kuo-Cheng Lu[6], Chi-Ming Chu[2], Fu-Huang Lin[2], Sen-Yeong Kao[2], Sui-Lung Su[2]*

1 Graduate Institute of Life Sciences, National Defense Medical Center, Taipei, Taiwan, ROC, **2** School of Public Health, National Defense Medical Center, Taipei, Taiwan, ROC, **3** Division of Nephrology, Department of Medicine, Tri-Service General Hospital, National Defense Medical Center, Taipei, Taiwan, ROC, **4** Division of Pathology, Tri-Service General Hospital, National Defense Medical Center, Taipei, Taiwan, ROC, **5** Division of Nephrology, Department of Medicine, Shuang Ho Hospital, Graduate Institute of Clinical Medicine, Taipei Medical University, New Taipei City, Taiwan, ROC, **6** Division of Nephrology, Department of Medicine, Cardinal Tien Hospital, School of Medicine, Fu Jen Catholic University, New Taipei City, Taiwan, ROC

Abstract

Background: Associations between angiotensin-converting enzyme (ACE) gene insertion/deletion (I/D) polymorphisms and chronic kidney disease (CKD) have been extensively studied, with most studies reporting that individuals with the D allele have a higher risk. Although some factors, such as ethnicity, may moderate the association between ACE I/D polymorphisms and CKD risk, gender-dependent effects on the CKD risk remain controversial.

Objectives: This study investigated the gender-dependent effects of ACE I/D polymorphisms on CKD risk.

Data sources: PubMed, the Cochrane library, and EMBASE were searched for studies published before January 2013.

Study eligibility criteria, participants, and interventions: Cross-sectional surveys and case–control studies analyzing ACE I/D polymorphisms and CKD were included. They were required to match the following criteria: age >18 years, absence of rare diseases, and Asian or Caucasian ethnicity.

Study appraisal and synthesis methods: The effect of carrying the D allele on CKD risk was assessed by meta-analysis and meta-regression using random-effects models.

Results: Ethnicity [odds ratio (OR): 1.24; 95% confidence interval (CI): 1.08–1.42] and hypertension (OR: 1.55; 95% CI: 1.04–2.32) had significant moderate effects on the association between ACE I/D polymorphisms and CKD risk, but they were not significant in the diabetic nephropathy subgroup. Males had higher OR for the association between ACE I/D polymorphisms and CKD risk than females in Asians but not Caucasians, regardless of adjustment for hypertension ($p<0.05$). In subgroup analyses, this result was significant in the nondiabetic nephropathy group. Compared with the I allele, the D allele had the highest risk (OR: 3.75; 95% CI: 1.84–7.65) for CKD in hypertensive Asian males.

Conclusions and implications of key findings: The ACE I/D polymorphisms may incur the highest risk for increasing CKD in hypertensive Asian males.

Editor: Michael Bader, Max-Delbrück Center for Molecular Medicine (MDC), Germany

Funding: The authors have no support or funding to report.

* E-mail: a131419@gmail.com

Introduction

The prevalence of chronic kidney disease (CKD) is approximately 10% in several countries [1–3]. CKD patients have high risk for cardiovascular disease and death [4]. Genetic factors, including ethnicity [5] and family history of disease [6,7], play a key role in CKD pathogenesis. Thus, it is desirable to identify candidate genes and evaluate their effects.

The renin–angiotensin system (RAS) regulates blood pressure and electrolyte balance [8]. Owing to the key role of angiotensin-converting enzyme (ACE) in RAS, ACE polymorphisms have frequently been investigated. One of the most important ACE polymorphisms is a 287-bp insertion/deletion in intron 16 (ACE

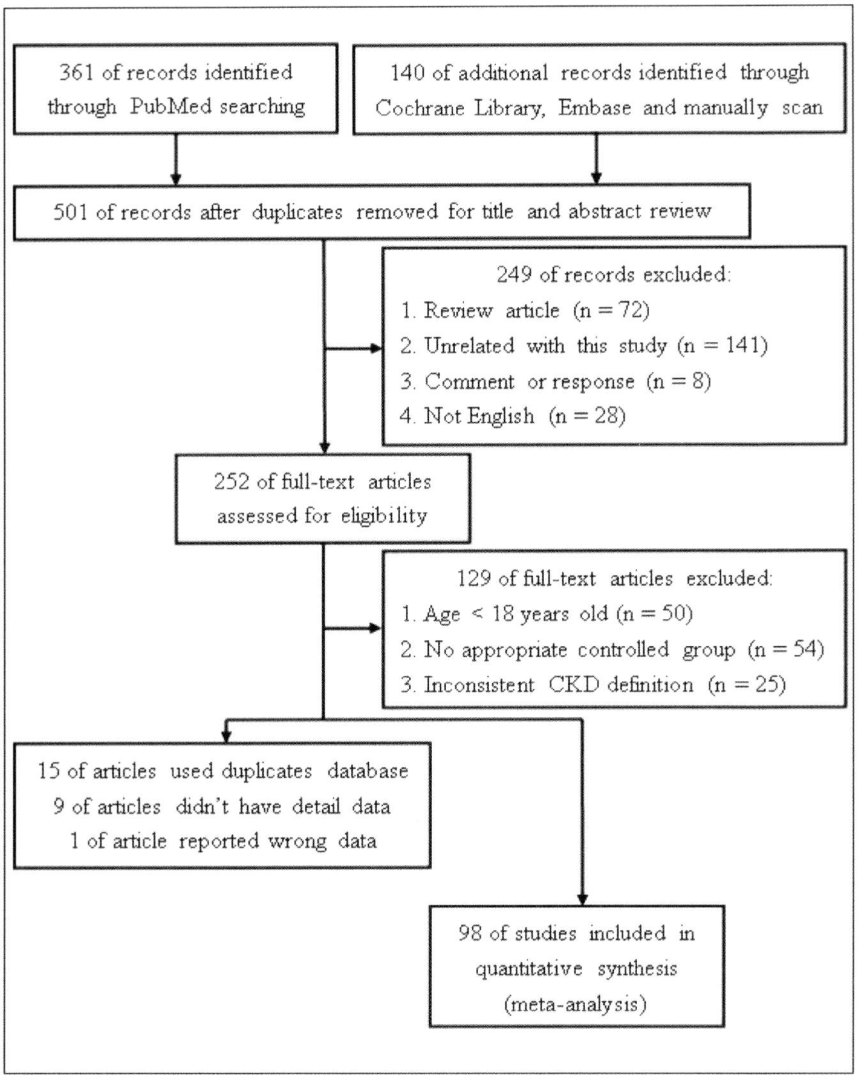

Figure 1. Flow diagram of identification process for eligible studies in this study. n: number of studies were deleted for aforementioned reasons.

I/D), and a previous study revealed a significant effect of this polymorphism on ACE gene expression [9]. Most studies have found that carriers of the D allele had a higher risk of CKD or end-stage renal disease (ESRD) than those of the I allele [10–12].

Because previous studies have found that gender and the DD genotype had an additive effect on blood ACE levels [13], we hypothesized that gender differences affect the relative risk of ACE I/D polymorphisms for CKD. Numerous studies of CKD or ESRD have reported appreciable, but not significant, gender-dependent effects of ACE I/D polymorphisms [14–19], but the populations used in these studies were of different ethnicities. Studies of Caucasian subjects have indicated additive effects of the D allele in females [14–16], but studies of Asian subjects have shown different results [17–19]. Although many previous meta-analysis studies investigating ACE I/D polymorphisms and CKD have been reported, but no studies have considered moderate effects of gender in our knowledge [10–12,20–22]. This study focused on general population without genetic abnormality or rare disorder, and we wanted to compare the risk of CKD in people with major allele (I allele) or minor allele (D allele) on ACE I/D. In addition, gender-dependent effects of ACE I/D polymorphisms on CKD risk was investigated.

Methods

Search Methods and Criteria for Considering Studies

The PRISMA 2009 Checklist was reported in Table S1. This study focused on the general population without genetic predisposing factors, and aimed to compare CKD risk between individuals carrying the major (I) and minor (D) alleles of ACE I/D. To identify relevant studies, English-language articles in MEDLINE, Cochrane Library and EMBASE were searched using relevant text words and medical subject headings that included all spellings of ACE I/D and CKD (the detailed search strategy is shown in Table S2). All articles published from the dates of inception of these medical databases to January 2013 were included. We manually scanned the reference lists of identified

Table 1. Characteristics of published studies included in this meta-analysis.

First author & year	Ethnicity	Study design	CKD type	Kidney function of case	Definition of case
Shaikh, 2012 [27]	Caucasian	CC	DN	non-ESRD	UAE >300 mg/day11
Rahimi, 2012 [28]	Caucasian	CS	DN	non-ESRD	ACR >30 mg/g
El-Baz, 2012 [29]	Caucasian	CS	DN	non-ESRD	ACR >30 mg/g
Zsom(1), 2011 [30]	Caucasian	CC	non-DN	non-ESRD	biopsy, ultrasound diagnosed & eGFR <60 ml/min/1.73 m^2
Zsom(2), 2011 [30]	Caucasian	CC	DN	non-ESRD	proteinuria & eGFR <60 ml/min/1.73 m^2
Al-Harbi, 2011 [31]	Caucasian	CC	DN	non-ESRD	no description
Jung, 2011 [32]	Asian	CC	GN	non-ESRD	biopsy diagnosed
Ali, 2011 [33]	Asian	CC	Comb	ESRD	doctor diagnosed
Huang, 2010 [34]	Asian	CC	GN	ESRD	biopsy diagnosed
Jayapalan, 2010 [35]	Asian	CS	DN	non-ESRD	ACR >30 mg/g or RRT
Mansoor, 2010 [14]	Caucasian	CS	DN	non-ESRD	albuminuria or RRT
Naresh, 2009 [36]	Asian	CC	DN	non-ESRD	no description
Ezzidi, 2009 [37]	Caucasian	CS	DN	non-ESRD	ACR >30 mg/g or eGFR <90 ml/min/1.73 m^2
Nikzamir, 2009 [38]	Caucasian	CS	DN	non-ESRD	UAE >30 mg/day
Anbazhagan, 2009 [39]	Asian	CC	Comb	ESRD	RRT
Ahluwalia, 2009 [40]	Asian	CC	DN	non-ESRD	UAE >200 μg/min, ACR >300 mg/g orRRT
Palomo-Piñón, 2009 [16]	Caucasian	CS	DN	non-ESRD	ACR >30 mg/g
Möllsten, 2008 [41]	Caucasian	CS	DN	non-ESRD	ACR >20 mg/g
Eroglu, 2008 [42]	Caucasian	CC	DN	non-ESRD	30 mg/day<UAE <300 mg/day
Arfa, 2008 [43]	Caucasian	CS	DN	non-ESRD	UAE >30 mg/day
Tripathi, 2008 [44]	Asian	CC	non-DN	ESRD	CCr <15 mL/min/1.73 m^2 & ultrasound diagnosedor CT
Movva, 2007 [45]	Asian	CC	DN	ESRD	SCr >1.5 mg/dL and UAE >30 mg/day
Uddin, 2007 [46]	Asian	CC	DN	ESRD	porteinuria
Buraczynska, 2006 [47]	Caucasian	CC	Comb	ESRD	RRT
So, 2006 [48]	Asian	CS	DN	non-ESRD	ACR >30 mg/g
Shestakova, 2006 [49]	Caucasian	CC	DN	non-ESRD	ACR >300 mg/g
Ng, 2006 [50]	Caucasian	CS	DN	non-ESRD	urinalyses positive, ACR >250 mg/g (men) or >355 mg/g (women)
Prasad, 2006 [51]	Asian	CC	DN	non-ESRD	SCr >3 mg/dL?ACR >200 mg/g
Degirmenci, 2005 [52]	Caucasian	CS	DN	ESRD	UAE >30 mg/day
van der Sman-de Beer, 2005 [53]	Caucasian	CC	Comb	non-ESRD	RRT
Park, 2005 [18]	Asian	CC	DN	ESRD	RRT
Canani, 2005 [54]	Caucasian	CS	DN	non-ESRD	UAE >20 μg/min
Fabris, 2005 [55]	Caucasian	CC	HN	non-ESRD	SCr >1.5 mg/dL
Lau, 2004 [56]	Asian	CC	GN	ESRD	biopsy diagnosed
Suzuki, 2004 [57]	Asian	CC	GN	non-ESRD	biopsy diagnosed
Stratta, 2004 [58]	Caucasian	CC	GN	non-ESRD	biopsy diagnosed
Lochynska, 2003 [59]	Caucasian	CC	GN	non-ESRD	biopsy diagnosed
Papp, 2003 [60]	Caucasian	CC	GN	ESRD	RRT
Aucella, 2003 [61]	Caucasian	CC	Comb	non-ESRD	RRT
Okuno, 2003 [62]	Asian	CS	DN	non-ESRD	UAE >10 μg/min
Ortiz, 2003 [63]	Caucasian	CC	non-DN	non-ESRD	CCr <50 mL/min/1.73 m^2
Hadjadj, 2003 [15]	Caucasian	CC	DN	non-ESRD	urinary albumin concentration >20 mg/L
Wang, 2003 [64]	Asian	CC	Comb	ESRD	RRT
Dixit, 2002 [65]	Caucasian	CC	GN	ESRD	biopsy diagnosed
Lee(1), 2002 [26]	Asian	CS	non-DN	non-ESRD	UAE >20 μg/min or ACR >20 mg/g
Lee(2), 2002 [26]	Asian	CS	DN	non-ESRD	UAE >20 μg/min or ACR >20 mg/g

Table 1. Cont.

First author & year	Ethnicity	Study design	CKD type	Kidney function of case	Definition of case
Losito, 2002 [66]	Caucasian	CC	Comb	ESRD	RRT
Yoon, 2002 [67]	Asian	CC	GN	non-ESRD	biopsy diagnosed
Fradin, 2002 [68]	Caucasian	CS	DN	non-ESRD	UAE >30 mg/day
Drouet, 2002 [69]	Caucasian	CC	GN	non-ESRD	biopsy diagnosed
Nicod, 2002 [70]	Caucasian	CC	Comb	non-ESRD	RRT
Araz, 2001 [71]	Caucasian	CS	DN	non-ESRD	ACR >30 mg/g
Azar, 2001 [72]	Caucasian	CC	DN	non-ESRD	UAE >30 mg/day
Lovati, 2001 [73]	Caucasian	CC	Comb	ESRD	RRT
Wang, 2001 [74]	Caucasian	CS	Comb	non-ESRD	CCr <60 mL/min/1.73 m^2
Taniwaki, 2001 [75]	Asian	CS	DN	non-ESRD	UAE >30 mg/day
Viswanathan, 2001 [76]	Asian	CC	DN	non-ESRD	proteinuria >500 mg/dL
Hadjadj, 2001 [77]	Caucasian	CS	DN	non-ESRD	urinary albumin concentration >20 mg/L
Wu, 2000 [78]	Asian	CC	DN	non-ESRD	no description
Hsieh, 2000 [79]	Asian	CC	DN	non-ESRD	proteinuria >500 mg/dL
van Ittersum, 2000 [80]	Caucasian	CS	DN	non-ESRD	UAE >30 mg/day
Tomino, 1999 [19]	Asian	CS	DN	non-ESRD	UAE >20 µg/min or ACR >30 mg/g
Solini, 1999 [81]	Caucasian	CS	DN	non-ESRD	Albuminuria
De Cosmo, 1999 [82]	Caucasian	CC	DN	non-ESRD	UAE >30 mg/day
Miura, 1999 [83]	Asian	CS	DN	non-ESRD	UAE >10 µg/min
Kuramoto, 1999 [84]	Asian	CS	DN	non-ESRD	UAE >15 µg/min
Huang, 1998 [85]	Caucasian	CS	DN	non-ESRD	UAE >30 mg/day
Walder, 1998 [86]	Caucasian	CC	DN	non-ESRD	UAE >30 mg/day
Freire, 1998 [87]	Caucasian	CS	DN	non-ESRD	UAE >30 mg/day
Grzeszczak, 1998 [88]	Caucasian	CS	DN	non-ESRD	ACR >1.9 mg/mol (men) or >2.8 mg/mol (women)
Young, 1998 [89]	Asian	CS	DN	non-ESRD	UAE >30 mg/day
Penno, 1998 [90]	Caucasian	CS	DN	non-ESRD	UAE >20 µg/min
Fernández-Llama, 1998 [91]	Caucasian	CS	HN	non-ESRD	UAE >20 µg/min
Frost, 1998 [92]	Caucasian	CS	DN	non-ESRD	UAE >30 mg/day
Pei, 1997 [93]	Caucasian	CS	GN	non-ESRD	biopsy diagnosed
Marre, 1997 [94]	Caucasian	CS	DN	non-ESRD	UAE >30 mg/day
Barnas, 1997 [95]	Caucasian	CS	DN	non-ESRD	UAE >30 mg/day
Ringel, 1997 [96]	Caucasian	CC	DN	non-ESRD	UAE >30 mg/day
Schmidt, 1997 [97]	Caucasian	CS	DN	non-ESRD	UAE >30 mg/day
Kawada, 1997 [98]	Asian	CC	Comb	ESRD	RRT
Kario, 1997 [99]	Asian	CS	HN	non-ESRD	UAE >15 µg/min
Nakajima, 1996 [17]	Asian	CS	DN	non-ESRD	ACR >30 mg/g
Chowdhury, 1996 [100]	Caucasian	CS	DN	non-ESRD	Albuminuria
McLaughlin, 1996 [101]	Caucasian	CC	Comb	non-ESRD	RRT or doctor diagnosed
Oh, 1996 [102]	Asian	CS	DN	non-ESRD	UAE >20 µg/min
Schmidt, 1996 [103]	Caucasian	CC	Comb	ESRD	RRT
Doi, 1996 [104]	Asian	CS	DN	non-ESRD	ACR >30 mg/g
Ohno, 1996 [105]	Asian	CS	DN	non-ESRD	ACR >10 mg/g
Mizuiri, 1995 [106]	Asian	CC	DN	non-ESRD	UAE >20 µg/min or RRT
Yorioka, 1995 [107]	Asian	CC	GN	non-ESRD	biopsy diagnosed
Fujisawa, 1995 [108]	Asian	CS	DN	non-ESRD	Albuminuria or RRT
Panagiotopoulos, 1995 [109]	Caucasian	CS	DN	non-ESRD	UAE >20 µg/min
Tarnow, 1995 [110]	Caucasian	CC	DN	non-ESRD	UAE >300 mg/day or biopsy diagnosed

Table 1. Cont.

First author & year	Ethnicity	Study design	CKD type	Kidney function of case	Definition of case
Schmidt, 1995 [111]	Caucasian	CC	GN	non-ESRD	biopsy diagnosed
Yoshida, 1995 [112]	Asian	CC	GN	non-ESRD	biopsy diagnosed
Dudley, 1995 [113]	Caucasian	CC	DN	non-ESRD	patients with urine in top tertile of the median UAE
Harden, 1995 [114]	Caucasian	CC	GN	non-ESRD	biopsy diagnosed
Doria, 1994 [115]	Caucasian	CC	DN	non-ESRD	UAE >30 μg/min
Marre, 1994 [116]	Caucasian	CS	DN	non-ESRD	UAE >30 mg/day
Powrie, 1994 [117]	Caucasian	CS	DN	non-ESRD	ACR >3 mg/mmol

CC: case control study; CS: cross-sectional survey; DN: diabetic nephropathy; non-DN: non diabetic nephropathy; GN: glomerulonephritis; HN: hypertensive nephropathy; Comb: combined; ESRD: only ESRD patients; non-ESRD: not only ESRD patients; UAE: urinary albumin excretion rate; ACR: Albumin creatinine ratio; eGFR: estimated glomerular filtration rate; CCr: creatinine clearance; RRT: renal replacement therapy; CT: computed tomography; SCr: serum creatinine.

trials and review articles to avoid missing any other relevant studies [10–12,20–22].

All related studies assessing the association between ACE I/D polymorphisms and CKD risk were considered for inclusion. The criteria for inclusion of a study were as follows: (1) cross-sectional surveys or case–control studies; (2) CKD defined according to the National Kidney Foundation: kidney damage by clinical diagnosis or a glomerular filtration rate <60 ml/min/1.73 m^2; (3) presence of a control group with normal kidney function; (4) study population age >18 years; (5) Asian or Caucasian ethnicity of the populations, and (6) articles providing detailed distribution of ACE genotypes. Studies investigating the relationships between genetic polymorphisms and other kidney diseases (lupus nephritis, polycystic kidney disease, endemic nephropathy, or reflux nephropathy) were excluded.

Data Extraction and Quality Assessment

Two reviewers (Chin Lin and Sui-Lung Su) independently extracted the data and assessed risk of bias. We recorded the first author's name, year of publication, ethnicity of the study population, kidney function of the cases, definition of the case group and its population characteristics (mean age, proportion of male subjects, body mass index, diabetes mellitus prevalence, hypertension prevalence, and ACE I/D genotype distribution). Ethnicity of the study population was categorized by study area. Subjects in the Arabian peninsula were classified as Caucasian because Arabs were the main race, and subjects in other regions of Asia (excluding Russia) were classified as Asian. Diabetes mellitus and hypertension were defined by plasma glucose level of > 126 mg/dL and systolic blood pressure of >140 mmHg. If the article did not report the prevalence of diabetes mellitus and hypertension or the definition did not match, we assumed a normal distribution of plasma glucose level and systolic blood pressure for calculation.

Estimating moderate effects is difficult in meta-analysis using case–control studies. Researchers prefer that studies provide stratified data or matching data, but previous studies have seldom reported these. Fortunately, the characteristics of case groups may be used to estimate moderate effects under the following two conditions: (1) outcomes were rare events, (2) the major independent variable and moderators were independent events.

For example, when the major independent variable is exposure, with values "yes" or "no," and the moderator is gender, with values "male" or "female," the variables p_1, p_2, p_3, and p_4 are the outcome prevalence of women without exposure, men without exposure, women with exposure, and men with exposure. The variable p_5 is the proportion of individuals with exposure in the whole population; p_6 is the proportion of men in the population without exposure; and p_7 is the proportion of men in the population with exposure.

When researchers wish to conduct a case–control study, they must survey the exposure proportion in the case and control groups to estimate the odds ratio (OR). The exposure proportions using a stratified view and ORs are as follows:

Exposure proportion among case women:

$$E_1 = \frac{p_3 p_5 (1-p_7)}{p_1(1-p_5)(1-p_6)+p_3 p_5(1-p_7)}$$

Exposure proportion among case men:

$$E_2 = \frac{p_4 p_5 p_7}{p_2(1-p_5)p_6+p_4 p_5 p_7}$$

Exposure proportion among control women:

$$E_3 = \frac{(1-p_3)p_5(1-p_7)}{(1-p_1)(1-p_5)(1-p_6)+(1-p_3)p_5(1-p_7)}$$

Exposure proportion among control men:

$$E_4 = \frac{(1-p_4)p_5 p_7}{(1-p_2)(1-p_5)p_6+(1-p_4)p_5 p_7}$$

OR in women: $OR_{women} = \dfrac{E_1(1-E_3)}{E_3(1-E_1)}$

OR in men: $OR_{men} = \dfrac{E_2(1-E_4)}{E_4(1-E_2)}$

Crude OR (simple combined):

$$OR_{crude} = \frac{((1-k_1)E_1+k_1E_2)((1-k_2)(1-E_3)+k_2(1-E_4))}{((1-k_2)E_3+k_2E_4)((1-k_1)(1-E_1)+k_1(1-E_2))}.$$

k_1 = proportion of males in the case group.

k_2 = proportion of males in the control group.

Two factors (k_1 and k_2) may affect the crude OR. However, when p_1, p_2, p_3, and p_4 are very rare and there is no association between the major independent variable and the moderator ($p_6 = p_7$),

$$E_3 = \lim_{p_1 \to 0} \lim_{p_3 \to 0} \left(\frac{(1-p_3)p_5(1-p_7)}{(1-p_1)(1-p_5)(1-p_6)+(1-p_3)p_5(1-p_7)} \right) = p_5$$

$$E_4 = \lim_{p_2 \to 0} \lim_{p_4 \to 0} \left(\frac{(1-p_4)p_5 p_7}{(1-p_2)(1-p_5)p_6+(1-p_4)p_5 p_7} \right) = p_5$$

Table 2. Quality score and description of studies' population in included studies.

First author & year	Quality score	Age (years)	Male (%)	BMI (kg/m²)	DM (%)	HT (%)	Case group			Control group		
							II	ID	DD	II	ID	DD
Shaikh, 2012 [27]	7	58	54	27	100	86	18	98	52	123	148	25
Rahimi, 2012 [28]	7	56	40	27	100	63	19	66	55	14	32	26
El-Baz, 2012 [29]	6	59	53		100		4	58	40	5	72	23
Zsom(1), 2011 [30]	4	64	55				39	88	68	44	110	46
Zsom(2), 2011 [30]	4	70	61		100		20	60	34	44	110	46
Al-Harbi, 2011 [31]	4	58	48	30	100	86	12	39	59	25	75	96
Jung, 2011 [32]	7	34	57			61	78	142	41	98	164	38
Ali, 2011 [33]	5	55	55	25	16	41	47	125	18	86	90	14
Huang, 2010 [34]	3	40	50			54	10	29	8	58	52	10
Jayapalan, 2010 [35]	7	60	38		100	42	77	77	21	31	31	19
Mansoor, 2010 [14]	6	53	31	27	100	29	27	45	12	65	102	33
Naresh, 2009 [36]	5	54	53	29	100	95	4	11	15	12	11	7
Ezzidi, 2009 [37]	7	60	46	28	100	50	88	260	167	152	196	54
Nikzamir, 2009 [38]	7	59	56	26	100	54	31	84	64	42	75	28
Anbazhagan, 2009 [39]	7	49	73		28	75	33	58	27	23	53	22
Ahluwalia, 2009 [40]	7	58	66	24	100	59	44	64	132	49	117	89
Palomo-Piñón, 2009 [16]	7	60	48	27	100	26	87	105	43	85	91	24
Möllsten, 2008 [41]	7	47	49		100	52	25	69	27	36	113	48
Eroglu, 2008 [42]	7	58	41	29	100	38	13	17	16	13	24	19
Arfa, 2008 [43]	7	62	43	29	100	68	9	41	40	6	24	21
Tripathi, 2008 [44]	6	36	88		0	69	53	72	55	379	148	42
Movva, 2007 [45]	6	57	70		100		47	88	39	74	74	27
Uddin, 2007 [46]	4	51	54		100	78	12	22	24	24	28	14
Buraczynska, 2006 [47]	8	51	56		19	78	174	346	228	112	268	140
So, 2006 [48]	6				100		407	364	93	549	526	150
Shestakova, 2006 [49]	6	26	48	23	100	26	15	35	13	24	30	12
Ng, 2006 [50]	7	61	61	32	100	48	47	148	96	32	83	52
Prasad, 2006 [51]	7	57	33		100	63	67	74	55	76	97	52
Degirmenci, 2005 [52]	4				100		6	25	12	19	47	30
van der Sman-de Beer, 2005 [53]	6	59	61	26	17	65	110	227	116	112	235	125
Park, 2005 [18]	5	60	58	23	100	83	27	49	27	30	51	7
Canani, 2005 [54]	6				100		66	181	126	120	308	181
Fabris, 2005 [55]	7	60	78	26	0	100	13	32	41	34	83	55
Lau, 2004 [56]	5	43	48				53	48	17	47	43	4
Suzuki, 2004 [57]	5	36	56				42	54	21	111	106	53
Stratta, 2004 [58]	5	50	67			39	23	50	44	29	76	66
Lochynska, 2003 [59]	5	42	74		0	0	13	32	5	20	45	35
Papp, 2003 [60]	4	49	46			65	11	25	14	34	83	33
Aucella, 2003 [61]	5	62	54		16	58	57	201	203	170	576	561
Okuno, 2003 [62]	7	78	50	20	100	31	1	8	3	21	12	5
Ortiz, 2003 [63]	6	56	59	22	0	100	9	71	81	17	66	46
Hadjadj, 2003 [15]	9	66	73	29	100	72	552	1468	1119	115	282	208
Wang, 2003 [64]	5	55	51	23	30	66	106	104	36	71	88	24
Dixit, 2002 [65]	7	24	55				12	26	9	3	24	13
Lee(1), 2002 [26]	8				0		20	45	12	330	277	66
Lee(2), 2002 [26]	8				100		117	137	40	208	170	39
Losito, 2002 [66]	6	67	61	25	14	50	27	81	52	22	84	63
Yoon, 2002 [67]	5	35	56		0	35	44	116	31	70	128	25

Table 2. Cont.

First author & year	Quality score	Age (years)	Male (%)	BMI (kg/m²)	DM (%)	HT (%)	Case group			Control group		
							II	ID	DD	II	ID	DD
Fradin, 2002 [68]	7	57	53	32	100	33	18	61	38	20	54	44
Drouet, 2002 [69]	6	44	77				16	46	63	13	28	36
Nicod, 2002 [70]	5	54	57	25			63	156	41	54	153	53
Araz, 2001 [71]	7	56	41	28	100	63	18	64	34	23	57	43
Azar, 2001 [72]	6	23	46		100		2	27	23	2	7	1
Lovati, 2001 [73]	7	54	57	25	12	51	63	156	41	69	195	63
Wang, 2001 [74]	8						28	99	41	313	662	311
Taniwaki, 2001 [75]	7	61	59	23	100	54	32	40	14	31	26	12
Viswanathan, 2001 [76]	7	57	66	26	100	64	17	45	24	10	8	5
Hadjadj, 2001 [77]	7	40	59	23	100	53	8	34	17	46	116	89
Wu, 2000 [78]	3	60	55		100		22	31	18	19	20	2
Hsieh, 2000 [79]	5	61	49	23	100	60	80	59	40	86	50	21
van Ittersum, 2000 [80]	6	55	59		100	80	23	33	13	53	86	49
Tomino, 1999 [19]	7	61	63		100		312	337	96	163	189	55
Solini, 1999 [81]	8	60	58	30	100	61	33	66	58	27	83	62
De Cosmo, 1999 [82]	7	43	61		100	42	23	76	73	18	53	65
Miura, 1999 [83]	7	36	34		100	21	36	49	13	35	58	10
Kuramoto, 1999 [84]	7	58	61	23	100	56	8	16	9	13	13	3
Huang, 1998 [85]	6				100		4	12	8	7	29	23
Walder, 1998 [86]	7	42	71		100	86	12	25	18	12	16	16
Freire, 1998 [87]	6	28	48		100	17	12	32	33	10	45	34
Grzeszczak, 1998 [88]	7	62		29	100	68	103	230	129	63	118	73
Young, 1998 [89]	7	56	34	25	100	73	23	30	3	26	20	8
Penno, 1998 [90]	5				100		15	38	23	62	258	114
Fernández-Llama, 1998 [91]	5				0	100	1	6	7	5	38	18
Frost, 1998 [92]	5				100		10	7	16	21	48	46
Pei, 1997 [93]	6	49	68				32	81	55	21	49	30
Marre, 1997 [94]	8	43	57	24	100	57	50	168	119	40	69	48
Barnas, 1997 [95]	6	47	70		100	48	9	27	14	15	21	4
Ringel, 1997 [96]	8	51	54	26	100	43	64	152	79	78	199	92
Schmidt, 1997 [97]	7	65	51	29	100	74	61	129	121	62	154	131
Kawada, 1997 [98]	5	59	62		22		89	89	30	84	96	28
Kario, 1997 [99]	6	72	41	25	0	100	42	62	29	86	98	16
Nakajima, 1996 [17]	6	56	64		100		37	50	14	18	19	4
Chowdhury, 1996 [100]	6	39	55		100	97	40	124	78	32	79	55
McLaughlin, 1996 [101]	4	42	57				114	366	312	75	203	93
Oh, 1996 [102]	6	35	42	19	100		12	9	10	11	10	7
Schmidt, 1996 [103]	5	55	58			63	27	51	28	21	38	36
Doi, 1996 [104]	7	62	51	22	100	55	50	85	29	56	56	12
Ohno, 1996 [105]	7	61	53	23	100	56	26	38	15	33	15	9
Mizuiri, 1995 [106]	6	54			100	90	11	51	19	11	11	9
Yorioka, 1995 [107]	5	33	44			6	27	13	8	46	47	10
Fujisawa, 1995 [108]	4				100		24	23	7	17	12	6
Panagiotopoulos, 1995 [109]	5	62	66		100		10	25	15	29	44	42
Tarnow, 1995 [110]	8	41	61	24	100	68	40	95	63	46	77	67
Schmidt, 1995 [111]	6	45	75			59	44	81	79	40	117	77
Yoshida, 1995 [112]	7	39	64			15	20	17	16	19	24	3
Dudley, 1995 [113]	7	53	67	29	100	58	29	82	47	35	87	36

Table 2. Cont.

First author & year	Quality score	Age (years)	Male (%)	BMI (kg/m^2)	DM (%)	HT (%)	Case group			Control group		
							II	ID	DD	II	ID	DD
Harden, 1995 [114]	5	35					19	41	40	17	42	39
Doria, 1994 [115]	5	29			100		15	35	24	20	41	16
Marre, 1994 [116]	6	39	60	23	100		4	35	23	15	28	19
Powrie, 1994 [117]	6	35	50	20	100		4	8	7	24	37	24

Quality score: result of quality assessed in each study (detailed data were shown in supplementary file); Age: mean age; Male: probability of male; BMI: mean body mass index; DM: prevalence of diabetes mellitus; HT: prevalence of hypertension; II: number of II genotype carries; ID: number of ID genotype carries; DD: number of DD genotype carries.

$$OR_{crude} = \frac{((1-k_1)E_1 + k_1E_2)(1-p_5)}{p_5((1-k_1)(1-E_1)+k_1(1-E_2))}$$

If moderate effects are present ($OR_{\text{women}} \neq OR_{\text{men}}$), the proportion of males in the case group (k_1) is the only factor that can affect the crude OR. In addition, the relationship between k_1 and log of odds ratio approximate the first order polynomial when above assumption were proper. We may accordingly use the characteristics of the case group to estimate the moderate effects in this study under the above assumptions.

Risk of bias was assessed by the following procedures suggested by the Newcastle–Ottawa Quality Assessment Scale [23] (shown in Table S3). This tool assesses studies with a focus on the following factors: (1) selection of study population, (2) comparability between the case and control groups, and (3) the exposure assessed. Each study received a score between 0 and 9. We investigated the relationship between the quality of studies and the estimation of risk.

Statistical Analysis

Variables are presented as means, proportions, or numbers as appropriate. Our meta-analysis examined the association between ACE I/D polymorphisms and CKD risk for each study by odds ratios (ORs) with 95% confidence intervals (CIs).

The τ^2 statistic estimated by the DerSimonian–Laird method was used for the assessment of heterogeneity, and a random-effects model based on the Mantel–Haenszel method was applied. Allele type, genotype, and dominant/recessive models were used to calculate the association between genetic polymorphism and CKD risk. This report displays results from the allele type model, unless estimates using a different model were obviously different. Egger's regression was used to test symmetry of pooled results. Prespecified subgroup analyses included the causes of CKD.

A moderate effect was defined as ratio between ORs in a stratified analysis. For example, if OR for the association between ACE I/D polymorphisms and CKD risk is 6 in the Asian group and 3 in the Caucasian group, the moderate effect of ethnicity will be 6/3 = 2. Possible moderators (ethnicity, age, gender, body mass index, diabetes mellitus, and hypertension) and study characteristic (quality score, study design, and kidney functions of cases) were tested by meta-regression. In multivariable analyses, we adjusted ethnicity because most previous studies have found significant moderate effects [10–12]. To assess the effect of ethnicity on gender-dependent effects, we investigated the interaction between gender and ethnicity. The interaction between other moderators and gender were also tested.

This study considered a p-value of <0.05 as significant for all analyses. Statistical analyses were carried out with R, version 2.15.0, using the "metafor" [24] and "meta" [25] packages.

Results

Screening Process

Our search strategy returned 501 papers (the identification process is shown in Figure 1). We excluded 249 papers after a preliminary search of titles and abstracts. An additional 129 papers were excluded after full-text articles were assessed, leaving 123 articles that matched our criteria. Of these, 15 used duplicate databases, 9 lacked detailed data, and 1 likely reported wrong data. In 98 of the studies finally included [14–19,26–117], 2 (Zsom et al. [30] and Lee et al. [26]) reported results of stratification, but studies by Zsom et al. [30] used a single control group. Accordingly, 99 populations were included in this meta-analysis, and their detailed data are shown in Tables 1 and 2.

Preliminary Pooled Analyses

Our meta-analysis showed that a significantly increased CKD risk was associated with the D allele compared with the I allele in each subgroup. Figure 2 shows that D allele carriers had an OR of 1.21 for risk of all-cause CKD compared with I allele carriers, and that these ORs were dissimilar in different ethnicities ($p = 0.002$). OR for CKD in Asian individuals carrying the D allele compared with those carrying the I allele was 1.40 (95% CI: 1.23–1.59), and in Caucasian individuals was 1.12 (95% CI: 1.04–1.21). A summary of the other results is shown in Table 3 and are very similar to those in Figure 2. In the allele type, genotype, and dominant/recessive models, individuals carrying the D allele showed higher CKD risk, and ORs were higher in Asians than in Caucasians. The heterogeneities were higher in Asian populations than in Caucasian populations in each subgroup.

Identifying Moderators of the Association between ACE I/D Polymorphisms and CKD Risk

Table 4 shows the assessment results of moderate effect on all-cause CKD using the allele type model. Compared with I allele carriers, D allele carriers had a higher OR for CKD risk in Asians than in Caucasians (OR of moderate effect: 1.24; 95% CI: 1.08–1.42). Hypertension also was a moderator (OR of moderate effect: 1.55; 95% CI: 1.04–2.32) and still had a significant moderate effect after adjusting ethnicity (OR of moderate effect: 1.57; 95% CI: 1.07–2.31). No additional moderators were significant after adjustment for ethnicity and hypertension (data not shown). In

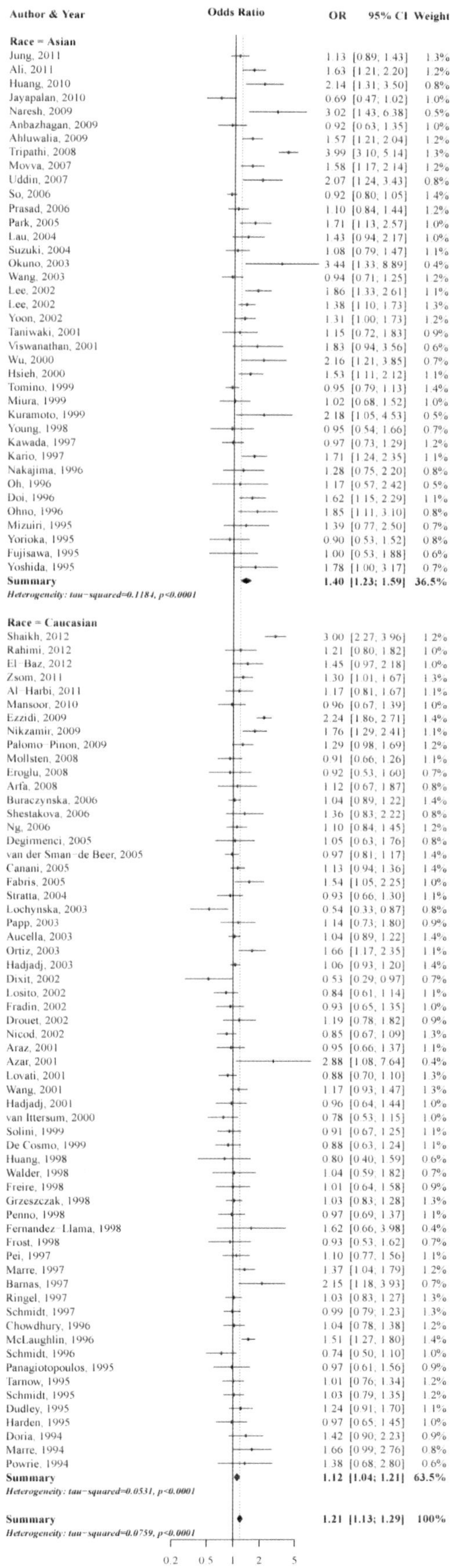

Figure 2. Forest plot of the association between ACE I/D and all-cause CKD using allele type model.

the final model of these analyses, τ^2 declined by 15.5% (crude: 0.097; after adjustment: 0.082) and p of Egger's regression test was not significant ($p = 0.258$). We did not find a significant gender-dependent effect.

In subgroup analyses of diabetic nephropathy, study design (OR for moderate effect: 1.21; 95% CI: 1.02–1.42) and body mass index (OR of moderate effect: 0.84; 95% CI: 0.70–1.00) had significant moderate effects on ACE I/D polymorphisms and diabetic nephropathy. After adjustment for ethnicity, the moderate effects of study design (OR of moderate effect: 1.19; 95% CI: 1.01–1.41) was still significant but that of body mass index (OR for moderate effect: 0.91; 95% CI: 0.73–1.13) was not (data not shown). The results of the nondiabetic nephropathy subgroup were similar to those for all-cause CKD, with ethnicity (OR of moderate effect: 1.69; 95% CI: 1.07–2.68) and hypertension (OR of moderate effect: 2.42; 95% CI: 1.19–4.93) the only two significant moderators in multivariable analyses (data not shown).

Estimated Gender-dependent Effects

Table 5 shows the interaction of ethnicity and gender. We found no significant interactions between the other variables and gender. Coefficients of interaction were significant for hypertension (p before adjustment for hypertension = 0.015; p after adjustment for hypertension = 0.003). No other moderators were significant when added to the final model. A proportion of 32.8% of heterogeneity (crude $\tau^2 = 0.100$; after adjustment, $\tau^2 = 0.068$) was caused by different ethnicity, gender probability, and prevalence of hypertension in the study population, and p of Egger's regression test was not significant ($p = 0.217$). Figure 3 shows OR of ACE I/D polymorphisms and CKD risk in different combination of ethnicity, gender, and hypertension status based on Model 2 in Table 5. A gender-dependent effect analysis showed the strongest association between the ACE I/D polymorphisms and CKD risk in Asian males with hypertension (OR: 3.75; 95% CI: 1.84–7.65) or without (OR: 2.42; 95% CI: 1.40–4.20).

Interaction of ethnicity and gender was borderline significant ($p = 0.056$) in the diabetic nephropathy subgroup, but was significant ($p = 0.030$) in the nondiabetic nephropathy subgroup. Although the result of symmetry assessment was significant in nondiabetic nephropathy subgroup (p of Egger's regression test = 0.032), it was noteworthy that 78.3% of heterogeneity (crude τ^2:0.166; after adjustment, τ^2:0.036) were caused by ethnicity, gender, and hypertension.

The symmetry of final models was shown in Figure 4. Funnel plots presented the association between residual and standard error based on results of Table 5, and each point represents a study. Egger's regression test indicated no evidence of publication bias among studies included into the final model this meta-analysis and diabetic nephropathy subgroup. The model in nondiabetic nephropathy subgroup was asymmetric, and it might be due to the study reported by Jung et al. [32]. We did sensitivity analyses leaving the article out (data not shown). The result of symmetry assessment was not significant (p of Egger's regression test = 0.245), and the coefficients in this model were still significant (p of interaction effect of ethnicity and gender = 0.002; p of moderate effect of hypertension <0.001). In addition, the τ^2 was 0 in this sensitivity model.

Table 3. Odds ratio of ACE I/D and all-cause CKD, diabetic nephropathy, non-diabetic nephropathy using assumption of allele type, genotype, dominant and recessive model.

Model	Ethnicity	All-cause CKD				Diabetic nephropathy				Non-diabetic nephropathy			
		n	OR	95% CI	τ^2	n	OR	95% CI	τ^2	n	OR	95% CI	τ^2
Allele type (D vs. I)	All studies	99	1.21	(1.13, 1.29)	0.076	65	1.23	(1.14, 1.33)	0.063	22	1.29	(1.06, 1.56)	0.166
	Asian	38	1.40	(1.23, 1.59)	0.118	24	1.36	(1.18, 1.56)	0.070	10	1.59	(1.17, 2.17)	0.212
	Caucasian	61	1.12	(1.04, 1.21)	0.053	41	1.17	(1.06, 1.29)	0.064	12	1.08	(0.91, 1.29)	0.054
Genotype-1 (DD vs. II)	All studies	99	1.44	(1.26, 1.64)	0.277	65	1.48	(1.26, 1.74)	0.249	22	1.67	(1.16, 2.41)	0.556
	Asian	38	1.87	(1.46, 2.38)	0.377	24	1.66	(1.27, 2.18)	0.230	10	2.77	(1.62, 4.75)	0.567
	Caucasian	61	1.25	(1.07, 1.46)	0.224	41	1.39	(1.14, 1.71)	0.275	12	1.11	(0.77, 1.60)	0.211
Genotype-2 (ID vs. II)	All studies	99	1.20	(1.10, 1.32)	0.098	65	1.26	(1.13, 1.40)	0.082	22	1.17	(0.92, 1.49)	0.206
	Asian	38	1.34	(1.14, 1.57)	0.152	24	1.31	(1.09, 1.57)	0.088	10	1.43	(0.99, 2.05)	0.259
	Caucasian	61	1.13	(1.02, 1.25)	0.062	41	1.23	(1.07, 1.42)	0.084	12	0.91	(0.74, 1.13)	0.570
Dominant (DD+ID vs. II)	All studies	99	1.28	(1.16, 1.41)	0.132	65	1.33	(1.19, 1.50)	0.110	22	1.30	(1.00, 1.69)	0.271
	Asian	38	1.48	(1.25, 1.74)	0.180	24	1.42	(1.19, 1.70)	0.095	10	1.66	(1.12, 2.45)	0.317
	Caucasian	61	1.17	(1.05, 1.31)	0.100	41	1.28	(1.10, 1.49)	0.130	12	1.01	(0.80, 1.27)	0.031
Recessive (DD vs. ID+II)	All studies	99	1.27	(1.15, 1.39)	0.090	65	1.26	(1.13, 1.42)	0.112	22	1.53	(1.18, 1.99)	0.262
	Asian	38	1.56	(1.28, 1.90)	0.227	24	1.42	(1.12, 1.79)	0.169	10	2.22	(1.42, 3.48)	0.369
	Caucasian	61	1.16	(1.04, 1.28)	0.090	41	1.21	(1.06, 1.37)	0.097	12	1.20	(0.92, 1.57)	0.118

Discussion

This study showed that CKD risk was higher in D allele carriers than in I allele carriers, and there was no strong evidence that analyses using different model assumptions might produce dissimilar results. Heterogeneity was higher in the Asian population than in the Caucasian population. Interaction between ACE I/D polymorphisms and hypertension exerted an additive effect on CKD risk. A gender-dependent effect of ACE I/D polymorphisms on CKD risk was clearly apparent in Asians but not in Caucasians.

The DD genotype showed higher gene expression and serum ACE levels than the ID genotype, followed by the II genotype [9,118]. High blood ACE levels may increase blood angiotensin II levels [8], and individuals with higher angiotensin II levels may have a higher CKD risk [119,120]. Previous studies showed that the association between ACE I/D polymorphisms and CKD risk might not be dominant or recessive [8,9,118]. Previous meta-analysis studies showed the supported results, they reported that DD genotype had higher risk of CKD than ID genotype, followed by the II genotype. We also observed the apparent linear association between numbers of D allele and odds ratios compared

Table 4. Moderator effects of allele type model (D vs. I) on all-cause CKD.

		Unadjusted		Adjusted ethnicity	
	n	OR	95% CI	OR	95% CI
Ethnicity (Caucasian is ref.)	99	1.24*	(1.08, 1.42)		
Study design (CS is ref.)	99	1.05	(0.92, 1.20)	1.03	(0.90, 1.18)
Quality score (per 1 score)	99	0.98	(0.93, 1.04)	0.99	(0.94, 1.05)
Kidney function of case (non-ESRD is ref.)	99	1.03	(0.87, 1.23)	0.97	(0.81, 1.16)
Age (per 10 years)	88	1.02	(0.95, 1.09)	1.01	(0.95, 1.08)
Male (per 100%)	84	1.48	(0.72, 3.01)	1.63	(0.81, 3.28)
BMI (per 5 kg/m^2)	45	0.86	(0.73, 1.03)	0.95	(0.78, 1.16)
DM (per 100%)	81	0.96	(0.78, 1.18)	0.99	(0.81, 1.22)
Hypertension (per 100%)	68	1.55*	(1.04, 2.32)	1.57*	(1.07, 2.31)

Depend variable: log odds ratio of ACE I/D and all-cause CKD using allele type model.
n: number of studies; OR: odds ratio for moderate effect; 95% CI: 95% confidence interval.
CS: cross-sectional study; non-ESRD: not only ESRD patients; Age: mean age; Male: probability of male; BMI: mean body mass index; DM: prevalence of diabetes mellitus; Hypertension: prevalence of hypertension.
*: $p<0.05$.

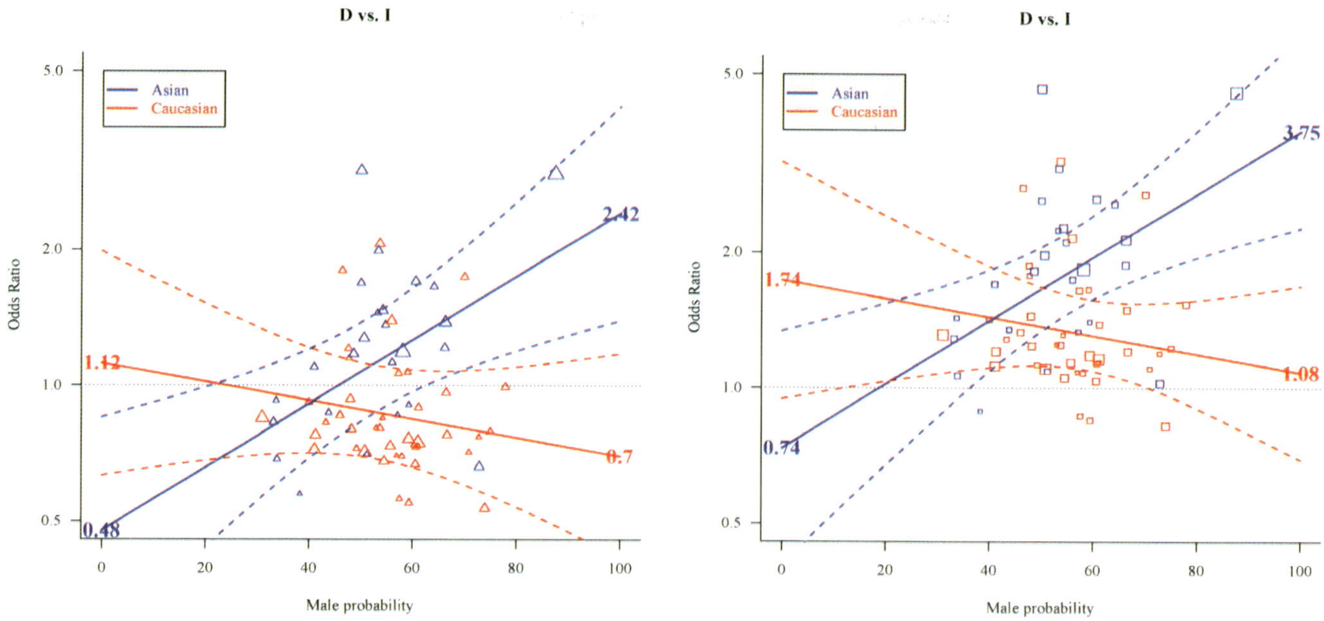

Figure 3. Gender-dependent effects of ACE I/D and all-cause CKD in each population. Left figure was showed the OR in people without hypertension; right figure was showed the odds ratio in patient with hypertension. Red triangle and square: individual studies in Caucasian; blue triangle and square: individual studies in Asian. Solid line: unbiased estimator of odds ratio; dashed line: 95% confidence interval of odds ratios. Estimated value of log odds ratio in individual studies without hypertension used following formula: observed log odds ratio – hypertension prevalence of study population×0.437 (according to Model 2 in Table 5) Estimated value of log odds ratio in individual studies with hypertension used following formula: observed log odds ratio+(1– hypertension prevalence of study population)×0.437 (according to Model 2 in Table 5).

the II genotype in genotype analyses [10–12,20–22]. The assumption of the allele type model in this association might be more reasonable, and it may thus be true that individuals carrying the D allele have a higher CKD risk.

Hypertension in some patients is due to a dysfunction of RAS such as abnormal secretion of renin, causing increased blood angiotensin I levels [121]. D allele carriers had higher ACE levels than I allele carriers [118], leading to more efficient conversion of angiotensin I to angiotensin II, resulting in CKD [119,120]. The mechanism may be an additive effect of hypertension and the D allele. An additive effect was significant in the nondiabetic group but not in the diabetic nephropathy subgroups. The blood levels of advanced glycation end products (AGE) diabetic patients may be high, possibly causing blood pressure increases [122]. We

Table 5. Three way interaction of Asian, male and ACE D allele on all-cause CKD, diabetic nephropathy and non-diabetic nephropathy.

	All-cause CKD				Diabetic nephropathy		Non-diabetic nephropathy	
	Model 1		Model 2					
	β	se	β	se	β	se	β	se
Intercept	0.297	0.275	0.115	0.291	0.090	0.369	−0.213	0.746
Race (Caucasian is ref.)	−0.697	0.391	−0.853*	0.402	−0.817	0.569	−1.080	0.816
Male (per 100%) €	−0.312	0.476	−0.470	0.501	−0.122	0.691	−0.349	1.050
Race×Male	1.662*	0.686	2.094*	0.715	2.064	1.082	2.666*	1.231
Hypertension (per 100%) €			0.437*	0.192	0.229	0.294	0.857*	0.245
τ^2	0.075		0.068		0.081		0.036*	
Egger's test	p = 0.097		p = 0.217		p = 0.385		p = 0.032	

Depend variable: log odds ratio of ACE I/D and CKD using allele type model.
β: coefficients in meta-regression; se: standard error of β.
Model 1: Hypertension was not included in independent variables.
Model 2: Hypertension was included in independent variables.
Egger's test: p-value of Egger's regression test.
€: references of parameters were 0%.
*: $p<0.05$.

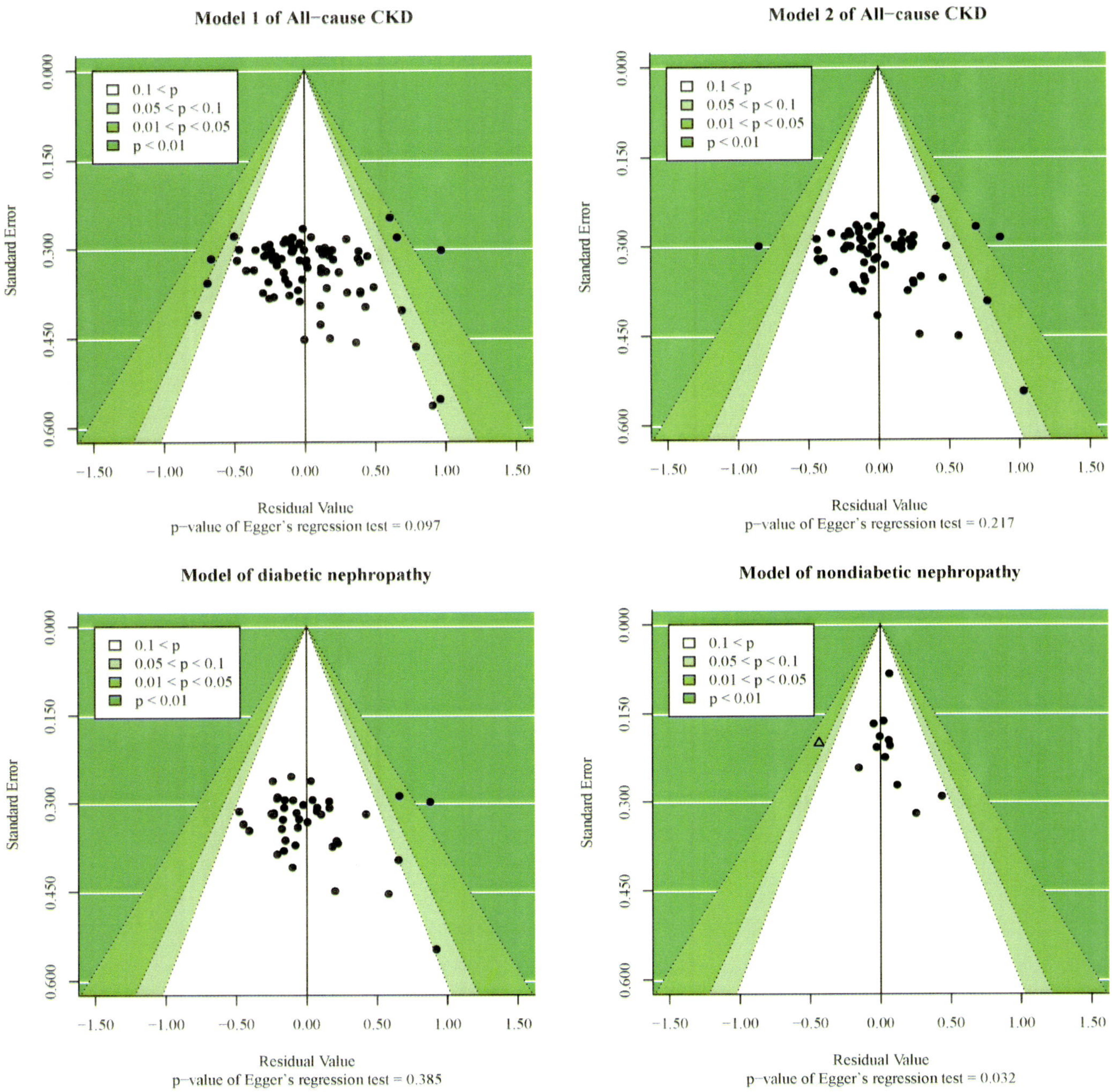

Figure 4. Funnel plot of three way interaction model in each subgroup. The model in nondiabetic nephropathy subgroup was asymmetric. The triangle in that plot was study reported by Jung et al. [32], and the p value of the student residual was less 0.05. After excluding this study, the p value of Egger's regression test was not significant ($p = 0.245$) and the moderate effect of interaction and hypertension were more significantly (p of interaction: 0.0304→0.0023; p of hypertension: 0.0005→<0.0001).

accordingly hypothesize that the probability of hypertension because of a dysfunction of RAS was higher in the nondiabetic nephropathy subgroup than in the diabetic nephropathy subgroup. Thus, the interaction between ACE I/D polymorphisms and hypertension was significant only in the nondiabetic nephropathy subgroup. This hypothesis may require further studies for confirmation.

We found a significant gender-dependent effect of ACE I/D polymorphisms on CKD risk in Asians. In previous studies in Asians, the ORs of the additive effect on the DD genotype of males were 2.94 and 1.41 in Japanese [17] and Koreans [18], respectively. Another study in Japan also reported a positive additive effect of the DD genotype of males [19]. Studies of Caucasians reported contrary results, with an interaction OR of 0.42 in Pakistan [14]. Another two studies in France [15] and Mexico [16] also showed an additive effect between the DD genotype and female gender but not male gender. Although the interaction tests in these studies were not significant, we could observe dissimilar gender-dependent effect in different ethnicity. Previous studies have also reported a different gender-dependent effect of ACE I/D polymorphisms on blood ACE levels in Asians and Caucasians. In a study conducted in China [13], differences in blood ACE levels between DD genotype and other genotypes among men were significantly greater than those in women. On the other hand, a study conducted in Germany [123] reported the opposite result.

Androgens may play a key role in this additive effect. A study has shown that in intact male rats and ovariectomized female rats that received testosterone for 5 weeks, the androgen may have contributed to the decrease in pressure natriuresis [124]. In an animal study, ACE activity was higher in male mice than in female mice, and this gender difference disappeared after gonadectomy [125]. In previous reports, sensitivity to androgens was stated to be higher in Caucasians than in Asians [126]. Blood androgen levels in Caucasians and Asians showed no significant differences [127,128]. On the basis of previous studies, we hypothesized that the dissimilar gender-dependent effect of ACE I/D polymorphisms on CKD risk in Caucasians and Asians might be accounted for by dissimilar sensitivity to androgens. The gender difference of male sex hormone utilization was higher in Asians than in Caucasians. Therefore, that the additive effect of the D allele and male gender was also higher in Asians than in Caucasians.

In subgroup analyses, the above additive effect was borderline significant in the diabetic nephropathy subgroup, but there was no evidence that diabetic mellitus might contribute to this additive effect. Although the additive effect also could explain why two populations with different ethnicities had different heterogeneity before adjustment for any moderators, the calculated risk ratio of ACE I/D polymorphisms on CKD risk may have been affected by the gender-dependent effect in Asians.

Our study had three limitations. First, we relied on tabular data rather than on individual patient data, possibly leading to an inflated standard error in pooled analyses. However, we still observed a significant gender-dependent effect difference in different ethnicities. Second, estimates of diabetes mellitus and hypertension prevalence did not factor in the effects of therapy for them. Some subjects having higher blood glucose and blood pressure may have taken drugs, leading to normal biochemical values in reports. Third, we may have missed unpublished data for the nondiabetic nephropathy subgroup. But the results of this subgroup were similar to the results of previous studies and we still observed a significant result excluding the greatest impact of symmetry study; therefore, there is no evidence to question their reliability.

In conclusion, CKD risk was higher with the D allele than with the I allele. Asian ethnicity and hypertension had positive moderate effects, and their effects were more likely to be higher in patients with nondiabetic nephropathy. A gender-dependent effect of ACE I/D polymorphisms on CKD risk was confirmed in Asians; the D allele showed 3.75-fold greater risk for CKD than the I allele in hypertensive Asian males. These results suggest that Asian males should be offered testing for defects in ACE I/D polymorphisms, especially if they are hypertensive. We suggest that physicians should provide specific protection to D-allele carriers, for example by administering ACE inhibitors to hypertensive patients.

Supporting Information

Table S1 PRISMA 2009 Checklist.

Table S2 Search strategies. Web sites and uniform resource locator: **MEDLINE**: http://www.ncbi.nlm.nih.gov/pubmed **Cochrane Library**: http://www.thecochranelibrary.com **Embase**: https://www.embase.com

Table S3 Quality assessment tool in this meta-analysis based on Wells et al. [23].

Author Contributions

Conceived and designed the experiments: CL HYY SLS. Performed the experiments: CL HYY SLS. Analyzed the data: CL. Contributed reagents/materials/analysis tools: CL CMC. Wrote the paper: CL HYY SLS. Critical review and comments: CCW HSL YFL KCL FHL SYK. Modify manuscript: CL HYY CCW HSL KCL SLS.

References

1. Coresh J, Selvin E, Stevens LA, Manzi J, Kusek JW, et al. (2007) Prevalence of chronic kidney disease in the United States. JAMA 298: 2038–2047.
2. Imai E, Horio M, Watanabe T, Iseki K, Yamagata K, et al. (2009) Prevalence of chronic kidney disease in the Japanese general population. Clin Exp Nephrol 13: 621–630.
3. Zhang L, Wang F, Wang L, Wang W, Liu B, et al. (2012) Prevalence of chronic kidney disease in China: a cross-sectional survey. Lancet 379: 815–822.
4. Go AS, Chertow GM, Fan D, McCulloch CE, Hsu CY (2004) Chronic kidney disease and the risks of death, cardiovascular events, and hospitalization. N Engl J Med 351: 1296–1305.
5. Li S, McAlpine DD, Liu J, Li S, Collins AJ (2004) Differences between blacks and whites in the incidence of end-stage renal disease and associated risk factors. Adv Ren Replace Ther 11: 5–13.
6. Tsai JC, Chen SC, Hwang SJ, Chang JM, Lin MY, et al. (2010) Prevalence and risk factors for CKD in spouses and relatives of hemodialysis patients. Am J Kidney Dis 55: 856–866.
7. McClellan WM, Warnock DG, Judd S, Muntner P, Patzer RE, et al. (2012) Association of family history of ESRD, prevalent albuminuria, and reduced GFR with incident ESRD. Am J Kidney Dis 59: 25–31.
8. Remuzzi G, Perico N, Macia M, Ruggenenti P (2005) The role of renin-angiotensin-aldosterone system in the progression of chronic kidney disease. Kidney Int Suppl: S57–65.
9. Mizuiri S, Hemmi H, Kumanomidou H, Iwamoto M, Miyagi M, et al. (2001) Angiotensin-converting enzyme (ACE) I/D genotype and renal ACE gene expression. Kidney Int 60: 1124–1130.
10. Qin YH, Zhou TB, Su LN, Lei FY, Huang WF, et al. (2011) Association between ACE polymorphism and risk of IgA nephropathy: a meta-analysis. J Renin Angiotensin Aldosterone Syst 12: 215–223.
11. Wang F, Fang Q, Yu N, Zhao D, Zhang Y, et al. (2012) Association between genetic polymorphism of the angiotensin-converting enzyme and diabetic nephropathy: a meta-analysis comprising 26,580 subjects. J Renin Angiotensin Aldosterone Syst 13: 161–174.
12. Zhou TB, Yin SS, Qin YH (2012) Association between angiotensin-converting enzyme insertion/deletion gene polymorphism and end-stage renal disease susceptibility. J Renin Angiotensin Aldosterone Syst [Epub ahead of print].
13. Zhang YF, Cheng Q, Tang NL, Chu TT, Tomlinson B, et al. (2013) Gender difference of serum angiotensin-converting enzyme (ACE) activity in DD genotype of ACE insertion/deletion polymorphism in elderly Chinese. J Renin Angiotensin Aldosterone Syst.
14. Mansoor Q, Bilal N, Qureshi S, Qureshi O, Javaid A, et al. (2010) Gender based disparities in ACE I/D polymorphism associated with progression of diabetic nephropathy in Pakistani patients with type 2 diabetes mellitus. International Journal of Diabetes and Metabolism 18: 67–71.
15. Hadjadj S, Gallois Y, Alhenc-Gelas F, Chatellier G, Marre M, et al. (2003) Angiotensin-I-converting enzyme insertion/deletion polymorphism and high urinary albumin concentration in French Type 2 diabetes patients. Diabet Med 20: 677–682.
16. Palomo-Pinon S, Gutierrez-Rodriguez ME, Diaz-Flores M, Sanchez-Barrera R, Valladares-Salgado A, et al. (2009) DD genotype of angiotensin-converting enzyme in type 2 diabetes mellitus with renal disease in Mexican Mestizos. Nephrology (Carlton) 14: 235–239.
17. Nakajima S, Baba T, Yajima Y (1996) Is ACE gene polymorphism a useful marker for diabetic albuminuria in Japanese NIDDM patients? Diabetes Care 19: 1420–1422.
18. Park HC, Choi SR, Kim BS, Lee TH, Kang BS, et al. (2005) Polymorphism of the ACE Gene in dialysis patients: overexpression of DD genotype in type 2 diabetic end-stage renal failure patients. Yonsei Med J 46: 779–787.

19. Tomino Y, Makita Y, Shike T, Gohda T, Haneda M, et al. (1999) Relationship between polymorphism in the angiotensinogen, angiotensin-converting enzyme or angiotensin II receptor and renal progression in Japanese NIDDM patients. Nephron 82: 139–144.
20. Zhou TB, Qin YH, Su LN, Lei FY, Huang WF, et al. (2011) The association between angiotensin-converting enzyme insertion/deletion gene variant and risk of focal segmental glomerulosclerosis: a systematic review and meta-analysis. J Renin Angiotensin Aldosterone Syst 12: 624–633.
21. Zhou TB, Yin SS, Liang R (2012) A meta-analysis of the association between angiotensin-converting enzyme insertion/deletion gene polymorphism and end-stage renal disease risk in IgA nephropathy patients. J Renin Angiotensin Aldosterone Syst [Epub ahead of print].
22. Yu ZY, Chen LS, Zhang LC, Zhou TB (2012) Meta-analysis of the relationship between ACE I/D gene polymorphism and end-stage renal disease in patients with diabetic nephropathy. Nephrology (Carlton) 17: 480–487.
23. Wells GA, Shea B, O'Connell D, Peterson J, Welch V, et al. (2002) The Newcastle-Ottawa Scale (NOS) for assessing the quality of nonrandomized-studies in meta-analysis. Available: www.ohri.ca/programs/clinical_epidemiology/oxford.asp. Accessed 2013 Aug 23.
24. Viechtbauer W (2010) Conducting meta-analyses in R with the metafor package. J Stat Softw 36: 1–48.
25. Schwarzer G (2012) meta: Meta-Analysis with R.
26. Lee YJ, Tsai JC (2002) ACE gene insertion/deletion polymorphism associated with 1998 World Health Organization definition of metabolic syndrome in Chinese type 2 diabetic patients. Diabetes Care 25: 1002–1008.
27. Shaikh R, Shahid SM, Nawab SN, Mansoor Q, Javaid A, et al. (2012) Distribution of ACE I/D polymorphism in the patients of diabetes and nephropathy in Pakistan. Int J Hum Genet 12: 133–138.
28. Rahimi Z, Vaisi-Raygani A, Rahimi Z, Parsian A (2012) Concomitant presence of endothelial nitric oxide 894T and angiotensin II-converting enzyme D alleles are associated with diabetic nephropathy in a Kurdish population from Western Iran. Nephrology 17: 175–181.
29. El-Baz R, Settin A, Ismaeel A, Khaleel AA, Abbas T, et al. (2012) MTHFR C677T, A1298C and ACE I/D polymorphisms as risk factors for diabetic nephropathy among type 2 diabetic patients. J Renin Angiotensin Aldosterone Syst 13: 472–477.
30. Zsom M, Fulop T, Zsom L, Barath A, Maroti Z, et al. (2011) Genetic polymorphisms and the risk of progressive renal failure in elderly Hungarian patients. Hemodial Int 15: 501–508.
31. Al-Harbi EM, Farid EM, Gumaa KA, Masuadi EM, Singh J (2011) Angiotensin-converting enzyme gene polymorphisms and T2DM in a case-control association study of the Bahraini population. Mol Cell Biochem 350: 119–125.
32. Jung ES, Kim SM, Cha RH, Oh YK, Kim YS, et al. (2011) Impact of polymorphisms of the genes encoding angiotensin II-forming enzymes on the progression of IgA nephropathy. Nephron Clin Pract 118: c122–129.
33. Ali A, Vasudevan R, Ismail P, Thiam Seong CL, Chakravarthi S (2011) Analysis of insertion/deletion polymorphisms of the angiotensin converting enzyme gene in Malaysian end-stage renal disease patients. J Renin Angiotensin Aldosterone Syst [Epub ahead of print].
34. Huang HD, Lin FJ, Li XJ, Wang LR, Jiang GR (2010) Genetic polymorphisms of the renin-angiotensin-aldosterone system in Chinese patients with end-stage renal disease secondary to IgA nephropathy. Chin Med J (Engl) 123: 3238–3242.
35. Jayapalan JJ, Muniandy S, Chan SP (2010) Null association between ACE gene I/D polymorphism and diabetic nephropathy among multiethnic Malaysian subjects. Indian J Hum Genet 16: 78–86.
36. Naresh VV, Reddy AL, Sivaramakrishna G, Sharma PV, Vardhan RV, et al. (2009) Angiotensin converting enzyme gene polymorphism in type II diabetics with nephropathy. Indian J Nephrol 19: 145–148.
37. Ezzidi I, Mtiraoui N, Kacem M, Chaieb M, Mahjoub T, et al. (2009) Identification of specific angiotensin-converting enzyme variants and haplotypes that confer risk and protection against type 2 diabetic nephropathy. Diabetes Metab Res Rev 25: 717–724.
38. Nikzamir A, Esteghamati A, Feghhi M, Nakhjavani M, Rashidi A, et al. (2009) The insertion/deletion polymorphism of the angiotensin-converting enzyme gene is associated with progression, but not development, of albuminuria in Iranian patients with type 2 diabetes. J Renin Angiotensin Aldosterone Syst 10: 109–114.
39. Anbazhagan K, Sampathkumar K, Ramakrishnan M, Gomathi P, Gomathi S, et al. (2009) Analysis of polymorphism in renin angiotensin system and other related genes in South Indian chronic kidney disease patients. Clin Chim Acta 406: 108–112.
40. Ahluwalia TS, Ahuja M, Rai TS, Kohli HS, Bhansali A, et al. (2009) ACE variants interact with the RAS pathway to confer risk and protection against type 2 diabetic nephropathy. DNA Cell Biol 28: 141–150.
41. Mollsten A, Kockum I, Svensson M, Rudberg S, Ugarph-Morawski A, et al. (2008) The effect of polymorphisms in the renin-angiotensin-aldosterone system on diabetic nephropathy risk. J Diabetes Complications 22: 377–383.
42. Eroglu Z, Cetinkalp S, Erdogan M, Kosova B, Karadeniz M, et al. (2008) Association of the angiotensinogen M235T and angiotensin-converting enzyme insertion/deletion gene polymorphisms in Turkish type 2 diabetic patients with and without nephropathy. J Diabetes Complications 22: 186–190.
43. Arfa I, Abid A, Nouira S, Elloumi-Zghal H, Malouche D, et al. (2008) Lack of association between the angiotensin-converting enzyme gene (I/D) polymorphism and diabetic nephropathy in Tunisian type 2 diabetic patients. J Renin Angiotensin Aldosterone Syst 9: 32–36.
44. Tripathi G, Sharma RK, Baburaj VP, Sankhwar SN, Jafar T, et al. (2008) Genetic risk factors for renal failure among north Indian ESRD patients. Clin Biochem 41: 525–531.
45. Movva S, Alluri RV, Komandur S, Vattam K, Eppa K, et al. (2007) Relationship of angiotensin-converting enzyme gene polymorphism with nephropathy associated with Type 2 diabetes mellitus in Asian Indians. J Diabetes Complications 21: 237–241.
46. Uddin M, Azam M, Chowdhury N, Akhteruzzaman S (2007) Angiotensin I-converting enzyme gene polymorphism in type 2 diabetic patients with nephropathy. J Med Sci 7: 682–685.
47. Buraczynska M, Ksiazek P, Drop A, Zaluska W, Spasiewicz D, et al. (2006) Genetic polymorphisms of the renin-angiotensin system in end-stage renal disease. Nephrol Dial Transplant 21: 979–983.
48. So WY, Ma RC, Ozaki R, Tong PC, Ng MC, et al. (2006) Angiotensin-converting enzyme (ACE) inhibition in type 2, diabetic patients– interaction with ACE insertion/deletion polymorphism. Kidney Int 69: 1438–1443.
49. Shestakova MV, Vikulova OK, Gorashko NM, Voronko OE, Babunova NB, et al. (2006) The relationship between genetic and haemodynamic factors in diabetic nephropathy (DN): Case-control study in type 1 diabetes mellitus (T1DM). Diabetes Res Clin Pract 74: S41–S50.
50. Ng DP, Placha G, Choo S, Chia KS, Warram JH, et al. (2006) A disease haplotype for advanced nephropathy in type 2 diabetes at the ACE locus. Diabetes 55: 2660–2663.
51. Prasad P, Tiwari AK, Kumar KM, Ammini AC, Gupta A, et al. (2006) Chronic renal insufficiency among Asian Indians with type 2 diabetes: I. Role of RAAS gene polymorphisms. BMC Med Genet 7: 42.
52. Degirmenci I, Kebapci N, Basaran A, Efe B, Gunes HV, et al. (2005) Frequency of angiotensin-converting enzyme gene polymorphism in Turkish type 2 diabetic patients. Int J Clin Pract 59: 1137–1142.
53. van der Sman-de Beer F, Verhagen C, Rombach SM, Boorsma P, van Manen JG, et al. (2005) ACE I/D polymorphism is associated with mortality in a cohort study of patients starting with dialysis. Kidney Int 68: 2237–2243.
54. Canani LH, Costa LA, Crispim D, Goncalves Dos Santos K, Roisenberg I, et al. (2005) The presence of allele D of angiotensin-converting enzyme polymorphism is associated with diabetic nephropathy in patients with less than 10 years duration of Type 2 diabetes. Diabet Med 22: 1167–1172.
55. Fabris B, Bortoletto M, Candido R, Barbone F, Cattin MR, et al. (2005) Genetic polymorphisms of the renin-angiotensin-aldosterone system and renal insufficiency in essential hypertension. J Hypertens 23: 309–316.
56. Lau YK, Woo KT, Choong HL, Zhao Y, Tan HB, et al. (2004) Renin-angiotensin system gene polymorphisms: its impact on IgAN and its progression to end-stage renal failure among Chinese in Singapore. Nephron Physiol 97: p1–8.
57. Suzuki H, Sakuma Y, Kanesaki Y, Eiro M, Asahi K, et al. (2004) Close relationship of plasminogen activator inhibitor-1 4G/5G polymorphism and progression of IgA nephropathy. Clin Nephrol 62: 173–179.
58. Stratta P, Bermond F, Guarrera S, Canavese C, Carturan S, et al. (2004) Interaction between gene polymorphisms of nitric oxide synthase and renin-angiotensin system in the progression of membranous glomerulonephritis. Nephrol Dial Transplant 19: 587–595.
59. Lochynska K, Ciechanowicz A, Pawlaczyk K, Oko A, Czekalski S (2003) Angiotensin-converting enzyme gene insertion/deletion polymorphism in newly diagnosed primary chronic glomerulonephritis. Adv Clin Exp Med 12: 161–165.
60. Papp F, Friedman AL, Bereczki C, Haszon I, Kiss E, et al. (2003) Renin-angiotensin gene polymorphism in children with uremia and essential hypertension. Pediatr Nephrol 18: 150–154.
61. Aucella F, Margaglione M, Vigilante M, Gatta G, Grandone E, et al. (2003) PAI-1 4G/5G and ACE I/D gene polymorphisms and the occurrence of myocardial infarction in patients on intermittent dialysis. Nephrol Dial Transplant 18: 1142–1146.
62. Okuno S, Utsugi T, Ohno T, Ohyama Y, Uchiyama T, et al. (2003) Angiotensin-converting enzyme gene polymorphism as a potent risk factor for developing microalbuminuria in Japanese patients with type 2 diabetes mellitus: a 9-year follow-up study. J Int Med Res 31: 290–298.
63. Ortiz MA, De Prado A, Donate T, Gallart L, Claramunt H, et al. (2003) Angiotensin-converting enzyme polymorphism gene and evolution of nephropathy to end-stage renal disease. Nephrology (Carlton) 8: 171–176.
64. Wang AY, Chan JC, Wang M, Poon E, Lui SF, et al. (2003) Cardiac hypertrophy and remodeling in relation to ACE and angiotensinogen genes genotypes in Chinese dialysis patients. Kidney Int 63: 1899–1907.
65. Dixit M, Mansur A, Dixit N, Gilman J, Santarina L, et al. (2002) The role of ACE gene polymorphism in rapidity of progression of focal segmental glomerulosclerosis. J Postgrad Med 48: 266–269; discussion 269.
66. Losito A, Kalidas K, Santoni S, Ceccarelli L, Jeffery S (2002) Polymorphism of renin-angiotensin system genes in dialysis patients–association with cerebrovascular disease. Nephrol Dial Transplant 17: 2184–2188.
67. Yoon HJ, Kim H, Kim HL, Lee SG, Zheng SH, et al. (2002) Interdependent effect of angiotensin-converting enzyme and platelet-activating factor acetylhy-

drolase gene polymorphisms on the progression of immunoglobulin A nephropathy. Clin Genet 62: 128–134.
68. Fradin S, Goulet-Salmon B, Chantepie M, Grandhomme F, Morello R, et al. (2002) Relationship between polymorphisms in the renin-angiotensin system and nephropathy in type 2 diabetic patients. Diabetes Metab 28: 27–32.
69. Drouet M, Aupetit C, Denizot Y, Bois M, Bridoux F, et al. (2002) Analysis of three genetic markers in IgA nephropathy patients from a single region. Clin Nephrol 57: 253–260.
70. Nicod J, Frey BM, Frey FJ, Ferrari P (2002) Role of the alpha-adducin genotype on renal disease progression. Kidney Int 61: 1270–1275.
71. Araz M, Yilmaz N, Gungor K, Okan V, Kepekci Y, et al. (2001) Angiotensin-converting enzyme gene polymorphism and microvascular complications in Turkish type 2 diabetic patients. Diabetes Res Clin Pract 54: 95–104.
72. Azar ST, Zalloua PA, Medlej R, Halabi G (2001) The DD genotype of the ACE gene polymorphism is associated with diabetic nephropathy in the type-1 diabetics. Endocr Res 27: 99–108.
73. Lovati E, Richard A, Frey BM, Frey FJ, Ferrari P (2001) Genetic polymorphisms of the renin-angiotensin-aldosterone system in end-stage renal disease. Kidney Int 60: 46–54.
74. Wang JG, Staessen JA, Tizzoni L, Brand E, Birkenhager WH, et al. (2001) Renal function in relation to three candidate genes. Am J Kidney Dis 38: 1158–1168.
75. Taniwaki H, Ishimura E, Matsumoto N, Emoto M, Inaba M, et al. (2001) Relations between ACE gene and ecNOS gene polymorphisms and resistive index in type 2 diabetic patients with nephropathy. Diabetes Care 24: 1653–1660.
76. Viswanathan V, Zhu Y, Bala K, Dunn S, Snehalatha C, et al. (2001) Association between ACE gene polymorphism and diabetic nephropathy in South Indian patients. JOP 2: 83–87.
77. Hadjadj S, Belloum R, Bouhanick B, Gallois Y, Guilloteau G, et al. (2001) Prognostic value of angiotensin-I converting enzyme I/D polymorphism for nephropathy in type 1 diabetes mellitus: a prospective study. J Am Soc Nephrol 12: 541–549.
78. Wu S, Xiang K, Zheng T, Sun D, Weng Q, et al. (2000) Relationship between the renin-angiotensin system genes and diabetic nephropathy in the Chinese. Chin Med J (Engl) 113: 437–441.
79. Hsieh MC, Lin SR, Hsieh TJ, Hsu CH, Chen HC, et al. (2000) Increased frequency of angiotensin-converting enzyme DD genotype in patients with type 2 diabetes in Taiwan. Nephrol Dial Transplant 15: 1008–1013.
80. van Ittersum FJ, de Man AM, Thijssen S, de Knijff P, Slagboom E, et al. (2000) Genetic polymorphisms of the renin-angiotensin system and complications of insulin-dependent diabetes mellitus. Nephrol Dial Transplant 15: 1000–1007.
81. Solini A, Giacchetti G, Sfriso A, Fioretto P, Sardu C, et al. (1999) Polymorphisms of angiotensin-converting enzyme and angiotensinogen genes in type 2 diabetic sibships in relation to albumin excretion rate. Am J Kidney Dis 34: 1002–1009.
82. De Cosmo S, Margaglione M, Tassi V, Garrubba M, Thomas S, et al. (1999) ACE, PAI-1, decorin and Werner helicase genes are not associated with the development of renal disease in European patients with type 1 diabetes. Diabetes Metab Res Rev 15: 247–253.
83. Miura J, Uchigata Y, Yokoyama H, Omori Y, Iwamoto Y (1999) Genetic polymorphism of renin-angiotensin system is not associated with diabetic vascular complications in Japanese subjects with long-term insulin dependent diabetes mellitus. Diabetes Res Clin Pract 45: 41–49.
84. Kuramoto N, Iizuka T, Ito H, Yagui K, Omura M, et al. (1999) Effect of ACE gene on diabetic nephropathy in NIDDM patients with insulin resistance. Am J Kidney Dis 33: 276–281.
85. Huang XH, Rantalaiho V, Wirta O, Pasternack A, Hiltunen TP, et al. (1998) Angiotensin-converting enzyme insertion/deletion polymorphism and diabetic albuminuria in patients with NIDDM followed Up for 9 years. Nephron 80: 17–24.
86. Walder B, Spanaus KS, Weinreich T, Sawicki PT, Widmer U (1998) Genetic heterogeneity in the renin-angiotensin system and the risk of diabetic nephropathy: Association with the angiotensinogen gene, but not with the ACE gene. J Clin Basic Cardiol 1: 55–58.
87. Freire MB, van Dijk DJ, Erman A, Boner G, Warram JH, et al. (1998) DNA polymorphisms in the ACE gene, serum ACE activity and the risk of nephropathy in insulin-dependent diabetes mellitus. Nephrol Dial Transplant 13: 2553–2558.
88. Grzeszczak W, Zychma MJ, Lacka B, Zukowska-Szczechowska E (1998) Angiotensin I-converting enzyme gene polymorphisms: relationship to nephropathy in patients with non-insulin dependent diabetes mellitus. J Am Soc Nephrol 9: 1664–1669.
89. Young RP, Chan JC, Critchley JA, Poon E, Nicholls G, et al. (1998) Angiotensinogen T235 and ACE insertion/deletion polymorphisms associated with albuminuria in Chinese type 2 diabetic patients. Diabetes Care 21: 431–437.
90. Penno G, Chaturvedi N, Talmud PJ, Cotroneo P, Manto A, et al. (1998) Effect of angiotensin-converting enzyme (ACE) gene polymorphism on progression of renal disease and the influence of ACE inhibition in IDDM patients: findings from the EUCLID Randomized Controlled Trial. EURODIAB Controlled Trial of Lisinopril in IDDM. Diabetes 47: 1507–1511.
91. Fernandez-Llama P, Poch E, Oriola J, Botey A, Coll E, et al. (1998) Angiotensin converting enzyme gene I/D polymorphism in essential hypertension and nephroangiosclerosis. Kidney Int 53: 1743–1747.
92. Frost D, Pfohl M, Clemens P, Haring HU, Beischer W (1998) Evaluation of the insertion/deletion ACE gene polymorphism as a risk factor for carotid artery intima-media thickening and hypertension in young type 1 diabetic patients. Diabetes Care 21: 836–840.
93. Pei Y, Scholey J, Thai K, Suzuki M, Cattran D (1997) Association of angiotensinogen gene T235 variant with progression of immunoglobin A nephropathy in Caucasian patients. J Clin Invest 100: 814–820.
94. Marre M, Jeunemaitre X, Gallois Y, Rodier M, Chatellier G, et al. (1997) Contribution of genetic polymorphism in the renin-angiotensin system to the development of renal complications in insulin-dependent diabetes: Genetique de la Nephropathie Diabetique (GENEDIAB) study group. J Clin Invest 99: 1585–1595.
95. Barnas U, Schmidt A, Illievich A, Kiener HP, Rabensteiner D, et al. (1997) Evaluation of risk factors for the development of nephropathy in patients with IDDM: insertion/deletion angiotensin converting enzyme gene polymorphism, hypertension and metabolic control. Diabetologia 40: 327–331.
96. Ringel J, Beige J, Kunz R, Distler A, Sharma AM (1997) Genetic variants of the renin-angiotensin system, diabetic nephropathy and hypertension. Diabetologia 40: 193–199.
97. Schmidt S, Strojek K, Grzeszczak W, Bergis K, Ritz E (1997) Excess of DD homozygotes in haemodialysed patients with type II diabetes. The Diabetic Nephropathy Study Group. Nephrol Dial Transplant 12: 427–429.
98. Kawada N, Moriyama T, Yokoyama K, Yamauchi A, Ando A, et al. (1997) Renin-angiotensin system component gene polymorphisms in Japanese maintenance haemodialysis patients. Nephrology 3: 521–526.
99. Kario K, Kanai N, Nishiuma S, Fujii T, Saito K, et al. (1997) Hypertensive nephropathy and the gene for angiotensin-converting enzyme. Arterioscler Thromb Vasc Biol 17: 252–256.
100. Chowdhury TA, Dronsfield MJ, Kumar S, Gough SL, Gibson SP, et al. (1996) Examination of two genetic polymorphisms within the renin-angiotensin system: no evidence for an association with nephropathy in IDDM. Diabetologia 39: 1108–1114.
101. McLaughlin KJ, Harden PN, Ueda S, Boulton-Jones JM, Connell JM, et al. (1996) The role of genetic polymorphisms of angiotensin-converting enzyme in the progression of renal diseases. Hypertension 28: 912–915.
102. Oh TG, Shin CS, Park KS, Kim SY, Cho BY, et al. (1996) Relationships between angiotensin I converting enzyme gene polymorphism and renal complications in Korean IDDM patients. Korean J Intern Med 11: 133–137.
103. Schmidt A, Kiener HP, Barnas U, Arias I, Illievich A, et al. (1996) Angiotensin-converting enzyme polymorphism in patients with terminal renal failure. J Am Soc Nephrol 7: 314–317.
104. Doi Y, Yoshizumi H, Yoshinari M, Iino K, Yamamoto M, et al. (1996) Association between a polymorphism in the angiotensin-converting enzyme gene and microvascular complications in Japanese patients with NIDDM. Diabetologia 39: 97–102.
105. Ohno T, Kawazu S, Tomono S (1996) Association analyses of the polymorphisms of angiotensin-converting enzyme and angiotensinogen genes with diabetic nephropathy in Japanese non-insulin-dependent diabetics. Metabolism 45: 218–222.
106. Mizuiri S, Hemmi H, Inoue A, Yoshikawa H, Tanegashima M, et al. (1995) Angiotensin-converting enzyme polymorphism and development of diabetic nephropathy in non-insulin-dependent diabetes mellitus. Nephron 70: 455–459.
107. Yorioka T, Suehiro T, Yasuoka N, Hashimoto K, Kawada M (1995) Polymorphism of the angiotensin converting enzyme gene and clinical aspects of IgA nephropathy. Clin Nephrol 44: 80–85.
108. Fujisawa T, Ikegami H, Shen GQ, Yamato E, Takekawa K, et al. (1995) Angiotensin I-converting enzyme gene polymorphism is associated with myocardial infarction, but not with retinopathy or nephropathy, in NIDDM. Diabetes Care 18: 983–985.
109. Panagiotopoulos S, Smith TJ, Aldred GP, Baker EJ, Jacklin CJ, et al. (1995) Angiotensin-converting enzyme (ACE) gene polymorphism in type II diabetic patients with increased albumin excretion rate. J Diabetes Complications 9: 272–276.
110. Tarnow L, Cambien F, Rossing P, Nielsen FS, Hansen BV, et al. (1995) Lack of relationship between an insertion/deletion polymorphism in the angiotensin I-converting enzyme gene and diabetic nephropathy and proliferative retinopathy in IDDM patients. Diabetes 44: 489–494.
111. Schmidt S, Stier E, Hartung R, Stein G, Bahnisch J, et al. (1995) No association of converting enzyme insertion/deletion polymorphism with immunoglobulin A glomerulonephritis. Am J Kidney Dis 26: 727–731.
112. Yoshida H, Mitarai T, Kawamura T, Kitajima T, Miyazaki Y, et al. (1995) Role of the deletion of polymorphism of the angiotensin converting enzyme gene in the progression and therapeutic responsiveness of IgA nephropathy. J Clin Invest 96: 2162–2169.
113. Dudley CR, Keavney B, Stratton IM, Turner RC, Ratcliffe PJ (1995) U.K. Prospective Diabetes Study. XV: Relationship of renin-angiotensin system gene polymorphisms with microalbuminuria in NIDDM. Kidney Int 48: 1907–1911.

114. Harden PN, Geddes C, Rowe PA, McIlroy JH, Boulton-Jones M, et al. (1995) Polymorphisms in angiotensin-converting-enzyme gene and progression of IgA nephropathy. Lancet 345: 1540–1542.
115. Doria A, Warram JH, Krolewski AS (1994) Genetic predisposition to diabetic nephropathy. Evidence for a role of the angiotensin I converting enzyme gene. Diabetes 43: 690–695.
116. Marre M, Bernadet P, Gallois Y, Savagner F, Guyene TT, et al. (1994) Relationships between angiotensin I converting enzyme gene polymorphism, plasma levels, and diabetic retinal and renal complications. Diabetes 43: 384–388.
117. Powrie JK, Watts GF, Ingham JN, Taub NA, Talmud PJ, et al. (1994) Role of glycaemic control in development of microalbuminuria in patients with insulin dependent diabetes. BMJ 309: 1608–1612.
118. Rigat B, Hubert C, Alhenc-Gelas F, Cambien F, Corvol P, et al. (1990) An insertion/deletion polymorphism in the angiotensin I-converting enzyme gene accounting for half the variance of serum enzyme levels. J Clin Invest 86: 1343–1346.
119. Wolf G, Neilson EG (1993) Angiotensin II as a renal growth factor. J Am Soc Nephrol 3: 1531–1540.
120. Ruiz-Ortega M, Lorenzo O, Suzuki Y, Ruperez M, Egido J (2001) Proinflammatory actions of angiotensins. Curr Opin Nephrol Hypertens 10: 321–329.
121. Kobori H, Nangaku M, Navar LG, Nishiyama A (2007) The intrarenal renin-angiotensin system: from physiology to the pathobiology of hypertension and kidney disease. Pharmacol Rev 59: 251–287.
122. Ahmed N (2005) Advanced glycation endproducts–role in pathology of diabetic complications. Diabetes Res Clin Pract 67: 3–21.
123. Biller H, Zissel G, Ruprecht B, Nauck M, Busse Grawitz A, et al. (2006) Genotype-corrected reference values for serum angiotensin-converting enzyme. Eur Respir J 28: 1085–1090.
124. Reckelhoff JF, Zhang H, Granger JP (1998) Testosterone exacerbates hypertension and reduces pressure-natriuresis in male spontaneously hypertensive rats. Hypertension 31: 435–439.
125. Lim YK, Retnam L, Bhagavath B, Sethi SK, bin Ali A, et al. (2002) Gonadal effects on plasma ACE activity in mice. Atherosclerosis 160: 311–316.
126. Ewing JA, Rouse BA (1978) Hirsutism, race and testosterone levels: comparison of East Asians and Euroamericans. Hum Biol 50: 209–215.
127. Setiawan VW, Haiman CA, Stanczyk FZ, Le Marchand L, Henderson BE (2006) Racial/ethnic differences in postmenopausal endogenous hormones: the multiethnic cohort study. Cancer Epidemiol Biomarkers Prev 15: 1849–1855.
128. Ellis L, Nyborg H (1992) Racial/ethnic variations in male testosterone levels: a probable contributor to group differences in health. Steroids 57: 72–75.

5

Predictive Significance of Kidney Myeloid-Related Protein 8 Expression in Patients with Obesity- or Type 2 Diabetes-Associated Kidney Diseases

Takashige Kuwabara[1], Kiyoshi Mori[1,2]*, Masato Kasahara[1,3], Hideki Yokoi[1], Hirotaka Imamaki[1], Akira Ishii[1], Kenichi Koga[1], Akira Sugawara[4], Shinji Yasuno[3], Kenji Ueshima[3], Takashi Morikawa[5], Yoshio Konishi[5], Masahito Imanishi[5], Akira Nishiyama[6], Kazuwa Nakao[1,2], Masashi Mukoyama[1]

1 Department of Medicine and Clinical Science, Kyoto University Graduate School of Medicine, Kyoto, Japan, **2** Medical Innovation Center, Kyoto University Graduate School of Medicine, Kyoto, Japan, **3** Department of EBM Research, Institute for Advancement of Clinical and Translational Science, Kyoto University Hospital, Kyoto, Japan, **4** Department of Nephrology, Osaka Red Cross Hospital, Osaka, Japan, **5** Division of Nephrology and Hypertension, Osaka City General Hospital, Osaka, Japan, **6** Department of Pharmacology, Kagawa University Medical School, Kagawa, Japan

Abstract

Background and Objective: We have reported that toll-like receptor 4 (TLR4) and one of its endogenous ligands, myeloid-related protein 8 (MRP8 or S100A8), play an important role in the progression of diabetic nephropathy in mice. The aim of this study was to evaluate significance of kidney MRP8 expression in patients with obesity- or type 2 diabetes-associated kidney diseases.

Methods: In diabetic, obese or control subjects, MRP8 mRNA and protein expression levels in renal biopsy samples were determined by real-time RT-PCR and immunohistochemistry ($n=28$ and 65, respectively), and their associations with baseline and prognostic parameters were analyzed. Effects of MRP8 upon pro-inflammatory gene expressions were examined using macrophages.

Results: Kidney MRP8 gene and protein expression levels were elevated in obese or diabetic groups compared to control group. Among all subjects, by univariate linear regression analysis, glomerular MRP8-positive cell count and tubulointerstitial MRP8-positive area at baseline were both, respectively, correlated not only with various known risk factors for diabetic nephropathy (such as systolic blood pressure, proteinuria and serum creatinine) but also with extent of glomerulosclerosis and tubulointerstitial fibrosis. Independent factors predicting urinary protein levels a year later were examined by multivariate analysis, and they included glomerular MRP8-positive cell count ($\beta=0.59$, $P<0.001$), proteinuria ($\beta=0.37$, $P=0.002$) and systolic blood pressure ($\beta=0.21$, $P=0.04$) at baseline, after adjustment for known risk factors. MRP8 protein expression was observed in CD68-positive macrophages and atrophic tubules. In cultured mouse macrophages, MRP8 protein induced proinflammatory cytokine expressions and also triggered auto-induction of MRP8 in a TLR4-dependent manner.

Conclusions: Glomerular MRP8 expression appears to be associated with progression of proteinuria in obese or type 2 diabetic patients, possibly by inducing inflammatory changes in macrophages through TLR4 signaling.

Editor: Utpal Sen, University of Louisville, United States of America

Funding: This work was supported in part by Grant-in-Aid for Diabetic Nephropathy and Nephrosclerosis Research from the Ministry of Health, Labour and Welfare of Japan (to KM), research grants from the Japanese Ministry of Education, Culture, Sports, Science and Technology (to TK, KM, and MM), from the Japan Foundation for Applied Enzymology (to TK) and from the Smoking Research Foundation (to MM). The funders had no role in study design, data collection and analysis, decision to publish, or preparation of the manuscript.

* E-mail: keyem@kuhp.kyoto-u.ac.jp

Introduction

Chronic inflammation plays an important role in the pathogenesis of diabetes or obesity and their cardiovascular complications [1]. Involvement of innate immune receptors and the endogenous ligands in the process of chronic inflammation has been implicated. Myeloid-related protein 8 (MRP8, also known as S100A8 or calgranulin A) was originally identified as a cytoplasmic calcium-binding protein in neutrophils and monocytes [2], and has become widely recognized as a potent endogenous ligand for toll-like receptor 4 (TLR4) in various diseases including septic shock, vascular and autoimmune disorders [3,4,5]. We have recently proposed that MRP8/TLR4 signaling plays an important role in hyperlipidemia-induced progression of diabetic nephropathy [6]. Glomerular macrophages and collecting duct cells are major sources of MRP8 in mouse models of diabetic nephropathy [6] and renal fibrosis [7], respectively. Plasma levels of MRP8, which usually forms a heterodimeric complex with a binding partner MRP14 in the bloodstream, are increased in obese subjects [8,9]. However, there have been no reports investigating renal expression of MRP8 in patients with obesity or type 2 diabetes and its association with renal prognosis.

The aim of this study was to determine mRNA and protein expression levels of MRP8 in the kidney of Japanese patients with diabetic nephropathy (DN), obesity-related glomerulopathy (ORG), minimal change nephrotic syndrome (MCNS) or minor glomerular abnormality (MGA), which were all diagnosed by renal biopsy, and to evaluate whether renal MRP8 expression can predict renal outcomes.

Materials and Methods

Ethics statement

The human study was conducted according to the principles expressed in the Declaration of Helsinki, and was approved by the Ethical Committees on Human Research of Kyoto University Graduate School of Medicine and Osaka City General Hospital, respectively. All participants gave written informed consent. The animal study protocol was approved by the Animal Research Committee of Kyoto University Graduate School of Medicine (Permit Number: Med Kyo 13318). All animal surgery was performed under sodium pentobarbital anesthesia, and all efforts were made to minimize suffering.

Study subjects

Proteinuric patients with obesity or type 2 diabetes who underwent renal biopsy were enrolled in this study. Patients with infectious disease, cancer, liver disease or collagen disease were excluded. Proteinuria was defined as urinary protein greater than 0.5 g/g creatinine or urinary albumin greater than 300 mg/g creatinine in at least two consecutive measurements. Obesity was defined as body mass index (BMI) greater than 25.0 (kg/m^2). Type 2 diabetes was diagnosed in accordance with the criteria of the World Health Organization. Biochemical measurements on admission for renal biopsy were used as baseline characteristics for cross-sectional analysis. Estimated glomerular filtration rate (eGFR) was calculated using a simplified prediction equation proposed by the Japanese Society of Nephrology: eGFR (ml/min/1.73 m^2) = 194 × [age (years)]$^{-0.287}$ × [serum creatinine (mg per dl)]$^{-1.094}$ ×0.739 (for females), which is a validated local modification of MDRD [10]. The serum concentrations of creatinine were measured using an enzymatic method.

For immunohistochemistry, 65 Japanese patients who underwent renal biopsy at Department of Medicine and Clinical Science, Kyoto University Hospital between 2000 and 2011 were analyzed. Biopsy-proven diagnoses of all patients during this period are listed in Table S1 in File S1. The subjects examined in this work included DN (n = 19), ORG (n = 10) and non-obese, non-diabetic control subjects who were diagnosed as MGA (n = 19) or MCNS (n = 17). Some cases in these categories were excluded because residual samples available contained less than 10 glomeruli. Definition of DN consisted of (1) more than 5 year duration after the onset of diabetes, (2) existence of micro- or macro-albuminuria, (3) compatible histopathological changes with DN such as glomerular basement membrane thickening, mesangial expansion, nodular sclerosis (Kimmelstiel-Wilson nodules) and/or arteriolar hyalinosis, and (4) exclusion of other causes for renal disorders [11]. ORG was defined morphologically as focal segmental glomerulosclerosis and/or glomerulomegaly in subjects having both obesity and proteinuria, whose definitions were described above [12,13].

For mRNA expression analysis, low quality samples, in which 18S ribosomal RNA (rRNA) levels were lower than the detection sensitivity limit by real-time RT-PCR, were excluded. Subjects enrolled consisted of 22 type 2 diabetic patients who underwent renal biopsy at Osaka City General Hospital between 2000 and 2010, and 6 non-diabetic control subjects, who had biopsy-proven MGA.

Tables 1 and 2 summarize the baseline clinical characteristics of the patients who were examined by immunohistochemical or gene expression analysis, respectively. For light microscopy, the tissue specimens were processed according to standard procedures. Sections were stained with haematoxylin-eosin, periodic acid-Schiff, periodic-acid methenamine silver or Masson trichrome (Fig. S1). The ratios of the number of glomeruli with global sclerosis among that of total glomeruli and the relative areas of tubulointerstitial fibrosis were evaluated independently by two pathologists unaware of diagnosis and clinical data.

Definition of renal outcomes

The following two prognostic indicators were examined by linear regression and logistic regression analyses, respectively: (1) the extent of proteinuria measured at one year post-biopsy, and (2) renal event defined as annual increase in serum creatinine by > 50% from baseline or initiation of chronic dialysis.

Immunohistochemistry

Immunohistochemistry of MRP8 and CD68 was carried out using kidney sections (thickness 4 μm) fixed with 4% buffered paraformaldehyde. After antigen retrieval by citrate buffer, kidney sections were incubated with 10% goat serum, followed by mouse anti-human MRP8 (1:100; BMA biomedicals, Augst, Switzerland) [14] or mouse anti-human CD68 antibodies (1:50; DAKO, Ely, UK), respectively. Primary antibodies were visualized with horseradish peroxidase-conjugated secondary antibody and 3,3-diaminobenzidine tetrahydrochloride (Dako USA, Carpinteria, CA). Nuclei were counterstained with hematoxylin. MRP8-positive cells were counted in more than 10 glomeruli, and MRP8-positive area in tubulointerstitium was measured quantitatively to obtain an average for each subject using MetaMorph 7.5 software (Molecular Devices, Downingtown, PA, USA). Co-localization of CD68- and MRP8-positive cells was evaluated with serial sections. There was neither MRP8 nor CD68 signal in negative controls stained without first antibody (Fig. S2). By preincubation of anti-MRP8 antibody with 20 molar excess of recombinant human MRP8 protein (Life Technologies, Carlsbad, CA, USA) at 4°C overnight, staining was markedly reduced, if not completely, further supporting the specificity of the antibody (Fig. S3).

Evaluation of mRNA expression

Frozen kidney sections were separated into glomeruli and non-glomerulus tissues by laser capture micro-dissection (LM200; Olympus, Tokyo, Japan) as previously described [15]. Total RNA was extracted with RNeasy mini kit (Qiagen, Tokyo, Japan). mRNA expression levels were determined by TaqMan real-time PCR (Applied Biosystems, Foster City, CA, USA) [16,17]. Expression levels of all genes were normalized by 18S rRNA (internal control) levels. See Table S2 in File S1 for primer and probe sequences. Eukaryotic 18S rRNA was detected with Pre-Developed TaqMan Assay Reagents (Applied Biosystems).

Table 1. Baseline clinical characteristics of patients at renal biopsy who were analyzed for MRP8 protein expression by immunohistochemistry.

	Non-obese, non-diabetic control				Between-group differences*
	MGA	MCNS	ORG	DN	
N	19	17	10	19	
Sex (male/female)	10/9	5/12	7/3	14/5	$\chi^2=8.1$, P=0.04
Age (years)	35.5±17.9	36.3±17.4	49.3±16.5	58.3±9.0	P<0.001
Diabetes duration (years)	-	-	-	11.3±6.7	-
BMI (kg/m^2)	19.7±2.1	23.7±3.3	32.0±5.6	24.7±3.5	P<0.001
HbA1c (NGSP, %)	5.6±0.1	5.8±0.2	6.0±0.7	7.1±1.5	P=0.04
Systolic blood pressure (mmHg)	112.2±11.4	113.0±10.2	129.3±10.4	149.4±17.2	P<0.001
Diastolic blood pressure (mmHg)	67.0±6.8	70.2±10.1	82.2±12.7	82.8±10.1	P<0.001
Urinary protein (g/g creatinine)	0.30±0.45	6.83±3.37	1.29±1.24	5.38±4.02	P<0.001
Creatinine (mg/dl)	0.66±0.14	0.68±0.15	0.84±0.23	1.45±0.66	P<0.001
eGFR (ml/min/1.73 m^2)	100.7±24.4	94.0±20.3	75.0±18.9	45.4±19.6	P<0.001
BUN (mg/dl)	13.3±3.7	13.5±6.8	15.6±4.6	23.9±10.3	P<0.001
Total protein (g/dl)	7.0±0.6	4.7±0.8	7.0±0.5	5.8±1.0	P<0.001
Albumin (g/dl)	4.3±0.4	2.2±0.8	4.1±0.6	3.2±0.8	P<0.001
Total cholesterol (mg/dl)	184.7±38.3	442.5±123.2	206.1±27.7	247.3±50.8	P<0.001
Triglyceride (mg/dl)	100.1±84.4	230.8±140.9	124.8±63.7	175.8±75.0	P=0.001
HDL cholesterol (mg/dl)	55.1±82.8	82.8±16.8	53.7±10.8	46.0±10.8	P<0.001
LDL cholesterol (mg/dl)	106.1±30.2	298.2±123.6	127.6±26.0	161.8±47.6	P<0.001
CRP (mg/dl)	0.3±0.9	0.3±0.8	0.3±0.2	0.1±0.2	NS
Global glomerulosclerosis (%)	2.2±4.2	2.5±4.5	22.9±15.9	33.2±17.4	P<0.001
Tubulointerstitial fibrosis (%)	0.6±1.4	0.1±0.5	15.5±9.5	38.6±18.6	P<0.001

MGA: minor glomerular abnormality, MCNS: minimal change nephrotic syndrome, ORG: obesity-related glomerulopathy, DN: diabetic nephropathy, BMI: body mass index, BUN: blood urea nitrogen, CRP: C-reactive protein. Data are means ± SD. *Overall differences between MGA, MCNS, ORG and DN groups were compared by ANOVA.

MRP8 treatment of macrophages

Bone marrow-derived macrophages were generated from wild-type or TLR4 knockout (KO) mice [18] on C57BL/6J genetic background (Oriental BioService, Kyoto, Japan) as described previously [6]. Briefly, following lysis of red blood cells, bone marrow cells were resuspended in medium containing 20% fetal calf serum and 50 ng/ml recombinant human macrophage colony-stimulating factor (Peprotech, Rocky Hill, NJ, USA), and cultured at 37°C in 5% CO_2 atmosphere. On day 7, macrophages were incubated with recombinant mouse MRP8 (Abnova, Taipei, Taiwan) or vehicle for 4 hours. Polymyxin B (25 μg/ml, Nacalai Tesque, Kyoto, Japan) was added to each well to minimize contamination of endotoxin as described previously [3,19]. No endotoxin was detected at any concentration of MRP8 tested here after incubation with 25 μg/ml of polymyxin B by ToxinSensor Chromogenic LAL Endotoxin Assay Kit (GenScript, Piscataway, NJ, USA). Total RNA from cells was extracted with RNeasy Mini Kit, and mRNA expression levels of interleukin-1 beta (IL-1β), tumor necrosis factor alpha (TNFα) and MRP8 were determined by TaqMan real-time RT-PCR. Expression levels of all genes were normalized by rodent GAPDH levels (internal control, Pre-Developed TaqMan Assay Reagents). Primer and Probe sequences for real-time PCR are listed in Table S2 in File S1.

Statistical analysis

Data are expressed as means ± SD, or means ±95% confidence interval (CI) when appropriate. For the comparison among four groups, one-way or two-way ANOVA with Bonferroni' post-hoc analysis was used, and categorical variables were compared using χ^2 test. Student's unpaired t-test was applied for comparison between two groups as appropriate. Spearman's correlation coefficients were estimated to determine associations between two variables. To examine the effects of baseline covariates determining the extent of glomerular or tubulointerstitial MRP8 expression or urinary protein levels one year after biopsy, univariate and multivariate linear regression analyses were performed. Logistic regression analysis was used to analyze explanatory variables predicting the occurrence of renal event. All data were analyzed using StatView 5.0 software (SAS Institute Inc., Cary, NC, USA). P values <0.05 were considered statistically significant.

Results

We compared MRP8 protein expression levels in the kidneys among DN, ORG and non-obese, non-diabetic control (MGA and MCNS) groups. Immunohistochemical analysis revealed that both glomerular MRP8-positive cell count (Fig. 1A) and tubulointerstitial MRP8-positive area (Fig. 1B) in DN were significantly larger than those in other groups including MGA, MCNS and ORG (P<

Table 2. Baseline clinical characteristics of patients at renal biopsy who were analyzed for MRP8 mRNA expression by real-time RT-PCR.

	MGA	DN	Between-group differences*
N	6	22	
Sex (male/female)	0/6	15/7	$\chi^2 = 8.8$, P = 0.003
Age (years)	38.3±10.4	57.0±11.1	P = 0.001
Diabetes duration (years)	-	14.1±6.8	-
RAS blockade (yes/no)	0/0	18/4	-
BMI (kg/m^2)	19.4±2.0	25.0±3.8	P = 0.002
HbA1c (NGSP, %)	-	7.9±2.0	-
Systolic blood pressure (mmHg)	111.2±13.5	157.9±30.1	P = 0.001
Diastolic blood pressure (mmHg)	67.3±9.0	86.8±11.7	P = 0.001
Urinary protein (g/g creatinine)	0.10±0.11	4.87±4.09	P = 0.009
Creatinine (mg/dl)	0.6±0.2	1.1±0.4	P = 0.004
eGFR (ml/min/1.73 m^2)	92.8±26.6	57.8±27.2	P = 0.009
Total protein (g/dl)	7.0±0.4	6.2±0.9	NS
Albumin (g/dl)	4.2±0.4	3.2±0.7	P = 0.002
Total cholesterol (mg/dl)	213.5±57.2	240.1±71.2	NS
Triglyceride (mg/dl)	172.0±161.4	241.0±137.7	NS
HDL cholesterol (mg/dl)	61.3±12.5	52.5±12.0	NS
LDL cholesterol (mg/dl)	117.8±33.6	137.3±59.1	NS

RAS: renin-angiotensin system. Data are means ± SD. *Differences between MGA and DN groups were compared by unpaired t-test.

0.01). ORG subjects also showed a tendency of elevated MRP8 expression compared to MGA and MCNS (Fig. 1A, 1B). Furthermore, glomerular MRP8 mRNA expression levels in DN subjects were significantly higher compared to non-DM control subjects (P<0.01, Fig. 1C). In non-glomerulus tissues, MRP8 mRNA expression levels were much lower than those in glomeruli, both in non-DM and DM groups. Abundant MRP8 protein expression in the tubulointerstitium of DN cases was not clearly reflected into increased mRNA expression, which may be partly caused by deposition of blood-derived proteins in the tubulointerstitium as discussed in the next section. As shown in representative photos (Fig. 1D–G, see Fig. S4 in detail), renal biopsy samples from MGA and MCNS subjects showed few MRP8-positive cells in glomeruli (Fig. 1D, 1E and Fig. S4). In ORG subjects, some MRP8-postive cells appeared in glomeruli and tubulointerstitium (Fig. 1F and Fig. S4). In DN subjects, marked increase of MRP8-expressing cells in glomeruli and significant expansion of MRP8-positive areas in the tubulointerstitium were observed in a focal manner (Fig. 1G and Fig. S4). Of note, MRP8-positive cells were absent in nodular sclerosing lesions of diabetic glomeruli (Fig. S4: DN case 2, 3) as described previously for sclerotic lesions in ANCA-associated glomerulonephritis [20]. Paired immunohistochemistry for CD68 and MRP8 in serial sections suggested that MRP8 signals were, at least in part, observed in macrophages expressing CD68 (Fig. 2), as we reported in a mouse model of diabetic nephropathy [6]. Besides, focally injured atrophic tubular epithelial cells also strongly expressed MRP8, which were surrounded by MRP8(+)-, CD68(+)-positive macrophages (Fig. 2, Fig S4: DN case 3-5). In the cases with nephrotic range proteinuria, MRP8 staining was also observed along brush borders of proximal tubules both in MCNS and DN cases (Fig. S4). Since sample number of mRNA expression was too small for multivariate analysis, the following analyses were performed using data from patients studied by immunohistochemistry.

The associations between kidney MRP8 signals and baseline clinical parameters at the time of renal biopsy were analyzed cross-sectionally (Table 3). By univariate analysis, glomerular and/or tubulointerstitial MRP8 protein expression was significantly correlated to age, systolic and diastolic blood pressures, urinary protein, serum levels of creatinine, BUN and HDL cholesterol, eGFR, and extent of global glomerulosclerosis and tubulointerstitial fibrosis. These parameters were further examined by multivariate analysis after excluding diastolic blood pressure, eGFR and BUN because of collinearity. Percentage of tubulointerstitial fibrosis was independently correlated with glomerular MRP8 signals ($\beta = 0.62$, adjusted P = 0.02) and tubulointerstitial MRP8 signals ($\beta = 0.85$, adjusted P<0.001), respectively. Additionally, tubulointerstitial MRP8 signals were also independently correlated with baseline proteinuria ($\beta = 0.20$, adjusted P = 0.01).

Scattered plot analyses between MRP8 signals in glomeruli or tubulointerstitium and clinical parameters indicated that MCNS group had a distinct distribution pattern from other groups, especially as to urinary protein and serum LDL cholesterol levels (Fig. S5A–D, S6A–D). Exclusion of MCNS group improved correlation between MRP8 signals and urinary protein or serum LDL-cholesterol levels (Fig. S5E–F, S6E–F). Therefore, we carried out sub-analysis excluding MCNS patients, and found that urinary protein was an independent factor correlated with glomerular MRP8 signals by multivariate analysis (Table 4; $\beta = 0.36$, adjusted P = 0.03).

Next, we performed linear regression or logistic regression analyses to identify explanatory factors predicting renal outcomes which were extent of proteinuria a year later and renal event within a year. Since there was a good association between glomerular and tubulointerstitial MRP8 signals (Fig. S7; R = 0.67,

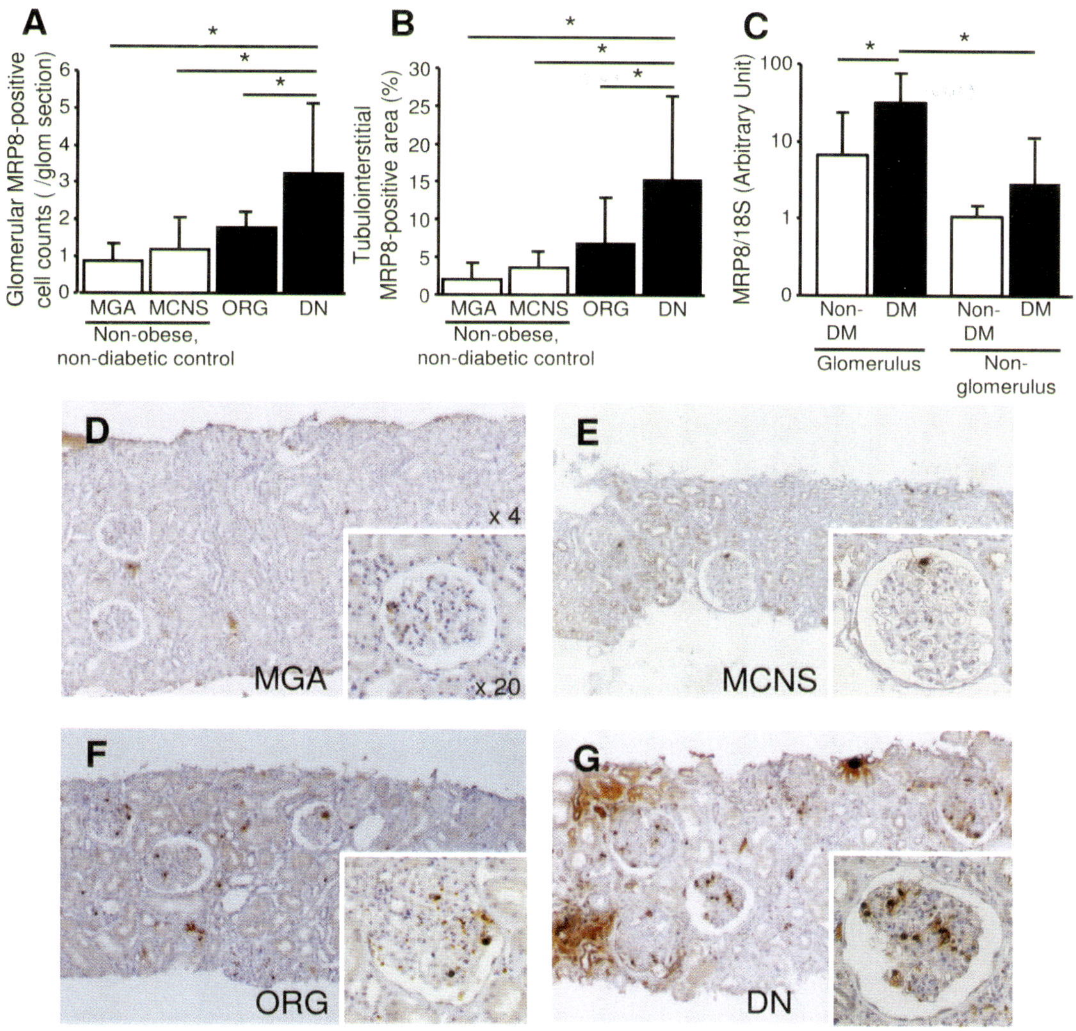

Figure 1. Immunohistochemical and mRNA analyses for MRP8 in kidney biopsy samples. Quantification of glomerular MRP8-positive cell count (A) and tubulointerstitial MRP8-positive area (B). mRNA expression of MRP8 in glomerular and non-glomerular fractions (C). Open bars: non-obese, non-diabetic controls which are MGA or MCNS, closed bars: ORG or DN (A–C). Representative pictures of MGA, MCNS, ORG and DN groups (D–G). MGA: minor glomerular abnormality, MCNS: minimal change nephrotic syndrome, ORG: obesity-related glomerulopathy, DN: diabetic nephropathy. *$P<0.01$.

$P<0.001$), these parameters were alternatively enrolled in further analyses. We evaluated association between baseline parameters and urinary protein at 1 year after renal biopsy by multiple regression analysis. As shown in Table 5, glomerular MRP8 signal ($\beta = 0.59$, adjusted $P<0.001$) was a predictive factor for the extent of proteinuria a year later, as well as baseline systolic blood pressure ($\beta = 0.21$, adjusted $P = 0.04$) and baseline proteinuria ($\beta = 0.37$, adjusted $P = 0.002$) were. These parameters were independent from other known diabetic nephropathy risk factors including renal dysfunction (serum creatinine) and extent of global sclerosis and tubulointerstitial fibrosis [11,21–24]. On the other hand, tubulointerstitial MRP8 signal ($\beta = 0.34$, adjusted $P = 0.09$) was not an independent predictive factor for urinary protein levels a year later. Renal events occurred in 7 patients (6 in DN and 1 in ORG cases) within a year after renal biopsy. By univariate analysis, not only extent of glomerulosclerosis and tubulointerstitial fibrosis, and glomerular and tubulointerstitial MRP8 signals, but also blood pressures, renal dysfunction and urinary protein levels at baseline were significant predictive factors for the occurrence of renal events. However, by multivariate analysis, there covariates were cancelled out by each other (Table S3 in File S1), likely due to high correlations among these parameters.

Finally, we examined the potency of MRP8 as an endogenous ligand for TLR4 using cultured macrophages. In bone marrow-derived macrophages from wild-type mice, MRP8 protein induced upregulation of proinflammatory cytokine genes such as IL-1β and TNFα and also triggered auto-induction of MRP8, in a dose-dependent manner between 10–1000 ng/ml. These effects of MRP8 were suppressed approximately by two-thirds in macrophages obtained from TLR4 KO mice ($P<0.01$) (Fig. 3).

Discussion

The present study has demonstrated that MRP8 is abundantly expressed in glomeruli and tubulointerstitium of patients with DN as compared to ORG and non-obese, non-diabetic control (MGA and MCNS). Furthermore, in ORG subjects, MRP8 expression

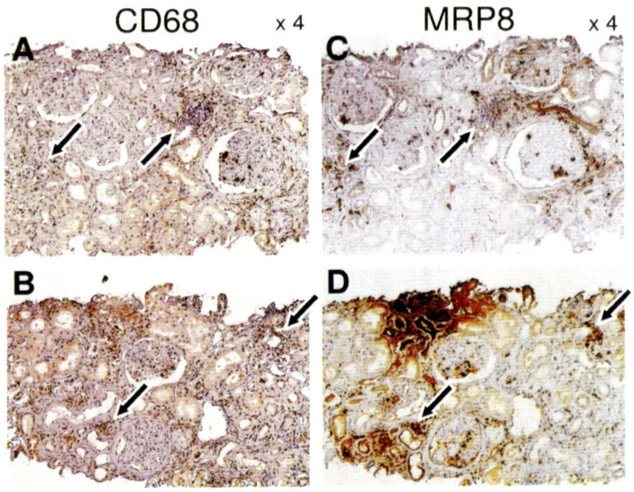

Figure 2. Localization of CD68 and MRP8 protein expression in serial sections of diabetic nephropathy cases. Expression of CD68 (A, B) and MRP8 expression (C, D) in paired renal specimens (A and C, or B and D). Arrows indicate colocalization of CD68 and MRP8 signals.

levels tended to be higher than MGA or MCNS subjects. In baseline cross-sectional investigation including all subjects, by univariate linear regression analysis, glomerular MRP8-positive cell count and tubulointerstitial MRP8-positive area were both, respectively, correlated not only with various known risk factors for diabetic nephropathy (such as systolic blood pressure, proteinuria and serum creatinine) but also with extent of glomerulosclerosis and tubulointerstitial fibrosis. By multivariate analysis, tubulointerstitial MRP8-positive area was significantly correlated with proteinuria and tubulointerstitial fibrosis. Glomerular MRP8-positive cell count was significantly correlated with tubulointerstitial fibrosis in the primary analysis, and with proteinuria in a sub-analysis excluding MCNS group. Immunohistochemistry indicated that MRP8 was expressed, at least partly, by CD68(+)-expressing macrophages and atrophic tubules. These findings raise a possibility that kidney MRP8 signals in glomeruli or tubulointerstitium may serve as novel markers of diabetic nephropathy.

In prognostic study, multivariate analysis revealed that urinary protein levels at a year after renal biopsy were independently associated with glomerular MRP8-positive cell count, urinary protein and systolic blood pressure at baseline. Of note, glomerular MRP8 expression showed the strongest correlation with urinary protein a year later ($\beta = 0.87$), even stronger than baseline urinary protein ($\beta = 0.78$), by univariate analysis. It is partly because glomerular MRP8 expression is not largely elevated in 'benign' forms of proteinuria such as ones observed in MCNS patients, whose levels of proteinuria are extremely high at diagnosis by renal biopsy but are usually resolved within a year after initiation of immunosuppressive therapy. These findings suggest that glomerular MRP8 expression may possess a unique predictive nature as a disease marker, which cannot be substituted by baseline proteinuria or routine pathological analysis evaluating

Table 3. Relationship between baseline clinical parameters and MRP8 signals.

	Glomerular MRP8-positive cell count				Tubulointerstitial MRP8-positive area			
	Univariate		Multivariate*		Univariate		Multivariate#	
	β	P	β	P	β	P	β	P
Sex (male)	0.21	0.09			0.16	0.20		
Age (y)	0.37	0.002	0.02	0.87	0.39	0.001	0.03	0.74
Diabetes duration (y)	0.28	0.14			0.33	0.08		
BMI (kg/m^2)	0.14	0.27			0.09	0.48		
HbA1c (NGSP, %)	0.11	0.52			0.04	0.82		
Systolic BP (mmHg)	0.62	<0.001	0.18	0.29	0.64	<0.001	−0.12	0.37
Diastolic BP (mmHg)	0.43	<0.001			0.42	<0.001		
Urinary protein (g/gCr)	0.37	0.003	0.18	0.07	0.43	<0.001	0.20	0.01
Creatinine (mg/dl)	0.60	<0.001	0.01	0.10	0.75	<0.001	0.20	0.08
eGFR (ml/min/1.73 m^2)	−0.49	<0.001			−0.70	<0.001		
BUN (mg/dl)	0.56	<0.001			0.71	<0.001		
Total protein (g/dl)	−0.16	0.21			−0.13	0.30		
Albumin (g/dl)	−0.22	0.09			−0.21	0.09		
T-chol (mg/dl)	−0.06	0.66			−0.04	0.76		
Triglyceride (mg/dl)	0.02	0.84			0.11	0.38		
HDL-chol (mg/dl)	−0.24	0.06			−0.28	0.03	−0.03	0.73
LDL-chol (mg/dl)	0.00	0.98			0.00	0.99		
CRP (mg/dl)	0.03	0.79			0.12	0.34		
Global GS (%)	0.52	<0.001	−0.17	0.40	0.61	<0.001	−0.27	0.07
TI fibrosis (%)	0.68	<0.001	0.62	0.02	0.80	<0.001	0.85	<0.001

Coefficient of determination (R^2) calculated with explanatory parameters enrolled in multiple regression analysis was 0.52* and 0.74#, respectively. y, years; BP, blood pressure; gCr, g creatinine; T-chol, total cholesterol; HDL-chol, HDL cholesterol; LDL-chol, LDL cholesterol; GS, glomerulosclerosis; TI, tubulointerstitial.

Table 4. Sub-analysis of relationship between baseline clinical parameters and MRP8 signals, after exclusion of MCNS group.

	Glomerular MRP8(+) cell count				Tubulointerstitial MRP8(+) area			
	Univariate		Multivariate*		Univariate		Multivariate#	
	β	P	β	P	β	P	β	P
Systolic BP (mmHg)	0.64	<0.001	0.16	0.38	0.63	<0.001	−0.16	0.23
Urinary protein (g/gCr)	0.70	<0.001	0.36	0.03	0.75	<0.001	0.47	<0.001
Creatinine (mg/dl)	0.62	<0.001	0.05	0.80	0.75	<0.001	0.24	0.09
Total protein (g/dl)	−0.51	<0.001	0.03	0.84	−0.49	<0.001	0.12	0.25
Triglyceride (mg/dl)	0.31	0.003			0.37	0.01		
HDL-chol (mg/dl)	−0.16	0.27			−0.20	0.18		
LDL-chol (mg/dl)	0.60	<0.001	0.13	0.35	0.52	0.001	−0.10	0.35
Global GS (%)	0.49	<0.001	−0.20	0.29	0.59	<0.001	−0.17	0.23
TI fibrosis (%)	0.68	<0.001	0.38	0.18	0.80	<0.001	0.70	0.002

R^2 was 0.60* and 0.77#, respectively. BP, blood pressure; gCr, g creatinine; HDL-chol, HDL cholesterol; LDL-chol, LDL cholesterol; GS, glomerulosclerosis; TI, tubulointerstitial.

Table 5. Multiple regression analysis for identification of factors predicting urinary protein levels 1 year after renal biopsy.

	Urinary protein 1-year after renal biopsy					
	Univariate		Multivariate			
			Model 1*		Model 2#	
	β	P	β	P	β	P
Sex (male)	−0.14	0.50				
Age (y)	−0.01	0.95				
Diabetes duration (y)	0.24	0.22				
BMI (kg/m$^{2)}$	−0.33	0.10				
HbA1c (NGSP, %)	0.08	0.70				
Systolic BP (mmHg)	0.43	0.03	0.21	0.04	0.30	0.10
Diastolic BP (mmHg)	0.07	0.73				
Urinary protein (g/gCr)	0.78	<0.001	0.37	0.002	0.55	0.002
Creatinine (mg/dl)	0.44	0.02				
eGFR (ml/min/1.73 m^2)	−0.56	0.003	−0.31	0.76	0.18	0.45
BUN (mg/dl)	0.46	0.02				
Total protein (g/dl)	−0.54	0.004				
Albumin (g/dl)	−0.69	<0.001				
T-chol (mg/dl)	0.66	<0.001				
Triglyceride (mg/dl)	0.18	0.38				
HDL-chol (mg/dl)	−0.02	0.91				
LDL-chol (mg/dl)	0.62	<0.001				
CRP (mg/dl)	−0.11	0.57				
Global glomerulosclerosis (%)	−0.05	0.79	−0.17	0.11	−0.31	0.06
Tubulointerstitial fibrosis (%)	0.43	0.02	−0.02	0.91	0.10	0.67
Glomerular MRP8(+) cell count	0.87	<0.001	0.59	<0.001		
Tubulointerstitial MRP8(+) area (%)	0.67	0.001			0.34	0.09

R^2 was 0.91* and 0.75#, respectively. y, years; BP, blood pressure; gCr, g creatinine; T-chol, total cholesterol; HDL-chol, HDL cholesterol; LDL-chol, LDL cholesterol.

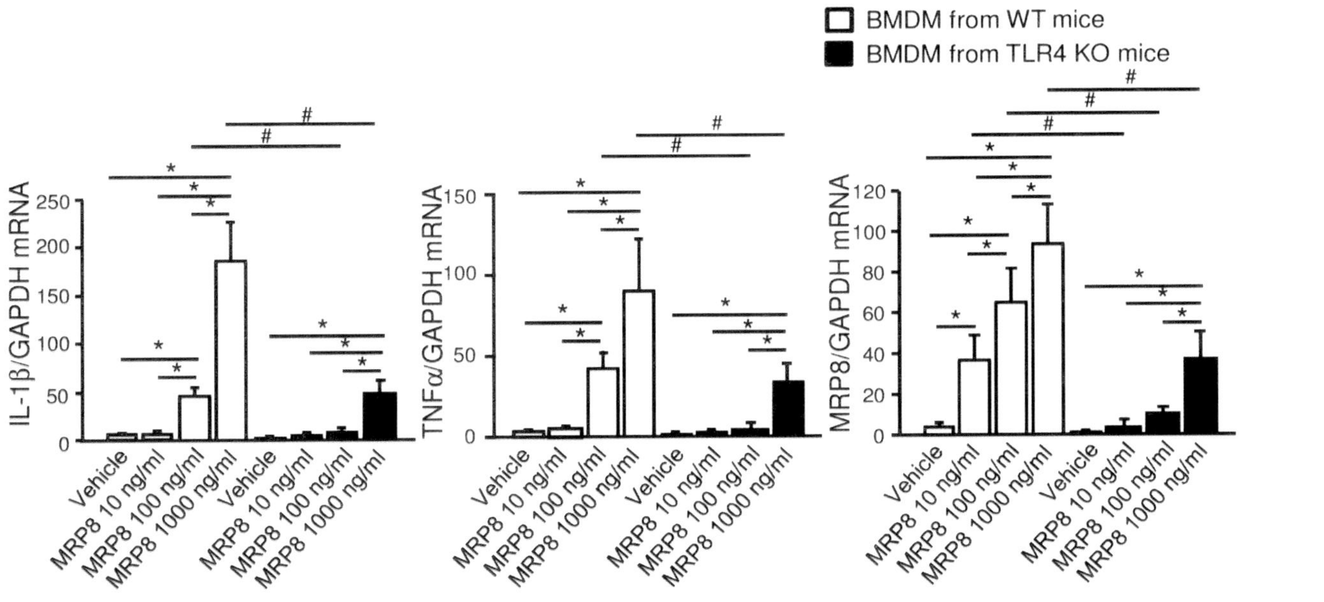

Figure 3. Effects of MRP8 upon bone marrow-derived macrophages. Bone marrow-derived macrophages (BMDM) were stimulated with recombinant mouse MRP8 for 4 hours. Error bars indicate 95% CI and statistical analyses were performed with log-transformed values. Two-way ANOVA revealed significant effects of genotypes, MRP8 concentrations and their interactions for expression of all 3 genes ($P<0.001$ for all comparisons). $n=4$. WT, wild-type; KO, knockout; IL-1β, interleukin 1 beta; TNFα, tumor necrosis factor alpha. *$P<0.01$ among different concentrations, $^{\#}P<0.01$ among genotypes.

global glomerulosclerosis and tubulointerstitial fibrosis. Moreover, we speculate that glomerular MRP8 expression is not a simple marker or bystander but an active player in glomerular injury as discussed below.

In another attempt of longitudinal study, logistic regression analysis failed to find out any independent predictors for the occurrence of renal event within a year. We speculate that this is partly because tubulointerstitial MRP8 expression and tubulointerstitial fibrosis were two potent predictors for renal event in univariate analysis but their significances were canceled by each other in multivariate analysis. These two parameters showed strong correlation ($R=0.68$, $P<0.001$) (Fig. S8), suggesting that these two parameters might be equivalent to predict renal event. Indeed, interstitial MRP8 expression showed quite similar pattern to interstitial fibrosis evaluated by Masson trichrome staining. Quantity of interstitial MRP8 largely depends on the positive signals in atrophic tubules rather than those in macrophages, whose feature differs from that of glomerular MRP8 in punctate distribution. Furthermore, small sample size, short observation period and few subjects who developed renal event might have reduced the detection power. Since MRP8 expression in tubular epithelial cells plays a causative role in the progression of tubulointerstitial inflammation in a mouse model of renal fibrosis [7], further analysis will be needed to clarify the role of tubulointerstitial MRP8 in DN.

In accordance with our previous study [6], MRP8 mRNA was upregulated predominantly in the glomerular fraction of human DN subjects as compared to control subjects with MGA. On the other hand, MRP8 protein expression was observed not only in the glomerulus but also in the tubulointerstitium. In this regard, it should be noted that there were two distinct patterns of MRP8 staining in the tubulointerstitium of DN. One was intense and focal staining in severely atrophic tubules. The other was mild staining distributed along the brush border of proximal tubules, which was also found in ORG and MCNS. The latter signals likely represent MRP8 protein derived from the blood and reabsorbed by proximal tubules, which should not be accompanied by increased MRP8 mRNA expression. Concerning proteins other than MRP8, we and others have recently reported similar phenomena of immunoreactive protein detection in the proximal tubules caused by reabsorption but not by renal synthesis [25,26]. On the other hand, since a little MRP8 staining remained in antibody absorption test, especially in glomerular exudative lesions and severely-scarred, fibrotic lesions around atrophic tubules, presence of non-specific signals cannot be completely negated (Fig. S3).

Glomerular MRP8 signals mainly showed punctuate pattern in DN subjects (Fig. 1, Fig. S4). Since both of CD68 and MRP8 were detected by mouse monoclonal antibodies, localization of these molecules were evaluated by serial sections, not by double-immunostaining. Staining patterns of MRP8 were compatible with those in other inflammatory renal disorders including IgA nephritis [27], membrano-proliferative glomerulonephritis [14], and ANCA-related glomerulonephritis [20], in which macrophages were suggested as a major source of MRP8, as we reported in a rodent model [6]. In addition, neutrophils could be considered as another source of MRP8 affecting vascular complications [28]. Currently, we are investigating the molecular mechanism why MRP8 is predominantly upregulated in myeloid-lineage cells infiltrating glomeruli. In vitro study revealed that MRP8 induced inflammatory cytokine expression and also potentiated expression of MRP8 itself in macrophages in a TLR4-dependent manner. Additionally, MRP8-positive cells were absent in nodular sclerosing lesion, suggesting that glomerular MRP8 might reflect on-going glomerular damage [20]. Importantly, a largest-scale human study reported that MRP8 gene expression in blood mononuclear cells of type 1 diabetic patients is significantly elevated in subjects with diabetic complications including nephropathy [29].

Since inhibition of renin-angiotensin system (RAS) is an important determinant of renal outcomes, we examined the effects of RAS blockade on kidney MRP8 expression. We found no significant difference in kidney MRP8 mRNA expression between DN patients treated with or without RAS blockade (Fig. S9), probably because cases treated with RAS blockade tended to have more severe hypertension and proteinuria than cases without RAS blockade.

In obese humans and mice, increased plasma MRP8/14 complex may reflect a degree of obesity and originate from adipocytes as well as leukocytes [8,9]. Our ORG cases had mild staining of MRP8 in proximal tubules, suggesting increased plasma levels of MRP8. In contrast, there was no significant correlation between tubulointerstitial MRP8 expression and body mass index (Fig. S6G). Therefore, local MRP8 expression in the kidney may serve better as a marker for renal injury rather than for obesity [8,9].

Our study has several limitations. Sample number of each group studied was small. Non-identical subjects were enrolled in the mRNA and immunohistochemical analyses. Since we only analyzed patients who underwent renal biopsy, the composition of patients investigated here may not reflect those in general type 2 diabetic patients or in general chronic kidney disease subjects. Although age was not retained as an independent factor associated with MRP8 signals in our data (Table 3), it is known that aging associates chronic inflammation [30]. The effects of age cannot be completely neglected. Although most MRP8 signals were lost in antibody absorption test, there were some positive signals remaining, which might be caused by a non-specific binding of the first antibody. As discussed above, investigation of renal MRP8 expression by renal biopsy helps us understand the pathophysiology and prognosis of chronic kidney diseases, especially associated with obesity and diabetes, but has a disadvantage for routine and repeated use in out-patient clinics.

In summary, the present study suggests that expression of MRP8 in the kidney reflects the current pathological status and also predicts renal outcomes in patients with obesity or type 2 diabetes. Further investigations studying urinary MRP8 levels among obese or diabetic patients in large scale may be warranted.

Supporting Information

Figure S1 Representative photos showing renal biopsy sections of a DN patient stained with (A) periodic acid-Schiff, (B) periodic-acid methenamine silver or (C) Masson trichrome. The ratio of the number of glomeruli with global sclerosis (arrows) among that of total glomeruli and the relative area of tubulointerstitial fibrosis were 33% and 65%, respectively, in this patient.

Figure S2 Immunohistochemistry for MRP8 and CD68 proteins in DN patients. Photos in the right column show negative control experiments without 1st antibody.

Figure S3 Antibody absorption test for MRP8 staining. PBS: phosphate buffered saline, rhMRP8: recombinant human MRP8.

Figure S4 Representative photos of MRP8 expression in MGA, MCNS, ORG and DN groups.

Figure S5 Correlation between glomerular MRP8-positive cell count and clinical parameters. The log-transformed values of MRP8 signals were used. The correlations were analyzed using all of 4 groups (A–D, G) or 3 groups excluding MCNS group (E, F). Open circles: minor glomerular abnormality (MGA), closed circles: minimal change nephrotic syndrome (MCNS), open triangles: obesity-related glomerulopathy (ORG), closed triangles: diabetic nephropathy (DN).

Figure S6 Correlation between tubulointerstitial MRP8-positive area and clinical parameters. The log-transformed values of MRP8 signals were used. These correlations were analyzed using all of the 4 groups (A–D, G) or 3 groups excluding MCNS group (E, F).

Figure S7 Correlation between glomerular and tubulointerstitial MRP8 expression. The log-transformed values of MRP8 signals were used.

Figure S8 Correlation between tubulointerstitial MRP8-positive area and tubulointerstitial fibrosis. The log-transformed values of MRP8 signals were used.

Figure S9 Renal mRNA expression of MRP8 in DN patients with or without renin-angiotensin blockade. N.S.: not significant. n = 15 (Yes), 6 (No). Among 22 DN cases, information about medication was not available in one patient.

File S1 Supporting Tables. Table S1, Pathological diagnoses of all cases who underwent renal biopsy at Department of Medicine and Clinical Science, Kyoto University Hospital between 2000 and 2011. Table S2, Primer and probe sequences for TaqMan real-time RT-PCR. Table S3, Logistic regression analysis for the occurrence of renal event within a year.

Acknowledgments

We gratefully acknowledge S. Tanaka for statistical advice, Y. Ogawa, N. Igarashi and C. Kimura for technical assistance, and A. Yamamoto and S Ogino for secretary assistance.

Author Contributions

Conceived and designed the experiments: TK KM MK HY MI AN KN MM. Performed the experiments: TK HI AI KK TM YK MI AN. Analyzed the data: TK KM MK HY AS SY KU KN MM. Contributed reagents/materials/analysis tools: TK KM. Wrote the paper: TK KM MM.

References

1. Donath MY, Shoelson SE (2011) Type 2 diabetes as an inflammatory disease. Nat Rev Immunol 11: 98–107.
2. Odink K, Cerletti N, Bruggen J, Clerc RG, Tarcsay L, et al. (1987) Two calcium-binding proteins in infiltrate macrophages of rheumatoid arthritis. Nature 330: 80–82.
3. Vogl T, Tenbrock K, Ludwig S, Leukert N, Ehrhardt C, et al. (2007) Mrp8 and Mrp14 are endogenous activators of Toll-like receptor 4, promoting lethal, endotoxin-induced shock. Nat Med 13: 1042–1049.
4. Croce K, Gao H, Wang Y, Mooroka T, Sakuma M, et al. (2009) Myeloid-related protein-8/14 is critical for the biological response to vascular injury. Circulation 120: 427–436.
5. Loser K, Vogl T, Voskort M, Lucken A, Kupas V, et al. (2010) The Toll-like receptor 4 ligands Mrp8 and Mrp14 are crucial in the development of autoreactive CD8+ T cells. Nat Med 16: 713–717.
6. Kuwabara T, Mori K, Mukoyama M, Kasahara M, Yokoi H, et al. (2012) Exacerbation of diabetic nephropathy by hyperlipidaemia is mediated by Toll-like receptor 4 in mice. Diabetologia 55: 2256–2266.

7. Fujiu K, Manabe I, Nagai R (2011) Renal collecting duct epithelial cells regulate inflammation in tubulointerstitial damage in mice. J Clin Invest 121: 3425–3441.
8. Sekimoto R, Kishida K, Nakatsuji H, Nakagawa T, Funahashi T, et al. (2012) High circulating levels of S100A8/A9 complex (calprotectin) in male Japanese with abdominal adiposity and dysregulated expression of S100A8 and S100A9 in adipose tissues of obese mice. Biochem Biophys Res Commun 419: 782–789.
9. Mortensen OH, Nielsen AR, Erikstrup C, Plomgaard P, Fischer CP, et al. (2009) Calprotectin—a novel marker of obesity. PLoS One 4: e7419.
10. Matsuo S, Imai E, Horio M, Yasuda Y, Tomita K, et al. (2009) Revised equations for estimated GFR from serum creatinine in Japan. Am J Kidney Dis 53: 982–992.
11. Gross JL, de Azevedo MJ, Silveiro SP, Canani LH, Caramori ML, et al. (2005) Diabetic nephropathy: diagnosis, prevention, and treatment. Diabetes Care 28: 164–176.
12. Kambham N, Markowitz GS, Valeri AM, Lin J, D'Agati VD (2001) Obesity-related glomerulopathy: an emerging epidemic. Kidney Int 59: 1498–1509.
13. Praga M, Morales E (2006) Obesity, proteinuria and progression of renal failure. Curr Opin Nephrol Hypertens 15: 481–486.
14. Kawasaki Y, Hosoya M, Takahashi A, Isome M, Tanji M, et al. (2005) Myeloid-related protein 8 expression on macrophages is a useful prognostic marker for renal dysfunction in children with MPGN type 1. Am J Kidney Dis 45: 510–518.
15. Nishiyama A, Konishi Y, Ohashi N, Morikawa T, Urushihara M, et al. (2011) Urinary angiotensinogen reflects the activity of intrarenal renin-angiotensin system in patients with IgA nephropathy. Nephrol Dial Transplant 26: 170–177.
16. Ogawa Y, Mukoyama M, Yokoi H, Kasahara M, Mori K, et al. (2012) Natriuretic peptide receptor guanylyl cyclase-A protects podocytes from aldosterone-induced glomerular injury. J Am Soc Nephrol 23: 1198–1209.
17. Yokoi H, Mukoyama M, Mori K, Kasahara M, Suganami T, et al. (2008) Overexpression of connective tissue growth factor in podocytes worsens diabetic nephropathy in mice. Kidney Int 73: 446–455.
18. Hoshino K, Takeuchi O, Kawai T, Sanjo H, Ogawa T, et al. (1999) Cutting edge: Toll-like receptor 4 (TLR4)-deficient mice are hyporesponsive to lipopolysaccharide: evidence for TLR4 as the Lps gene product. J Immunol 162: 3749–3752.
19. Suganami T, Tanimoto-Koyama K, Nishida J, Itoh M, Yuan X, et al. (2007) Role of the Toll-like receptor 4/NF-kappaB pathway in saturated fatty acid-induced inflammatory changes in the interaction between adipocytes and macrophages. Arterioscler Thromb Vasc Biol 27: 84–91.
20. Pepper RJ, Hamour S, Chavele KM, Todd SK, Rasmussen N, et al. (2013) Leukocyte and serum S100A8/S100A9 expression reflects disease activity in ANCA-associated vasculitis and glomerulonephritis. Kidney Int 83: 1150–1158.
21. Ravid M, Brosh D, Ravid-Safran D, Levy Z, Rachmani R (1998) Main risk factors for nephropathy in type 2 diabetes mellitus are plasma cholesterol levels, mean blood pressure, and hyperglycemia. Arch Intern Med 158: 998–1004.
22. Adler AI, Stratton IM, Neil HA, Yudkin JS, Matthews DR, et al. (2000) Association of systolic blood pressure with macrovascular and microvascular complications of type 2 diabetes (UKPDS 36): prospective observational study. Bmj 321: 412–419.
23. Ruggenenti P, Remuzzi G (1998) Nephropathy of type-2 diabetes mellitus. J Am Soc Nephrol 9: 2157–2169.
24. Taft JL, Nolan CJ, Yeung SP, Hewitson TD, Martin FI (1994) Clinical and histological correlations of decline in renal function in diabetic patients with proteinuria. Diabetes 43: 1046–1051.
25. Matsusaka T, Niimura F, Shimizu A, Pastan I, Saito A, et al. (2012) Liver angiotensinogen is the primary source of renal angiotensin II. J Am Soc Nephrol 23: 1181–1189.
26. Kuwabara T, Mori K, Mukoyama M, Kasahara M, Yokoi H, et al. (2009) Urinary neutrophil gelatinase-associated lipocalin levels reflect damage to glomeruli, proximal tubules, and distal nephrons. Kidney Int 75: 285–294.
27. Kawasaki Y, Suyama K, Go H, Imamura T, Ushijima Y, et al. (2009) Accumulation of macrophages expressing myeloid-related protein 8 associated with the progression of sclerotic changes in children with IgA nephropathy. Tohoku J Exp Med 218: 49–55.
28. Nagareddy PR, Murphy AJ, Stirzaker RA, Hu Y, Yu S, et al. (2013) Hyperglycemia promotes myelopoiesis and impairs the resolution of atherosclerosis. Cell Metab 17: 695–708.
29. Jin Y, Sharma A, Carey C, Hopkins D, Wang X, et al. (2013) The Expression of Inflammatory Genes Is Upregulated in Peripheral Blood of Patients with Type 1 Diabetes. Diabetes Care.
30. Longo VD, Finch CE (2003) Evolutionary medicine: from dwarf model systems to healthy centenarians? Science 299: 1342–1346.

Elevated Soluble VEGF Receptor sFlt-1 Correlates with Endothelial Injury in IgA Nephropathy

Ya-Ling Zhai[1,2,3,4], Li Zhu[1,2,3,4]*, Su-Fang Shi[1,2,3,4], Li-Jun Liu[1,2,3,4], Ji-Cheng Lv[1,2,3,4], Hong Zhang[1,2,3,4]

1 Renal Division, Department of Medicine, Peking University First Hospital, Beijing, China, **2** Peking University Institute of Nephrology, Beijing, China, **3** Key Laboratory of Renal Disease, Ministry of Health of China, Beijing, China, **4** Key Laboratory of Chronic Kidney Disease Prevention and Treatment (Peking University), Ministry of Education, Beijing, China

Abstract

Background: Endothelial injury, which may present clinically as hypertension, proteinuria and increased von Willebrand Factor (vWF) level, is a common manifestation in IgA nephropathy (IgAN). However, causal factors for endothelial injury in IgAN are not completely understood. An imbalance of vascular endothelial growth factor/Soluble fms-like tyrosine kinase-1 (VEGF/sFlt-1) has been observed in many diseases with endothelial dysfunction, including pre-eclampsia and diabetic retinopathy, but whether it contributes to endothelial injury in IgAN requires further exploration.

Methods: Initially, 96 IgAN patients and 22 healthy volunteers were enrolled as a discovery cohort. VEGF/sFlt-1, sFlt-1 and VEGF levels were compared between patients with IgAN and healthy volunteers to explore the underlying factors that contribute to endothelial injury in IgAN. The identified contributor (sFlt-1) was further confirmed in a replication cohort, which included 109 IgAN patients and 30 healthy volunteers. Correlations of sFlt-1 with hypertension, proteinuria, Oxford-E score and plasma vWF were further evaluated in the combined 205 patients with IgAN.

Results: VEGF/sFlt-1 levels were significantly lower in IgAN patients than healthy volunteers (0.33 ± 0.27 *vs.* 0.43 ± 0.22, $p=0.02$) in the discovery cohort. Within the ratio, plasma sFlt-1 levels were significantly elevated (101.18 ± 25.19 *vs.* 79.73 ± 18.85 pg/ml, $p<0.001$), but plasma VEGF levels showed no significant differences. Elevated sFlt-1 levels in the replication cohort were confirmed in IgAN patients (93.40 ± 39.78 *vs.* 71.92 ± 15.78 pg/ml, $p<0.001$). Plasma sFlt-1 levels in IgAN patients correlated with proteinuria (severe (>3.5 g/d) *vs.* moderate (1–3.5 g/d) *vs.* mild (<1 g/d) proteinuria: 115.95 ± 39.09 *vs.* 99.89 ± 28.55 *vs.* 83.24 ± 33.92 pg/ml; severe *vs.* mild: $p<0.001$, moderate *vs.* mild $p=0.001$, severe *vs.* moderate: $p=0.014$), hypertension (with *vs.* without hypertension: 107.87 ± 31.94 *vs.* 87.32 ± 32.76 pg/ml, $p=0.015$) and vWF levels ($r=0.161$, $p=0.021$).

Conclusions: The present study found elevated sFlt-1 in IgAN patients and further identified its correlation with proteinuria, hypertension and vWF levels. These results suggested that elevated sFlt-1 contributes to endothelial injury in IgAN.

Editor: Maria Pia Rastaldi, Fondazione IRCCS Ospedale Maggiore Policlinico & Fondazione D'Amico per la Ricerca sulle Malattie Renali, Italy

Funding: This work was supported by the National Natural Science Foundation for Innovative Research Groups of China (Grant No. 81021004) and by the National Natural Science Foundation for Youths of China (Grants No. 81000297 and 81200515). The funders had no role in study design, data collection and analysis, decision to publish, or preparation of the manuscript.

* Email: funnyzhuli@bjmu.edu.cn

Background

IgA nephropathy (IgAN) is the most common primary glomerulonephritis worldwide[1]. The peak age of the clinical onset of IgAN is during the second and third decade of life[2]. Approximately half of the IgAN patients present with hypertension or a history of hypertension at disease onset despite their young age[3], and some patients present with secondary malignant hypertension[4]. Recently, Karoui et al. reported frequent (up to 53%) thrombotic microangiopathy (TMA) lesions in IgAN patients that may occur in normotensive patients with near-normal renal histology, which excluded severe hypertension or advanced renal disease as sole causes and left the underlying pathophysiological mechanisms undetermined[5]. Moreover, many studies show that plasma von Willebrand Factor (vWF), a specific marker for endothelial cells injury, is abnormal in patients with IgAN, who exhibit elevated levels or defective molecules[6,7]. The high prevalence of hypertension, frequently observed TMA and elevated circulating vWF indicate vascular endothelial injury in IgAN. However, the underlying mechanism has not been discovered.

Soluble fms-like tyrosine kinase-1 (sFlt-1 or sVEGFR-1) is a soluble splice variant of the vascular endothelial growth factor (VEGF) receptor, which is produced by several tissues. sFlt-1 lacks a transmembrane and cytoplasmic domain, and it negatively regulates the actions of VEGF, a highly specific mitogen for vascular endothelial cells, by binding free circulating VEGF and occupying the VEGF receptor. VEGF and sFlt-1 constitute a balance of angiogenic and anti-angiogenic factors in human circulation[8–10]. An imbalance between an angiogenic agent

(VEGF) and an anti-angiogenic factor (sFlt-1), as reflected by VEGF/sFlt-1, has been reported in many diseases[11–13]. Pre-eclampsia is the most popular condition. The elevated sFlt-1 in pre-eclampsia patients leads to widespread endothelial dysfunction and clinical findings of proteinuria and hypertension, which are often observed in many glomerular diseases. Angiogenic imbalance was also reported in diabetic retinopathy patients, and this imbalance was further associated with the fate of diabetic macular edema[14]. Kim et al. found that the urinary excretion of sFlt-1 increased at a relatively early stage in diabetic nephropathy, and it was associated with urinary albumin excretion[12]. Recently, Di et al. reported that excess sFlt-1 was associated with endothelial dysfunction in CKD patients, which implies the involvement of an angiogenic imbalance in kidney disease[15].

Few studies have explored the mechanism of vascular endothelial injury in IgA nephropathy. Our previous studies found that the prevalence of anti-endothelial cell antibodies (AECA) was higher in IgAN patients with severe intra-renal arterial lesions and malignant hypertension[16,17]. AECA cannot explain all of the endothelial dysfunction in patients with IgAN. Therefore, we speculated that the presence of other risk factors, such as an angiogenic imbalance of VEGF/sFlt-1, may be involved in these processes. The present study investigated whether patients with IgAN exhibited imbalanced VEGF and sFlt-1 expression and whether this imbalance contributed to endothelial injury in IgAN.

Subjects and Methods

Study population

Two independent cohorts, a discovery cohort and replication cohort, were included in the present study (Figure S1). In the discovery cohort, 96 plasma-available IgAN patients (diagnosed in 2006–2007) and 22 healthy volunteers with normal urine analysis and blood pressure were enrolled. The replication cohort included 109 plasma-available IgAN patients (diagnosed in 2011–2012) and 30 healthy volunteers.

The granular deposition of IgA in the glomerular mesangium using immunofluorescence detection and the deposition of electron-dense material in the mesangium using ultra-structural examination confirmed the diagnosis of IgAN. Detailed clinical and laboratory examinations excluded patients with Henoch-Schonlein purpura, systemic lupus erythematosus, and chronic hepatic diseases.

Plasma (EDTA anticoagulated) was collected, on the morning that IgAN patients received a renal biopsy or the healthy volunteers were included in the study. Plasma samples were divided into aliquots and stored at −80°C for measurements of sFlt-1, VEGF and vWF levels. Blood pressure and 24-hour urine protein excretion at the time of renal biopsy were collected from medical records. Hypertension was defined as the average of two blood pressure readings on a single occasion with a systolic blood pressure $>$140 mmHg or diastolic blood pressure $>$90 mmHg or patients who reported use of antihypertensive medication. The estimated glomerular filtration rate (eGFR) was evaluated using the Modified Glomerular Filtration Rate Estimating Equation for Chinese[18]. Percutaneous renal biopsy was performed in every IgAN patient. The severity of renal lesions of patients with IgAN was graded according to the Oxford classifications[19,20]. Biopsy adequacy was defined as a minimum of 8 glomeruli available for light microscopy examination. Two renal pathologists blinded to the clinical data scored the renal histopathology from all patients using 4 pathological variables: mesangial hypercellularity (M), segmental glomerulosclerosis (S), endocapillary hypercellularity (E) and tubular atrophy/interstitial fibrosis (T).

The study protocol was approved by the Medical Ethics Committee of Peking University First Hospital and informed written consent was obtained from every participant.

Detection of plasma sFlt-1, VEGF and vWF

The plasma levels of sFlt-1 and VEGF were detected using commercial ELISA kits according to the manufacturer's specifications (R&D Systems, Minneapolis, MN, USA). Plasma levels of vWF were determined using ELISA as previously described[16]. Briefly, ELISA plates were coated with rabbit anti-human vWF polyclonal antibodies (DAKO, Denmark) at 4°C overnight. After blocking, diluted (1:50) test plasma was added, and vWF was detected with horseradish peroxidase (HRP)-conjugated rabbit anti-human vWF polyclonal antibodies (DAKO, Denmark). Individual vWF levels were determined from OD450 values within the linear range of the standard curve via comparison to values obtained from dilutions of purified vWF (Calbionchem, Germany)

Statistical Analysis

Descriptive statistical analyses were performed with SPSS10.0 software (SPSS Inc., USA). Continuous variables were compared by the unpaired Student's t test or ANOVA (ANalysis Of VAriance between groups). Dichotomous and polychromous data were analysed by the $\chi 2$ test. The Spearman correlation was used to analyze correlation. Results were expressed as means ± SD or median (IQR). A p value of less than 0.05 was considered statistically significant.

Results

Clinical and pathological manifestations of IgAN patients

The present study enrolled a total of 205 IgAN patients, including 96 patients in the discovery cohort and 106 patients in the replication cohort. We confirmed that none of these patients received anticoagulant therapy because low molecular weight heparin administration increases circulating sFlt-1 levels[21]. The clinical and pathological manifestations were comparable between patients in the discovery and replication cohorts. The primary clinical and pathological manifestations of patients are summarized in Table 1. Within the 205 IgAN patients, 132 patients were male and 73 patients were female. The average age at renal biopsy was 32.77±10.09 years old, and 47.32% (97/205) of patients presented with hypertension. The proteinuria levels were 1.40 (0.84, 2.76) g/d. The eGFR levels of patients in this group were 82.15±38.65 ml/min/1.73 m^2. According to the Oxford classification, 83.41% (171/205) of the patients were grade M1, 20.98% (43/205) were grade E1, 44.39% (91/205) were grade S1, 36.10% (74/205) were grade T1, and 18.05% (37/205) were grade T2.

Identification of elevated sFlt-1 in IgAN patients in the discovery cohort

Gender distribution and age were not significantly different between the enrolled IgAN patients and healthy volunteers in the discovery cohort. VEGF/sFlt-1 levels (ratio) were significantly lower in IgAN patients than healthy volunteers (IgAN *vs.* healthy volunteers: 0.33±0.27 *vs.* 0.43±0.22, p = 0.02), which indicated an imbalance of pro-angiogenesis and anti-angiogenesis. The VEGF levels were comparable in the two groups (IgAN *vs.* healthy volunteers: 31±27.12 *vs.* 31.86±13.92 pg/ml, p = 0.213), but plasma sFlt-1 levels were significantly elevated in IgAN patients (IgAN *vs.* healthy volunteers: 101.18±25.19 *vs.* 79.73±18.85 pg/ml, p<0.001), which indicated that elevated sFlt-1 contributed to endothelial injury in IgAN (Table 2).

Table 1. Clinical and pathological manifestations of enrolled IgAN patients.

Characteristics	Mean ± SD (IQR or percentage)		
	Discovery cohort	Replication cohort	combined cohort
Age (year)	32.94±9.96	32.62±10.25	32.77±10.09
Gender (male)	65/96 (67.71%)	67/109 (61.47%)	132/205 (64.39%)
Hypertension (%)			
with hypertension	45/96 (46.87%)	52/109 (47.71%)	97/205 (47.32%)
without hypertension	51/96 (53.13%)	57/109 (52.29%)	108/205 (52.68%)
Initial proteinuria (g/day, median, IQR)	1.59 (0.93, 3.22)	1.26 (0.79,2.47)	1.40 (0.84,2.76)
<1 (%)	26/96 (27.08%)	42/109 (38.53%)	70/205 (34.15%)
1–3.5 (%)	48/96 (50%)	54/109 (49.54%)	102/205 (49.76%)
≥3.5 (%)	22/96 (22.92%)	13/109 (11.93%)	33/205 (16.09%)
eGFR (ml/min per 1.73 m^2)	77.27±37.26	86.44±39.58	82.15±38.65
Oxford classification (%)			
M score			
M0	16/96 (16.67%)	18/109 (16.51%)	34/205 (16.59%)
M1	80/96 (83.33%)	91/109 (83.49%)	171/205 (83.41%)
E score			
E0	72/96 (75%)	90/109 (82.57%)	162/205 (79.02%)
E1	24/96 (25%)	19/109 (17.43%)	43/205 (20.98%)
S score			
S0	62/96 (64.58%)	52/109 (47.71%)	114/205 (55.61%)
S1	34/96 (35.42%)	57/109 (52.29%)	91/205 (44.39%)
T score			
T0	63/96 (65.63%)	31/109 (28.44%)	94/205 (45.85%)
T1	15/96 (15.62%)	59/109 (54.13%)	74/205 (36.10%)
T2	18/96 (18.75%)	19/109 (17.43%)	37/205 (18.05%)

Validation of elevated sFlt-1 in IgAN patients in the replication cohort

We enrolled another independent cohort (the replication cohort) to confirm our identification of elevated sFlt-1 in IgAN patients. sFlt-1 levels in IgAN patients in the replication cohort were significantly higher than healthy volunteers (93.40±39.78 *vs.* 71.92±15.78 pg/ml, p<0.001; Figure 1), which was similar to the discovery cohort.

Correlations between elevated sFlt-1 and endothelial injury in patients with IgAN

In pre-eclampsia, a disease resulting from an obvious angiogenic imbalance, proteinuria and hypertension implicate the endothelium as the target of the disease[11]. We included proteinuria and hypertension as evaluations of endothelial injury to explore the factors involved in endothelial injury in IgAN. Moreover, the newly proposed Oxford-MEST histological classification for IgAN uses E scores to evaluate endocapillary proliferation. Therefore we

Table 2. Plasma sFlt-1, VEGF, VEGF/sFlt-1 levels of enrolled IgAN patients and healthy volunteers in the discovery cohort.

	Healthy volunteers	IgAN patients	p-value
Number	22	96	
Age (y)	32.64±6.69	32.94±9.96	0.864
Gender (M/F)	14/8	65/31	0.714
VEGF/sFlt-1	0.43±0.22	0.33±0.27	0.02
sFlt-1 (pg/ml)	79.73±18.85	101.18±25.19	<0.001
VEGF (pg/ml)	31.86±13.92	31.31±27.12	0.213

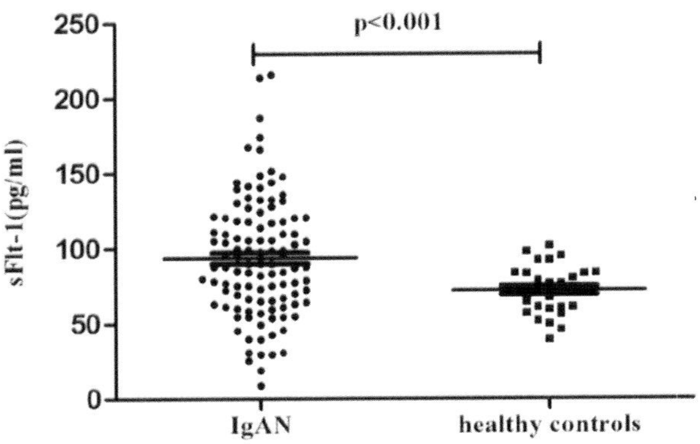

Figure 1. Validation of sFlit-1 levels in the replication cohort. Scatter plot showing the distribution of sFlt-1 levels in IgAN patients and healthy volunteers in the replication cohort. Patients with IgAN showed significantly elevated sFlt-1 levels compared to healthy volunteers.

used Oxford-E scores to evaluate the histological endothelial injury. Furthermore, vWF, a widely agreed biochemical marker for endothelial injury, was also used. We included proteinuria, hypertension, histological E scores and plasma vWF levels as parameters to evaluate endothelial injury in the present study.

Proteinuria. A correlation was observed between plasma sFlt-1 and proteinuria in IgAN patients. Patients with mild proteinuria (<1 g/d) showed lower plasma sFlt-1 levels compared to patients with moderate (1–3.5 g/d) and severe proteinuria (> 3.5 g/d) (severe *vs.* moderate *vs.* mild: 115.95±39.09 *vs.* 99.89±28.55 *vs.* 83.24±33.92 pg/ml, severe *vs.* mild: p<0.001, moderate *vs.* mild: p = 0.001, severe *vs.* moderate: p = 0.014) (Figure 2).

Hypertension. We found elevated plasma sFlt-1 levels in IgAN patients. IgAN patients with hypertension presented with significantly elevated sFlt-1 levels compared to patients without (107.87±31.94 *vs.* 87.32±32.76 pg/ml, p = 0.015) and healthy volunteers (107.87±31.94 *vs.* 75.06±17.55 pg/ml, p<0.001). Furthermore, IgAN patients without hypertension also showed higher sFlt-1 levels than healthy volunteers (107.87±31.94 *vs.* 75.06±17.55 pg/ml, p = 0.001) (Figure 2). These results indicated a correlation between plasma sFlt-1 and clinical hypertension in IgAN patients.

E scores of Oxford classification. No correlation was observed between Oxford-E scores and sFlt-1. IgAN patients with scores of E0 and E1 did not show significantly different plasma sFlt-1 levels (E1 *vs.* E0: 92.13±25.68 *vs.* 98.35±35.71 pg/ml, p = 0.20) (Figure 2).

Von Willebrand Factor. We first investigated the correlation between sFlt-1 and vWF. sFlt-1 was positively correlated with vWF in IgAN patients (r = 0.161, p = 0.021), which is a specific endothelial injury marker (Figure 2).

We next compared plasma vWF levels between patients and volunteers. IgAN patients showed significantly higher vWF levels than healthy volunteers (11.08±12.16 *vs.* 7.48±7.72 μg/ml, p = 0.003) (Figure 3), in accordance with sFlt-1. Furthermore, correlations between vWF and proteinuria, hypertension, and Oxford-E score were also analyzed. IgAN patients with mild proteinuria showed lower levels of vWF than patients with moderate proteinuria (mild *vs.* moderate: 7.78±6.34 *vs.* 10.01±9.58 μg/ml, p = 0.066) and severe proteinuria (mild *vs.* severe: 7.78±6.34 *vs.* 18.96±19.80 μg/ml, p<0.001). Patients with moderate proteinuria had significantly lower vWF levels than patients with severe proteinuria (10.01±9.58 *vs.* 18.96±19.80 μg/ml, p = 0.002) (Figure 3). Patients with hypertension showed significantly higher levels of vWF than patients without hypertension (14.92±15.07 *vs.* 7.63±7.26 μg/ml, p<0.001) and healthy volunteers (14.92±15.07 *vs.* 7.48±7.72 μg/ml, p<0.001), but there was no difference between IgAN patients without hypertension and healthy volunteers (7.63±7.26 *vs.* 7.48±7.72 μg/ml, p = 0.44) (Figure 3). IgAN patients with scores of E0 and E1 did not show significantly different plasma vWF levels (E1 *vs.* E0: 11.61±12.90 *vs.* 10.94±11.99 pg/ml, p = 0.518) (Figure 3).

Our results indicated that elevated sFlt-1 levels in IgAN patients were significantly correlated with the well-proven endothelial injury marker, vWF.

Plasma vWF levels, but not sFlt-1 levels, correlated with eGFR

Renal excretion greatly influences many circulating elements. Therefore, we further investigated the correlation of elevated sFlt-1 and vWF with eGFR in patients with IgAN, whose renal excretion function is often impaired. Our data showed that plasma vWF levels were negatively correlated with eGFR in IgAN patients (r = −0.286, p<0.001; Figure 4), but no correlation between sFlt-1 and eGFR was observed (r = −0.057, p = 0.414; Figure 4).

Discussion

IgA nephropathy is a common, complex disease with variable manifestations. Endothelial dysfunction, which is observed in a considerable proportion of patients with IgAN, is one of these manifestations, but the mechanism that leads to this dysfunction is not clear. The present study explored the underlying mechanism of endothelial injury in IgAN patients and identified an angiogenic imbalance of VEGF/sFlt-1 in IgAN patients for the first time.

VEGF is a potent mitogen for endothelial cells, and it plays a central role in maintaining the integrity of the endothelial lining. sFlt-1, also known as soluble VEGFR-1, acts as a VEGF antagonist. The ratio of VEGF/sFlt-1 is often used to evaluate the balance of angiogenesis. It is very interesting that both sFlt-1 and VEGF/sFlt-1, but not VEGF, were significantly different between IgAN patients and healthy volunteers in the present study. These results implied that elevated sFlt-1 may be the most important contributor to the angiogenic imbalance in IgAN, which is different from diabetic nephropathy and pre-eclampsia in which both a decreased VEGF and increased sFlt-1 have been reported[11,22]. Elevated sFlt-1 in patients with IgAN was further confirmed in an independent replication cohort in our study. Another important thing to note is that, sFlt-1 levels are significantly elevated to over 3000 pg/ml in patients with pre-eclampsia. Even in normal-term pregnancy women, the sFlt-1 levels were already 10 times higher than healthy volunteers[11]. The placenta is the main source of elevated sFlt-1[23], although one recent study found that platelet-monocyte aggregate-derived sFlt-1 also contributed to the pathogenesis of pre-eclampsia [24]. The sFlt-1 levels in patients with IgAN were elevated slightly but significantly compared to pre-eclampsia. Further in depth studies are required to identify the source and the variance of elevated sFlt-1 in IgAN.

We further explored the correlations of elevated sFlt-1 with proteinuria, hypertension, Oxford-E scores and vWF levels (Figure S1). Previous studies in animal models and humans have proven the importance of VEGF signaling in maintaining the integrity of glomerular filtration barrier[25,26]. A defective survival of glomerular endothelial cells would occur in the absence of VEGF signaling, which leads to proteinuria. Our study found that IgAN

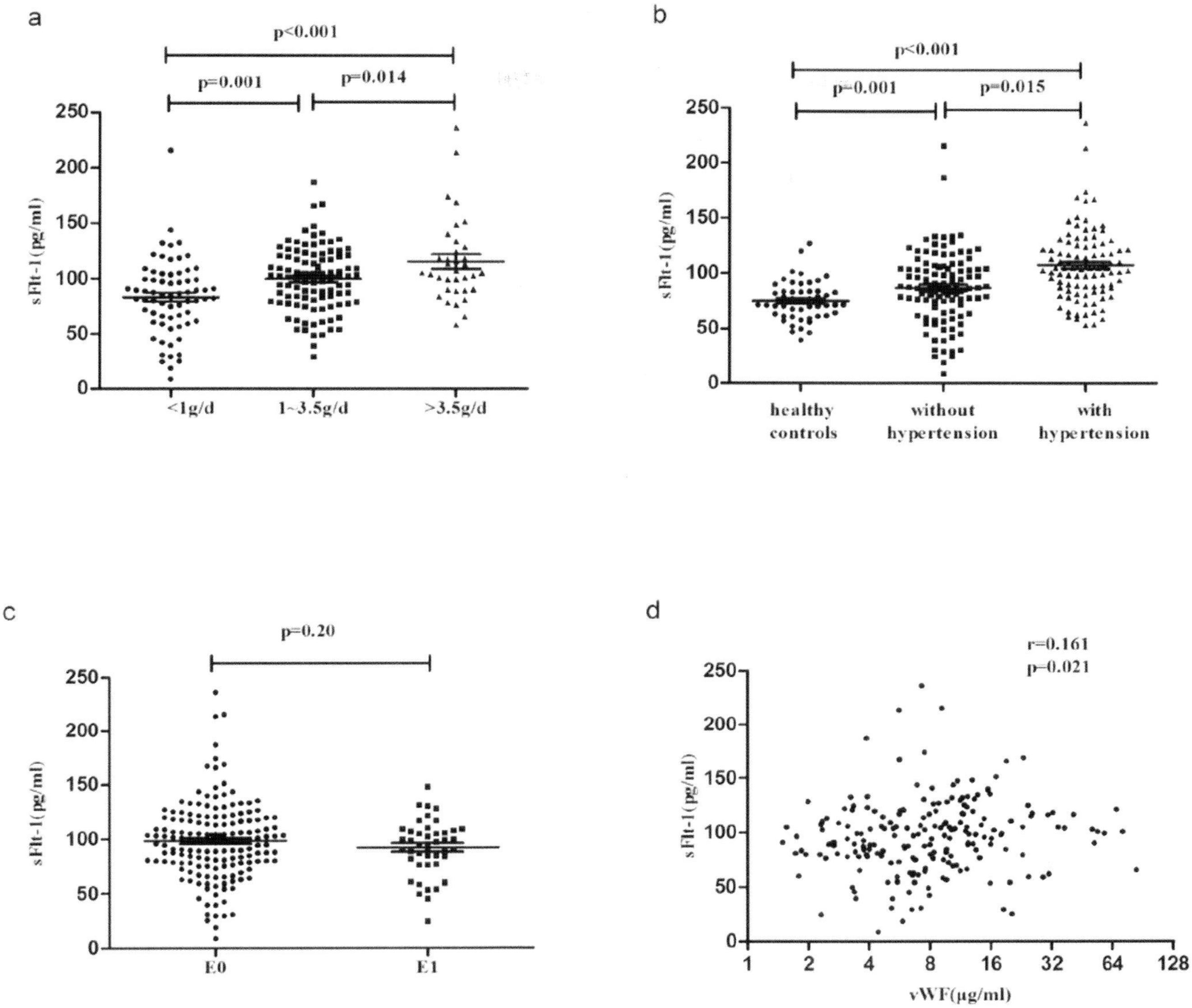

Figure 2. Correlations of sFlt-1 with proteinuria, hypertension, Oxford-E score and vWF levels. a. Scatter plot showing the distribution of sFlt-1 levels in IgAN patients according to different degrees of proteinuria. Patients with mild proteinuria (<1 g/d) showed lower plasma sFlt-1 compared to patients with moderate (1–3.5 g/d) and severe proteinuria (>3.5 g/d). **b**. Scatter plot showing the distribution of sFlt-1 levels of IgAN patients according to hypertension. IgAN patients with hypertension presented significantly higher sFlt-1 levels than patients without hypertension and healthy volunteers. Furthermore, IgAN patients without hypertension also showed higher sFlt-1 levels than healthy volunteers. **c**. Scatter plot showing the distribution of sFlt-1 levels in IgAN patients according to Oxford-E score. The sFlt-1 levels were similar in the E1 group compared to the E0 group. **d**. Scatter plot showing the correlation between sFlt-1 and vWF levels. Plasma sFlt-1 levels were significantly correlated with vWF levels.

patients with severe proteinuria had higher sFlt-1, and IgAN patients with mild proteinuria had lower sFlt-1. These results imply the following underlying mechanism: increased sFlt-1, through its inhibition of VEGF, interfered with glomerular endothelial survival, and finally destroyed the glomerular filtration barrier to result in proteinuria.

Except for renal endothelial injury, VEGF signaling dysfunction can also lead to systemic endothelial injury. Maynard et al. reported that sFlt-1 administration to pregnant rats induced hypertension and glomerular endotheliosis[11].We found a correlation between increased sFlt-1 and hypertension in our population, which suggested that elevated sFlt-1 might be a factor of systemic endothelial cell injury.

A correlation between plasma sFlt-1 levels and Oxford-E scores was not observed in the present study. We grouped patients into groups with hypertension and without hypertension, and correlations were not found in either group (Figure S2). Similarly, vWF levels also failed to show correlations with Oxford-E scores. We have some considerations at this point. At first, the E score was a semi-quantitative pathological parameter, and although it worked well for the prediction of prognosis, it might not be sensitive enough to evaluate variations of endothelial injury in IgAN. Secondly, Oxford-E scores were evaluated mainly in the endocapillary hypercellularity, which may have limited power for these scores to reflect the sFlt-1-induced endothelial injury for decreased endothelial survival. Thirdly, it would be more

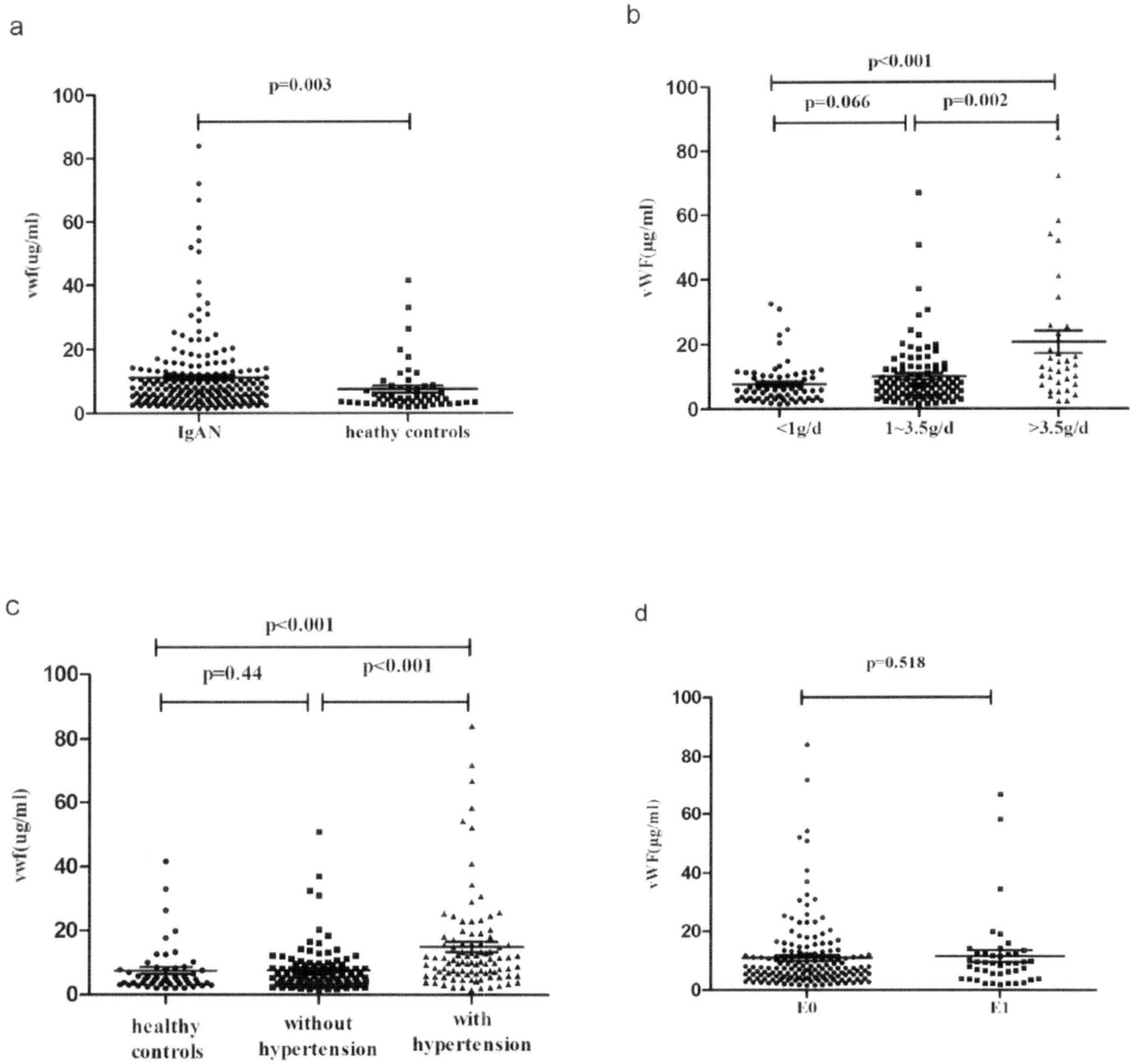

Figure 3. Correlations of vWF with proteinuria, hypertension and Oxford-E score. a. Scatter plot showing the distribution of vWF levels in IgAN patients and healthy volunteers. IgAN patients showed significantly higher vWF levels than healthy volunteers. **b**. Scatter plot showing the distribution of vWF levels of IgAN patients according to different degrees of proteinuria. Patients with mild proteinuria (<1 g/d) showed lower plasma sFlt-1 levels compared to patients with moderate (1–3.5 g/d) and severe proteinuria (>3.5 g/d). **c**. Scatter plot showing the distribution of vWF levels in IgAN patients with or without hypertension. IgAN patients with hypertension presented significantly higher vWF levels than patients without hypertension and healthy volunteers. However, IgAN patients without hypertension showed similar vWF levels compared to healthy volunteers. **d**. Scatter plot showing the distribution of sFlt-1 levels of IgAN patients according to Oxford-E score. The sFlt-1 levels were similar in the E1 group compared with the E0 group.

reasonable to analyze the correlation of Oxford-E scores with local sFlt-1 levels rather than plasma sFlt-1 levels because there may be some difference.

vWF is a well-known marker for endothelial dysfunction. Our present study observed elevated vWF levels in patients with IgAN, which also correlated with clinical proteinuria and hypertension in IgAN and confirmed the existence of endothelial injury in IgAN. Moreover, sFlt-1 levels were positively correlated with vWF in our patients with IgAN, which provided direct evidence to suggest sFlt-1 as a causal factor for endothelial injury in IgAN.

Plasma vWF levels are widely used as a biomarker for endothelial injury in several conditions. We found a negative correlation of vWF levels with eGFR in our patients with IgAN. However, sFlt-1 levels seemed not influenced by eGFR. Therefore, sFlt-1 might be a more suitable biomarker for endothelial injury

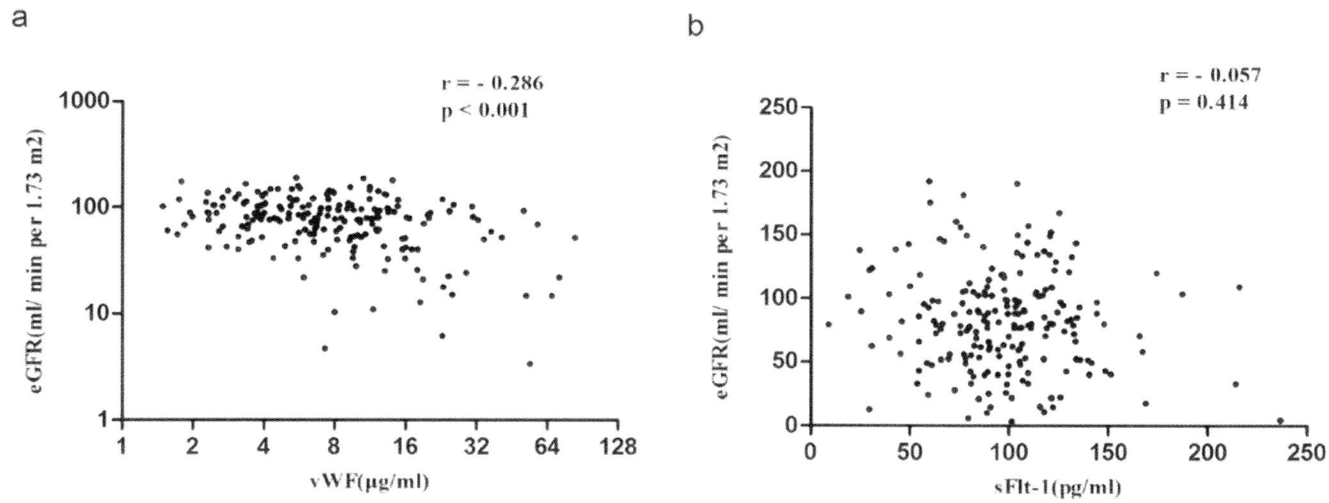

Figure 4. Correlation of vWF and sFlt-1 levels with eGFR. a. Plasma vWF levels were negatively correlated with eGFR. **b**. Plasma sFlt-1 levels showed no correlation with eGFR.

for patients with chronic kidney diseases, especially those patients with impaired renal function.

Notably, our present study was a cross-sectional study. We only detected the sFlt-1 levels on the day of renal biopsy for patients with IgAN. Therefore, we cannot currently evaluate the variability of sFlt-1 measurements over time. The identification of sFlt-1 as a correlated biomarker for endothelial injury in our study will be of great clinical importance for investigating sFlt-1 levels in a follow-up population of IgAN patients.

In conclusion, the present study found elevated sFlt-1 in IgAN patients for the first time and further identified its correlation with proteinuria, hypertension and vWF levels. Our results suggest elevated sFlt-1 as one of the contributors to endothelial injury in IgA nephropathy.

Supporting Information

Figure S1 Flow chart showing the process of the present study. VEGF/sFlt-1, sFlt-1 and VEGF levels were firstly compared in discovery cohort between 96 patients with IgAN and 22 healthy volunteers. Next, the identified contributor (sFlt-1) was confirmed in a replication cohort (109 IgAN patients, 30 healthy volunteers). At last, the correlations of sFlt-1 with hypertension, proteinuria, Oxford-E score and plasma vWF, were evaluated in the combined 205 patients with IgAN.

Figure S2 sFlt-1 levels in patients with E1 and E0 in hypertension group and without hypertension group. In patients with IgAN, sFlt-1 levels were similar in those with Oxford-E1 and Oxford-E0, either in hypertension group (**a**) or without hypertension group (**b**).

Acknowledgments

We are very grateful to all the blood donors.

Author Contributions

Conceived and designed the experiments: LZ HZ. Performed the experiments: YLZ SFS. Analyzed the data: LJL JCL. Contributed reagents/materials/analysis tools: LJL JCL. Wrote the paper: LZ HZ.

References

1. D'Amico G (1987) The commonest glomerulonephritis in the world: IgA nephropathy. Q J Med 64: 709–27.
2. Barratt J, Feehally J (2005) IgA nephropathy. J Am Soc Nephrol 16: 2088–97.
3. Woo KT, Wong KS, Lau YK, Chiang GS, Lim CH (1988) Hypertension in IgA nephropathy. Ann Acad Med Singapore 17: 583–88.
4. Chen Y, Tang Z, Yang G, Shen S, Yu Y, et al. (2005) Malignant hypertension in patients with idiopathic IgA nephropathy. Kidney Blood Press Res 28: 251–58.
5. El KK, Hill GS, Karras A, Jacquot C, Moulonguet L, et al. (2012) A clinicopathologic study of thrombotic microangiopathy in IgA nephropathy. J Am Soc Nephrol 23: 137–48.
6. Hernandez E, Toledo T, Alamo C, Mon C, Rodicio JL, et al. (1997) Elevation of von Willebrand factor levels in patients with IgA nephropathy: effect of ACE inhibition. Am J Kidney Dis 30: 397–403.
7. Bertaglia G, Ossi E, Casonato A, Miglietta A, Forino M, et al. (1997) Von Willebrand factor abnormalities in IgA nephropathy. Nephrol Dial Transplant 12: 474–79.
8. Kendall RL, Wang G, Thomas KA (1996) Identification of a natural soluble form of the vascular endothelial growth factor receptor, FLT-1, and its heterodimerization with KDR. Biochem Biophys Res Commun 226: 324–28.
9. Shibuya M (2006) Vascular endothelial growth factor receptor-1 (VEGFR-1/Flt-1): a dual regulator for angiogenesis. Angiogenesis 9: 225–30, 231.
10. Wu FT, Stefanini MO, Mac GF, Kontos CD, Annex BH, et al. (2010) A systems biology perspective on sVEGFR1: its biological function, pathogenic role and therapeutic use. J Cell Mol Med 14: 528–52.
11. Maynard SE, Min JY, Merchan J, Lim KH, Li J, et al. (2003) Excess placental soluble fms-like tyrosine kinase 1 (sFlt1) may contribute to endothelial dysfunction, hypertension, and proteinuria in preeclampsia. J Clin Invest 111: 649–58.
12. Kim NH, Oh JH, Seo JA, Lee KW, Kim SG, et al. (2005) Vascular endothelial growth factor (VEGF) and soluble VEGF receptor FLT-1 in diabetic nephropathy. Kidney Int 67: 167–77.
13. Belgore FM, Blann AD, Li-Saw-Hee FL, Beevers DG, Lip GY (2001) Plasma levels of vascular endothelial growth factor and its soluble receptor (SFlt-1) in essential hypertension. Am J Cardiol 87: 805–07, A9.
14. Javanmard SH, Hasanpour Z, Abbaspoor Z, Naderian GA, Jahanmard M (2012) Aqueous concentrations of VEGF and soluble VEGF receptor-1 in diabetic retinopathy patients. J Res Med Sci 17: 1124–27.
15. Di Marco GS, Reuter S, Hillebrand U, Amler S, Konig M, et al. (2009) The soluble VEGF receptor sFlt1 contributes to endothelial dysfunction in CKD. J Am Soc Nephrol 20: 2235–45.
16. Zhang JJ, Jiang L, Liu G, Wang SX, Zou WZ, et al. (2008) Elevation of serum von Willebrand factor and anti-endothelial cell antibodies in patients with immunoglobulin A nephropathy are associated with intrarenal arterial lesions. Nephrology (Carlton) 13: 712–20.

17. Jiang L, Zhang JJ, Lv JC, Liu G, Zou WZ, et al. (2008) Malignant hypertension in IgA nephropathy was not associated with background pathological phenotypes of glomerular lesions. Nephrol Dial Transplant 23: 3921–27.
18. Ma YC, Zuo L, Chen JH, Luo Q, Yu XQ, et al. (2006) Modified glomerular filtration rate estimating equation for Chinese patients with chronic kidney disease. J Am Soc Nephrol 17: 2937–44.
19. Roberts IS, Cook HT, Troyanov S, Alpers CE, Amore A, et al. (2009) The Oxford classification of IgA nephropathy: pathology definitions, correlations, and reproducibility. Kidney Int 76: 546–56.
20. Cattran DC, Coppo R, Cook HT, Feehally J, Roberts IS, et al. (2009) The Oxford classification of IgA nephropathy: rationale, clinicopathological correlations, and classification. Kidney Int 76: 534–45.
21. Hagmann H, Bossung V, Belaidi AA, Fridman A, Karumanchi SA, et al. (2014) Low-molecular weight heparin increases circulating sFlt-1 levels and enhances urinary elimination. PLoS One 9: e85258.
22. Karalliedde J, Gnudi L (2011) Endothelial factors and diabetic nephropathy. Diabetes Care 34 Suppl 2: S291–96.
23. Clark DE, Smith SK, He Y, Day KA, Licence DR, et al.(1998)A vascular endothelial growth factor antagonist is produced by the human placenta and released into the maternal circulation. Biol Reprod 59: 1540–48.
24. Major HD, Campbell RA, Silver RM, Branch DW, Weyrich AS(2014)Synthesis of sFlt-1 by platelet-monocyte aggregates contributes to the pathogenesis of preeclampsia. Am J Obstet Gynecol In press.
25. Keedy VL, Sandler AB (2007) Inhibition of angiogenesis in the treatment of non-small cell lung cancer. Cancer Sci 98: 1825–30.
26. Sugimoto H, Hamano Y, Charytan D, Cosgrove D, Kieran M, et al. (2003) Neutralization of circulating vascular endothelial growth factor (VEGF) by anti-VEGF antibodies and soluble VEGF receptor 1 (sFlt-1) induces proteinuria. J Biol Chem 278: 12605–08.

7

TWEAK Promotes Peritoneal Inflammation

Ana Belen Sanz[1,4]*, Luiz Stark Aroeira[2], Teresa Bellon[3], Gloria del Peso[3,4], Jose Jimenez-Heffernan[5], Beatriz Santamaria[1¤], Maria Dolores Sanchez-Niño[3,4], Luis Miguel Blanco-Colio[1], Manuel Lopez-Cabrera[4,6], Marta Ruiz-Ortega[1,4,7], Jesus Egido[1,7,8], Rafael Selgas[3,4,7,8], Alberto Ortiz[1,4,7,8]

1 Laboratory of Nephrology, IIS-Fundacion Jimenez Diaz, Madrid, Spain, **2** Department of Immunology, Instituto de Investigación Biomédica de Vigo (IBIV), Vigo, Pontevedra, Spain, **3** Department of Nephrology, IDIPAZ, Madrid, Spain, **4** REDinREN, Madrid, Spain, **5** Hospital Universitario de la Princesa, Madrid, Spain, **6** Centro Biologia Molecular Severo Ochoa, Madrid, Spain, **7** Universidad Autonoma de Madrid, Madrid, Spain, **8** IRSIN, Madrid, Spain

Abstract

Peritoneal dialysis (PD) is complicated by peritonitis episodes that cause loss of mesothelium and eventually sclerosing peritonitis. An improved understanding of the molecular contributors to peritoneal injury and defense may increase the therapeutic armamentarium to optimize peritoneal defenses while minimizing peritoneal injury. There is no information on the expression and function of the cytokine TWEAK and its receptor Fn14 during peritoneal injury. Fn14 expression and soluble TWEAK levels were measured in human PD peritoneal effluent cells or fluids with or without peritonitis. Fn14 expression was also analyzed in peritoneal biopsies from PD patients. Actions of intraperitoneal TWEAK were studied in mice in vivo. sTWEAK levels were increased in peritoneal effluent in PD peritonitis. Effluent sTWEAK levels correlated with the number of peritoneal macrophages ($r = 0.491$, $p = 0.002$). Potential TWEAK targets that express the receptor Fn14 include mesothelial cells and macrophages, as demonstrated by flow cytometry of peritoneal effluents and by analysis of peritoneal biopsies. Peritoneal biopsy Fn14 correlated with mesothelial injury, fibrosis and inflammation, suggesting a potential deleterious effect of TWEAK/Fn14. In this regard, intraperitoneal TWEAK administration to mice promoted peritoneal inflammation characterized by increased peritoneal effluent MCP-1, Fn14 and $Gr1^+$ macrophages, increased mesothelial Fn14, MCP-1 and CCL21 expression and submesothelial tissue macrophage recruitment. Taken together these data suggest that the TWEAK/Fn14 system may promote inflammation and tissue injury during peritonitis and PD.

Editor: Bernhard Ryffel, French National Centre for Scientific Research, France

Funding: This work was supported by FIS PS09/00447, PI08/1564, PI10/00234, MS12/03262, FEDER funds ISCIII-RETIC REDinREN/RD06/0016, RD12/0021, Comunidad de Madrid (Fibroteam S2010/BMD-2321, S2010/BMD-2378). Programa Intensificación Actividad Investigadora (ISCIII/Agencia Laín-Entralgo/CM) to AO, Programa Estabilización Investigadores to LB-C, Miguel Servet to ABS, Sara Borrell to BS, MDSN. The funders had no role in study design, data collection and analysis, decision to publish, or preparation of the manuscript.

* E-mail: asanz@fjd.es

¤ Current address: Instituto de Investigaciones Biomedicas "Alberto Sols", CSIC-UAM, Madrid, Spain

Introduction

Peritonitis is a potentially devastating disease occurring in the context of abdominal visceral injury, cirrhosis, peritoneal dialysis (PD) and others. PD is a renal replacement therapy modality that is marred by episodes of bacterial infection, leading to localized inflammation evidenced as peritonitis [1]. Moreover, dialysis solutions can themselves induce sterile peritoneal inflammation [2,3]. PD represents an interesting human model of inflammation since the technique allows repeated non-invasive access to the peritoneal cavity, allowing both monitoring of the inflammatory process as well as therapy by local delivery of drugs [4]. Peritoneal inflammation is characterized by local upregulation of several cytokines, macrophage recruitment, and collagen synthesis by mesothelial cells and fibroblasts leading to loss of peritoneal membrane integrity and fibrosis. Both acute and chronic peritoneal inflammation may lead to PD technique failure [5]. In some cases PD-associated chronic peritoneal inflammation may result in sclerosing peritonitis [6]. Sclerosing peritonitis is a fatal form of peritoneal inflammation characterized by a fibrous thickening of the peritoneum. Understanding the role of the different players involved may help design strategies to limit inflammation-mediated tissue injury without compromising anti-bacterial defenses.

Tumor necrosis factor-like weak inducer of apoptosis (TWEAK, TNFSF12) is a member of the TNF superfamily of structurally-related cytokines. TWEAK may modulate cell death, proliferation, inflammation and angiogenesis [7–10]. Fibroblast growth factor-inducible 14 (Fn14) is the functional TWEAK receptor. Fn14 expression is strongly induced during tissue injury, repair and remodeling [11]. Cells can express full-length membrane-anchored TWEAK (mTWEAK) and secrete a soluble form (sTWEAK), and both bind and activate Fn14 [11]. sTWEAK levels in serum/plasma or urine may have biomarker value in inflammatory diseases, such as atherosclerosis, lupus nephritis and chronic kidney disease [12–14]. The role of TWEAK in inflammation has been described in the central nervous system, cardiovascular injury and kidney disease [15–20], but there is no information on the expression and role of TWEAK and Fn14 during human infection or peritoneal inflammation.

We have now explored the expression of TWEAK and Fn14 during human peritoneal infection and in vivo effects of TWEAK on peritoneal inflammation. We report that sTWEAK levels are

Table 1. Clinical characteristics of PD patients with peritonitis providing peritoneal effluent samples.

Patient	Age (years)	Sex	Cause of ESRD	Peritonitis number for the patient	Culture results	Duration of peritonitis (days)	Catheter removal	PD vintage at time of peritonitis (months)
1	76	Male	Nephroangiosclerosis	7th	*Enterococcus faecalis*	2	Yes	62
				8th	*Klebsiella*	2	No	65
				9th	*Klebsiella*	2	No	66
2	59	Male	Glomerulonephritis	3rd	*Escherichia coli*	7	No	30
3	64	Male	Nephroangiosclerosis	1st	*Streptococcus salivarius*	3	No	11
4	72	Female	Interstitial	1st	*Streptococcus*	2	No	19
5	30	Female	Vasculitis	1a	*Campylobacter fetus*	2	No	6
6	71	Male	Nephroangiosclerosis	3rd	*Escherichia coli*	16	Yes	13
7	84	Male	Unknown	1st	*Bacteroides fragilis*	4	No	5
8	71	Male	Glomerulonephritis	2nd	*Streptococcus salivarius*	2	No	13
				3rd	*Staphylococcus coagulase negative*	5	No	15
9	74	Male	Unknown	1st	*Staphylococcus epidermidis*	2	No	9
10	48	Male	Unknown	1st	Sterile	3	No	-
11	48	Male	Unknown	1st	*Streptococcus*	4	No	0.5
12	50	Female	Unknown	4th	*Klebsiella*	5	No	37
13	25	Male	Interstitial	1st	*Staphylococcus aureus*	4	No	3
14	65	Female	Unknown	2nd	*Candida*	7	Yes	12

ESRD: End-stage renal disease.

Table 2. Clinical characteristics of stable PD patients without peritonitis in the prior 3 months providing peritoneal effluent samples.

Patient	Age	Sex	Cause of ESRD
1	30	Female	Vasculitis
2	30	Female	Unknown
3	60	Female	Polycystic kidneys
4	57	Male	Nephroangiosclerosis
5	76	Male	Diabetes type II
6	58	Female	Interstitial
7	29	Male	Glomerulonephritis
8	29	Male	Glomerulonephritis

ESRD: End-stage renal disease.

increased in effluents from PD patients with peritonitis and correlate with effluent macrophage number. Fn14 expression is also increased in cells from peritonitis effluents and local tissue Fn14 expression correlates with mesothelial injury in human peritoneal biopsies. Finally, intraperitoneal TWEAK injection in mice promotes peritoneal inflammation and increases macrophages in peritoneal effluents and in the peritoneal tissue. These results support a role of TWEAK in peritoneal injury and inflammatory cell recruitment and suggest that TWEAK may be a biomarker of peritoneal inflammation during PD.

Materials and Methods

Human samples

Human samples were obtained following a protocol approved by the IDIPAZ Ethics Committee and informed consent was obtained. Peritoneal effluent samples were obtained from patients undergoing chronic PD in the course of a peritonitis episode (n = 14) or from stable PD patients without peritonitis in the prior 3 months and without any other cause systemic inflammation (Non-peritonitis group; n = 8). The characteristics of study participants are presented in **Tables 1 and 2**. Human peritoneum biopsy samples were obtained at the time of transplantation or abdominal surgery from 9 patients without evidence of systemic inflammation (**Table 3**). PD patients were stable at the time of biopsy, with no recent peritonitis. An experienced pathologist (JJH) scored the biopsies blinded as to the nature of the sample and following a previously established peritoneal injury score. This score assesses 3 items (mesothelial integrity, peritoneal fibrosis and peritoneal inflammation) in a 0–3 scale for a total possible maximum score of 9 for most severely injured samples [21]. In this regard, in the present manuscript, the published score was modified in order to assign a score of 3 (rather than 0) to the most severe mesothelial injury (loss of mesothelium) and a score of 0 (rather than 3) to mesothelial integrity.

ELISA

sTWEAK levels in human peritoneal effluent were determined with a commercially available enzyme-linked immunosorbent assay (ELISA) kit (BMS2006INST; Bender MedSystems, Vienna, Austria). MCP-1 levels in murine peritoneal lavages were measured by commercial ELISA (BD Pharmingen, NJ).

Table 3. Clinical characteristics of patients providing peritoneal biopsy samples.

Patient	Age (years)	Sex	Cause of ESRD	PD vintage (months)	MTC Cr (ml/min)	4.25% glucose UF (ml/4 h)	Mesothelial integrity	Fibrosis	Chronic inflammation	Peritoneal injury score
1	53	M	ND	Non-ESRD	ND	ND	0	1	0	1
2	59	M	Tubulointerstitial Nephritis	HD	ND	ND	0	0	0	0
3	68	M	Glomerulonephritis	12	8.7	600	0	0	0	0
4	27	M	Unknown	8	10.4	900	0	1	0	1
5	55	F	Glomerulonephritis	21	8.9	600	2	0	0	2
6	34	M	Glomerulonephritis	4	6.3	870	2	1	2	5
7	25	F	Glomerulonephritis	52	6.6	850	3	2	2	7
8	32	M	Interstitial	23	13.7	480	2	1	1	4
9	50	F	Unknown	37	10.8	310	2	2	2	6

ND: no data. ESRD: End-stage renal disease.
HD: hemodialysis. M: male, F: female.

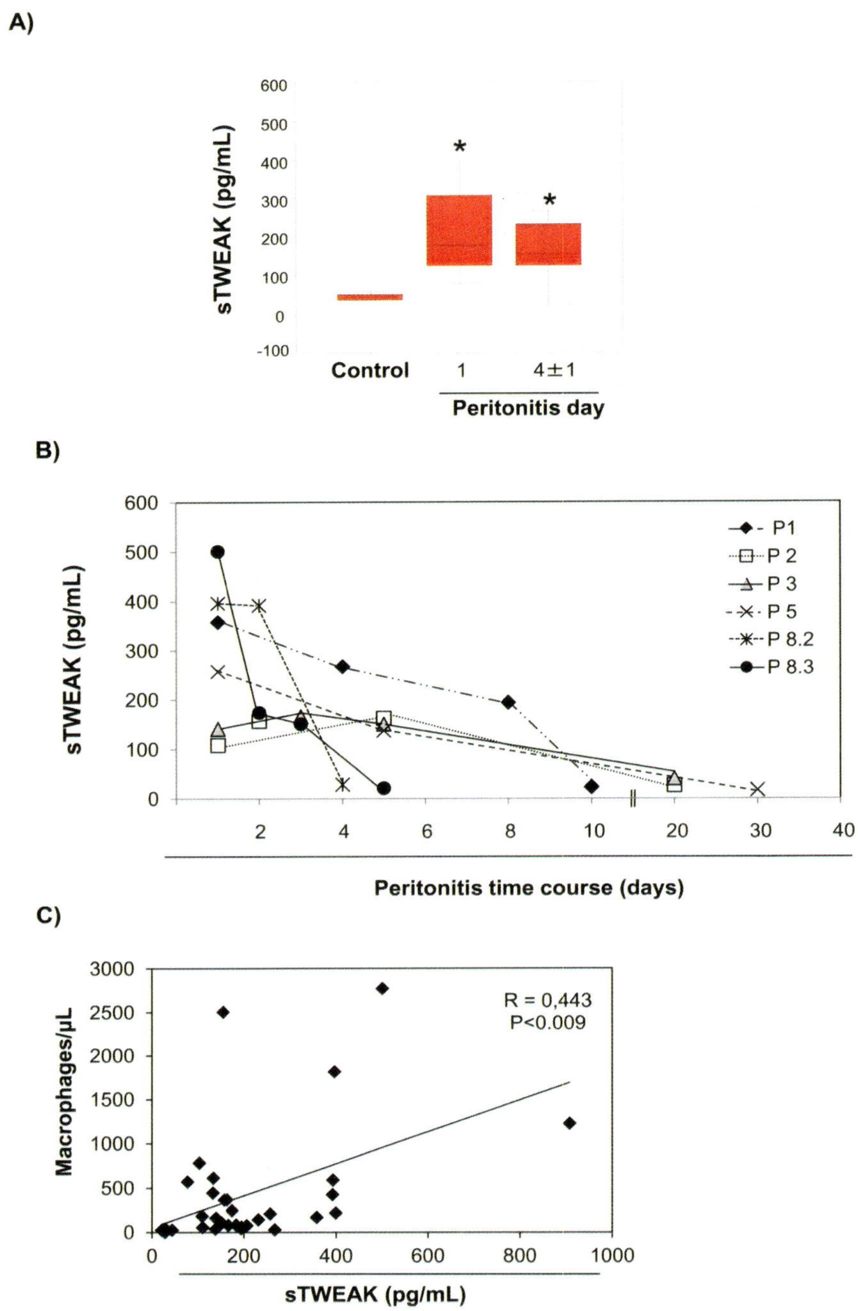

Figure 1. Increased peritoneal effluent sTWEAK in PD peritonitis. A) sTWEAK levels were measured in peritoneal effluents from PD patients with peritonitis (days 1 and 4±1) or without peritonitis. Clinical data in tables 1 and 2. *$p<0.002$ vs non-peritonitis. **B**) Evolution of sTWEAK levels through the peritonitis episode in 6 individual patients with at least three samples that cover the whole peritonitis episode. sTWEAK levels decrease when peritonitis resolves. Peritonitis episodes correspond to those presented in table 1. **C**) Scatter plot showing the significant positive correlation between sTWEAK levels and the number of peritoneal macrophages in peritoneal effluents during 17 episodes of peritonitis in PD patients.

Mesothelial cell cultures

The study was approved by the clinical ethics committee of IIS-Fundación Jiménez Díaz and written informed consent was obtained. Human omental mesothelial cells (HOMC) were obtained from omentum from 6 non-PD patients who underwent unrelated elective abdominal surgery [22,23].

Western blot

Cell samples were homogenized in lysis buffer (50 mM TrisHCl, 150 mM NaCl, 2 mM EDTA, 2 mM EGTA, 0.2% Triton X-100, 0.3% NP-40, 0.1 mM PMSF and 1 μg/ml pepstatin A) then separated by 12% SDS-PAGE under reducing conditions [20]. After electrophoresis, samples were transferred to PVDF membranes (Millipore), blocked with 5% skimmed milk in PBS/0.5% v/v Tween 20 for 1 hr, washed with PBS/Tween, and

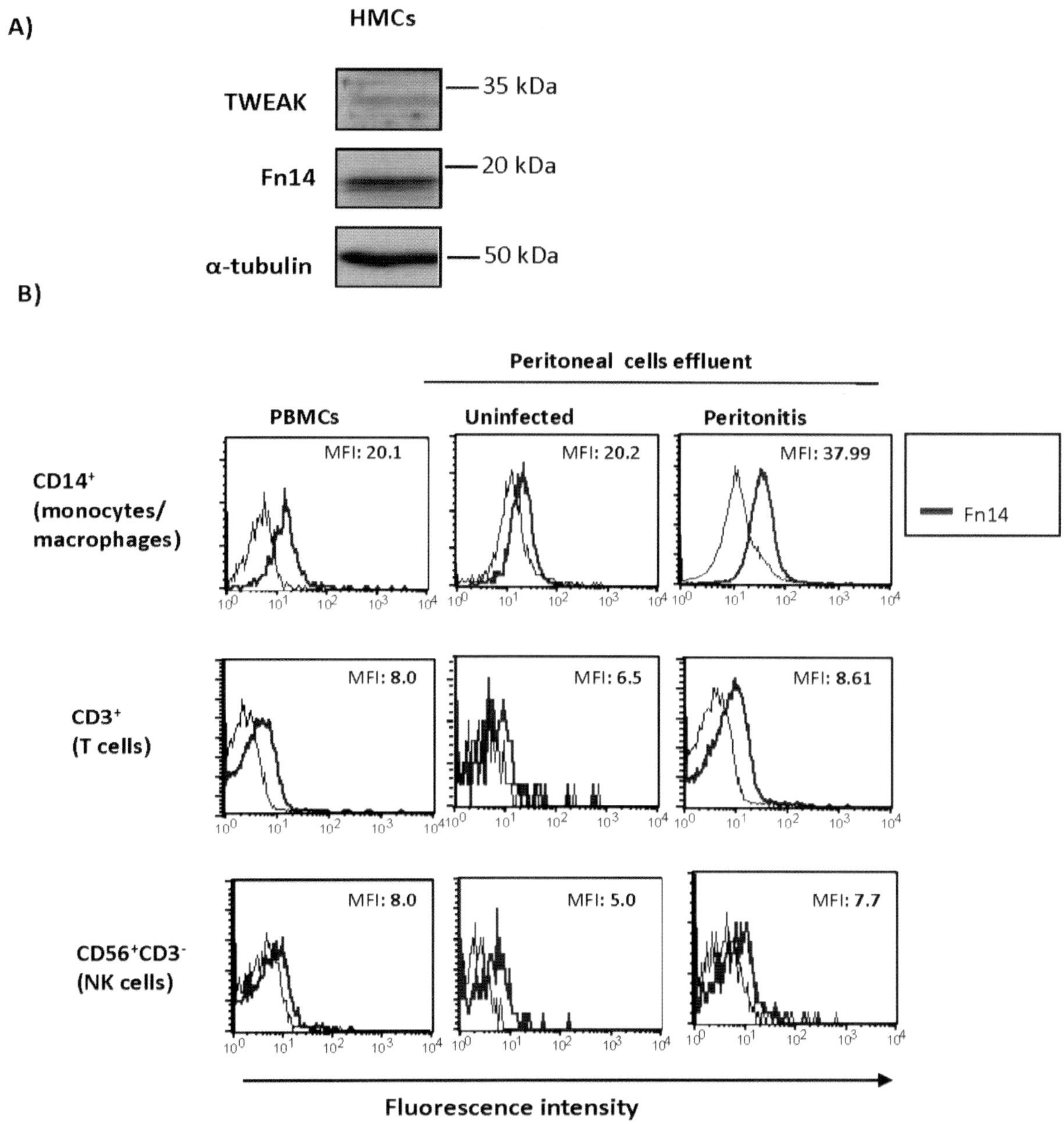

Figure 2. Fn14 is expressed by cultured human mesothelial cells and by leukocytes in peritoneal effluents from PD patients. A) Cultured human mesothelial cells (HMC) express Fn14 and TWEAK as assessed by western blot. Representative images of three different experiments. **B**) Fn14 expression was analyzed by flow cytometry in peripheral blood and peritoneal effluent leucocytes. Cells were stained with Fn14-PE and monocyte/macrophages, T cells and NK cells were identified with anti-CD14, anti-CD3 and anti-CD56 antibodies respectively within the appropriate gates according to FSC and SSC parameters. Controls for the technique were stained with isotype immunoglubulin. Peripheral blood mononuclear cells (PBMCs) were used as positive controls for leukocyte population markers. Numbers within histograms indicate mean fluorescence intensity (MFI) for Fn14 staining. Note increased Fn14 expression mainly in peritoneal macrophages from patients with peritonitis.

incubated with rabbit polyclonal anti-Fn14 (1:1000, Cell Signaling, Danvers, MA) and rabbit polyclonal anti-TWEAK (1:500, Santa Cruz Biotechnology, Santa Cruz, CA) diluted in 5% BSA. Blots were washed with PBS/Tween and incubated with appropriate horseradish peroxidase-conjugated secondary antibody (1:2000, Amersham, Aylesbury, UK). After washing with PBS/Tween blots were developed with the chemiluminescence method (ECL) (Amersham). Blots were then probed with mouse monoclonal anti-α-tubulin antibody (1:2000, Sigma) and levels of expression were corrected for minor differences in loading.

Fn14 immunofluorescence colocalization in human peritoneum biopsies

The general procedures have been previously described [24]. Antigenic epitope retrieval was performed in 3 μm thick sections of paraffin-embedded tissue using a PTlink device (with a high pH solution, 95°C, 20 min). Tissue slides were incubated overnight at

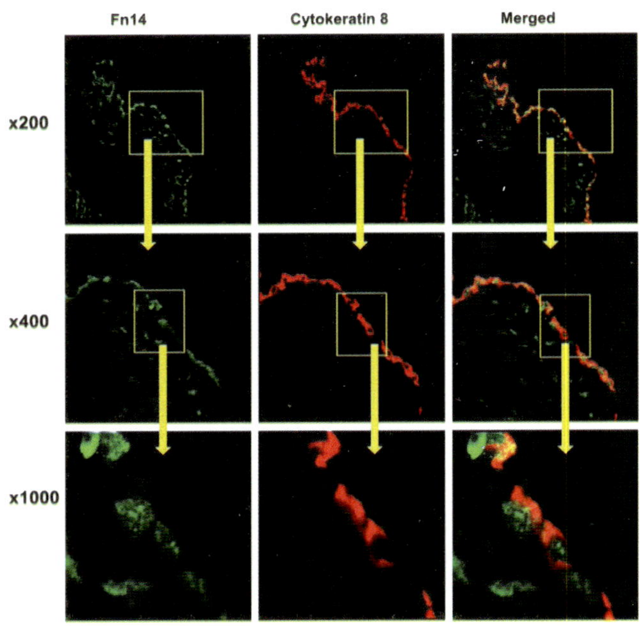

Figure 3. Colocalization of Fn14 and mesothelial cell markers in human preserved peritoneum. Human non-infected peritoneum from stable chronic PD patient with preserved mesothelium was stained with both anti-Fn14 antibody (green) and anti-cytokeratin 8 antibody (red). Mesothelial cells (red) express Fn14 (green). Confocal microscopy. Original magnification x200, detail x400 and x1000.

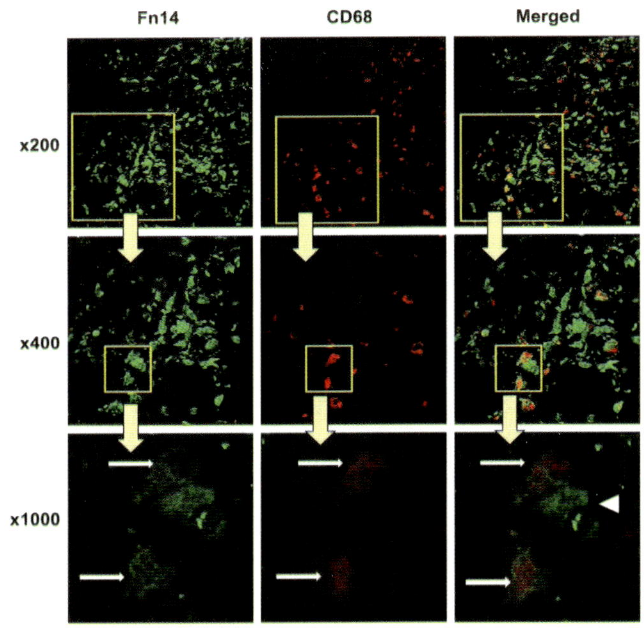

Figure 4. CD68 positive macrophages express Fn14 in human injured peritoneum. Human peritoneum biopsies from non-infected, stable, chronic PD patients were stained with both anti-Fn14 antibody (green) and anti-CD68 antibody (red). $CD68^+$ macrophages (red) are among the submesothelial cells that express Fn14 (green)(white arrows). Additional submesothelial cells express Fn14 (arrowhead). Confocal microscopy. Original magnification x200, detail x400 and x1000.

4°C with the primary antibodies, rabbit polyclonal anti-Fn14 (1:100, Cell Signaling) and mouse monoclonal anti-cytokeratin 8 (1:60, Santa Cruz Biotechnology) or mouse monoclonal anti-CD68 (Dako Diagnostics, Barcelona, Spain). Slides were then washed with PBS and incubated with anti-rabbit Alexa488 and anti-mouse Alexa 633 conjugated secondary antibodies (1:300, Invitrogen, Carlsbad, CA).

Fn14 immunohistochemistry

In human peritoneum biopsies antigenic epitope retrieval was performed in 3 μm thick sections of paraffin-embedded tissue using a PTlink device (with a high pH solution, 95°C, 20 min). Endogenous peroxidase was blocked by incubation in 3% H2O2/methanol (1:1) at 25°C for 30 minutes [25]. Slides were incubated in PBS with 4% bovine serum albumin (BSA) and 1% horse serum, for 1 hour at 37°C to reduce nonspecific background staining, and then incubated overnight at 4°C with rabbit polyclonal anti-Fn14 (1:100, Cell Signaling) in PBS, 4% BSA, 1% serum. After washing with PBS, sections were incubated with a secondary biotin-labeled antibody, washed and developed with AB streptavidin-complex. Finally, sections were washed and stained with DAB (Dako Diagnostics). Sections were counterstained with Carazzi's hematoxylin. Negative controls included incubation with isotype IgG. Fn14 staining was evaluated by a quantitative scoring system, Image-Pro Plus software (Media cybernetics, MD) in 12 randomly selected fields (x20) per sample by an observer blinded as to eh nature of the samples.

In murine samples antigenic epitope retrieval was performed in 5 μm thick sections of paraffin-embedded tissue using a PTlink device (with a high pH solution, 95°C, 20 min). Tissue slices were incubated for 30 min at room temperature with the primary antibody, rabbit polyclonal anti-Fn14 (1:100, Cell Signaling), goat polyclonal anti-MCP-1 (1:500, Santa Cruz), goat polyclonal anti-CCL21 (1:150, R&D Systems, Minneapolis, MN) and rat polyclonal anti-F4/80 (1:10000, Serotec) [20]. For immunohistochemical staining Envision FLEX + visualization system was used, in a DAKO Autostainerplus platform. Tissue sections were subsequently counterstained with hematoxylin. Same sections were incubated without the primary antibody as negative controls.

Animal model

Studies were conducted in accord with the NIH Guide for the Care and Use of Laboratory Animals. C57BL6 female mice (12- to 14-week-old) (IFFA-CREDO, Barcelona, Spain) received 0.75 μg/human recombinant TWEAK (Millipore, Billerica, MA) or saline (n = 5 per group) intraperitoneally. Mice were killed 4 h or 24 h after injection. The dose of TWEAK was calculated based on in vitro experiments for an extracellular volume of 7.5 ml/mouse [19].The dose had been validated in prior animal experiments, where the time course of systemic TWEAK actions were explored with focus on the kidney. To determine peritoneal production of chemokines, the peritoneal cavity was lavaged with two ml saline immediately after mice were euthanised. The solution (murine peritoneal lavage) was centrifuged and the supernatant was separated into small aliquots and stored at −80°C and the pellet containing cells was used for flow cytometry analysis and for RT-PCR. After sacrifice parietal peritoneum was collected, fixed in neutral-buffered formalin and embedded in paraffin [26].

Flow cytometry

Human peripheral blood mononuclear cells, human peritoneal effluent cells and murine peritoneal effluent cells were analyzed by flow cytometry.

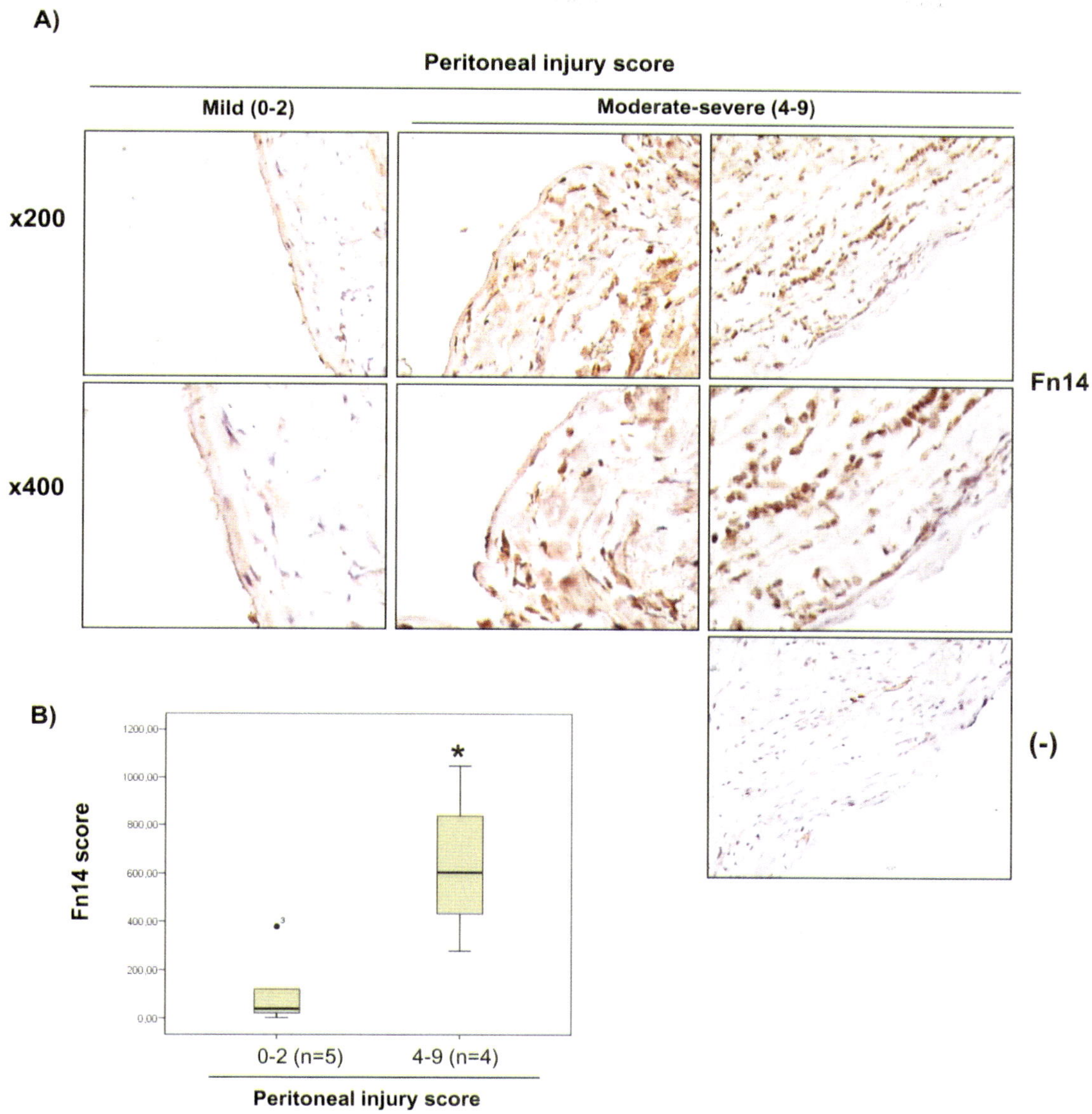

Figure 5. Increased Fn14 protein expression in peritoneal biopsies from non-infected patients. A) Fn14 immunohistochemistry in peritoneal tissue from non-infected, stable, chronic PD patients with different degrees of injury. Representative images from each group. Controls for the technique are stained with nonspecific immunoglobulin (Ig (-)). **B**) Quantification of Fn14 protein expression in peritoneal biopsies from non-infected patients. Fn14 staining was higher in patients with a more severe peritoneal histological injury score that evaluated mesothelial integrity, peritoneal fibrosis and peritoneal inflammation (**table 3**)[32]. Mean ± SEM *$p<0.04$, n = 4–5 patients per group.

Cells were isolated from PD effluents by centrifugation at 500 g for 15′ at 4°C. PBMCs from healthy control donors were prepared by Ficoll-Hypaque (Amersham Pharmacia Biotech, Sweden) density gradient centrifugation. The following mAb were used for flow cytometry analysis of surface molecules: CD3-PerCP, CD14-FITC, CD56-APC (BD Biosciences) and Fn14-PE (eBioscience). Cells were pre-incubated with 50 µg/mL human IgG to prevent binding to FcR and stained according to standard protocols. Analysis was performed in a FACScalibur cytometer with ProQuest software (BD Bioscience).

Cells from murine peritoneal effluent were analyzed by flow cytometry using the following antibodies: anti-mouse CD4 PE and Alexa Fluor® 488-labelled anti-mouse CD8a for T cells. F4/80 PE-Cy7, Gr1 APC, CD14 FITC and CD11b PE for macrophages (BD Biosciences, San Diego, USA). Macrophages were defined as CD11b+F4/80+ cells and Gr1+ macrophages as CD11b+F4/80+Gr1+ cells. Neutrophils were defined as Gr1+/F4/80- cells.

RNA extraction and Real-Time Polymerase Chain Reaction

Total RNA was extracted from cells and tissue by the TRI Reagent method (Sigma) and 1 µg of RNA was reverse transcribed with High Capacity cDNA Archive Kit (Applied Biosystems, Foster City, CA). Pre-developed primer and probe assays for Fn14, and GAPDH (human) were from Applied (Applied Biosystems). Quantitative PCR was performed by 7500 Real Time PCR

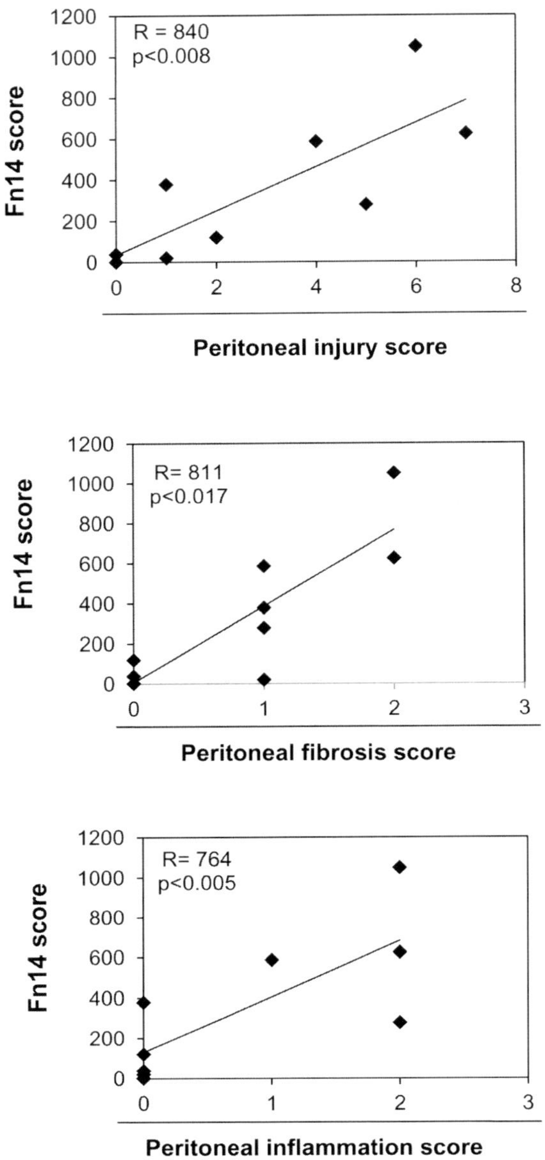

Figure 6. Fn14 protein expression in peritoneal tissue correlates with peritoneal injury, fibrosis and inflammation in humans. Scatter plot showing the significant positive correlation between Fn14 expression in peritoneal tissue from non-infected patients (n = 9) and histological peritoneal injury, peritoneal fibrosis and peritoneal inflammation scores.

System with the Prism 7000 System SDS Software (Applied Biosystems) and RNA expression of different genes was corrected for GAPDH [27].

Statistical analysis

Non-normally distributed variables were expressed as median (interquartile range), and normally distributed variables were expressed as mean ± SEM. $p<0.05$ was considered to be statistically significant. Mann–Whitney tests were used to compare the results between two groups. Spearman rank correlation was used to determine correlations between two variables. Statistical analysis was performed with SPSS software package version 11.0.

Results

sTWEAK concentrations are increased in peritoneal effluent from PD peritonitis

sTWEAK levels were measured in peritoneal effluents from PD patients during and after peritonitis episodes. General characteristic of the studied populations are summarized in **tables 1 and 2**. Peritoneal effluent sTWEAK levels were increased in patients with peritonitis between day 1 and day 4±1 compared with patients without peritonitis (**Figure 1.A**). Moreover, peritoneal effluent sTWEAK levels decreased when peritonitis was resolving (**Figure 1.B**) and correlated with the number of peritoneal effluent macrophages (**Figure 1.C**). However, no correlation was found between sTWEAK and peritoneal effluent neutrophils, indeed the number of peritoneal effluent neutrophils rapidly decreases after initiation of antibiotic therapy in PD patients (**Figure S1**).These data indicate that sTWEAK could be a biomarker for severity of local inflammation in a model of human infection, peritonitis. TNFα levels were undetectable in these samples (not shown).

Fn14 is expressed by cultured human mesothelial cells and by PD peritoneal effluent leukocytes

Fn14 is the only known signal-transducing TWEAK receptor. Thus, we evaluated cell types potentially responsive to TWEAK by assessing the expression of Fn14. Cultured human mesothelial cells express Fn14 (**Figure 2.A**). Mesothelial cells may also be a source of TWEAK (**Figure 2.A**). In addition, Fn14 expression is increased in monocytes/macrophages ($CD14^+$) present in peritoneal effluents from PD patients with peritonitis compared to patients without peritonitis (**Figure 2.B**). This result suggests that mesothelial cells or monocytes/macrophages might be responsive to TWEAK during peritonitis.

Increased Fn14 expression in peritoneal biopsies from chronic PD patients

Next we checked whether the cell culture observation of Fn14 expression by mesothelial cells was relevant in vivo. We immunolocalized Fn14 in peritoneal biopsies from subjects in table 3. Fn14 colocalized with mesothelial cell markers in peritoneal biopsies with preserved histological features, including a preserved mesothelial monolayer (**Figure 3**), confirming the cell culture observation that mesothelial cells express Fn14 (**Figure 2.A**). However, in human PD-induced peritoneal injury, Fn14 colocalized with CD68 positive macrophages and was not present in the demesothelized peritoneal membrane (**Figure 4**). Additional submesothelial cell types also expressed Fn14.

Next, we quantified Fn14 expression in peritoneal biopsies. Peritoneal tissue samples were classified by a histological peritoneal injury score that quantified mesothelial integrity, fibrosis and inflammation (**Table 3**). Histological tissue injury was classified as mild (peritoneal injury score 0-2) or moderate-severe (score 4–9). Local peritoneal Fn14 expression was increased in patients with peritoneal injury (**Figure 5**). Fn14 expression correlated with peritoneal injury score (a composite of mesothelial integrity, peritoneal fibrosis and peritoneal inflammation), peritoneal fibrosis and peritoneal inflammation (**Figure 6**).

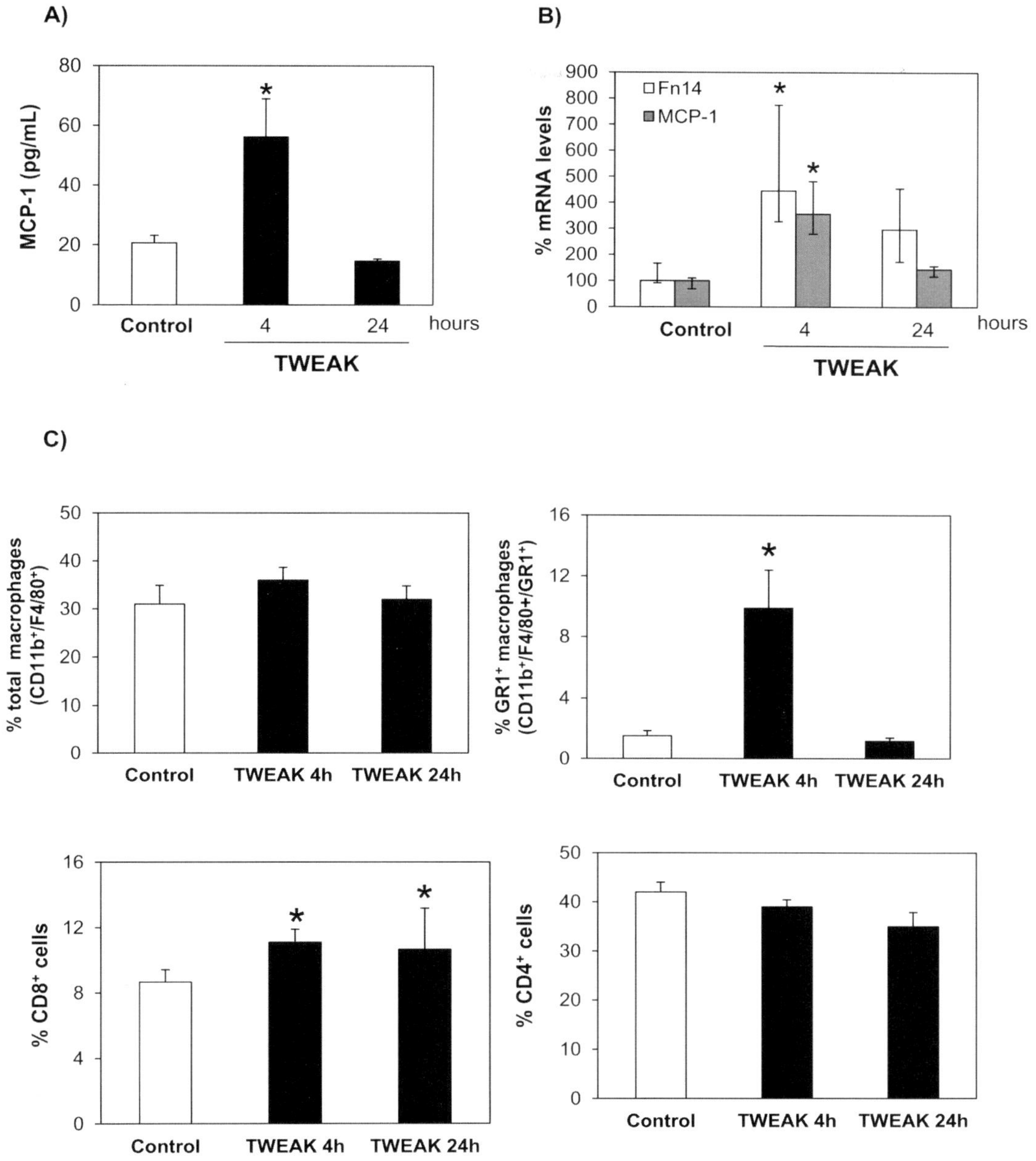

Figure 7. TWEAK increases inflammatory mediators in murine peritoneal effluents. A) MCP-1 protein levels were quantified by ELISA in peritoneal lavage of mice that had received intraperitoneal TWEAK or vehicle (control). Mean $\pm$ SEM of 5 animals per group. *p<0.001 vs control. **B**) MCP-1 and Fn14 mRNA levels measured in peritoneal lavage cells. Median (25th to 75th percentile) of 5 animals per group. *p<0.03. **C**) Quantification by flow cytometry of inflammatory cells present in murine peritoneal lavage. Mean $\pm$ SEM of 5 animals per group. *p<0.05. Macrophages were defined as CD11b+F4/80+ cells and Gr1+ macrophages as CD11b+F4/80+Gr1+ cells.

Intraperitoneal TWEAK promotes peritoneal inflammation in mice

The association between TWEAK/Fn14 expression and inflammation in humans begets the question whether TWEAK promotes inflammation or inflammation increases TWEAK. We next explored TWEAK actions on the peritoneal effluent and the peritoneal tissue in vivo. Intraperitoneal TWEAK administration to mice increased peritoneal lavage monocyte chemotatic protein 1 (MCP-1) levels (**Figure 7.A**), peritoneal lavage cell expression of MCP-1 and Fn14 mRNA (**Figure 7.B**), and the percentage of $Gr1^+$ macrophages, the murine equivalent to activated human $CD14^+$ macrophages that express the CCR2 receptor for MCP-1 [28] (**Figure 7.C**). Moreover, TWEAK mildly increased the percentage of $CD8^+$ cells (**Figure 7.C**) and neutrophils (**Figure S2**). Changes in peritoneal cell distribution or chemokine levels following a single TWEAK injection were observed at early time points (4 hours) and had returned to baseline or were decreasing at 24 h. This time-course is consistent with previously described time-courses of TWEAK or TNF-induced inflammation in other organs such as the kidney [19].

TWEAK also increased peritoneal tissue Fn14 mRNA expression as assessed by quantitative RT-PCR (**Figure 8.A**). Immunohistochemistry showed Fn14 expression in mesothelial cells and

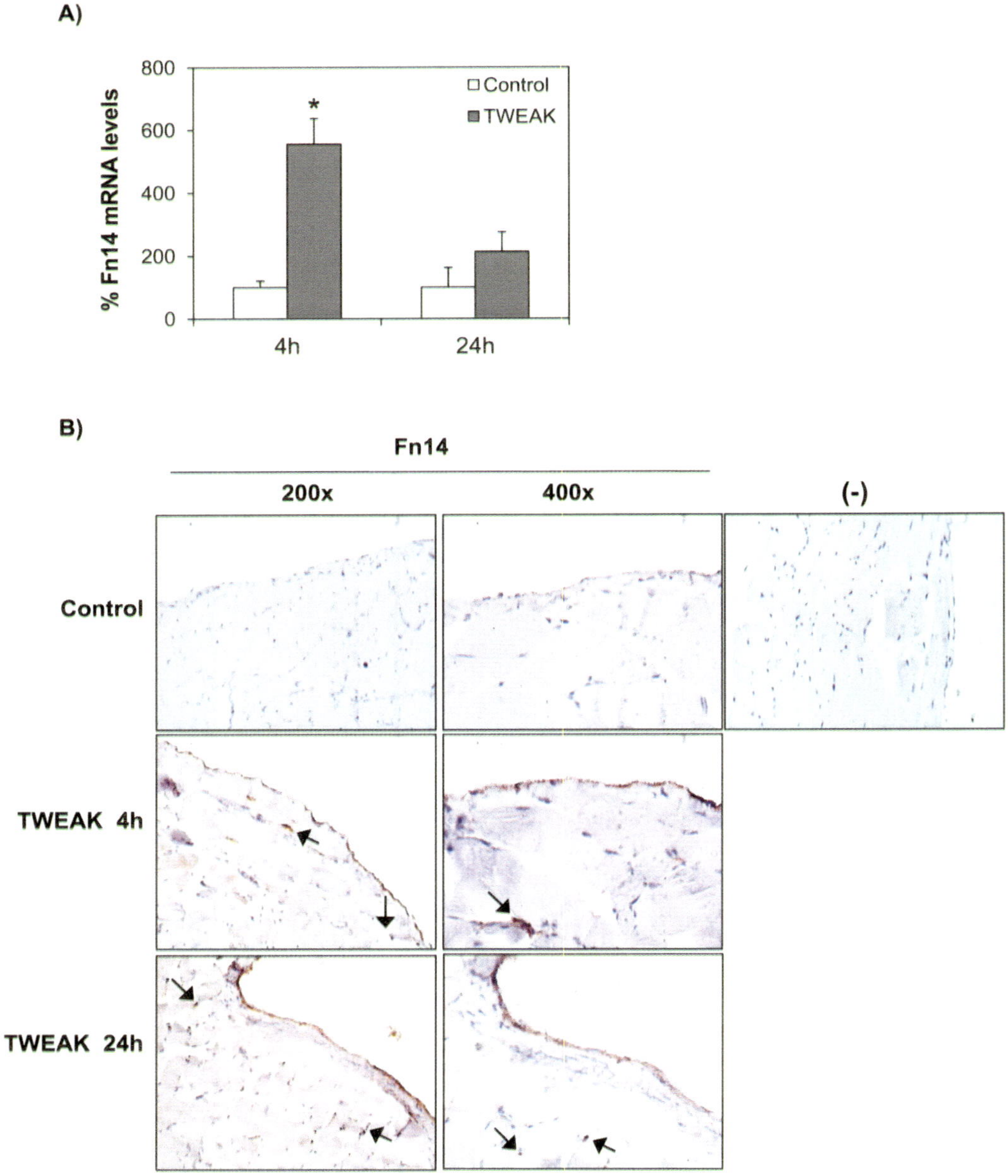

Figure 8. TWEAK increases Fn14 expression in murine peritoneal tissue in vivo. A) Intraperitoneal TWEAK administration increased Fn14 mRNA in peritoneal tissue. Mean ± SEM of 5 animals per group. *p<0.02. **B**) Fn14 immunohistochemistry. TWEAK administration increased Fn14 expression in mesothelial cells and submesothelial infiltrating cells (arrows). Controls for the technique are stained with nonspecific Ig (-). Images representative of 5 animals per group.

in infiltrating submesothelial cells (**Figure 8.B**), as was the case for human peritoneal biopsies (**Figure 3, 4**). TWEAK also increased peritoneal tissue MCP-1 and CCL21 mRNA expression (**Figure 9**). These chemokines were chosen for analysis because they represent canonical and non-canonical NFKB activation by TWEAK, respectively [29], and they are relevant for peritoneal injury since MCP-1 attracts macrophages and CCL21 attracts fibrocytes [30]. Upregulation of peritoneal tissue Fn14 and MCP-1 mRNA was observed earlier (4 hours) than CCL21 mRNA upregulation (24 hours). This time course is similar to that observed in the kidney of TWEAK-treated mice [19,20]. Likewise, immunohistochemistry disclosed increased MCP-1 and CCL21 protein in peritoneal tissue of mice treated with TWEAK (**Figure 10**). Mesothelial cells expressed the chemokines, indicating that these Fn14-expressing cells are key peritoneal responders to TWEAK stimulation. Moreover, TWEAK promoted tissue macrophage recruitment (**Figure 10**). Macrophage infiltration was observed in the sub-mesothelial region, next to Fn14- and chemokine-expressing mesothelial cells.

Discussion

The main findings are high sTWEAK levels in peritoneal effluents during human peritonitis, a correlation of peritoneal tissue Fn14 receptor expression with peritoneal injury in long-term PD, and the observation that in vivo TWEAK activates Fn14-

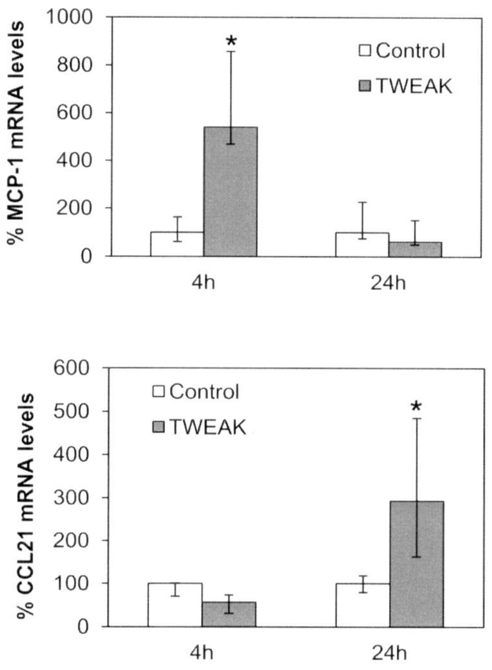

Figure 9. TWEAK promotes murine peritoneal tissue chemokine mRNA expression *in vivo*. MCP-1 and CCL21 mRNA levels measured by RT-PCR in murine peritoneal tissue 4 and 24 hours following TWEAK administration. Median (25th to75th percentile) of 5 animals per group. $^{*}p<0.05$.

expressing cells mesothelial cells and promotes peritoneal inflammation in mice. These findings identify sTWEAK as a potential biomarker and therapeutic target in peritoneal inflammation. This observation may be of interest to other forms of bacterial peritonitis and to chronic peritoneal injury associated with PD. Moreover, the findings could apply to tissue injury in the course of other human bacterial infections.

The nature of PD allows repeated non-invasive access to events taking place in the peritoneal cavity. Thus, PD is a human model which allows the monitoring of inflammatory events in vivo during infection or in the long-term course of sterile inflammation. Findings in the human PD model may be representative of events in other conditions characterized by bacterial infection or sterile inflammation and may guide the development of hypothesis and studies on the role of specific molecules in these events. We have taken advantage of this model to identify high levels of sTWEAK in peritoneal effluents during peritonitis episodes and to study the potential role of en excess of this cytokine in the peritoneal cavity.

While our study draws attention to the potential of sTWEAK as a biomarker in peritoneal inflammation, the design does not allow definition of a specific role of sTWEAK in monitoring of peritoneal inflammation and in assessing potential outcomes that might guide therapeutic decision-making regarding intensification or change of antibiotic therapy or the decision to remove the peritoneal catheter. However, further studies should address these possibilities. A role in this respect may be envisioned since another candidate indicator of the severity of inflammation, TNFα, could not be detected in these samples. We did not address the sources of peritoneal effluent sTWEAK in humans in vivo, but cell culture results presented here and a literature review suggest that both mesothelial cells and macrophages are potential sources [31].

Inflammation is a physiological response to bacterial aggression. In the course of peritonitis multiple inflammatory mediators are released locally [32–35]. For some of them functional evidence of their link to tissue injury has been provided [23,36–40]. Thus, TGFβ1 promotes peritoneal fibrosis and dysfunction [37,39], PDGF-B promotes angiogenesis [38], IL-6 and its soluble receptor (sIL-6R) control the pattern of leukocyte recruitment during peritoneal inflammation [40] and the IFNγ/TNFα combination promotes mesothelial cell apoptosis [23]. Indeed, a single episode of very severe peritonitis may cause irreversible peritoneal fibrosis. It is thus necessary to understand the different contributors to peritoneal inflammation. Our results indicate that during peritoneal inflammation mesothelial cells upregulate the TWEAK receptor Fn14 and that TWEAK activates mesothelial cells to promote the expression of chemokines dependent on both canonical and non-canonical NFκB activation [19,20] to attract macrophages into the peritoneal cavity and peritoneal tissue. Although we did not specifically explore non-canonical vs canonical NFκB activation in the present work, the time-course of gene expression of the canonical NFκB target MCP-1 and of the non-canonical NFκB target CCL21 observed in vivo in mice is consistent with prior studies supporting the involvement of these pathways in upregulation of these specific chemokines [20]. Indeed, the transient, self-limited nature of MCP-1 upregulation is characteristic of canonical NFκB response elicited by a single exposure to TWEAK or TNF [29]. Macrophages are the key targets of the chemotactic activity of MCP-1. In this regard, the observed increase in the percentage of $Gr1^{+}$ peritoneal lavage macrophages coinciding with peak MCP-1 levels is consistent with the inflammatory nature of these macrophages. $Gr1^{+}$ macrophages express the MCP-1 receptor CCR2 and activate integrins, increasing their ability to roll on endothelial cell and migrate into inflamed tissue [41]. TWEAK may also directly activate macrophages, since Fn14 expression is upregulated in macrophages during peritonitis. Among CCL21 targets, fibrocytes are of particular interest. These are circulating fibroblast precursors that are attracted by CCL21 and may contribute to peritoneal fibrosis [30]. In this regard, Fn14 expression in human peritoneum correlated with the peritoneal fibrosis score. In mice, intraperitoneal TWEAK also transiently increased peritoneal lavag neutrophils, although the effect was milder than on macrophages. In this regard, no correlation between peritoneal effluent sTWEAK and macrophages was observed in human PD peritonitis, suggesting that factors other than TWEAK are more important in recruiting neutrophils or that neutrophil contribution to sTWEAK levels is minor.

In several animal models TWEAK has consistently shown to promote further inflammation and tissue injury during sterile inflammation. This has been observed in kidney, vascular and central nervous system disease [15–20,42,43]. The association between Fn14 expression and histological peritoneal injury scores in chronic, non-infected PD patients suggests that TWEAK may also have such a role in long-term PD peritoneal injury. Current ongoing clinical trials are testing the tissue protective action of neutralizing anti-TWEAK antibodies during sterile inflammation (http://clinicaltrials.gov/show/NCT00771329, accessed on March 23, 2013, http://clinicaltrials.gov/ct2/show/NCT01499355, accessed on October 23, 2013). The results of these trials will guide the potential evaluation of this therapeutic tool in the PD context. In this regard, TWEAK has additional actions of potential relevance for peritoneal injury which we have not addressed. Thus, TWEAK has a pro-angiogenic role and angiogenesis has been associated with peritoneal dysfunction. However, the role of TWEAK/Fn14 during infection has not been adequately characterized. A potential contribution of sTWEAK to

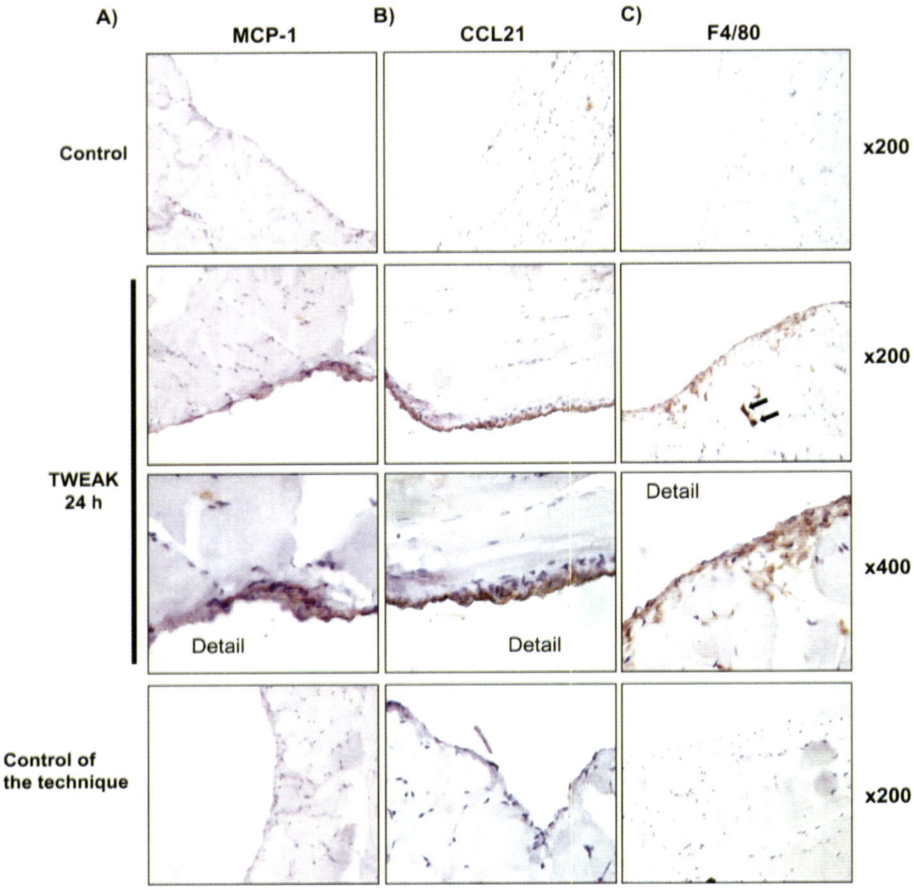

Figure 10. TWEAK induces chemokine protein expression and peritoneal inflammation in mice *in vivo*. A and B) Increased MCP-1 (**A**) and CCL21 (**B**) protein expression in mesothelium from mice 24 h after TWEAK injection. **C**) F4/80 antigen immunohistochemistry. An increased number of submesothelial macrophages stained with F4/80 were noted 24 h after TWEAK injection (arrows). Controls for the technique are stained with nonspecific Ig. Images representative images of 5 animals per group.

peritoneal defense during acute peritonitis, probably by favoring leukocyte recruitment, cannot be excluded.

In conclusion, TWEAK and its receptor are highly expressed in the peritoneum under diverse pathological circumstances and they promote inflammation. Further studies are needed to explore the biomarker and therapeutic potential of these findings.

Supporting Information

Figure S1 Human peritoneal effluent sTWEAK levels do not correlate with peritoneal effluent neutrophils. A) Neutrophil counts rapidly decrease in peritoneal effluents from PD patients after initiation of antibiotic therapy. Mean ± SEM. Clinical data in table 1. $^*p<0.002$ vs day 1. **B)** Scatter plot showing the negative correlation between sTWEAK levels and the number of peritoneal neutrophils in peritoneal effluents during 17 episodes of peritonitis in PD patients.

Figure S2 TWEAK induces transient neutrophil recruitment in murine peritoneal effluents. Quantification by flow cytometry of neutrophils present in murine peritoneal lavage. Mean ± SEM of 5 animals per group. $^*p<0.008$ vs control. Neutrophils were defined as $Gr1^+/F4/80^-$ cells.

Acknowledgments

We thank Susana Carrasco for technical assistance.

Author Contributions

Conceived and designed the experiments: LSA ABS AO. Performed the experiments: ABS LSA MDSN LBC TB BS. Analyzed the data: ABS AO GDP JJH MRO. Contributed reagents/materials/analysis tools: RS JE GDP JJH. Wrote the paper: ABS LSA AO MLC.

References

1. Santamaría B, Sanz A, Justo P, Catalán M, Sánchez-Niño MD, et al. (2006) Peritoneal defence—lessons learned which apply to diabetes complications. Nephrol Dial Transplant 21 Suppl 2: ii12–15.
2. Flessner MF (2007) Inflammation from sterile dialysis solutions and the longevity of the peritoneal barrier. Clin Nephrol 68: 341–348.
3. Lai KN, Leung JC (2010) Inflammation in peritoneal dialysis. Nephron Clin Pract 116: c11–18.
4. Blake PG (2010) Peritonitis and catheter guidelines—a 2010 update. Perit Dial Int 30: 391–392.

5. Yung S, Chan TM (2012) Pathophysiological changes to the peritoneal membrane during PD-related peritonitis: the role of mesothelial cells. Mediators Inflamm 2012: 484167.
6. Merkle M, Wörnle M (2012) Sclerosing peritonitis: a rare but fatal complication of peritoneal inflammation. Mediators Inflamm 2012: 709673.
7. Campbell S, Michaelson J, Burkly L, Putterman C (2004) The role of TWEAK/Fn14 in the pathogenesis of inflammation and systemic autoimmunity. Front Biosci 9: 2273–2284.
8. Harada N, Nakayama M, Nakano H, Fukuchi Y, Yagita H, et al. (2002) Pro-inflammatory effect of TWEAK/Fn14 interaction on human umbilical vein endothelial cells. Biochem Biophys Res Commun 299: 488–493.
9. Chicheportiche Y, Chicheportiche R, Sizing I, Thompson J, Benjamin CB, et al. (2002) Proinflammatory activity of TWEAK on human dermal fibroblasts and synoviocytes: blocking and enhancing effects of anti-TWEAK monoclonal antibodies. Arthritis Res 4: 126–133.
10. Tran NL, McDonough WS, Savitch BA, Sawyer TF, Winkles JA, et al. (2005) The tumor necrosis factor-like weak inducer of apoptosis (TWEAK)-fibroblast growth factor-inducible 14 (Fn14) signaling system regulates glioma cell survival via NFkappaB pathway activation and BCL-XL/BCL-W expression. J Biol Chem 280: 3483–3492.
11. Winkles JA (2008) The TWEAK-Fn14 cytokine-receptor axis: discovery, biology and therapeutic targeting. Nat Rev Drug Discov 7: 411–425.
12. Blanco-Colio LM, Martin-Ventura JL, Muñóz-García B, Orbe J, Páramo JA, et al. (2007) Identification of soluble tumor necrosis factor-like weak inducer of apoptosis (sTWEAK) as a possible biomarker of subclinical atherosclerosis. Arterioscler Thromb Vasc Biol 27: 916–922.
13. Schwartz N, Su L, Burkly LC, Mackay M, Aranow C, et al. (2006) Urinary TWEAK and the activity of lupus nephritis. J Autoimmun 27: 242–250.
14. Yilmaz MI, Carrero JJ, Ortiz A, Martín-Ventura JL, Sonmez A, et al. (2009) Soluble TWEAK plasma levels as a novel biomarker of endothelial function in patients with chronic kidney disease. Clin J Am Soc Nephrol 4: 1716–1723.
15. Desplat-Jégo S, Varriale S, Creidy R, Terra R, Bernard D, et al. (2002) TWEAK is expressed by glial cells, induces astrocyte proliferation and increases EAE severity. J Neuroimmunol 133: 116–123.
16. Muñoz-García B, Madrigal-Matute J, Moreno JA, Martin-Ventura JL, López-Franco O, et al. (2011) TWEAK-Fn14 interaction enhances plasminogen activator inhibitor 1 and tissue factor expression in atherosclerotic plaques and in cultured vascular smooth muscle cells. Cardiovasc Res 89: 225–233.
17. Muñoz-García B, Moreno JA, López-Franco O, Sanz AB, Martín-Ventura JL, et al. (2009) Tumor necrosis factor-like weak inducer of apoptosis (TWEAK) enhances vascular and renal damage induced by hyperlipidemic diet in ApoE-knockout mice. Arterioscler Thromb Vasc Biol 29: 2061–2068.
18. Sanz AB, Sanchez-Niño MD, Izquierdo MC, Jakubowski A, Justo P, et al. (2009) Tweak induces proliferation in renal tubular epithelium: a role in uninephrectomy induced renal hyperplasia. J Cell Mol Med 13: 3329–3342.
19. Sanz AB, Justo P, Sanchez-Niño MD, Blanco-Colio LM, Winkles JA, et al. (2008) The cytokine TWEAK modulates renal tubulointerstitial inflammation. J Am Soc Nephrol 19: 695–703.
20. Sanz AB, Sanchez-Niño MD, Izquierdo MC, Jakubowski A, Justo P, et al. (2010) TWEAK activates the non-canonical NFkappaB pathway in murine renal tubular cells: modulation of CCL21. PLoS One 5: e8955.
21. Del Peso G, Jiménez-Heffernan JA, Bajo MA, Aroeira LS, Aguilera A, et al. (2008) Epithelial-to-mesenchymal transition of mesothelial cells is an early event during peritoneal dialysis and is associated with high peritoneal transport. Kidney Int Suppl: S26–33.
22. Catalan MP, Subirá D, Reyero A, Selgas R, Ortiz-Gonzalez A, et al. (2003) Regulation of apoptosis by lethal cytokines in human mesothelial cells. Kidney Int 64: 321–330.
23. Santamaría B, Benito-Martin A, Ucero AC, Aroeira LS, Reyero A, et al. (2009) A nanoconjugate Apaf-1 inhibitor protects mesothelial cells from cytokine-induced injury. PLoS One 4: e6634.
24. Sanchez-Niño MD, Sanz AB, Lorz C, Gnirke A, Rastaldi MP, et al. (2010) BASP1 promotes apoptosis in diabetic nephropathy. J Am Soc Nephrol 21: 610–621.
25. Sanchez-Niño MD, Sanz AB, Ihalmo P, Lassila M, Holthofer H, et al. (2009) The MIF receptor CD74 in diabetic podocyte injury. J Am Soc Nephrol 20: 353–362.
26. Aroeira LS, Loureiro J, González-Mateo GT, Fernandez-Millara V, del Peso G, et al. (2008) Characterization of epithelial-to-mesenchymal transition of mesothelial cells in a mouse model of chronic peritoneal exposure to high glucose dialysate. Perit Dial Int 28 Suppl 5: S29–33.
27. Moreno JA, Izquierdo MC, Sanchez-Niño MD, Suárez-Alvarez B, Lopez-Larrea C, et al. (2011) The inflammatory cytokines TWEAK and TNFα reduce renal klotho expression through NFκB. J Am Soc Nephrol 22: 1315–1325.
28. Tacke F, Randolph GJ (2006) Migratory fate and differentiation of blood monocyte subsets. Immunobiology 211: 609–618.
29. Sanz AB, Sanchez-Niño MD, Ramos AM, Moreno JA, Santamaria B, et al. (2010) NF-kappaB in renal inflammation. J Am Soc Nephrol 21: 1254–1262.
30. Sakai N, Wada T, Yokoyama H, Lipp M, Ueha S, et al. (2006) Secondary lymphoid tissue chemokine (SLC/CCL21)/CCR7 signaling regulates fibrocytes in renal fibrosis. Proc Natl Acad Sci U S A 103: 14098–14103.
31. Sanz AB, Sanchez-Niño MD, Ortiz A (2011) TWEAK, a multifunctional cytokine in kidney injury. Kidney Int 80: 708–718.
32. Dasgupta MK, Larabie M, Halloran PF (1994) Interferon-gamma levels in peritoneal dialysis effluents: relation to peritonitis. Kidney Int 46: 475–481.
33. Brauner A, Hylander B, Wretlind B (1996) Tumor necrosis factor-alpha, interleukin-1 beta, and interleukin-1 receptor antagonist in dialysate and serum from patients on continuous ambulatory peritoneal dialysis. Am J Kidney Dis 27: 402–408.
34. Zemel D, Imholz AL, de Waart DR, Dinkla C, Struijk DG, et al. (1994) Appearance of tumor necrosis factor-alpha and soluble TNF-receptors I and II in peritoneal effluent of CAPD. Kidney Int 46: 1422–1430.
35. McLoughlin RM, Witowski J, Robson RL, Wilkinson TS, Hurst SM, et al. (2003) Interplay between IFN-gamma and IL-6 signaling governs neutrophil trafficking and apoptosis during acute inflammation. J Clin Invest 112: 598–607.
36. Margetts PJ, Kolb M, Yu L, Hoff CM, Holmes CJ, et al. (2002) Inflammatory cytokines, angiogenesis, and fibrosis in the rat peritoneum. Am J Pathol 160: 2285–2294.
37. Loureiro J, Aguilera A, Selgas R, Sandoval P, Albar-Vizcaíno P, et al. (2011) Blocking TGF-β1 protects the peritoneal membrane from dialysate-induced damage. J Am Soc Nephrol 22: 1682–1695.
38. Cina D, Patel P, Bethune JC, Thoma J, Rodriguez-Lecompte JC, et al. (2009) Peritoneal morphological and functional changes associated with platelet-derived growth factor B. Nephrol Dial Transplant. 24: 448–457.
39. Margetts PJ, Kolb M, Galt T, Hoff CM, Shockley TR, et al. (2001) Gene transfer of transforming growth factor-beta1 to the rat peritoneum: effects on membrane function. J Am Soc Nephrol 12: 2029–2039.
40. Hurst SM, Wilkinson TS, McLoughlin RM, Jones S, Horiuchi S, et al. (2001) Il-6 and its soluble receptor orchestrate a temporal switch in the pattern of leukocyte recruitment seen during acute inflammation. Immunity 14: 705–714.
41. Qian BZ, Li J, Zhang H, Kitamura T, Zhang J, et al. (2011) CCL2 recruits inflammatory monocytes to facilitate breast-tumour metastasis. Nature 475: 222–225.
42. Xia Y, Campbell SR, Broder A, Herlitz L, Abadi M, et al. (2012) Inhibition of the TWEAK/Fn14 pathway attenuates renal disease in nephrotoxic serum nephritis. Clin Immunol 145: 108–121.
43. Michaelson JS, Wisniacki N, Burkly LC, Putterman C (2012) Role of TWEAK in lupus nephritis: a bench-to-bedside review. J Autoimmun 39: 130–142.

8

The Alternative Pathway of Complement Activation May Be Involved in the Renal Damage of Human Anti-Glomerular Basement Membrane Disease

Rui Ma[1,2], Zhao Cui[1]*, Shui-Yi Hu[1], Xiao-Yu Jia[1], Rui Yang[1], Xin Zheng[1], Jie Ao[1], Gang Liu[1], Yun-Hua Liao[2], Ming-Hui Zhao[1,3]

1 Renal Division, Department of Medicine, Peking University First Hospital, Peking University Institute of Nephrology, Key Laboratory of Renal Disease, Ministry of Health of China, Key Laboratory of Chronic Kidney Disease Prevention and Treatment (Peking University), Ministry of Education of China, Beijing, China, **2** Renal Division, Department of Medicine, First Affiliated Hospital of Guangxi Medical University, Nanning, Guangxi Zhuang Autonomous Region, China, **3** Peking-Tsinghua Center for Life Sciences, Beijing, China

Abstract

Linear deposition of IgG and complement 3 (C3) along glomerular basement membrane (GBM) is generally revealed in the kidneys of human anti-GBM disease. Our recent studies demonstrated the pathogenic role of complement activation in renal damage of this disease. However, the pathways of complement activation were still paradoxical. In this study, renal biopsy tissues from 10 patients with anti-GBM disease were used to investigate the pathways of complement activation by detecting the deposition of various complement components, including C1q, factor B, factor P (properdin), mannose-binding lectin (MBL), C3d, C4d and C5b-9, using immunohistochemistry and immunofluorescence. We found that C1q, factor B, properdin, C3d, C4d and C5b-9 were detected in all the glomeruli of our patients, along GBM with a linear and/or granular staining pattern. Furthermore, C1q, factor B and properdin co-localized well with C5b-9. The properdin also co-localized well with C3d. However, the deposition of MBL was diffusive in mesangium, GBM, Bowman's capsule and within crescents and was not co-localized with C5b-9 but partially co-localized with C4d. The intensity of factor B deposition (3.3 vs. 1.2, $P<0.001$) and C5b-9 deposition (3.2 vs. 1.6, $P<0.001$) was significantly stronger in the glomeruli with crescent formation, compared with the glomeruli without crescents. The complement system is overall activated via both the alternative pathway and classical pathway in the kidneys of human anti-GBM disease. The alternative pathway might play an important role in complement activation induced renal damage.

Editor: Suzan H. M. Rooijakkers, University Medical Center Utrecht, Netherlands

Funding: This work was supported by a grant of Chinese 973 project (No. 2012CB517702), a grant from Natural Science Fund of China to the Innovation Research Group (81321064) and a grant of National Natural Science Fund of China (81370801). The funders had no role in study design, data collection and analysis, decision to publish, or preparation of the manuscript.

* E-mail: cuizhao@bjmu.edu.cn

Introduction

Anti-glomerular basement membrane (GBM) disease is a rare but life-threatening autoimmune disease, which clinically manifests rapidly progressive glomerulonephritis with or without pulmonary hemorrhage [1,2]. IgG autoantibodies against the non-collagenous domain of $\alpha3$ chain of type IV collagen on GBM [$\alpha3$(IV)NC1] have been proven to be pathogenic in the disease [3,4]. The presence of circulating anti-GBM autoantibodies and linear deposition of IgG along glomerular capillary wall (GCW) are the characteristics of this disease [2]. In the renal biopsy of patients, linear deposition of IgG is often accompanied by complement 3 (C3) deposits, also on GCW in linear or granular staining pattern, which indicates that complement activation is involved in the kidney injury [5]. Our recent study in human anti-GBM disease also identified that the plasma level of the terminal component of complement activation, C5b-9, also named as membrane attack complex, was closely associated with the severity of kidney damage and was the predictor for renal failure during patient follow up [6].

The pathways of complement activation in anti-GBM disease are largely studied by passive injection of heterologous antibodies against GBM. This model in mice with complete deficiency of C3 or C4 revealed a protective effect of C3 deficiency more than that of C4 deficiency, which suggests the involvement of classical pathway and/or lectin pathway, and the involvement of alternative pathway in the complement activation [7,8,9]. However, none of the three pathways is clearly identified or excluded. In human anti-GBM disease, the pathways of complement activation are also poorly understood. Although anti-GBM disease is a well-known autoantibody induced disease, C1q, the key component of classical pathway, is seldom found deposit in the renal biopsy specimens [5]. In the present study, we investigated the deposition of various complement components in the renal biopsy specimens from patients with anti-GBM disease, with the aim to clarify the pathways of complement activation in the kidney injury of human anti-GBM disease.

Table 1. The species, dilutions and sources of primary antibodies for the detection of each complement component.

Complements	Species	Dilutions	Sources
C1q	Mouse anti-human monoclonal	1:4000 (IHC)	Abcam, Cambridge, UK
		1:400 (IF)	
Factor B	Mouse anti-human monoclonal	1:50	Quidel, San Diego, CA, USA
Properdin	Mouse anti-human monoclonal	1:50	Lifespan Biosciences, WA, USA
MBL	Mouse anti-human monoclonal	1:30	Abcam, Cambridge, UK
C3d	Rabbit anti-human polyclonal	1:1000 (IHC)	Dako A/S, Copenhagen, Denmark
		1:100 (IF)	
C4d	Rabbit anti-human polyclonal	1:400 (IHC)	Abcam, Cambridge, UK
		1:40 (IF)	
C5b-9	Mouse anti-human monoclonal	1:50 (IHC)	Abcam, Cambridge, UK
	Rabbit anti-human polyclonal	1:20 (IF)	

MBL: mannose-binding lectin, IHC: immunohistochemistry, IF: immunofluorescence.

Materials and Methods

Patients

Consecutive renal biopsy tissues were collected from 10 patients with anti-GBM disease admitted in Peking University First Hospital from 2002 to 2007. All the 10 patients had a positive test for circulating anti-GBM autoantibodies by enzyme-linked immunosorbent assay (ELISA) using purified bovine α(IV)NC1 as solid phase antigen, with confirmation of antibody specificity by ELISA against recombinant human α3(IV)NC1. Patients with any other coexisting diseases such as membranous nephropathy were excluded. The clinical data were collected from medical records. As complement activation has been considered to be not involved in minimal change disease, renal biopsy specimens from 5 such patients were used as disease control. Renal tissues obtained from the normal part of a nephrectomized kidney due to renal carcinoma were used as normal control. Each patient gave written inform consent when renal biopsy was performed and this study was in compliance of the Declaration of Helsinki and approved by the ethics committee of Pecking University first hospital.

Renal Histopathology

Renal biopsy was performed at the time of diagnosis. For light microscopy, paraffin sections were stained with haematoxylin and eosin, periodic acid-schiff, periodic acid-silver methenamine and Masson's trichrome. For electron microscopy, biopsy materials were fixed in glutaraldehyde, postfixed in osmium tetroxide, dehydrated in graded acetone and embedded in Epon 812 resin. Ultrathin sections were stained with uranyl acetate and lead citrate, and examined by a transmission electron microscope JEM-1230 (JEOL, Tokyo, Japan). For direct immunofluorescence, frozen sections were examined by fluorescent microscope (Nikon, Tokyo, Japan) after staining with fluorescein isothiocyanate (FITC) -conjugated antibodies specific for human IgG, IgM, IgA, C3c, C1q, fibrinogen and albumin (Dako A/S, Copenhagen, Denmark).

Detection of Renal Deposition of Complement Components by Immunohistochemistry

Staining of single complement component was performed by immunohistochemistry as our previously described [10]. To investigate the complement activation, immunohistochemical staining was performed for C1q, factor B, C3d, C4d and C5b-9 using primary antibodies listed in Table 1. 10% formalin-fixed, paraffin embedded renal tissues was cut into 4 μm sections. After deparaffinized in xylene and rehydrated in grading alcohols, sections were incubated in 3% H_2O_2 for 10 min at room temperature and in dark to quench endogenous peroxidase activity. Appropriate pretreatments for antigen retrieval were predetermined. Pepsin pretreatment consisted of 0.4% pepsin (Zhongshan Golden Bridge Biotechnology, Beijing, China) to sections for 45 min at 37°C. Proteinase K pretreatment consisted of 0.5 mg/ml proteinase K (Roche, Switzerland) to sections for 10 min at 37°C. After pretreatments, all sections were blocked non-specific staining for 30 min at room temperature with 3% bovine serum albumin, and then incubated with primary antibody overnight at 4°C. All the antibodies' optimal dilutions were predetermined by means of titration on renal sections from patients with lupus nephritis and IgA nephropathy. Dako EnVision HRP (Dako A/S, Copenhagen, Denmark) was used as detection system, which was an avidin-free two-step indirect method with goat anti-rabbit and goat anti-mouse immunoglobulins conjugated with horseradish peroxidase as secondary antibodies. The secondary antibodies were incubated for 30 min at 37°C and the sections were developed in fresh hydrogen peroxide plus 3-3-diaminobenzidine tetrahydrochloride solution for 1 min. Finally, the sections were counterstained with hematoxylin, differentiated with acid alcohol, dehydrated and cleared in alcohols and xylene, and coverslipped with permount. The sections were examined by light microscopy. As negative controls, normal rabbit IgG or normal mouse IgG replaced the primary antibodies.

Detection of Renal Deposition of Complement Components by Immunofluorescence Using Laser Scanning Confocal Microscopy

Sections were cut into 5 μm slides from frozen renal biopsy tissues and then air-dried for 25 min at room temperature and fixed in −20°C pre-cooled acetone for 10 min at 4°C. After washed three times with phosphate buffered saline, sections were incubated in 3% bovine serum albumin for 30 min at room temperature. Mouse antibodies against C1q, factor B, properdin and MBL were incubated overnight at 4°C as primary antibodies, respectively (Table 1). FITC-labeled goat anti-mouse IgG

Table 2. The demographic, clinical and pathological parameters of patients with anti-GBM disease.

Patient	Gender	Age	pulmonary hemorrhage	SCr (μmol/L)	Anti-GBM antibodies in circulation (U/mL)	ANCA	Percentage of crescents in glomeruli	Routine direct immunofluorescence						
								IgG	IgA	IgM	C3c	C1q	FRA	Alb
1	Male	23	+	581	33	–	100%	3+ (GCW)	–	–	–	–	–	–
2	Male	23	+	224	13	–	90%	3+ (GCW)	–	–	3+ (GCW)	–	–	–
3	Male	20	+	551	21	–	100%	3+ (GCW)	–	–	3+ (GCW)	–	–	–
4	Male	59	–	427	13	–	82%	+ (GCW)	–	–	2+ (Ms)	–	–	–
5	Male	22	–	269	96		84%	–	–	–	–	–	–	–
6	Male	66	–	796	116	+	100%	2+ (GCW)	–	–	–	–	–	–
7	Male	62	+	955	176	+	100%	3+ (GCW)	–	+ (Ms)	3+ (GCW)	+ (GCW)	3+ (GCW)	–
8	Female	30	–	682	60	–	100%	2+ (GCW)	–	+ (Ms)	2+ (Ms)	–	+ (Ms)	–
9	Female	21	+	614	113	–	100%	3+ (GCW)	–	–	–	–	–	–
10	Female	21	+	475	60	–	91%	–	–	–	–	–	+ (Ms)	–

SCr: serum creatinine, ANCA: anti-neutrophil cytoplasmic antibodies, FRA: fibrinogen related antigens, Alb: albumin, GCW: glomerular capillary wall, Ms: mesangium.
This study included two patients with negative staining for linear IgG, possibly because of the severe destruction of glomerular capillary walls. The diagnosis was confirmed by the detection of anti-GBM IgG in serum and linear IgG staining on paraffin tissue by immunofluorescence.

(Zhongshan Golden Bridge Biotechnology, Beijing, China) diluted 1:30, was used as secondary antibodies for 30 min at 37°C. Next, rabbit anti-C5b-9 antibodies were added to the sections with C1q, factor B, properdin and MBL; rabbit anti-C3d antibodies were added to the sections with properdin; rabbit anti-C4d antibodies were added to the sections with MBL for 60 min at 37°C (Table 1). Tetramethylrhodamine isothiocyanate (TRITC) -labeled goat anti-rabbit IgG (Zhongshan Golden Bridge Biotechnology, Beijing, China) diluted 1:30, was used as secondary antibodies for 30 min at 37°C. The sections were air-dried in dark, mounted with citifluor (Zhongshan Golden Bridge Biotechnology, Beijing, China), and visualised using a fluorescence microscopy (Nikon 80i, Tokyo, Japan) and a confocal microscope (Olympus viewer 1000, Tokyo, Japan). Renal tissue sections from patients with lupus nephritis and IgA nephropathy were used as positive controls. As negative controls, normal rabbit IgG or normal mouse IgG replaced the primary antibodies.

Criteria for Semiquantitative Scoring

Two pathologists evaluated all sections separately, blinded to each other and the patients' data. Differences in scoring between the two pathologists were resolved by re-reviewing the sections and coming to a consensus.

The intensity of GCW staining of complement components was evaluated at 400× magnification and scored on a scale of 0 to 4+: 0, no staining; 1, mild staining; 2, moderate staining; 3, moderate-high staining; and 4, high staining on a high-power field.

Co-localization of different complement components was judged by merging of the green fluorescence of FITC and the red fluorescence of TRITC.

Statistical Analysis

Differences in quantitative parameters between groups were assessed using Student *t*-test (for normally distributed data) or nonparametric test (for non-normally distributed data). Differences in semiquantitative data were tested using Kruskal Wallis H one-way analysis and Mann-Whitney U test. Differences in qualitative data were compared using Chi square test. Pearson's correlation test was used to measure the correlation between two normally distributed variables. Spearman's correlation test was used to measure the correlation between two non-normally distributed variables or one normally with one non-normally distributed variable. All statistical analyses were two-tailed and $P<0.05$ was considered as significant. Analysis was performed using SPSS statistical software package, version 13.0 (SPSS Inc., Chicago, IL, USA).

Results

Demographic, clinical and pathological data of patients with anti-GBM disease

The demographic, clinical and pathological parameters of the 10 patients with anti-GBM disease were listed in Table 2. Among them, 7 were male and 3 were female with a median age of 23 years (range, 20–66 years). 6 (60%) patients had pulmonary hemorrhage and presented as Goodpasture syndrome. The mean level of serum creatinine was 557.4±224.2 μmol/L at presentation. 2 (20%) patients had positive ANCA, both with specificity for MPO.

All the 10 patients received renal biopsy with an average of 29.3±12.4 glomeruli seen in each section. All the patients were diagnosed as crescentic glomerulonephritis (over 50% of the glomeruli had larger crescents) with a mean percentage of crescent formation in 85.3±14.6% of the glomeruli. The percentage of

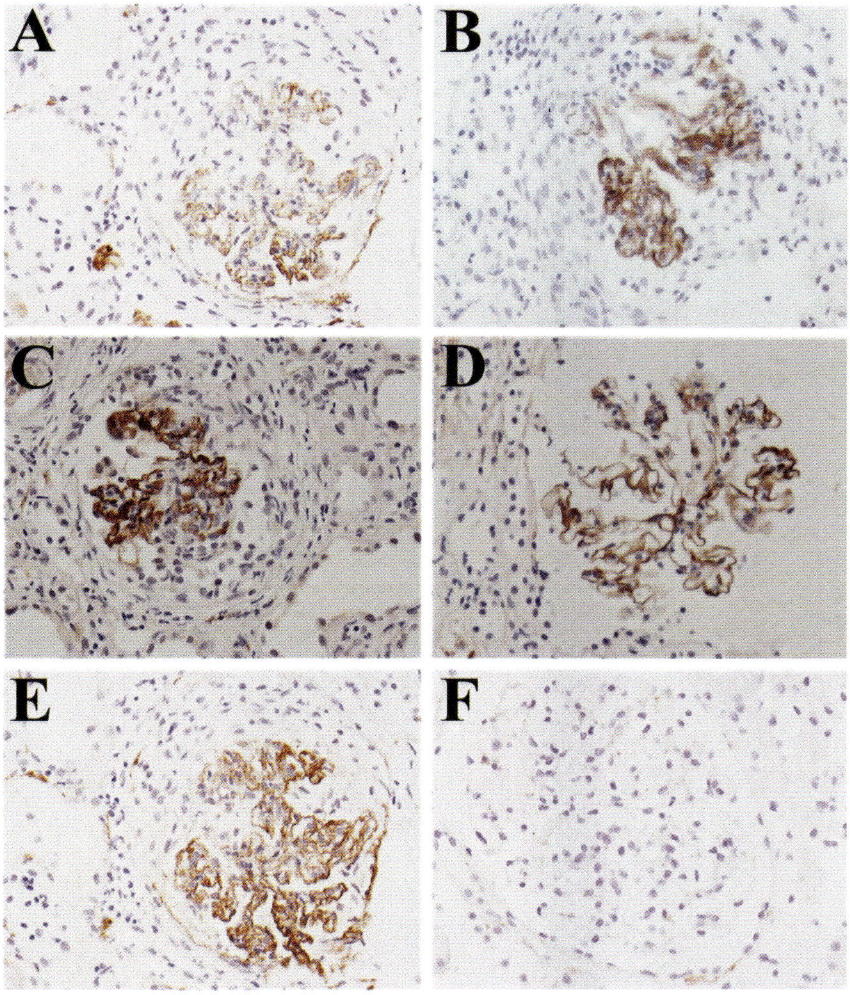

Figure 1. Complement components C5b-9, C3d, C4d, C1q and factor B were detected on paraffin sections of renal tissues from patients with anti-GBM disease by immunohistochemistry (magnification ×400). A: C5b-9 linear deposition along the glomerular capillary wall (Patient #7); B: C3d linear deposition along the capillary wall (Patient #2); C: C4d linear deposition along the capillary wall (Patient #5); D: C1q linear deposition along the capillary wall (Patient #1); E: factor B linear deposition along the capillary wall (Patient #7); F: all the complement components above were negative in the renal tissues from patients with minimal change disease.

crescents in glomeruli was positively correlated with the concentration of serum creatinine at presentation ($r = 0.83$, $P = 0.003$). Routine direct immunofluorescence showed that linear IgG deposition along GBM was detected in eight (80%) patients with fluorescence intensity +~3+ on the scale of 0 to 4+. Five (50%) patients had linear or granular C3c deposition along GBM with fluorescence intensity 2+~3+. Only one patient had mild deposition of C1q along GBM.

Deposition of Complement Components in Glomeruli

C5b-9. C5b-9, also called membrane attack complex, represents the terminal product of complement activation. The number of glomeruli scored per biopsy of paraffin sections was 5.8±2.3 (range 2–9) in immunohistochemistry staining. C5b-9 was detected clearly in a linear pattern along the GCW in 29 (100%) glomeruli of all the 10 patients, and in several glomeruli along the tubular basement membrane (Figure 1A). Occasionally, C5b-9 was found in the mesangial regions or the small artery walls in a mild granular pattern. The intensity of C5b-9 staining was scored as 1 (2/29 glomeruli), 2 (6/29 glomeruli), 3 (15/29 glomeruli) and 4 (6/29 glomeruli) (Table 3). Compared with the glomeruli without crescent formation, the intensity of C5b-9 deposition was much stronger (3.2 vs. 1.6, $P<0.001$) in glomeruli with crescent formation. No deposit of C5b-9 was found in renal biopsy specimens from patients with minimal change disease or normal control renal tissue.

C3d. The number of glomeruli scored for C3d per biopsy of paraffin sections was 6.6±3.8 (range 2–10). C3d was detected clearly in a linear or granular pattern along the GCW of 33 (100%) glomeruli of all the 10 patients (Figure 1B). The intensity of C3d was scored as 1 (4/33 glomeruli), 2 (4/33 glomeruli), 3 (17/33 glomeruli) and 4 (8/33 glomeruli) (Table 3). No correlation was found between the intensity of C3d deposition and the clinical characteristics of patients.

C4d. The number of glomeruli scored for C4d per biopsy of paraffin sections was 8.8±4.2 (range 4–15). C4d could be detected clearly along the GCW in a linear pattern (Figure 1C). 50/53 (94.3%) glomeruli were positive for C4d deposition, with the

Table 3. The deposition of complement components in glomeruli of patients with anti-GBM disease.

Complement	Glomeruli per section (mean±SD)	Glomerular capillary walls, n (%)	Mesangial regions, n (%)	Crescents, n (%)	Bowman's capsules, n (%)	Scores			
						1	2	3	4
C5b-9	5.8±2.3	29/29 (100%)	12/29(41.4%)	0/29(0%)	3/29(10.3%)	2/29	6/29	15/29	6/29
C3d	6.6±3.8	33/33(100%)	7/33(21.2%)	0/29(0%)	0/29(0%)	4/33	4/33	17/33	8/33
C4d	8.8±4.2	50/53(94.3%)	5/53(9.4%)	0/53(0%)	0/53(0%)	6/50	11/50	29/50	4/50
C1q	7.6±3.6	76/76(100%)	13/76(17.1%)	0/76(0%)	55/76(72.4%)	13/76	39/76	20/76	4/76
MBL	3.3±1.0	13/13(100%)	13/13(100%)	9/13(69%)	10/13(76.9%)	0/13	3/13	10/13	0/13
Factor B	4.2±2.3	21/21(100%)	7/21(33.3%)	0/21(0%)	0/21(0%)	2/21	4/21	15/21	0/21
Properdin	3.0±1.0	9/9(100%)	3/9(33.3%)	0/9(0%)	0/9(0%)	0/9	0/9	9/9	0/9

SD: standard deviation, MBL: mannose-binding lectin.

intensity scored as 1 (6/50 glomeruli), 2 (11/50 glomeruli), 3 (29/50 glomeruli) and 4 (4/50 glomeruli) (Table 3). We found no correlation between the intensities of C4d deposition and the clinical features of patients.

C1q. C1q represents the classical pathway of complement activation. The number of glomeruli scored for C1q per biopsy of paraffin sections was 7.6±3.6 (range 4–13). C1q linear deposition could be found along the GCW and the Bowman's capsules in 76 (100%) glomeruli of all the 10 patients (Figure 1D). The intensity was scored as 1 (13/76 glomeruli), 2 (39/76 glomeruli), 3 (20/76 glomeruli) and 4 (4/76 glomeruli) (Table 3). We found no correlation between the intensities of C1q deposition and the clinical features of patients.

MBL. MBL represents the lectin pathway of complement activation. The number of glomeruli scored for MBL per biopsy of frozen sections was 3.3±1.0 (range 2–4) using immunofluorescence. MBL diffusive deposition could be detected along GCW, in mesangial regions and in crescents in a linear or granular pattern (Figure 2A). 13/13 (100%) glomeruli in frozen sections were positive for MBL deposition, with the intensity scored as 1 (0/13 glomeruli), 2 (3/13 glomeruli), 3 (10/13 glomeruli) and 4 (0/13 glomeruli) (Table 3). We found no correlation between the intensities of MBL deposition and the clinical features of patients.

Factor B and Properdin. Factor B and properdin both represent the alternative pathway of complement activation. The number of glomeruli scored for factor B per biopsy of paraffin sections was 4.2±2.3 (range 2–8) using immunohistochemistry. Factor B deposition could be detected along GCW in a linear and granular pattern (Figure 1E). 21/21 (100%) glomeruli were all positive for factor B deposition, with the intensity scored as 1 (2/21 glomeruli), 2 (4/21 glomeruli), 3 (15/21 glomeruli) and 4 (0/21 glomeruli) (Table 3). The intensity of factor B deposition was related with the crescent formation in glomeruli. The intensity of factor B deposition was significantly stronger in the glomeruli with crescent formation (3.3 vs. 1.2, $P<0.001$), compared with the glomeruli without crescent.

The number of glomeruli scored for properdin per biopsy of frozen sections was 3.0±1.0 (range 2–4) using immunofluorescence. Properdin deposition showed a linear deposition on GCW in all patients (Figure 2B). 9/9 (100%) glomeruli were positive for properdin deposition, with the intensity scored as 1 (0/9 glomeruli), 2 (0/9 glomeruli), 3 (9/9 glomeruli) and 4 (0/9 glomeruli) (Table 3). All the glomeruli had crescent formation.

Co-localization of Complement Components by Immunofluorescence

By immunofluorescence and laser scanning confocal microscopy, the positive staining of IgG, C5b-9, C4d, C3d, C1q, MBL, factor B and properdin was further confirmed on the glomeruli of patients with anti-GBM disease (Figure 3).

IgG co-localized with C3d exactly along the GCW (Figure 3A–C). C1q, factor B and properdin co-localized with C5b-9 exactly along the GCW too (Figure 3D–L). Furthermore, properdin co-localized with C3d along the GCW (Figure 3M–O). As for MBL, it was found just partially co-localized with C4d (Figure 3S–U), but was not co-localized with C5b-9 at all (Figure 3P–Q).

In this study, we detected all the three pathways of complement activation, which included seven kinds of complement components. Confocal microscopy was also performed for all the three pathways. These examinations consumed lots of sections from the renal biopsy tissues, which made the renal tissues not sufficient for all the detections on all the ten patients. The staining for C1q was performed for all patients, while C4d for six patients, C5b-9, C3d

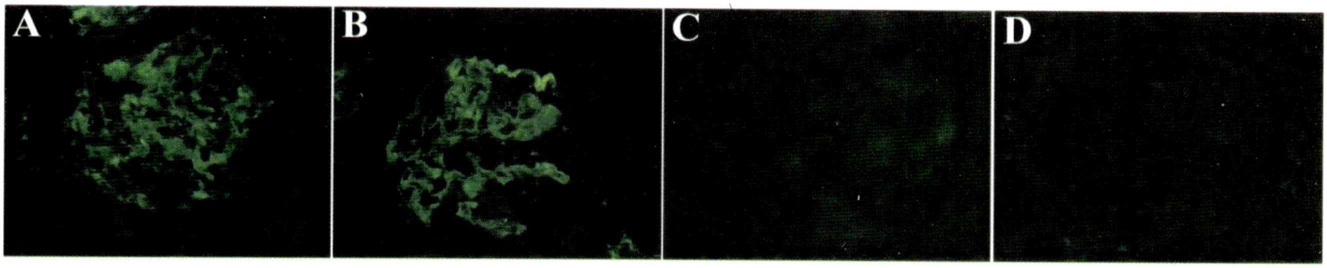

Figure 2. Complement components MBL and properdin were detected on frozen renal tissues from patients with anti-GBM disease by immunofluorescence (magnification ×400). A: MBL diffusive granular deposition on the glomerular capillary wall, mesangial region and crescent in the glomeruli (Patient #4); B: properdin linear deposition along the capillary wall (Patient #10); C: MBL were negative in the renal tissues from patients with minimal change disease; D: Properdin was negative in the renal tissues from patients with minimal change disease.

and factor B for five patients, MBL for four patients and properdin for three patients.

Discussion

In our present study, C3d deposition on glomerular capillary wall was shown in each glomerulus of all patients with anti-GBM disease, even in those C3c negative cases, which indicated that the complement system was activated after the binding of anti-GBM IgG to the target antigens. C3c is in free state and C3d binds covalently via thiolester bond on the membrane of activated site [11]. Thus C3c indicates the ongoing complement activation while C3d can be detected not only at the active lesions but also where after complement activation [12]. In the current study, the general finding of C3d deposition on the capillary wall reflects the activation of complement system during the renal damage process of human anti-GBM disease.

C3 can be activated via the classical, the lectin or the alternative pathway. Classical pathway is initiated with C1q binding to the immune complex. We detected C1q deposition along the glomerular capillary wall in each patient. The same result was found on C4d, the later component of classical activation. Furthermore, C1q deposition co-localized well with C5b-9, the terminal complement complex. These findings indicate the participation of classical pathway in the complement activation of human anti-GBM disease. This was also proven using the C1q knockout mice, in which the kidney injury and C3 deposition caused by the induction of heterologous anti-GBM antibodies were attenuated in comparison with the wild type mice [8]. The absence of C1q in routine direct immunofluorescence on renal biopsy examination is commonly observed, not simply in anti-GBM disease, which may be explained by the following reasons. Unlike C3d and C4d, C1q does not bind covalently to its ligands, which results in its short half-life time *in vivo* and easy to be cleared by macrophages [13]. Also, the lack of anti-C1q antibody in the disease could not display the local stabilizing effect for C1q deposition as it does in lupus nephritis [14].

Factor B and properdin are unique factors needed in the alternative complement pathway. In the present study, we identified the deposition of factor B and properdin along the glomerular capillary wall in each patient. Furthermore, the deposition of factor B and properdin both co-localized well with C5b-9. Properdin could co-localize with C3d as well. These findings indicate the activation of alternative pathway. Bb is a split product after factor B activation, which makes our detection more definite for the indication of alternative complement activation [15]. Properdin is a positive regulation protein, which binds to the C3 convertase, C3bBb, and protects it from the cleavage effects of factor H and factor I [16]. In C4 knockout mice, which lack an intact classical pathway and lectin pathway, the injection of heterologous anti-GBM antibodies could still produce almost the same degree of proteinuria as compared with the wild type mice [8]. These findings provide evidence for the involvement of alternative complement activation in anti-GBM disease.

MBL is the key molecule in the activation of lectin pathway [17,18,19]. We did find the deposition of MBL in our patients; however, the staining appeared diffusively, not only on the glomerular capillary wall, but also in the mesangial region, Bowman's capsule and even within the crescents. In addition, MBL could not co-localize with C5b-9 and just partially co-localized with C4d, which indicates that the lectin pathway may be not involved in the complement activation of human anti-GBM disease. The reason for MBL deposition, we suggested, should attribute to its general binding to the carbohydrate ligands, including mannose and N-acetylglucosamine, which were greatly exposed during the glomerular damage of the disease.

In this current study, we found a positive correlation between the intensity of factor B deposition and the crescent formation in glomeruli. The staining intensity of factor B was much stronger in glomeruli with crescents. Our recent study on the circulating complement also found a positive correlation between the plasma level of factor B and the severity of kidney injury. Thus it is implied indirectly that the alternative complement activation might play a pathogenic role in the renal damage of the disease. The pathogenic role of the alternative pathway can only be demonstrated in a GBM model using properdin-deficient and C1q-deficient animals. When properdin-deficient animals show reduced proteinuria and glomerular injury, this may clearly proves that the alternative pathway is pathogenic. However, at this stage this is still for debate.

The alternative pathway might exert the pathogenic role through the following processes. Firstly, the classical pathway is triggered by anti-GBM antibody bindings; then the activation and generation of inflammatory molecules might be further amplified by the alternative pathway [20,15]. In an arthritis model, Ji et al [21] have shown that the alternative pathway is critical for the recruitment and/or activation of polymorphonuclear leukocytes and development of arthritis, while the classical pathway are entirely dispensable for the effect phase of arthritis. Indeed, the alternative pathway may participate in 80% of total complement activation and be both required and sufficient for tissue injury [22,23,24]. Secondly, properdin itself can act as the pathogen recognition protein, binds to the apoptotic cells and target surfaces, and then initiates and amplifies the alternative complement activation [25,26,27,28]. All these characteristics may

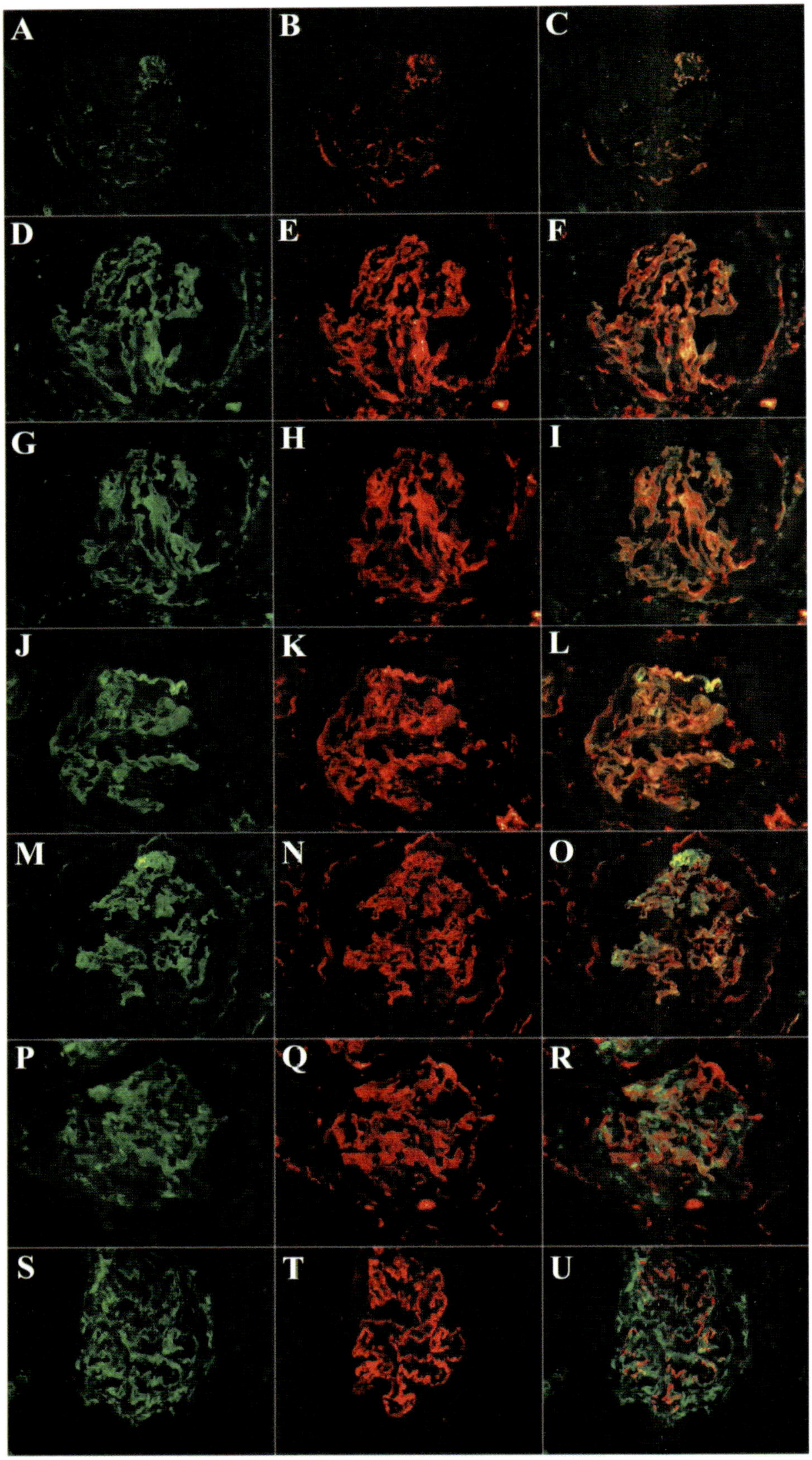
A
B
C
D
E
F
G
H
I
J
K
L
M
N
O
P
Q
R
S
T
U

Figure 3. Co-localization of various complement components were detected in frozen sections by immunofluorescence using laser confocal microscopy (magnification ×400). A: IgG linear deposition along the glomerular capillary wall; B: C3d granular deposition along the glomerular capillary wall in the same section; C: IgG and C3d co-localized completely; D: C1q linear deposition along the glomerular capillary wall; E: C5b-9 granular deposition along the glomerular capillary wall in the same section; F: C1q and C5b-9 co-localized completely; G: factor B linear deposition along the glomerular capillary wall; H: C5b-9 granular deposition along the glomerular capillary wall in the same section; I: factor B and C5b-9 co-localized completely; J: properdin linear deposition along the glomerular capillary wall; K: C5b-9 granular deposition along the glomerular capillary wall in the same section; L: properdin and C5b-9 co-localized completely; M: properdin linear deposition along the glomerular capillary wall; N: C3d granular deposition along the glomerular capillary wall in the same section; O: properdin and C3d co-localized completely; P: MBL diffusive deposition; Q: C5b-9 granular deposition along the glomerular capillary wall in the same section; R: MBL and C5b-9 could not co-localize; S: MBL diffusive deposition; T: C4d granular deposition along the glomerular capillary wall in the same section; U: MBL and C4d partially co-localized along the glomerular capillary wall.

contribute to the pathogenic role of alternative pathway in the kidney injury of human anti-GBM disease.

In conclusion, the present study demonstrates that the complement system is overall activated, via the classical pathway and the alternative pathway, in the kidney of human anti-GBM disease. The alternative complement activation might play a pathogenic role in the process of renal damage.

Acknowledgments

The technical support by Miao Wang was greatly appreciated.

Author Contributions

Conceived and designed the experiments: ZC MHZ. Performed the experiments: RM SYH XYJ RY. Analyzed the data: RM. Contributed reagents/materials/analysis tools: XZ JA GL YHL. Wrote the paper: RM.

References

1. Cui Z, Zhao MH, Xin G, Wang HY (2005) Characteristics and prognosis of Chinese patients with anti-glomerular basement membrane disease. Nephron Clin Pract 99: c49–55.
2. Kluth DC, Rees AJ (1999) Anti-glomerular basement membrane disease. J Am Soc Nephrol 10: 2446–2453.
3. Segelmark M, Hellmark T, Wieslander J (2003) The prognostic significance in Goodpasture's disease of specificity, titre and affinity of anti-glomerular-basement-membrane antibodies. Nephron Clin Pract 94: c59–68.
4. Lerner RA, Glassock RJ, Dixon FJ (1999) The role of anti-glomerular basement membrane antibody in the pathogenesis of human glomerulonephritis. J Am Soc Nephrol 10: 1389–1404.
5. Fischer EG, Lager DJ (2006) Anti-glomerular basement membrane glomerulonephritis: a morphologic study of 80 cases. Am J Clin Pathol 125: 445–450.
6. Ma R, Cui Z, Liao YH, Zhao MH (2013) Complement Activation Contributes to the Injury and Outcome of Kidney in Human Anti-glomerular Basement Membrane Disease. J Clin Immunol 33: 172–178.
7. Sheerin NS, Springall T, Carroll MC, Hartley B, Sacks SH (1997) Protection against anti-glomerular basement membrane (GBM)-mediated nephritis in C3- and C4-deficient mice. Clin Exp Immunol 110: 403–409.
8. Otten MA, Groeneveld TW, Flierman R, Rastaldi MP, Trouw LA, et al. (2009) Both complement and IgG fc receptors are required for development of attenuated antiglomerular basement membrane nephritis in mice. J Immunol 183: 3980–3988.
9. Hebert MJ, Takano T, Papayianni A, Rennke HG, Minto A, et al. (1998) Acute nephrotoxic serum nephritis in complement knockout mice: relative roles of the classical and alternate pathways in neutrophil recruitment and proteinuria. Nephrol Dial Transplant 13: 2799–2803.
10. Xing GQ, Chen M, Liu G, Heeringa P, Zhang JJ, et al. (2009) Complement activation is involved in renal damage in human antineutrophil cytoplasmic autoantibody associated pauci-immune vasculitis. J Clin Immunol 29: 282–291.
11. Sahu A, Lambris JD (2001) Structure and biology of complement protein C3, a connecting link between innate and acquired immunity. Immunol Rev 180: 35–48.
12. Schulze M, Pruchno CJ, Burns M, Baker PJ, Johnson RJ, Couser WG (1993) Glomerular C3c localization indicates ongoing immune deposit formation and complement activation in experimental glomerulonephritis. Am J Pathol 142: 179–187.
13. Daha MR (1989) Possible mechanisms of degradation of C1q in vivo and in vitro: role of macrophages. Behring Inst Mitt : 42–46.
14. Trouw LA, Groeneveld TW, Seelen MA, Duijs JM, Bajema IM, et al. (2004) Anti-C1q autoantibodies deposit in glomeruli but are only pathogenic in combination with glomerular C1q-containing immune complexes. J Clin Invest 114: 679–688.
15. Lachmann PJ (2009) The amplification loop of the complement pathways. Adv Immunol 104: 115–149.
16. Hourcade DE (2006) The role of properdin in the assembly of the alternative pathway C3 convertases of complement. J Biol Chem 281: 2128–2132.
17. Hisano S, Matsushita M, Fujita T, Iwasaki H (2005) Activation of the lectin complement pathway in Henoch-Schonlein purpura nephritis. Am J Kidney Dis 45: 295–302.
18. Hisano S, Matsushita M, Fujita T, Takeshita M, Iwasaki H (2007) Activation of the lectin complement pathway in post-streptococcal acute glomerulonephritis. Pathol Int 57: 351–357.
19. Roos A, Rastaldi MP, Calvaresi N, Oortwijn BD, Schlagwein N, et al. (2006) Glomerular activation of the lectin pathway of complement in IgA nephropathy is associated with more severe renal disease. J Am Soc Nephrol 17: 1724–1734.
20. Harboe M, Mollnes TE (2008) The alternative complement pathway revisited. J Cell Mol Med 12: 1074–1084.
21. Ji H, Ohmura K, Mahmood U, Lee DM, Hofhuis FM, et al. (2002) Arthritis critically dependent on innate immune system players. Immunity 16: 157–168.
22. Elliott MK, Jarmi T, Ruiz P, Xu Y, Holers VM, Gilkeson GS (2004) Effects of complement factor D deficiency on the renal disease of MRL/lpr mice. Kidney Int 65: 129–138.
23. Hietala MA, Jonsson IM, Tarkowski A, Kleinau S, Pekna M (2002) Complement deficiency ameliorates collagen-induced arthritis in mice. J Immunol 169: 454–459.
24. Holers VM, Girardi G, Mo L, Guthridge JM, Molina H, et al. (2002) Complement C3 activation is required for antiphospholipid antibody-induced fetal loss. J Exp Med 195: 211–220.
25. Spitzer D, Mitchell LM, Atkinson JP, Hourcade DE (2007) Properdin can initiate complement activation by binding specific target surfaces and providing a platform for de novo convertase assembly. J Immunol 179: 2600–2608.
26. Kemper C, Mitchell LM, Zhang L, Hourcade DE (2008) The complement protein properdin binds apoptotic T cells and promotes complement activation and phagocytosis. Proc Natl Acad Sci U S A 105: 9023–9028.
27. Xu W, Berger SP, Trouw LA, de Boer HC, Schlagwein N, et al. (2008) Properdin binds to late apoptotic and necrotic cells independently of C3b and regulates alternative pathway complement activation. J Immunol 180: 7613–7621.
28. Gaarkeuken H, Siezenga MA, Zuidwijk K, van Kooten C, Rabelink TJ, et al. (2008) Complement activation by tubular cells is mediated by properdin binding. Am J Physiol Renal Physiol 295: F1397–1403.

Prognosis in IgA Nephropathy: 30-Year Analysis of 1,012 Patients at a Single Center in Japan

Takahito Moriyama*, Kayu Tanaka, Chihiro Iwasaki, Yasuko Oshima, Ayami Ochi, Hiroshi Kataoka, Mitsuyo Itabashi, Takashi Takei, Keiko Uchida, Kosaku Nitta

Department of Medicine, Kidney Center, Tokyo Women's Medical University, Tokyo, Japan

Abstract

Background: Little is known about the long-term prognosis of patients with IgA nephropathy (IgAN).

Methods: This retrospective cohort analysis evaluated clinical and histological findings at the time of renal biopsy, initial treatment, patient outcomes over 30 years, and risk factors associated with progression in 1,012 patients diagnosed with IgAN at our center since 1974.

Results: Of the 1,012 patients, 40.5% were male. Mean patient age was 33±12 years and mean blood pressure was 122±17/75±13 mmHg. Mean serum creatinine concentration was 0.89±0.42 mg/dL, and mean estimated glomerular filtration rate (eGFR) was 78.5±26.2 ml/min/1.73 m^2. Mean proteinuria was 1.19±1.61 g/day, and mean urinary red blood cells were 36.6±35.3/high-powered field. Histologically, mesangial hypercellularity was present in 47.6% of patients, endothelial hypercellularity in 44.3%, segmental sclerosis in 74.6%, and tubular atrophy/interstitial fibrosis in 28.8% by Oxford classification. Initial treatment consisted of corticosteroids in 26.9% of patients, renin-angiotensin-aldosterone system inhibitor in 28.9%, and tonsillectomy plus steroids in 11.7%. The 10-, 20-, and 30-year renal survival rates were 84.3, 66.6, and 50.3%, respectively. Tonsillectomy plus steroids dramatically improved renal outcome. Cox multivariate regression analysis showed that higher proteinuria, lower eGFR, and higher uric acid at the time of renal biopsy were independent risk factors for the development of end stage renal disease (ESRD).

Conclusions: IgAN is not a benign disease, with about 50% of patients progressing to ESRD within 30 years despite treatment.

Editor: Ivan Cruz Moura, Institut national de la santé et de la recherche médicale (INSERM), France

Funding: The authors have no support or funding to report.

* E-mail: takamori@kc.twmu.ac.jp

Introduction

Mesangial proliferative glomerulonephritis with mesangial deposition of immunoglobulin A (IgA) and IgG, now recognized as IgA nephropathy (IgAN) was first described in 1968 [1]. Since then, the mechanism of onset and progression of this disease have been described, along with treatment modalities, patient prognosis, and risk factors. Although IgAN was initially regarded as a benign disease, a study in the 1990s reported that about 40% of patients with IgAN progressed to end stage renal disease (ESRD) within 20 years [2,3]. Since the first report, in 1986, showing that steroid therapy had a beneficial effect in patients with IgAN [4], steroids have been frequently used to treat IgAN patients with massive proteinuria (>1 g/day), active histological findings such as crescent formation, and normal renal function. A randomized controlled trial in 1999 found that steroid pulse therapy could decrease amount of proteinuria and improve patient prognosis [5]. Moreover, steroid pulse therapy was found to have long term efficacy in these patients [6] and has been widely recognized as the most effective treatment for IgAN. Since a retrospective analysis in 2001 found that the combination of tonsillectomy plus steroid pulse therapy induced complete remission of proteinuria and hematuria and prevented deterioration of renal function [7], the number of institutions in Japan performing tonsillectomy plus steroid pulse therapy in patients with IgAN has dramatically increased [8,9]. Although these intensive therapies may improve the prognosis of patients with IgAN, the mechanisms underlying the onset and progression of IgAN, the risk factors for progression and the long term prognosis of these patients have not been determined. Indeed, despite intensive treatment, many patients with IgAN progress to ESRD.

This retrospective cohort study was performed to analyze the long term outcomes in patients with IgAN and their prognosis over 30 years. We therefore analyzed clinical and histological findings at renal biopsy and risk factors for progression in 1,012 IgAN patients diagnosed at our institution.

Materials and Methods

Ethics statement

This cohort study was conducted in accordance with the Declaration of Helsinki, and approved by the Medical Ethics

Table 1. Clinical and laboratory findings at renal biopsy.

Variables	Values
Clinical Findings	
Sex	410/602 (Male/Female)
Age	32.9±12.0 years
Body Mass Index	21.6±3.1 kg/m^2
Systolic Blood Pressure	121.7±17.1 mmHg
Diastolic Blood Pressure	74.6±12.8 mmHg
Mean arterial Pressure	90.4±12.8 mmHg
Interval from onset	5.8±6.6 years
Observation period	7.9±7.1 years
Laboratory Findings	
Total Protein	6.69±0.73 g/dl
Serum Albumin	3.92±0.53 g/dl
Blood Urea Nitrogen	15.8±5.7 mg/dl
Serum Creatinine	0.89±0.42 mg/dl
eGFR	78.5±26.2 ml/min/1.73m^2
Uric Acid	5.71±1.62 mg/dl
Total Cholesterol	197.3±48.5 mg/dl
HDL Cholesterol	56.4±16.7 mg/dl
Triglyceride	123.7±82.2 mg/dl
IgG	1158.1±341.2 mg/dl
IgA	325.1±126.6 mg/dl
IgM	144.7±75.7 mg/dl
CH50	40.6±8.4 mg/dl
C3	87.5±35.2 mg/dl
C4	29.0±15.5 mg/dl
Urinary protein excretion	1.19±1.61 g/day
U-RBC	36.6±35.3 counts/HF

Table 2. Histological findings (glomerular lesions and Oxford classification).

Glomerular lesions	Values
Number of glomeruli	16.1±10.4 (number)
Global Sclerosis	15.5±16.6 %
Segmental Sclerosis or Adhesion	13.6±13.7 %
Crescent	9.12±12.3 %
Cellular or Fibro-Cellular	6.72±10.5 %
Fibrous	2.25±5.76 %
Oxford Classification [number/(%)]	**Values [number(%)]**
Mesangial hypercellularity: M0/M1	449/408 (52.4/47.6%)
Endocapillary hypercellularity: E0/E1	477/380 (55.7/44.3%)
Segmental glomerulosclerosis: S0/S1	218/639 (25.4/74.6%)
Tubular atrophy/Interstitial fibrosis: T0/T1/T2	610/197/50 (71.2/23.0/5.8%)
Not evaluated	155 (15.3%)

Committee of Tokyo Women's Medical University (#2962). Written informed consent for renal biopsy was obtained from all patients and for use of clinical data at the time of renal biopsy and subsequent histological data was obtained from all recent patients.

Patients

Between 1974 and 2011, 1,012 patients at Tokyo Women's Medical University were diagnosed with primary IgAN by renal biopsy. IgAN was diagnosed based on light microscopic findings of mesangial proliferative changes, immunofluorescence findings of mesangial IgA and C3 deposition, and electron microscopic findings of electron-dense deposits in the mesangial area. Patients were observed for a mean 7.9±7.1 years (maximum 36 years); 4 patients died during the observation period.

Histological evaluation of renal biopsy specimens

All renal biopsy specimens were obtained by percutaneous needle biopsy. The specimens were fixed in 10% phosphate-buffered formalin (pH 7.2), embedded in paraffin, and cut into 4-µm-thick sections. The sections were stained with hematoxylin and eosin, periodic acid–Schiff, silver methenamine, and Masson trichrome and examined by light microscopy. The percentage of glomerular lesions, such as global sclerosis, segmental sclerosis or adhesion, cellular or fibrocellular crescents, and fibrous crescents, were evaluated. The histological findings were also graded according to the Oxford classification [11,12], which scored four key pathological features in each specimen. (i) Mesangial hypercellularity was scored as M0 if >50% of glomeruli had fewer than three cells per mesangial area or M1 if >50% of glomeruli had more than three cells per mesangial area. (ii) Segmental glomerulosclerosis was scored as absent (S0) or present (S1). (iii) Endocapillary hypercellularity was scored as absent (E0) or present (E1). (iv) Tubular atrophy/interstitial fibrosis score was based on the ratio of tubular atrophy/interstitial fibrosis in the total interstitium and scored as T0 (0–25%), T1 (26–50%), or T2 (>51%). Biopsies containing fewer than 8 glomeruli were excluded from analysis.

Demographic and clinical data

Patient sex, age, body mass index (BMI), systolic blood pressure (S-BP), diastolic blood pressure (D-BP), mean arterial pressure (MAP), and time from onset of IgAN were recorded. In Japan, a large proportion of the population can receive free annual medical examinations, including annual urinary screening. These screenings are regularly performed in school, the workplace, and in municipal facilities. These screenings enable recognition of the onset of IgAN as the first manifestation of a urinary abnormality or a finding of macrohematuria. Laboratory data included serum total protein, albumin, creatinine, uric acid, total cholesterol, HDL-cholesterol, triglyceride, IgG, IgA, IgM, C3, and C4 concentrations; blood urea nitrogen concentration; estimated glomerular filtration rate (eGFR), CH50 activity; urinary protein excretion (U-Prot), and urinary red blood cells (U-RBC). These clinical and laboratory findings were measured at the time of renal biopsy. Time to progression to ESRD, defined as requiring dialysis or renal transplantation, and the risk factors associated with progression to ESRD were also evaluated. Initial treatment, defined as treatment performed during the first year after renal biopsy, and renal survival rate relative to treatment were evaluated. The eGFR was calculated by the modified isotope dilution mass spectorometry – modification of diet in renal disease (IDMS-MDRD) study for Japanese [$eGFR = 194 \times S\text{-}Cre^{-1.094} \times age^{-0.287} \times 0.739$ (if female)] [10].

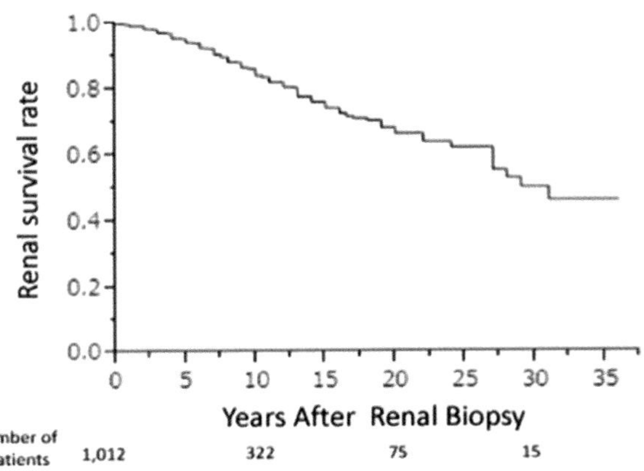

Figure 1. Cumulative renal survival rate from renal biopsy until ESRD in all 1,012 patients with IgAN.

Table 3. Initial treatment of individual patients.

Treatment	Values [number (%)]
Corticosteroid	272 (26.9%)
Steroid combined with tonsillectomy	119 (11.7%)
Tonsillectomy without steroid	15 (1.5%)
Steroid with Immunosuppressing agents	15 (1.5%)
RAS inhibitors	293 (28.9%)
Anti-platelet agents/anti coagulation	600 (59.3%)
EPA	159 (15.7%)
PE/DFPP	3 (0.3%)
No therapy	154 (15.2%)
Unknown	60 (5.9%)

RAS, renin angiotensin system; EPA, eicosapentaenoic acid; PE, plasma exchange; DFPP, double filtration plasmapheresis.

Statistical analysis

Data are presented as means ± standard deviation (SD) and were analyzed using JMP 10.0.1 (SAS Institute, Cary, NC, USA). Cumulative renal survival rates until ESRD were calculated according to the Kaplan–Meier method and compared using the log rank test. Univariate and multivariate Cox regression analysis were used to evaluate the risk of deterioration to ESRD. In univariate analyses, sex (male/female) was regarded as a categorical variable, whereas age, BMI, MAP, interval from onset, eGFR, serum albumin, uric acid, total cholesterol, U-Prot, U-RBC, IgA, IgA/C3 and histological grading were regarded as quantitative variables. Multivariate analysis included the factors differing significantly in univariate analysis. The results of these univariate and multivariate analyses are expressed as hazard ratios (HRs) with 95% confidence intervals (CIs). In all analyses, $P<0.05$ was considered statistically significant.

Results

Clinical findings at the time of renal biopsy

Table 1 shows the clinical characteristics at the time of renal biopsy. Of the 1,012 patients, 40.5% were male. Mean patient age was 32.9±12.0 years, with 41% aged 20–29 years and 25% aged 30–39 years. Mean S-BP was 121.7±17.1 mmHg and mean D-BP was 74.6±12.8 mmHg. Mean MAP was 90.4±12.8 mmHg and 79% of IgAN patients had a MAP below 100 mmHg. Mean interval from IgAN onset to renal biopsy was 7.9±7.1 years. We found that renal biopsies were obtained from 32% of patients within 2 years of IgAN onset and from 21% 10 years after onset.

Table 1 also shows laboratory data at the time of renal biopsy. Mean total protein concentration was 6.69±0.73 g/dl, and mean serum albumin concentration was 3.92±0.53 g/dl. Of these patients, 6% had serum albumin concentrations <3.0 g/dl and 12% had serum albumin concentrations between 3.0 and 3.5 g/dl, with the remainder having serum albumin concentrations over 3.5 g/dl. The mean eGFR was 78.5±26.2 ml/min/1.73m^2, with 46% of patients having eGFR over 80 ml/min/1.73m^2, 30% between 60 and 80 ml/min/1.73m^2, 19% between 40 and 60 ml/min/1.73m^2, and 5% between 20 and 40 ml/min/1.73m^2. Mean serum total cholesterol and triglyceride concentrations were 197.3±48.5 mg/dl and 123.7±82.2 mg/dl, respectively. Mean IgA concentration was 325.1±126.6 mg/dl, with 28% of patients having IgA concentrations between 300 and 400 mg/dl, and 23% >400 mg/dl. Mean U-Prot was 1.19±1.61 g/day, with 62% of patients having less than 1 g/day, 30% between 1 and 3 g/day, and 9% over 3 g/day. Mean U-RBC was 36.6±35.3 counts/high powered field (HPF), with 51% of patients having <25/HPF, 20% having between 25 and 50 counts/HPF, 4% having between 50 and 100 counts/HPF, and 20% having >100 counts/HPF.

Histological findings

Table 2 shows the histological findings in samples taken from patients with IgAN. The mean number of glomeruli per renal biopsy was 16.1±10.4. Over 8 glomeruli were present in biopsy specimens from 858 patients and these samples were used to evaluate glomerular lesions and Oxford classification. Global sclerosis was observed in a mean 15.5±16.6% of samples, segmental sclerosis or adhesion in 13.6±13.7%, cellular or fibrocellular crescents in 6.72±10.5%, and a fibrous crescent in 2.25±5.76%. According to the Oxford classification, 47.6% of samples were classified as M1, 44.3% as E1, 74.6% as S1, 23.0% as T1 and 5.8% as T2.

Initial treatment

Table 3 shows the initial treatment of patients with IgAN. We found that 272 patients (26.9%) received corticosteroids; 119 (11.7%) received corticosteroid therapy combined with tonsillectomy; 15 (1.5%) underwent tonsillectomy alone; 15 (1.5%) received immunosuppressive agents such as cyclophosphamide, mizoribine, and rituximab; 293 (28.9%) received a renin-angiotensin-aldosterone system inhibitor; 600 (59.3%) received an antiplatelet/anticoagulation agent; 159 (15.7%) received eicosapentaenoic acid; 3 (0.3%) underwent plasma exchange or double filtration plasmapheresis; and 169 (16.7%) received no treatment.

Long term outcome of IgA nephropathy

The cumulative 10-, 20- and 30-year renal survival rates, from renal biopsy to ESRD, were 84.3%, 66.6%, and 50.3%, respectively. The 36-year renal survival rate was 46.4% (Figure 1).

Outcome according to initial treatment

The cumulative renal survival rate relative to initial treatment is shown in Figure 2. The 8.5-year cumulative survival rate in patients treated with steroids plus tonsillectomy was 100%, the 17-year survival rate in patients treated with tonsillectomy was 100%, the 20-year survival rate in patients treated with steroids plus an immunosuppressive agent was 57.6%, and the 25-year survival rate in patients treated with steroids was 41.4%. The 35-year renal survival rates in patients treated with conservative therapy (RAS inhibitors and/or anti-platelet agents/anti-coagulation therapy, and/or EPA) and in untreated patients were 42.0% and 64.5%, respectively. The difference among groups was statistically significant (P = 0.0011).

Univariate and multivariate analysis of factors associated with ESRD

Univariate analysis found that male gender, higher age, higher BMI, higher MAP, lower eGFR, lower serum albumin, higher uric acid, higher total cholesterol, higher U-Prot, higher IgA/C3, and higher T level on the Oxford classification were associated with a risk of progression to ESRD. Multivariate Cox regression analysis showed that lower eGFR (HR, 1.93; 95% CI, 1.47–2.56; P< 0.0001), higher uric acid concentration (HR, 1.24; 95% CI, 1.054–1.48, P = 0.0176), and higher U-Prot (HR, 1.34; 95% CI 1.07–1.69, P = 0.0116) were independent factors predicting

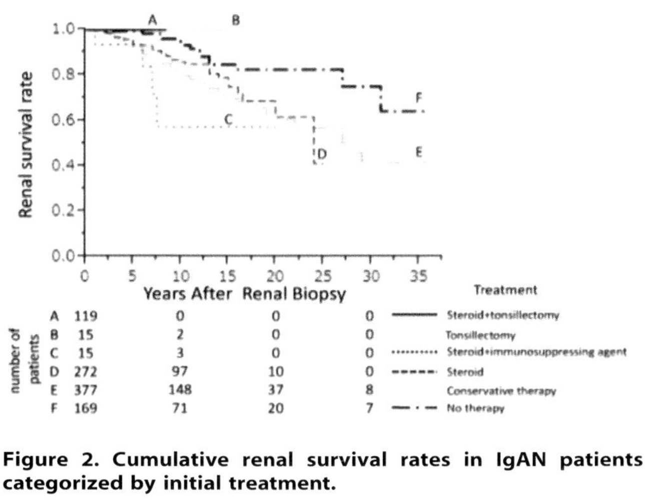

Figure 2. Cumulative renal survival rates in IgAN patients categorized by initial treatment.

Table 4. Univariate and multivariate analysis of risk factors associated with ESRD in patients diagnosed with IgAN.

	HR	95% CI	P value
Univariate Analysis			
male (vs. female)	1.76	1.25–2.49	0.0013
Age (10 year increase)	1.25	1.09–1.44	0.0031
BMI (1 kg/m^2 increase)	1.10	1.04–1.16	0.0012
MAP (10 mmHg increase)	1.44	1.27–1.65	<0.0001
Interval from onset (1 year increase)	1.02	0.99–1.05	0.0763
eGFR (20ml/min decrease)	2.22	1.86–2.67	<0.0001
Serum Albumin (1 g/dl decrease)	1.99	1.71–2.30	<0.0001
Uric Acid (1 mg/dl increase)	1.57	1.39–1.77	<0.0001
T-Cho (30 mg/dl increase)	1.44	1.26–1.64	<0.0001
U-Prot (1g/day increase)	1.69	1.53–1.86	<0.0001
U-RBC (20/HPF increase)	1.02	0.92–1.13	0.6851
IgA (100 mg/dl increase)	1.09	0.93–1.27	0.2833
IgA/C3 (1 increase)	1.16	1.00–1.35	0.0460
Oxford classification M1(vs. M0)	1.35	0.94–1.97	0.1039
Oxford classification E1 (vs. E0)	1.30	0.89–1.91	0.1733
Oxford classification S1 (vs. S0)	1.23	0.81–1.92	0.3455
Oxford classification T (1 increase)	2.38	1.91–3.20	<0.0001
Multivariate Analysis			
male (vs. female)	1.16	0.72–1.90	0.5390
Age (10 year increase)	0.84	0.67–1.03	0.0992
BMI (1 kg/m^2 increase)	0.93	0.85–1.01	0.0781
MAP (10 mmHg increase)	1.14	0.94–1.38	0.1755
eGFR (20ml/min decrease)	1.93	1.47–2.56	<0.0001
Alb (1 g/dl decrease)	1.24	0.92–1.66	0.1627
Uric Acid (1 mg/dl increase)	1.24	1.04–1.48	0.0176
T-Cho (30 mg/dl increase)	1.17	0.96–1.42	0.1105
U-Prot (1g/day increase)	1.34	1.07–1.69	0.0116
IgA/C3 (1 increase)	1.17	0.96–1.42	0.1111
Oxford classification T (1 increase)	1.06	0.75–1.50	0.7318

HR, hazard ratio; CI, confidence interval; BMI, body mass index; MAP, mean arterial pressure; eGFR, estimated glomerular filtration rate; T-Cho, total cholesterol; U-Prot, urinary protein excretion; U-RBC, urinary red blood cells; IgA, immunoglobulin A.

progression to ESRD (Table 4). Kaplan–Meier analysis showed that cumulative renal survival rates were significantly higher in patients with higher than lower eGFR (Figure 3a), in patients with lower than higher U-Prot (Figure 3b), and in patients with lower than higher uric acid concentration (Figure 3d; P<0.0001 each). Cumulative survival, however, did not differ significantly according to the degree of hematuria (Figure 3c, P=0.1122). Kaplan–Meier analysis also showed that the cumulative renal survival rate was significantly higher in patients diagnosed with IgAN over the last 20 years than during the previous 20 years (75.2% vs. 59.0 %, P=0.0002; Figure 4).

Discussion

IgAN is the most common type of chronic glomerulonephritis worldwide [13]. Although slowly progressive over decades, IgAN is not a benign disease. Since IgAN was first described over 40 years ago, patients with this disease have been treated with oral steroids [4,14,15], steroid pulse therapy [5,6], tonsillectomy [7,16,17], renin-angiotensin aldosterone system inhibitors [18–20], eicosapentaenoic acid [21], statins [22] and combinations of these agents [23]. Although these agents were found to improve short and intermediate term renal outcomes, less is known about very long term outcomes in these patients. In this retrospective analysis, we showed that the 10-, 20-, 30-, and 36-year cumulative renal survival rates were 84.3%, 66.6%, 50.3% and 46.4%, respectively, findings similar to those reported previously for up to 20 years. For example, a study of 282 patients in France showed that the cumulative 10- and 20-year renal survival rates from biopsy to S-Cre >1.5 mg/dl were 84% and 64%, respectively [2]. A study of 502 patients in Japan reported that the 10- and 20-year cumulative survival rates from onset of IgAN until ESRD were 85% and 61%, respectively [3], and a study of 1,155 patients in China found that the 10- and 20-year cumulative renal survival rates until eGFR < 15 ml/min/1.73m^2 were 83% and 64%, respectively [24]. In addition, a study of 1,364 patients in Korea reported that the cumulative 10- and 20-year survival rates from renal biopsy until ESRD or death were 79.8% and 66.9%, respectively [25]. These findings, however, suggested that treatment may not improve

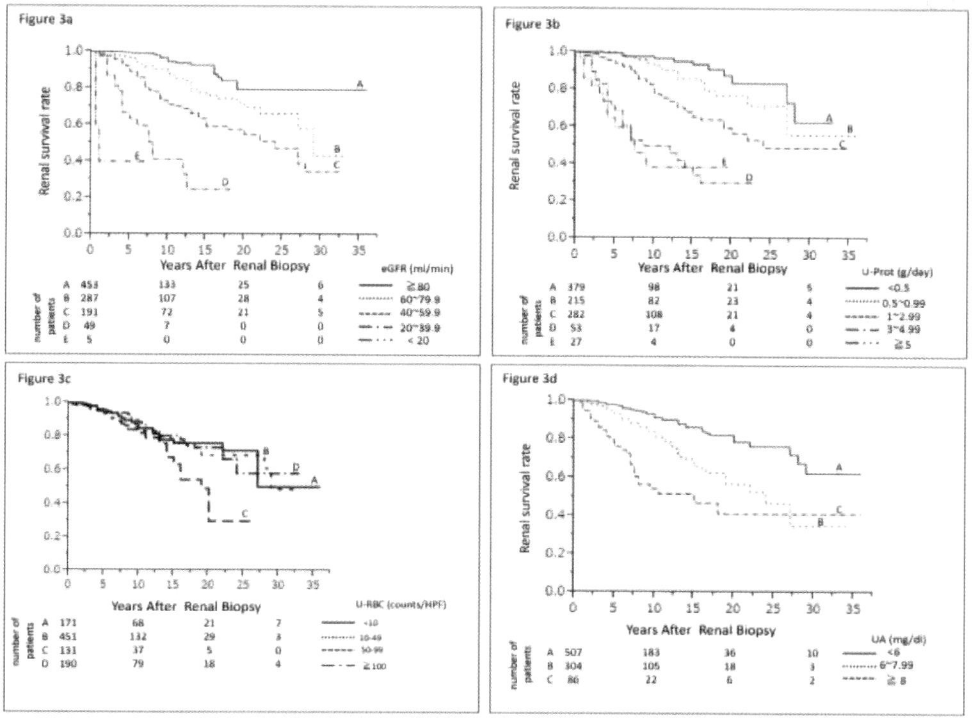

Figure 3. Cumulative renal survival rates in IgAN patients categorized by eGFR, U-Prot, U-RBC and uric acid concentration. (a) The 30-year survival rates of patients with eGFR >80 ml/min/1.73m^2, between 80 and 60 ml/min/1.73m^2, and between 60 and 40 ml/min/1.73m^2 were 80.1%, 43.1%, and 34.6%, respectively. The survival rates of patients with eGFR between 40 and 20 ml/min/1.73m^2 and <20 ml/min/1.73m^2 were 24.8% over 18 years and 40.0% over 7 years, respectively. The difference among groups was statistically significant (P<0.0001). (b) The 30-year renal survival rates of patients with U-Prot <0.5 g/day, between 0.5 and 1 g/day, and between 1 and 3 g were 62.6%, 55.6%, and 49.0%, respectively. The survival rates of patients with U-Prot between 3 and 5 g/day and >5 g/day were 29.9% over 20 years and 34.4% over 15 years, respectively. The difference among groups was statistically significant (P<0.0001). (c) The 30-year renal survival rates of patients with U-RBC <10 counts/HF, between 10 and 49 counts/HF, and ≥100 counts/HF were 50.2, 49.0, and 41.7%. The survival rates of patients with U-RBC between 50 and 99 counts/HF was 29.6% over 25 years. The difference among groups was not statistically significant (P = 0.1122). (d) The 30-year renal survival rates of patients with uric acid <6 mg/dl, between 6 and 8 mg/dl, and >8 mg/dl were 62.3, 35.1, and 41.2%, respectively (P<0.0001).

prognosis in patients with IgAN because renal survival rates had not increased dramatically over time. We therefore compared renal survival rates in patients diagnosed with IgAN between 1974 and 1991 and those diagnosed between 1992 and 2011, finding

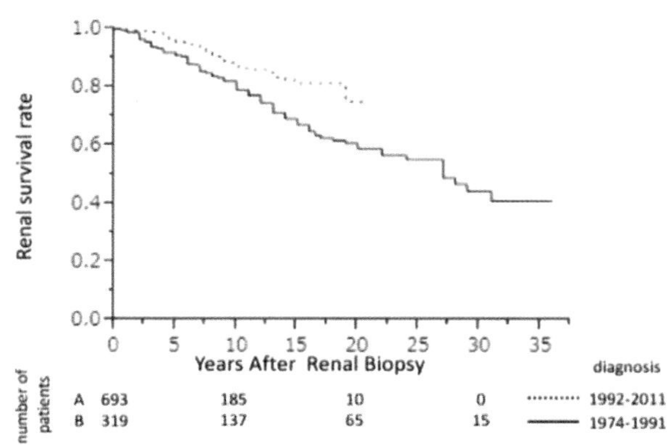

Figure 4. Renal survival rates in IgAN patients diagnosed between 1974 and 1991 and between 1992 and 2001. The 10 year (86.6% vs. 79.1%) and 20 year (75.2% vs. 59.0%) renal survival rates were significantly higher in patients diagnosed between 1992 and 2011 than in between 1974 and 1991 (P = 0.0002).

that the 20-year survival rate was significantly higher in the latter than in the former group (75.2% vs. 59.0%, P = 0.0002). Similar findings were reported previously [23], confirming that treatment of IgAN improved renal outcomes. Beginning in 2004, patients in our institution have been treated with a combination of steroids with tonsillectomy, with none of the 119 patients treated since 2004 progressing to ESRD. This result, indicating that steroid therapy combined with tonsillectomy improves renal outcomes dramatically, was similar to previous findings [7]. In contrast, 169 patients (16.7% of all patients) received no treatment at the time of renal biopsy, because their clinical and histological findings were mild. These patients had a mean eGFR of 80.9±24.7 ml/min/1.73m^2 and a mean U-Prot of 0.60±0.69 g/day, with 43.3% classified as M1, 23.3% as E1, 54.1% as S1, 15.8% as T1, and 3.3% as T2. Interestingly, their renal survival rate was better than that of the patients who received steroids, immunosuppressive agents, or conservative therapy as initial treatment, although 35.6% progressed to ESRD in 35 years. These results indicate that, despite their mild clinical and histological findings at the time of renal biopsy, some patients with IgAN progressed to ESRD. Furthermore, careful observation of all IgAN patients is needed, regardless of findings at the time of renal biopsy. Moreover, in our cohort, median (interquartile range) U-Prot (0.68 (0.3–1.305) vs. 0.77 (0.225–1.55) g/day, P = 0.0037) and U-RBC (20 (10–50) vs. 30 (10–100) counts/HF, P<0.0001) were significantly lower and eGFR (80.3 (61.7–99.3) vs. 70.9 (58.5–88.3) ml/min/1.73m^2, P<

0.0001) was significantly higher in patients diagnosed between 1992 and 2011 than in those diagnosed between 1974 and 1991. These findings indicated that more recently diagnosed patients had milder disease at the time of renal biopsy and a better overall prognosis.

In our cohort, about 60% of patients diagnosed as IgAN were female, which contrasts with worldwide findings. We suspected that this may have been due to the name of our institution, Tokyo *Women's* Medical University, which may have attracted more female than male patients. More women than men were found to undergo underwent renal biopsy [13], with several reports from Japan yielding results similar to ours [8,23,31]. In addition, two reports from Asia, evaluating over 1,000 IgAN patients, found that the gender distribution was even [24,25]. The frequency of IgAN in Japan was similar to that of other nations in East Asia, but different from that of other regions in the world [13]. These results indicated that specific genetic and ethnic backgrounds may be related to gender distribution of this disease. Using the Oxford classification, we found that 47.6% of patients could be classified as M1, 44.3% as E1, 74.6% as S1, 23.0% as T1, and 5.8% as T2, although including criteria different from those of the original Oxford classification. We selected all patients diagnosed with IgAN in our institution, including patients with U-Prot <0.5 g/day or eGFR <30 ml/min/1.74^2, patient not selected by the original Oxford classification. Except for M1, however, the distribution of patients in our cohort was similar to that of the cohort from the original Oxford classification, in which 81% of patients were classified as M1, 42% as E1, 76% as S1, 30% as T1, and 5% as T2 [11,12]. The lower percentage of our patients classified as M1 may have been due to the large percentage of patients with mild IgAN, defined as U-Prot <0.5 g/day.

Multivariate Cox regression analysis showed that risk factors associated with deterioration to ESRD were impaired renal function and severe proteinuria at the time of renal biopsy, findings similar to those of previous reports [2,3,23,24,25]. Kaplan–Meier analysis also indicated that renal function and proteinuria affected renal outcome. Acute deterioration of renal function after 25 years was observed in patients with very low proteinuria (<0.5 g/day). The renal survival rate, which was 83.4% at 25 years after renal biopsy, decreased to 73.0% at 27 years and 62.6% at 28 years. However, only nine patients were available for follow-up after 25 years in patients with low proteinuria, with two of these nine patients progressing to ESRD. One of these two patients had diabetic nephropathy and the other had multiple organ failure with severe infection, suggesting that, in the absence of these complications, their renal function may not have deteriorated after 25 years. Other risk factors reported associated with ESRD included uncontrolled hypertension [3,23,24,25] and severe histological damage [3,23,25], although none of these was significant in our analysis. We also found that age, sex, hematuria, IgA/C3 ratio and serum albumin were not associated with deterioration to ESRD. Kaplan–Meier analysis also indicated that hematuria did not affect renal outcome. Interestingly, uric acid concentration was a risk factor for progression to ESRD by multivariate Cox regression analysis and Kaplan–Meier analysis. Indeed, higher uric acid concentration has been associated with glomerular damage [26,27], tubulointerstitial change [26,27,28], and vascular damage [26], as well as with poor prognosis [24,26,27,29], and it was independent from renal function [24,27], further suggesting the importance of controlling uric acid concentration in patients with IgAN.

Univariate analysis showed that the only Oxford classification associated with patient prognosis was T grade (HR 2.38, 95% CI 1.91–3.20, P<0.0001), whereas M, E, and S grades were not. Following multivariate analysis, however, T grade was no longer prognostic, whereas clinical factors, such as lower eGFR, higher U-Prot, and higher uric acid were powerful predictors of renal deterioration. Similar findings have been observed in several other studies. For example, Kaplan–Meier analysis showed no significant differences in renal survival rate in patients assorted by M, E, and S grades, with T grade being the only Oxford classification predictive of renal outcome [30]. Another study reported that higher T grade and extracapillary lesions were risk factors for progression to ESRD, as were lower eGFR, higher U-Prot and the absence of steroid treatment, whereas M, E, and S grades were not [31]. Multivariate analysis showed that the most powerful predictor of renal outcome was renal function at biopsy, with eGFR, U-Prot and hypertension being prognostic; in contrast, none of the Oxford classifications was predictive of progression to ESRD [32]. Although Oxford classification is recognized as useful in predicting renal outcomes, these findings suggest that the Oxford classification be evaluated in prospective, large sized, worldwide validation studies.

Our study had several limitations, including the relatively low number of patients followed-up. Of the 1,012 patients who underwent of renal biopsy, only about 30% could be evaluated at 10 years, and only 6% at 20 years. Loss of patients with milder disease to follow-up, with more severely ill patients remaining under observation, may have biased our results towards more severe outcomes. In conclusion, we assessed long term renal survival in patients with IgAN, as well as evaluating factors associated with renal survival. We found that about 50% of patients with IgAN developed ESRD within 30 years. Higher U-Prot, lower eGFR, and higher uric acid were independent risk factors for the development of ESRD.

Author Contributions

Conceived and designed the experiments: TM HK MI TT KU KN. Performed the experiments: TM KT CI YO AO. Analyzed the data: TM KT CI YO AO. Contributed reagents/materials/analysis tools: TM TT KN. Wrote the paper: TM.

References

1. Berger J, Hinglais N (1968) Intercapillary deposits of IgA-IgG. J Urol Nephrol 74: 694–695.
2. Alamartine E, Sabatier JC, Guerin C, Berliet JM, Berthoux F (1991) Prognostic factors in mesangial IgA glomerulonephritis: an extensive study with univariate and multivariate analysis. Am J Kidney Dis 18: 12–19.
3. Koyama A, Igarashi M, Kobayashi M (1997) Coworkers of the research group on progressive renal disease. Natural history and risk factors for immunoglobulin A nephropathy in Japan. Am J Kidney Dis 29: 526–532.
4. Kobayashi Y, Hiki Y, Kokubo T, Tateno S (1996) Steroid therapy during the early stage of progressive IgA nephropathy. A 10-year follow-up study. Nephron 72: 237–242.
5. Pozzi C, Bolasco PG, Fogazzi GB, Andrulli S, Altieri P, et al. (1999) Corticosteroids in IgA nephropathy: a randomized controlled trial. Lancet 353: 883–887.
6. Pozzi C, Andrulli S, Del Vecchio L, Melis P, Fogazzi GB, et al. (2004) Corticosteroid effectiveness in IgA nephropathy: long-term results of a randomized, controlled trial. J Am Soc Nephrol 15: 157–163.
7. Hotta O, Miyazaki M, Furuta T, Tomioka S, Chiba S, et al. (2001) Tonsillectomy and steroid pulse therapy significantly impact on clinical remission in patients with IgA nephropathy. Am J Kidney Dis 38: 736–743.
8. Miura N, Imai H, Kikuchi S, Hayashi S, Endoh M, et al. (2009) Tonsillectomy and steroid pulse (TSP) therapy for patients with IgA nephropathy: a nationwide

survey of TSP therapy in Japan and an analysis of the predictive factors or resistance to TSP therapy. Clin Exp Nephrol 13: 460–466.

9. Matsuzaki K, Suzuki Y, Nakata J, Sakamoto N, Horikoshi S, et al. (2013) Nationwide survey on current treatments for IgA nephropathy in Japan. Clin Exp Nephrol, in press.
10. Matsuo S, Imai E, Horio M, Yasuda Y, Tomita K, et al. (2009) Revised equation for estimated GFR from serum creatinine in Japan: Am J Kidney Dis 53: 982–992.
11. A Working Group of the International IgA Nephropathy Network and the Renal Pathology Society (2009) the Oxford Classification of IgA Nephropathy: rationale, clinicopathological correlations, and classification. Kidney Int 76: 534–545.
12. A Working Group of the International IgA Nephropathy Network and the Renal Pathology Society (2009) the Oxford Classification of IgA Nephropathy: pathology definitions, correlations, and reproducibility. Kidney Int 76: 546–556.
13. Moriyama T, Suzuki K, Sugiura H, Itabashi M, Tsukasa M, et al. (2010) Frequency of renal disease in Japan: An analysis of 2,404 renal biopsies at a single center. Nephron Clin Pract 115: c227–c236.
14. Moriyama T, Honda K, Nitta K, Yumura W, Nihei H (2004) The effectiveness of steroid therapy for patients with advanced IgA nephropathy and impaired renal function: Clin Exp Nephrol 8: 237–242.
15. Moriyama T, Nakayama K, Iwasaki C, Ochi A, Tsuruta Y, et al. (2012) Severity of nephrotic IgA nephropathy according to the Oxford classification: Int Urol Nephrol 44: 1177–1184.
16. Ochi A, Moriyama T, Takei T, Uchida K, Nitta K (2013) Comparison between steroid pulse therapy alone and in combination with tonsillectomy for IgA nephropathy: Int Urol Nephrol 45: 469–476.
17. Kamei D, Moriyama T, Takei T, Wakai S, Nitta S (2013) Comparison between consecutive and intermittent steroid pulse therapy combined with tonsillectomy for clinical remission of IgA nephropathy: Clin Exp Nephrol: In press.
18. Moriyama T, Amamiya N, Ochi A, Tsuruta Y, Shimizu A, et al. (2011) Long-term beneficial effects of angiotensin-converting enzyme inhibitor and angiotensin receptor blocker therapy for patients with advanced immunoglobulin A nephropathy and impaired renal function: Clin Exp Nephrol 15: 700–707.
19. Moriyama T, Amemiya N, Ochi A, Tsuruta S, Shimizu A, et al. (2011) Comparison of steroids and angiotensin receptor blockers for patients with advanced IgA nephropathy and impaired renal function: Am J Nephrol 34: 233–240.
20. Moriyama T, Nakayama K, Ochi A, Amemiya N, Tsuruta Y, et al. (2012) Comparison of inhibitors of renin-angiotensin-aldosterone system (RAS) and combination therapy of steroids plus RAS inhibitors for patients with advanced immunoglobulin A nephropathy and impaired renal function: Clin Exp Nephrol 16: 231–237.
21. Moriyama T, Iwasaki C, Tanaka K, Ochi A, Shimizu A, et al. (2013) Effects of combination therapy with renin-angiotensin system inhibitors and eicosapentaenoic acid on IgA nephropathy: Intern Med 52: 193–199.
22. Moriyama T, Oshima Y, Tanaka K, Iwasaki C, Ochi A, et al. (2013) Statin stabilize the renal function of IgA nephropathy: Ren Fail: In press.
23. Komatsu H, Fujimoto S, Hara S, Fukuda A, Fukudome K, et al. (2009) Recent therapeutic strategies improve renal outcome in patients with IgA nephropathy. Am J Nephrol 30: 19–25.
24. Le W, Liang S, Hu Y, Deng K, Bao H, et al. (2012) Long-term renal survival and related risk factors in patients with IgA nephropathy: results from a cohort of 1155 cases in a Chinese adult population. Nephrol Dial Transplant 27: 1479–1485.
25. Lee H, Kim DK, Oh KH, Joo KW, Kim YS, et al. (2012) Mortality of IgA nephropathy patients: a single center experience over 30 years. PLOS One 7: e51225.
26. Cheng GY, Liu DW, Zhang N, Tang L, Zhao ZZ, et al. (2013) Clinical and prognostic implications of serum uric acid levels on IgA nephropathy: a cohort study of 348 cases with a mean 5-year follow up. Clin Nephrol 80: 40–46.
27. Ohno I, Hosoya T, Gomi H, Ichida K, Okabe H, et al. (2001) Serum uric acid and renal prognosis in patients with IgA nephropathy. Nephron 87: 333–339.
28. Myllmäki J, Honkanen T, Syrjänen J, Helin H, Rantala I, et al. (2005) Uric acid correlates with the severity of histopathological parameters in IgA nephropathy. Nephrol Dial Transplant 20: 89–95.
29. Shi Y, Chen W, Jalal D, Li Z, Chen W, et al. (2012) Clinical outcome of hyperuricemia in IgA nephropathy: A retrospective cohort study and randomized controlled trial. Kidney Blood Press Res 35: 153–160.
30. Yau T, Korbet AM, Schwartz MM, Cimbaluk DJ (2011) The Oxford classification of IgA nephropathy: a retrospective analysis: Am J Nephrol 34: 435–444.
31. Katafuchi R, Ninomiya T, Nagata M, Mitsuki K, Hiraoka H (2011) Validation study of Oxford classification of IgA nephropathy: The significance of extracapillary proliferation: Clin J Am Soc Nephrol 6: 2806–2813.
32. Alamartine E, Sauron C, Laurent B, Sury A, Seffert A, et al. (2011) The use of Oxford Classification of IgA nephropathy to predict renal survival: Clin J Am Soc Nephrol 6: 2384–2388.

10

Diffuse Glomerular Nodular Lesions in Diabetic Pigs Carrying a Dominant-Negative Mutant Hepatocyte Nuclear Factor 1-Alpha, an Inheritant Diabetic Gene in Humans

Satoshi Hara[1,4], Kazuhiro Umeyama[2], Takashi Yokoo[3], Hiroshi Nagashima[2], Michio Nagata[1]*

1 Department of Kidney and Vascular Pathology, University of Tsukuba, Tsukuba, Japan, **2** Meiji University International Institute for Bio-Resource Research, Kawasaki, Japan, **3** Division of Nephrology and Hypertension, Department of Internal Medicine, The Jikei University School of Medicine, Tokyo, Japan, **4** Division of Rheumatology, Department of Internal Medicine, Kanazawa University of Graduate School of Medicine, Kanazawa, Japan

Abstract

Glomerular nodular lesions, known as Kimmelstiel-Wilson nodules, are a pathological hallmark of progressive human diabetic nephropathy. We have induced severe diabetes in pigs carrying a dominant-negative mutant hepatocyte nuclear factor 1-alpha (HNF1α) P291fsinsC, a maturity-onset diabetes of the young type-3 (MODY3) gene in humans. In this model, glomerular pathology revealed that formation of diffuse glomerular nodules commenced as young as 1 month of age and increased in size and incidence until the age of 10 months, the end of the study period. Immunohistochemistry showed that the nodules consisted of various collagen types (I, III, IV, V and VI) with advanced glycation end-product (AGE) and N^{ε}-carboxymethyl-lysine (CML) deposition, similar to those in human diabetic nodules, except for collagen type I. Transforming growth factor-beta (TGF-β) was also expressed exclusively in the nodules. The ultrastructure of the nodules comprised predominant interstitial-type collagen deposition arising from the mesangial matrices. Curiously, these nodules were found predominantly in the deep cortex. However, diabetic pigs failed to show any of the features characteristic of human diabetic nephropathy; e.g., proteinuria, glomerular basement membrane thickening, exudative lesions, mesangiolysis, tubular atrophy, interstitial fibrosis, and vascular hyalinosis. The pigs showed only Armanni-Ebstein lesions, a characteristic tubular manifestation in human diabetes. RT-PCR analysis showed that glomeruli in wild-type pigs did not express endogenous HNF1α and HNF1β, indicating that mutant HNF1α did not directly contribute to glomerular nodular formation in diabetic pigs. In conclusion, pigs harboring the dominant-negative mutant human MODY3 gene showed reproducible and distinct glomerular nodules, possibly due to AGE- and CML-based collagen accumulation. Although the pathology differed in several respects from that of human glomerular nodular lesions, the somewhat acute and constitutive formation of nodules in this mammalian model might provide information facilitating identification of the principal mechanism underlying diabetic nodular sclerosis.

Editor: Leighton R. James, University of Florida, United States of America

Funding: This work was partially supported by Grants-in-Aid for Scientific Research (C) (#23500505) from the Ministry of Education, Culture, Sports, Science and Technology/Japan Society for the Promotion of Science (HN). The funders had no role in study design, data collection and analysis, decision to publish, or preparation of the manuscript.

* E-mail: nagatam@md.tsukuba.ac.jp

Introduction

Diabetic nephropathy is the leading cause of end-stage renal disease [1,2]. Glomerular nodular lesions, known as Kimmelstiel-Wilson nodules, are a pathological hallmark of human diabetic nephropathy. In 1936 Kimmelstiel and Wilson first described intercapillary glomerulosclerosis as a sign of advanced diabetic glomerular changes [3]. The presence of glomerular nodular lesions is known to be associated with poor renal outcome [4,5].

Although investigated extensively, the morphogenesis of diabetic glomerular nodules remains to be determined. One major reason for this is a lack of animal models that accurately represent the nodules typically present in humans. Some rodent models of diabetes show segmental mesangial expansion and glomerular basement membrane (GBM) thickening, but few exhibit distinct glomerular nodular lesions [6]. To date, the four representative diabetic rodent models with glomerular nodules are: endothelial nitric oxide synthase (eNOS) knockout *db/db* mice [7], receptor for advanced glycation end products (RAGE)/megsin/inducible nitric oxide synthase (iNOS) overexpressing transgenic mice [8], monocrotaline-treated Otsuka Long-Evans Tokushima Fatty (OLETF) rats [9] and BTBR *ob/ob* mice [10]. eNOS knockout *db/db* mice developed focal nodular glomerulosclerosis at 26 weeks of age [7]. RAGE/megsin/iNOS overexpressing transgenic mice also showed nodular-like lesions in 30–40% of glomeruli at 16 weeks of age [8]. Monocrotaline-treated OLETF rats showed a few nodular-like lesions at 50 weeks of age [9]. BTBR *ob/ob* mice showed diffuse but rare nodular mesangial sclerosis at 20 weeks of age [10]. These rodent models suggest that diabetic conditions in rodents do not lead to reproducible formation of diffuse glomerular nodular lesions. In addition, although two diabetic pig models—streptozotocin-induced diabetic pigs and INS^{C94Y} transgenic pigs—were created, both failed to reproduce diabetic kidney manifestations [11,12,13]. Thus, it may be more appropriate to create a diabetic mammalian model with the same genetic mutations present in human diabetes that exhibits diabetic renal complications similar to those in humans.

In humans, several forms of diabetes are associated with genetic mutations. Maturity-onset diabetes of the young type-3 (MODY3) is an early onset, non-insulin-dependent form of diabetes characterized by autosomal-dominant inheritance [14]. Those suffering from MODY3 have insufficient insulin secretion, resulting in a similar pathophysiology to that seen in human type-2 diabetes [14,15]. Hepatocyte nuclear factor 1-alpha (HNF1α) is the transcription factor believed to be responsible for MODY3 [14,15]. It is expressed in the liver, pancreas, proximal tubules, stomach, and small intestine [15,16,17]. The most common mutation in the HNF1α gene is the result of a cytosine (C) nucleotide insertion into a poly-C tract around codon 291 (designated as P291fsinsC), which causes frameshift-mutation-mediated deletion of the transactivation domain [14,15].

We have successfully created diabetic pigs carrying the dominant-negative mutant HNF1αP291fsinsC gene that is responsible for severe hyperglycemia with decreasing numbers of pancreatic beta cells [18]. Using these transgenic animals, in the present study we investigated the sequence of morphological events that leads to glomerular nodular lesions in diabetic nephropathy based on the human MODY3 gene. We expected the components and processes of glomerular nodular lesions in diabetic pigs to resemble those in human diabetic nephropathy.

Materials and Methods

Animals

All animal experiments were approved by the Institutional Animal Care and Use Committee of Meiji University (IACUC-09-006). As described previously, focus was on the use of transgenic pigs carrying a dominant-negative mutant HNF1α gene [18]. In short, a transgenic pig carrying an expression vector for the mutant human HNF1α cDNA (HNF1αP291fsinsC) was used. The transgene construct consisted of the enhancer for an immediate-early gene of human cytomegalovirus, followed by a porcine insulin promoter, the human HNF1αP291fsinsC cDNA, a SV40 poly-adenylation signal and a chicken β-globin insulator. Transgenic pigs carrying this cDNA were produced as reported elsewhere [19].

Study protocol

One transgenic and three wild-type pigs were used for biochemical and histological analyses through kidney biopsy. Tests were conducted at monthly intervals until the animals were 10 months of age. For histological analyses, autopsy of additional three transgenic and three wild-type pigs was conducted at 19 weeks of age.

Biochemical analysis

Serum and urine were collected each month after birth until completion of the study. The following biochemical parameters were measured: blood urea nitrogen, creatinine, plasma glucose, total protein, total cholesterol, triglycerides, aspartate aminotransferase, alanine aminotransferase and 1,5-anhydroglucitol. Urine was also analyzed in terms of total protein/creatinine and albumin/creatinine.

Histochemistry of renal sections

For kidney biopsy, the animals were anesthetized by an intramuscular injection of ketamine (11 mg/kg, Fujita Pharmaceutical Co., Ltd., Tokyo, Japan), with isoflurane (DS Pharma Animal Health Co., Ltd., Osaka, Japan) inhalation for maintenance. After the kidney location was confirmed using an ultrasonic pulse-echo technique, specimens were obtained using a Bard Monopty disposable biopsy needle (18 G×20 cm, Bard Biopsy Systems, Tempe, AZ, USA). Kidney specimens were fixed with 4% paraformaldehyde for paraffin sections or 2% glutaraldehyde for electron microscopy. For kidney autopsy, the animals were anesthetized by an intramuscular injection of 1% mafoprazine (0.5 mg/kg, DS Pharma animal Health Co., Ltd.) and intravenous injection of pentobarbital (Kyoritsu Seiyaku Corporation, Tokyo, Japan). After the animals were sacrificed by exsanguination through cutting cervical artery under anesthesia, kidney tissues were dissected and fixed with 4% paraformaldehyde for paraffin sections.

Paraffin sections were processed for periodic acid–Schiff (PAS) staining, periodic acid–methenamine-silver (PAM) staining, Masson's trichrome (MT) staining and immunostaining. Specific primary antibodies were as follows: mouse anti-collagen I antibody (1:50; Abcam, Cambridge, UK), rabbit anti-collagen III antibody (1:400; Abcam), rabbit anti-collagen IV antibody (1:50; Abcam), mouse anti-collagen V antibody (1:50; Abcam), rabbit anti-collagen VI antibody (1:50; Abcam), rabbit anti-advanced glycation end products (AGE) antibody (1:250; Abcam), mouse anti-N^{ε}-carboxymethyl-lysine (CML) antibody (1:500; TransGenic Inc., Ltd., Kumamoto, Japan) and rabbit anti-transforming growth factor beta-1 (TGF-β1) (V) antibody (1:100; Santa Cruz Biotechnology Inc., Santa Cruz, CA, USA). For immunostaining, antigen retrieval was performed using a microwave (10 mM citrate buffer; pH 6.0) (collagen I) or 100 µg/mL proteinase K (collagen III, IV, V, and VI). Thereafter, primary antibodies were incubated in an EnVision labeled polymer-HRP (Dako, Glostrup, Denmark) or Histofine kit (Nichirei Bioscience Inc., Tokyo, Japan) followed by reaction with peroxidase-conjugated streptavidin (Nichirei). Peroxidase activity was visualized using a liquid diaminobenzidine substrate (Dako). Hematoxylin was used to stain nuclei.

Distribution of glomeruli with nodular lesions

To estimate the prevalence of glomeruli with nodular lesions between the superficial and deep cortexes, sections representing the entire depth of the cortex were subdivided into three zones of equal width: the superficial, middle and deep cortex. The proportion of glomeruli with nodules in each sample was calculated and compared between the superficial and deep cortexes in autopsy specimens of transgenic and wild-type pigs at 19 weeks of age (60–240 glomeruli per kidney per animal).

Measurement of glomerular tuft area

To estimate glomerular tuft area between the superficial and deep cortexes, sections representing the entire depth of the cortex were subdivided into three zones of equal width: the superficial, middle and deep cortex. The glomerular tuft area in each sample was calculated using NanoZoomer 2.0-RS (Hamamatsu Photonics K.K., Hamamatsu, Japan) and compared between the superficial and deep cortexes in autopsy specimens of transgenic and wild-type pigs at 19 weeks of age (69–393 glomeruli per kidney per animal).

Table 1. Analysis of biochemical parameters in transgenic (Tg) and wild-type (WT) pigs at age 1, 5 and 10 months.

	1 month old		5 months old		10 months old	
	Tg (n = 1)	WT (n = 3)	Tg (n = 1)	WT (n = 3)	Tg (n = 1)	WT (n = 1)
Blood urea nitrogen (mmol/l)	13.6	2.71±0.43	10.8	5.07±0.43	9.35	4.53
Plasma glucose (mmol/l)	33.3	6.11±0.03	>33.3	5.87±0.40	26.0	5.51
Creatinine (μmol/l)	53.0	61.9±0.0	35.4	88.4±8.8	26.5	115
Total protein (g/l)	54.0	48.0±1.0	63.0	62.0±0.0	72.0	68.0
Total cholesterol (mmol/l)	11.6	2.95±0.18	1.86	2.00±0.05	1.09	1.66
Triglycerides (mmol/l)	1.69	0.26±0.03	>5.60	0.50±0.10	4.35	0.17
Asperate aminotransferase (IU/l)	23.0	43.0±6.4	128	21.7±1.0	51.0	21.0
Alanine aminotransferase (IU/l)	38.0	31.0±2.3	68.0	33.3±0.7	62.0	32.0
1,5-anhydroglucitol (μg/ml)	2.8	8.8±0.3	1.1	9.6±0.7	2.5	6.7
Urinary protein/creatinine (g/gCr)	<0.20	0.24*	0.72	0.47±0.31	0.45	<0.20
Urinary albumin/creatinine (g/gCr)	<0.10	0.16*	1.41	0.77±0.59	0.23	<0.1

Aberrations: Tg = transgenic pigs; WT = wild-type pigs; *: n = 1.

Thickness of the glomerular basement membrane

In biopsy specimens of pigs at 4 weeks and 5 months of age, 2% glutaraldehyde-fixed kidney cortex tissue was visualized by transmission electron microscopy. GBM thickness was estimated by measurements at five random capillaries in one glomerulus per animal. In each capillary, a series of five photographs were taken at 12,000× magnification, a grid was overlaid on the photograph, and GBM thickness was measured at the points intersecting the grid, with the exception of paramesangial areas. This method is a modified version of that of Hudkins, *et al.* [10].

Glomerular isolation, RNA isolation and reverse transcription PCR (RT-PCR)

To evaluate HNF1α or HNF1β expression, RT-PCR was performed using isolated glomeruli from one wild-type pig at 4 weeks of age. The animal was anesthetized using isoflurane (DS Pharma Animal Health Co., Ltd.) and perfused with phosphate-buffered saline (PBS). The kidneys, liver and heart were then removed. Using the renal artery, the kidneys were perfused with a 1 mg/mL iron powder in PBS. They were then minced into 1-mm^3 pieces and passed through a 100-μm cell strainer. Finally, glomeruli containing the iron powder were isolated using a magnetic particle concentrator. Total RNA was extracted from the isolated glomeruli, liver, and heart using the RNeasy Mini Kit (Qiagen, Hilden, Germany). RNA was quantified using a Nanodrop 1000 spectrophotometer (Thermo Fisher Scientific K.K., Rockford, IL). Total RNA (1 μg) was reverse-transcribed using the Thermoscript RT-PCR System (Life Technologies Corporation, Carlsbad, CA, USA) into first-strand cDNA. Then, 10 ng of cDNA template and 0.25 mmol/l of sequence-specific primers were used to perform RT-PCR. Primer sequences (5′ to 3′) were as follows: HNF1α forward: CACAGTCTGCTGAG-CACAGA

HNF1α reverse: TTGGTGGTGTCGGTGATGAG

HNF1β forward: AGAGGGAGGCCTTAGTGGAG

HNF1β reverse: GAGAGGGGCGTCATGATGAG

The liver and heart were used as positive and negative controls, respectively.

Statistical analysis

Mann-Whitney *U* tests using StatView-J 5.0 (Adept Scientific, Acton, MA, USA) were performed for comparison of the glomerular nodular distribution and glomerular tuft area. Data are shown as means ± standard errors (SE). *P*-values were calculated from the data. Statistical significance was considered at p-values < 0.05.

Results

Transgenic pigs carrying a dominant-negative mutant HNF1α gene showed severe diabetic mellitus

The biochemical parameters of a single transgenic pig were compared with those of three wild-type pigs over a 10-month period (Table 1). Body weight was lower in transgenic pigs than in wild-type pigs (Figure S1A). In transgenic pigs, the plasma glucose levels were elevated to 22.2–33.3 mmol/L as early as 11 days after birth. This hyperglycemia persisted until 10 months of age (Figure S1B). 1,5-Anhydroglucitol, which reflects the increase in plasma glucose levels during the past several days, was at low levels, indicating severe diabetes mellitus (Figure S1C). In 1-month-old pigs, total cholesterol was high, but decreased after 2 months of age. In contrast, triglycerides were elevated throughout the lifespan of the pigs, which is a symptom also observed in humans with diabetic mellitus. However, serum creatinine levels were within the normal range and no proteinuria was detected in transgenic pigs until 10 months of age.

Transgenic pigs exhibited characteristic diffuse glomerular nodular lesions

Kidney autopsy revealed distinct glomerular nodular lesions at age 19 weeks in all three transgenic pigs (Figure 1A). These nodules were diffuse and acellular, consisting of abnormal matrices. Matrices were slightly evident by PAS staining, strongly by PAM staining, and appeared as a distinct blue color by MT staining. This staining pattern points to the abundance of collagen fibers in the nodules. Numerous nodules formed within an individual glomerulus and were distributed throughout with no discernible pattern. However, more were present in the deep cortex than in the superficial cortex (86.6±7.73 *vs.* 30.6±12.2%) ($p = 0.0495$; Figure 1B). Additionally, the glomerular tuft area in

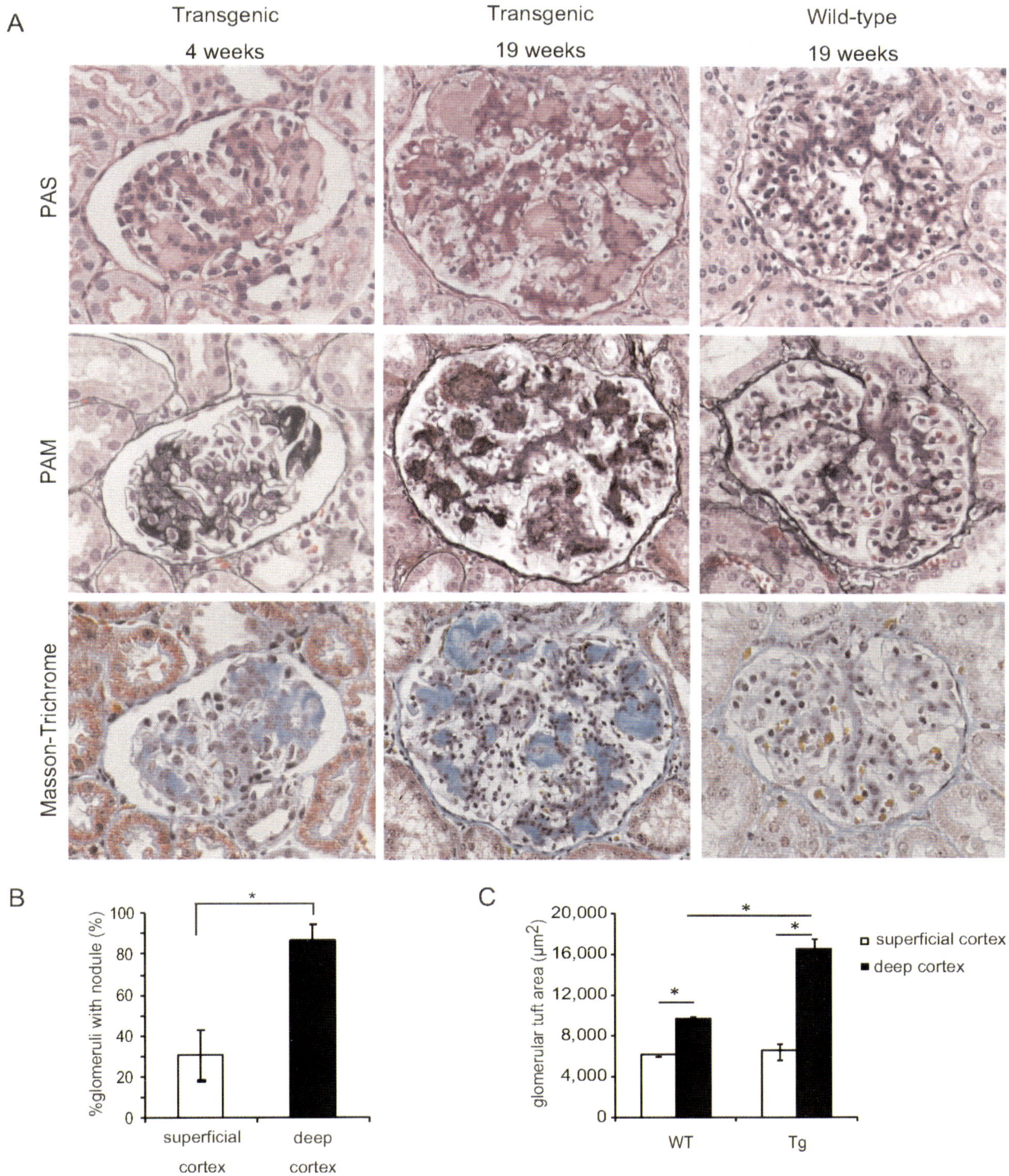

Figure 1. Renal pathological findings at age 4 and 19 weeks in transgenic pigs. A) In transgenic pigs, mesangial expansion commenced as early as 4 weeks. At 19 weeks, distinct glomerular nodules had formed. Magnification: 400×. **B**) The number of glomeruli with nodules as a fraction of the total number was compared between the superficial cortex and deep cortex. **C**) Glomerular tuft area in superficial and deep cortexes was compared between wild-type pigs and transgenic pigs. Transgenic pigs; n = 3, wild-type pigs; n = 3. *$P < 0.05$. WT = wild-type pigs; Tg = transgenic pigs.

the deep cortex was significantly larger in transgenic pigs than in wild-type pigs (16,566±983 *vs.* 9,694±224 μm^2; $p = 0.0495$), but was not significantly different in the superficial cortex (6,616±588 *vs.* 6,166±80 μm^2; $p = 0.8273$; Figure 1C). This unique distribution of nodules and glomerular tuft size suggested that glomerular

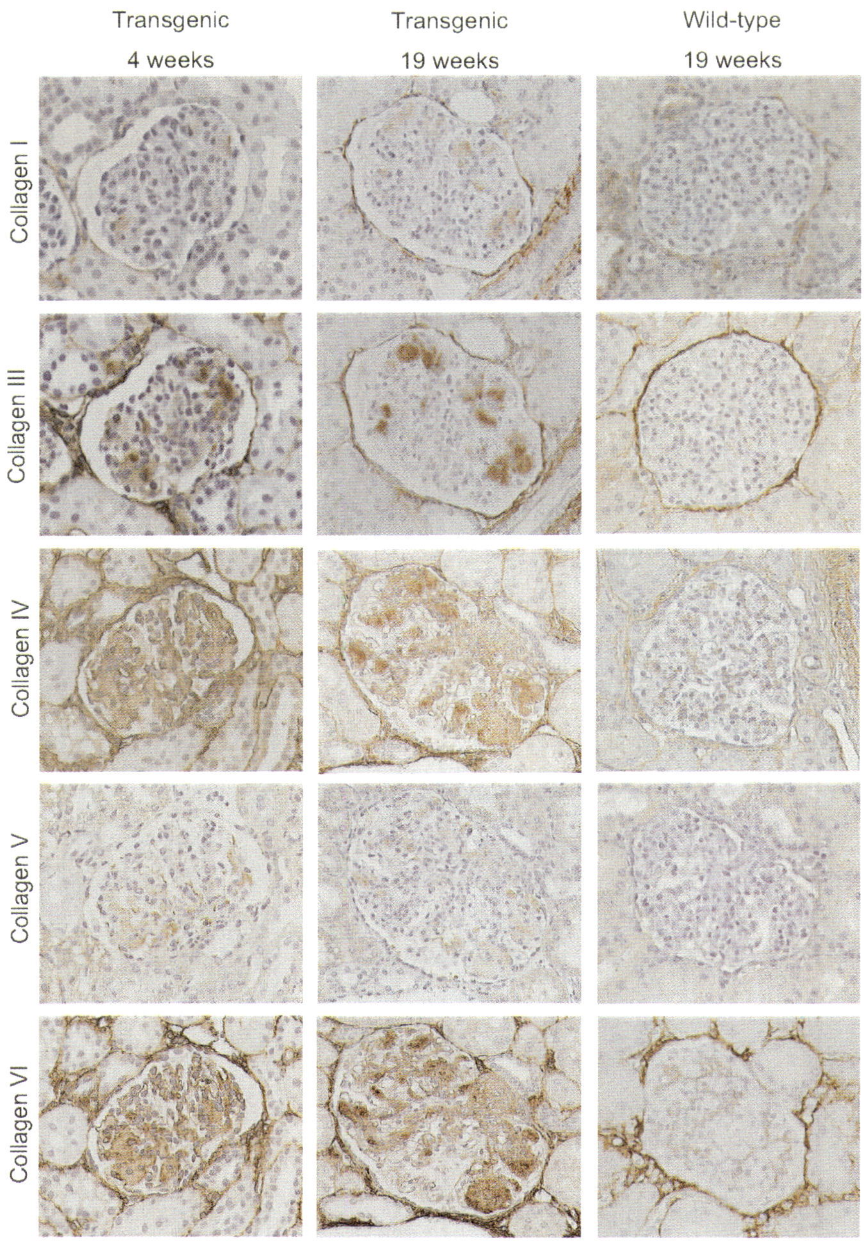

Figure 2. Immunostaining for collagen types I, III, IV, V and VI at age 4 weeks (left) and 19 weeks (middle) in transgenic pigs, and 19 weeks in wild-type pigs (right). In transgenic pigs, collagen types I, III, IV, V and VI were accumulated in the nodules as early as 4 weeks. Collagen types III, IV and VI were strongly positive. Magnification: 400×.

hyperfiltration might contribute to formation of nodules in transgenic pigs.

Immunostaining revealed that the nodules consisted of various types of collagen, including types I, III, IV, V and VI (Figure 2). Collagen types III, IV and VI were present at high concentrations, whereas collagen types I and V were relatively less abundant. AGE, CML and TGF-β1 were also detected in the nodules (Figure 3). AGE tended to be found at the margins of the nodule. CML and TGF-β1 were localized in the nodules in the same patterns as seen in human diabetic nephropathy [20,21,22].

To monitor the sequence of nodular formation, monthly kidney biopsies were performed until the age of 10 months. Mesangial expansions were formed as early as 4 weeks of age and contained the abnormal matrices similar to those seen in transgenic pigs at 19 weeks of age (Figure 1A). Thereafter, the matrices expanded gradually with age. Collagen fibers and AGE deposition were exclusively associated from the early evolution to the end of the study period (Figures 2 and 3). Glomerular nodular lesions did not lead to segmental glomerulosclerosis or active adhesion.

Another major histological development was the vacuolization of the cytoplasm of epithelial cells in the proximal tubules, resembling Armanni-Ebstein lesions (Figure S2) [23]. The frequency of mesangiolysis and exudative lesions was low (~1 per 200 glomeruli). Other diabetic changes normally seen in

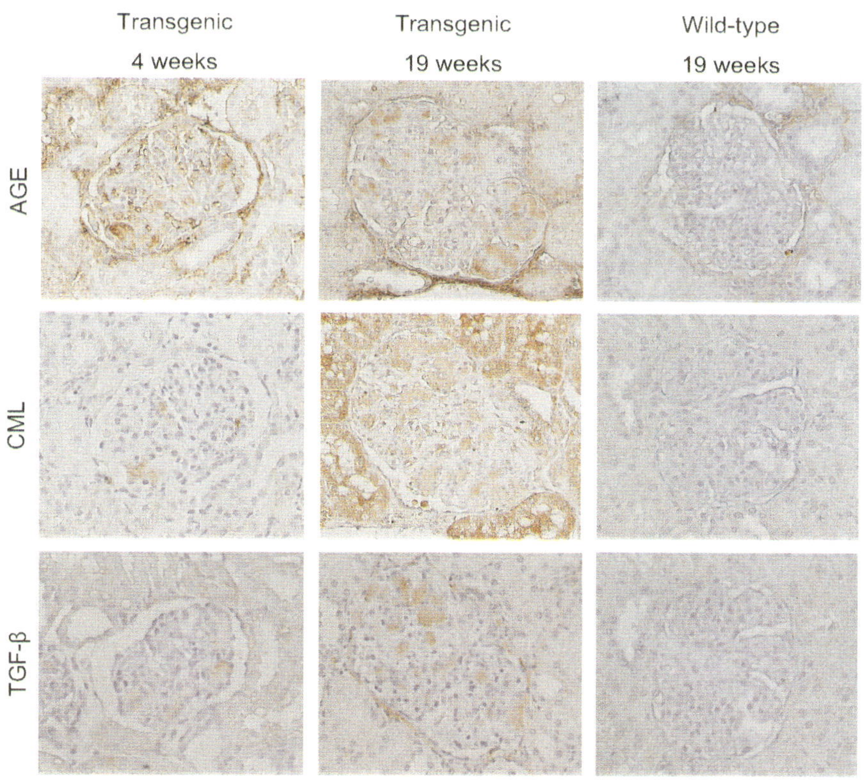

Figure 3. Immunostaining for AGE, CML and TGF-β at age 4 weeks (left) and 19 weeks (middle) in transgenic pigs, and 19 weeks in wild-type pigs (right). In transgenic pigs, AGE, CML and TGF-β accumulated in the glomerular nodules as early as 4 weeks. Magnification: 400×. AGE = advanced glycation end product; CML = N^{ε}-carboxymethyl-lysine; TGF-β = transforming growth factor-beta.

humans were absent from the pig models, including tubular atrophy, interstitial fibrosis and arteriolar hyalinosis.

Glomerular nodular lesions consisted of interstitial forms of fibril collagen

To determine whether glomerular nodular lesions were associated with the typical diabetic changes found in humans, biopsy specimens from animals at 4 weeks and 5 months of age were visualized by electron microscopy. At 4 weeks, bright fibers began to appear in the mesangial matrices (Figure 4A and B), accompanied by lipid particles and cell debris. At a high magnification, the fibers were seen to closely resemble interstitial types of collagen, being of 46-nm diameter with a 50-nm cross-striation cycle (Figure 4E). These collagens were found predominantly around mesangial cells, suggesting that this was their point of origin (Figure 4A). Within 5 months the fibers had accumulated in the mesangium and had expanded to nodular formations (Figure 4C). This nodule expansion encroached upon capillary lumens and caused them to become occluded. A subendothelial widening, accompanied by a loss of endothelial fenestration and occasional mesangial interposition, was also noted (Figure 4D). The GBM thickness of the transgenic pigs was not different from that of wild-type pigs at both 4 weeks and 5 months of age (4 weeks: 163 nm in transgenic pigs *vs.* 186±10.3 nm in wild-type pigs, 5 months: 194 nm in transgenic pigs *vs.* 181±5.2 nm in wild-type pigs) (Figure 4F).

Endogenous HNF1α and HNF1β were absent from the glomeruli of wild-type pigs

RT-PCR for HNF1α and HNF1β in the glomeruli of wild-type pigs at 4 weeks of age was performed to determine whether insertion of the dominant-negative mutant HNF1αP291fsinsC gene contributed to the development of glomerular nodular lesions by inhibiting endogenous HNF1α or HNF1β function in glomerular cells. Both HNF1α and HNF1β were absent from the isolated glomeruli, but were expressed in the positive control liver tissue (Figure 5A and B). Therefore, the dominant-negative mutant HNF1αP291fsinsC gene insertion did not contribute directly to the glomerular nodular formation in transgenic pigs.

Discussion and Conclusions

Our pig model carrying a dominant-negative human MODY3 gene is the first to show reproducible diffuse glomerular nodular lesions in a mammalian model of diabetes. The ability to perform repeat kidney biopsies was a great advantage in terms of understanding the *in vivo* morphological events involved in glomerular nodular formation.

Glomerular nodular lesions in our diabetic pigs were characterized by monotonous accumulation of interstitial forms of collagen fibrils in the mesangium. Initially, small nodules were detected as early as 1 month of age and developed diffusely until 10 months of age. Notably, these were basically acellular round nodules without mesangial proliferation, inflammatory infiltrates or mesangiolysis, (cold nodule); this differs from human diabetic nodules. Immunostaining for various collagens revealed predominantly collagen type III, IV, V and VI in our model, similar to in

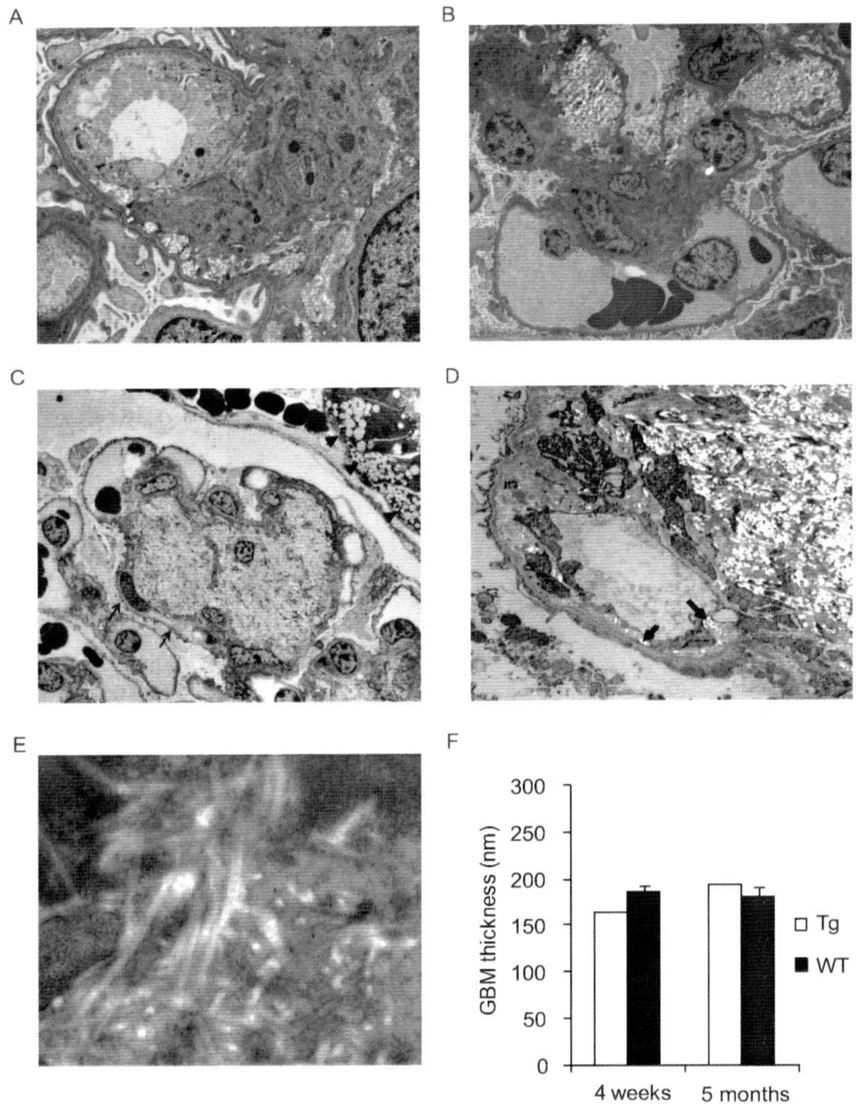

Figure 4. Transmission electron microscopy at age 4 weeks (A,B,E) and 5 months (C,D) in transgenic pigs. A) In 4-week-old transgenic pigs, mesangial widening is associated with fiber deposition in the mesangial matrices. Magnification: 2,000×. **B**) Fibers accumulated at mesangial areas, forming early lesion. Magnificat on: 500×. **C**) At 5 months, established glomerular nodules showed that mesangial areas and capillary lumens are filled with bright fibers (arrows). Vacuolations of proximal tubules were also seen (arrowheads). Magnification: 300×. **D**) Subendothelial widening with loss of endothelial fenestration and mesangial interposition are shown. Note that collagen is also found in the subendothelial spaces (arrows). Magnification: 1,500×. **E**) The nodules consist of fibril collagens with cross striation, indicating interstitial-type forms of collagen fibrils. Magnification: 10,000×. **F**) Thickness of glomerular basement membranes in transgenic pigs was no different from those in wild-type pigs at 4 weeks and 5 months old. Transgenic pigs; n = 1, wild-type pigs; n = 3. Tg = transgenic pigs; WT = wild-type pigs; GBM = glomerular basement membrane.

human diabetic nodules [24,25]. However, our diabetic nodules also exhibited collagen type I deposition, which is unusual in human diabetic nephropathy [24,25,26]. Electron microscopy showed a distinct interstitial collagen type, which appeared to be a mixture of types I, III and V collagen, as the main component. This was synthesized in the mesangial cells in the early stage, and tended to expand toward the corresponding capillary lumina, finally resulting in nodular sclerosis.

Although the detailed sequence of events leading to nodular formation, and the structure of the nodules, in this model may not be identical to that in humans with type-2 diabetes, the nodules expressed AGEs from a young age AGEs are produced by non-enzymatic glycation under hyperglycemia, and glomerular AGE deposition is an important characteristic of nodular morphogenesis in human diabetes [21,27,28]. Specifically, CML is the major AGE accumulated in nodular lesions [20,21]. Glomerular AGEs stimulate extracellular matrix production by mesangial cells through reactive oxygen species (ROS)-promoted TGF-β expression [27,28,29,30]. Glomerular ROS production was caused by AGE-mediated RAGE upregulation or glucose metabolism [27,28,30,31]. In this regard, early onset exclusive AGE deposition and TGF-β1 expression in the nodules of diabetic pigs suggest AGE-mediated collagen synthesis in mesangial cells under a persistent hyperglycemic condition. The differences in nodular morphogenesis and its collagen composition between our model and human diabetic nephropathy suggest that the mesangial

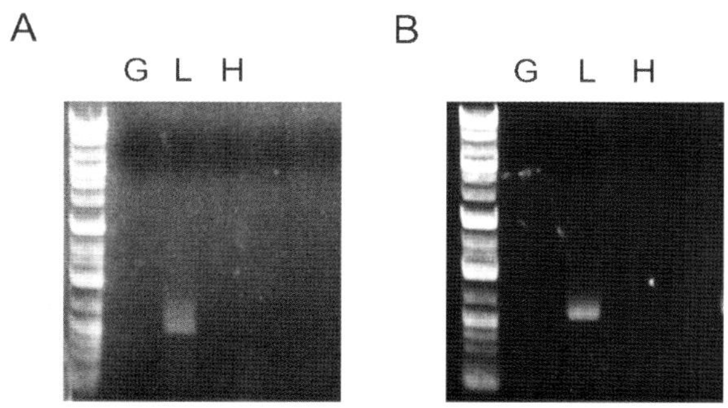

Figure 5. Reverse transcription-PCR for endogenous HNF1α and HNF1β in wild-type pigs at 4 weeks of age. Both HNF1α (**A**) and HNF1β (**B**) were negative in isolated glomeruli. Liver was used as a positive control, and heart as a negative control. G = isolated glomeruli; L = liver; H = heart.

cellular response in these species is different under diabetic conditions. Several reports of nodular sclerosis in the diabetic rodent model support this explanation.

In addition to the mesangial changes under hyperglycemia, our model suggests the involvement of unique hemodynamic factors in nodular morphogenesis. Glomerular hyperfiltration or hypertrophy promotes diabetic nephropathy; however, whether glomerular hemodynamic effects accelerate the formation of diabetic nodules in humans remains controversial. Accordingly, the present study showed that glomerular nodular lesions in diabetic pigs were localized predominantly in the deep cortex. Notably, glomeruli were significantly larger in the deep cortex of diabetic pigs compared to in that of wild-type pigs, but were unchanged in the superficial cortex of both groups. These observations suggest that glomerular hemodynamic effects also promote formation of glomerular nodular lesions in diabetic pigs. Similarly, diabetic nephropathy was accelerated in eNOS-knockout mice, attenuated by improvement of eNOS activity in *db/db* mice [32,33], and antihypertensive therapy alone significantly suppressed the development of nodular lesions and mesangiolysis in diabetic eNOS-knockout mice [34]. Based on these reports and our current findings, our results suggest the involvement of glomerular hypertension in nodular lesion formation in diabetes. Therefore, prominent glomerular hyperfiltration and hypertrophy may be the basis of glomerular nodule development in our diabetic pig model.

The inserted dominant-negative human MODY gene might have stimulated mesangial matrix synthesis by inhibiting endogenous HNF1α or HNF1β function, regardless of the diabetic milieu. Typically, HNF1α functions as a homodimer or a heterodimer with the structurally related protein HNF1β [14,15,35]. Thus, a dominant-negative mutant HNF1αP291fsinsC should inhibit HNF1α or HNF1β by forming an inactive heterodimer at the site of endogenous HNF1α or HNF1β expression. The RT-PCR study confirmed that mutant HNF1αP291fsinsC could not interact with endogenous HNF1α and HNF1β in the glomeruli of transgenic pigs. This supports the notion that the diabetic milieu, but not the genetic alteration, promotes glomerular nodular formation in the pig model.

Our diabetic pig model lacks several diabetic renal features characteristic of human diabetic nephropathy; e.g., proteinuria, GBM thickening, exudative lesions, tubular atrophy, interstitial fibrosis and arteriolar hyalinosis. Furthermore, the glomeruli did not undergo glomerulosclerosis. These results suggest that our model does not accurately reproduce human diabetic nephropathy, even in pigs carrying the human MODY3 gene. In addition to the species difference in the cellular response to hyperglycemia, a possible explanation for this discrepancy is that we were unable to monitor the histology for a sufficiently long period because due to the relatively short lifespan of the pigs. In addition, the mechanism of nodular formation is considered to be different from that of other diabetic kidney lesions. Nevertheless, this pig model indicated that glomerular nodules could form independently of diabetic complications.

In conclusion, this was the first report of distinct and reproducible glomerular nodular lesions in transgenic pigs carrying a dominant-negative HNF1α mutation of the human MODY3 gene. Although there were several differences compared to the pathology of human glomerular nodular lesions, the somewhat acute and constitutive formation of nodules in the mammalian models might provide information that will facilitate identification of the principal mechanism underlying glomerular nodular formation.

Supporting Information

Figure S1 Body weight and diabetic parameter changes over time. A) Body weight was lower in transgenic pigs than in wild-type pigs. **B**) Plasma glucose was at a high level in transgenic pigs. **C**) 1,5-Anhydroglucitol was at a low level in transgenic pigs. Tg = transgenic pigs (n = 1); WT = wild-type pigs (up to 6 months of age, n = 3; 6–10 months of age, n = 1).

Figure S2 Armanni-Ebstein lesions in diabetic pigs at 19 weeks of age. Transgenic pigs revealed vacuolation of proximal tubules known as Armanni-Ebstein lesions. Note that distal tubules and the collecting duct are intact. **A**) Magnification: 100×. **B**) Magnification: 400×.

Author Contributions

Conceived and designed the experiments: KU HN. Performed the experiments: KU TY SH. Analyzed the data: SH TY MN. Contributed reagents/materials/analysis tools: SH TY KU HN MN. Wrote the paper: SH KU MN.

References

1. Nakai S, Iseki K, Itami N, Ogata S, Kazama JJ, et al. (2012) An overview of regular dialysis treatment in Japan (as of 31 December 2010). Ther Apher Dial 16: 483–521.
2. White SL, Chadban SJ, Jan S, Chapman JR, Cass A (2008) How can we achieve equity in provision of renal replacement therapy? Bull World Health Organ 86: 229–237.
3. Kimmelstiel P, Wilson C (1936) Intercapillary Lesions in the Glomeruli of the Kidney. Am J Pathol 12: 83–98.7.
4. Hong D, Zheng T, Jia-qing S, Jian W, Zhi-hong L, et al. (2007) Nodular glomerular lesion: a later stage of diabetic nephropathy? Diabetes Res Clin Pract 78: 189–195.
5. Heaf JG, Løkkegaard H, Larsen S (2001) The relative prognosis of nodular and diffuse diabetic nephropathy. Scand J Urol Nephrol 35: 233–238.
6. Brosius FC 3rd, Alpers CE, Bottinger EP, Breyer MD, Coffman TM, et al. (2009) Mouse models of diabetic nephropathy. J Am Soc Nephrol 20: 2503–2512.
7. Zhao HJ, Wang S, Cheng H, Zhang MZ, Takahashi T, et al. (2006) Endothelial nitric oxide synthase deficiency produces accelerated nephropathy in diabetic mice. J Am Soc Nephrol 17: 2664–2669.
8. Inagi R, Yamamoto Y, Nangaku M, Usuda N, Okamoto H, et al. (2006) A severe diabetic nephropathy model with early development of nodule-like lesions induced by megsin overexpression in RAGE/iNOS transgenic mice. Diabetes 55: 356–366.

9. Furuichi K, Hisada Y, Shimizu M, Okumura T, Kitagawa K, et al. (2011) Matrix metalloproteinase-2 (MMP-2) and membrane-type 1 MMP (MT1-MMP) affect the remodeling of glomerulosclerosis in diabetic OLETF rats. Nephrol Dial Transplant 26: 3124–3131.
10. Hudkins KL, Pichaiwong W, Wietecha T, Kowalewska J, Banas M, et al. (2010) BTBR ob/ob mutant mice model progressive diabetic nephropathy. J Am Soc Nephrol 21: 1533–1542.
11. Larsen MO, Wilken M, Gotfredsen CF, Carr RD, Svendsen O, et al. (2002) Mild streptozotocin diabetes in the Göttingen minipig. A novel model of moderate insulin deficiency and diabetes. Am J Physiol Endocrinol Metab 282: E1342–1351.
12. Bellinger DA, Merricks EP, Nichols TC (2006) Swine models of type 2 diabetes mellitus: insulin resistance, glucose tolerance, and cardiovascular complications. ILAR J 47: 243–258.
13. Renner S, Braun-Reichhart C, Blutke A, Herbach N, Emrich D, et al. (2013) Permanent neonatal diabetes in INS(C94Y) transgenic pigs. Diabetes 62: 1505–1511.
14. Yamagata K, Oda N, Kaisaki PJ, Menzel S, Furuta H, et al. (1996) Mutations in the hepatocyte nuclear factor-1α gene in maturity-onset diabetes of the young (MODY3). Nature 384: 455–458.
15. Yamagata K (2003) Regulation of pancreatic β-cell function by the HNF transcription network: lessons from maturity-onset diabetes of the young (MODY). Endocr J 50: 491–499.
16. Pontoglio M, Barra J, Hadchouel M, Doyen A, Kress C, et al. (1996) Hepatocyte nuclear factor 1 inactivation results in hepatic dysfunction, phenylketonuria, and renal Fanconi syndrome. Cell 84: 575–585.
17. Pontoglio M (2000) Hepatocyte nuclear factor 1, a transcription factor at the crossroads of glucose homeostasis. J Am Soc Nephrol 11: S140–S143.
18. Umeyama K, Watanabe M, Saito H, Kurome M, Tohi S, et al. (2009) Dominant-negative mutant hepatocyte nuclear factor 1alpha induces diabetes in transgenic-cloned pigs. Transgenic Res 18: 697–706.
19. Umeyama K, Honda K, Matsunari H, Nakano K, Hidaka T, et al. (2013) Production of diabetic offspring using cryopreserved epididymal sperm by in vitro fertilization and intrafallopian insemination techniques in transgenic pigs. J Reprod Dev 59: 599–603.
20. Tanji N, Markowitz GS, Fu C, Kislinger T, Taguchi A, et al. (2000) Expression of advanced glycation end products and their cellular receptor RAGE in diabetic nephropathy and nondiabetic renal disease. J Am Soc Nephrol 11: 1656–1666.
21. Horie K, Miyata T, Maeda K, Miyata S, Sugiyama S, et al. (1997) Immunohistochemical colocalization of glycoxidation products and lipid peroxidation products in diabetic renal glomerular lesions. Implication for glycoxidative stress in the pathogenesis of diabetic nephropathy. J Clin Invest 100: 2995–3004.
22. Yamamoto T, Nakamura T, Noble NA, Ruoslahti E, Border WA (1993) Expression of transforming growth factor beta is elevated in human and experimental diabetic nephropathy. Proc Natl Acad Sci U S A 90: 1814–1818.
23. Ritchie S, Waugh D (1957) The pathology of Armanni-Ebstein diabetic nephropathy. Am J Pathol 33: 1035–1057.
24. Nerlich A, Schleicher E (1991) Immunohistochemical localization of extracellular matrix components in human diabetic glomerular lesions. Am J Pathol 139: 889–899.
25. Makino H, Shikata K, Wieslander J, Wada J, Kashihara N, et al. (1994) Localization of fibril/microfibril and basement membrane collagens in diabetic glomerulosclerosis in type 2 diabetes. Diabet Med 11: 304–311.
26. Glick AD, Jacobson HR, Haralson MA (1992) Mesangial deposition of type I collagen in human glomerulosclerosis. Hum Pathol 23: 1373–1379.
27. Renner S, Braun-Reichhart C, Blutke A, Herbach N, Emrich D, et al. (2001) Biochemistry and molecular cell biology of diabetic complications. Nature 414: 813–820.
28. Yamagishi S, Matsui T (2010) Advanced glycation end products, oxidative stress and diabetic nephropathy. Oxid Med Cell Longev 3: 101–108.
29. Fukami K, Ueda S, Yamagishi S, Kato S, Inagaki Y, et al. (2004) AGEs activate mesangial TGF-β-Smad signaling via an angiotensin II type I receptor interaction. Kidney Int 66: 2137–2147.
30. Mason RM, Wahab NA (2003) Extracellular matrix metabolism in diabetic nephropathy. J Am Soc Nephrol 14: 1358–1373.
31. Yan SD, Schmidt AM, Anderson GM, Zhang J, Brett J, et al. (1994) Enhanced cellular oxidant stress by the interaction of advanced glycation end products with their receptors/binding proteins. J Biol Chem 269: 9889–9897.
32. Kanetsuna Y, Takahashi K, Nagata M, Gannon MA, Breyer MD, et al. (2007) Deficiency of endothelial nitric-oxide synthase confers susceptibility to diabetic nephropathy in nephropathy-resistant inbred mice. Am J Pathol 170: 1473–1484.
33. Cheng H, Wang H, Fan X, Paueksakon P, Harris RC (2012) Improvement of endothelial nitric oxide synthase activity retards the progression of diabetic nephropathy in db/db mice. Kidney Int 82: 1176–1183.
34. Kosugi T, Heinig M, Nakayama T, Connor T, Yuzawa Y, et al. (2009) Lowering blood pressure blocks mesangiolysis and mesangial nodules, but not tubulointerstitial injury, in diabetic eNOS knockout mice. Am J Pathol 174: 1221–1229.
35. Mendel DB, Hansen LP, Graves MK, Conley PB, Crabtree GR (1991) HNF-1 alpha and HNF-1 beta (vHNF-1) share dimerization and homeo domains, but not activation domains, and form heterodimers in vitro. Genes Dev 5: 1042–1056.

11

The Diagnosis Accuracy of PLA2R-AB in the Diagnosis of Idiopathic Membranous Nephropathy: A Meta-Analysis

Yu Du[1], Junhua Li[1], Fan He[1], Yongman Lv[1], Wei Liu[1], Ping Wu[2], Jiao Huang[3], Sheng Wei[3], Hongyu Gao[1]*

1 Department of Nephrology, Tongji hospital affiliated to Tongji medical college, Huazhong University of Science and Technology, Wuhan, Hubei, China, **2** Department of Pathophysiology, Tongji Medical College, Huazhong University of Science and Technology, Wuhan, Hubei, China, **3** Department of Epidemiology and Biostatistics, School of Public Health, Tongji Medical College, Huazhong University of Science and Technology, Wuhan, Hubei, China

Abstract

Background: The presence of antibodies against the M-type phospholipase A2 receptor (PLA2R-AB) is considered to be a promising serological diagnostic biomarker of idiopathic membranous nephropathy (iMN). However, controversy remains about the diagnostic accuracy of serum PLA2R-AB testing. Here, we performed a comprehensive meta-analysis to assess the overall diagnostic value of serum PLA2R-AB testing in iMN detection.

Methods: PubMed, Embase, and CNKI (Chinese National Knowledge Infrastructure) were searched for relevant original articles through January 31, 2014. The summary sensitivity, specificity, positive likelihood ratio, negative likelihood ratio and diagnostic odds ratio (DOR) were estimated using the bivariate model. The heterogeneity among studies was explored by subgroup and meta-regression analysis.

Results: 9 articles, including 15 studies, were eventually identified with a total of 2212 patients. The summary sensitivity of all studies is 78% (95% CI: 66% to 87%) and the specificity is 99% (95% CI: 96% to 100%). The summary positive and negative likelihood ratios are 96.1 (95% CI, 19.5 to 472.1) and 0.22 (95% CI: 0.14 to 0.35), respectively. The DOR is 437 (95%CI, 74 to 2592). The subgroup analysis and meta-regression suggest the test interval is the main source of heterogeneity.

Conclusions: Serum PLA2R-AB testing is a useful tool to detect iMN. In addition, considering the high heterogeneity and potential publication bias, further high quality studies are needed in the future.

Editor: Ariela Benigni, IRCSS - Istituto di Ricerche Farmacologiche Mario Negri, Italy

Funding: This work was supported by the National Natural Science Foundation of China (grants 81100498 to JL and 81100481 to HG). The funder had no role in study design, data collection and analysis, decision to publish, or preparation of the manuscript.

* Email: gaohongyu2010@gmail.com

Introduction

Membranous nephropathy (MN) is one of the leading causes of nephritic syndrome in adults [1]. The disease is characterized by the formation of subepithelial immune deposits and complement mediated proteinuria [2,3]. Approximately 80% of all cases are referred to as 'idiopathic' MN (iMN) because they have no known etiology. The remaining 20–25% cases of MN are classified as 'secondary' cases due to their association with co-morbid clinical conditions such as systemic lupus erythematodes (SLE), cancer, viral or bacterial infection, and/or drug intoxication [4,5]. In order to substantially improve the management and clinical outcome of patients with MN, it is extremely important to ensure reliable differential diagnoses between idiopathic and secondary MN [2,6].

The M-type phospholipase A2 receptor (PLA2R) was recently identified as a major target antigen in autoimmune idiopathic membranous nephropathy [7]. Several studies have indicated that about 70–80% of patients with iMN tested positive for circulating antibodies against PLA2R(PLA2R-AB). Conversely, patients with secondary MN or other proteinuric disease tested negative for PLA2R-AB [8]. Since the level of PLA2R-AB correlates with clinical disease activity, it could be used to monitor a patient's response to treatment. This suggests that serum PLA2R-AB may serve as promising alternative diagnostic biomarker for iMN [7,9,10].

Compared with histological examination, serological testing for circulating PLA2R-AB is both more convenient and safer than traditional pathological examination. While a renal biopsy is invasive and may cause glomerular injury or other more serious complications, testing serum PLA2R-AB provides a quick disease detection method for clinicians. However, a series of prior studies showed that serum PLA2R-AB diagnoses were conflicting and could be extremely varied. For example, the sensitivity of PLA2R-AB tests ranged from 52% to 98.4% across all current studies [11–15]. Although PLA2R-AB may be a new tool for iMN diagnosis, its efficacy still remains controversial. Therefore, to comprehensively assess the diagnostic value of serum PLA2R-AB testing for iMN, we undertook the present meta-analysis to assess the overall diagnostic sensitivity and specificity of PLA2R-AB testing in patients with idiopathic membranous nephropathy.

Materials and Methods

Search strategy and study selection

PubMed, Embase, and CNKI (Chinese National Knowledge Infrastructure) were searched to identify eligible studies published prior to January 1st, 2014. The search terms used were "phospholipase A2 receptor antibody", "PLA2R AB" and "membranous nephropathy". Studies were also identified by the references cited in selected articles and were then searched manually. Two reviewers (YD and JH) independently determined study eligibility and disagreement between reviewers was resolved by consensus.

Selection criteria

Studies were included in the current meta-analysis if they met the following criteria: (1) evaluation of the accuracy of PLA2R-AB testing on iMN diagnosis; (2) estimation of the sensitivity and specificity of the PLA2R-AB test; and (3) using of biopsy test results as a gold standard. Cases were excluded from this study for the following reason(s) (1): were a case report, review, letter, editorial, or comment; (2) had not performed any tests on serum levels of the PLA2R antibody; or (3) did not provide sufficient data. If studies had overlapping subjects, only the study with the largest sample size was included in the final analysis. Finally, since immunosuppressive therapy could affect the serum levels of PLA2R-AB, patients who received immunosuppressive therapy were excluded from our meta-analysis.

Data extraction and quality assessment of studies

Two reviewers independently reviewed the articles and extracted the following data from all eligible publications: first author, year of publication, total number of patients, race, mean age, proportion of females, test methods, sensitivity, specificity, funding source and methodological quality.

The methodological quality of studies was evaluated independently by two reviewers (YD and JH) with the quality assessment of diagnostic accuracy studies (QUADAS) tool [16]. Component analysis was performed by creating a proportional bar graph for each of the 14 individual criteria. Each item was scored 'yes' if reported, 'no' if not reported, or 'unclear' if there were insufficient data to make a definitive assessment.

Data analysis

A random-effects model was used to calculate the average sensitivity, specificity, positive likelihood ratio, negative likelihood ratio, and diagnostic odds ratio (DOR) across studies. A summary receiver operator characteristic (SROC) curve was then used to plot the consistency of results among all studies as well as the accuracy of the test. Both the χ^2-test and I^2 were used to detect statistically significant heterogeneity. Subgroup analyses were performed to identify factors which may be sources of heterogeneity. Such factors included: race, type of controls (e.g. patients with other kidney disease versus healthy controls), sample size, PLA2R-AB testing methods (e.g. Western blotting versus indirect immunofluorescence), test time intervals (e.g. testing simultaneously with the biopsy test versus testing after the biopsy test), and funding sources (e.g. sponsorship from government or corporate monies). These factors were then included as covariates in a meta-regression analysis to determine if they were statistically significant sources of heterogeneity. Lastly, a sensitivity analysis was conducted to assess the influence of each study on the overall parameter estimates.

A funnel plot and the effective sample size regression test for asymmetry were used to explore potential publication biases [17]. All analyses were performed in *mdias* module in Stata 10.0 (College Station, TX, USA).

Results

Study characteristics

As shown in Figure 1, there were 70 potentially relevant articles found in our search. Forty-two articles met exclusion criteria (22 reviews, 6 editorials, 5 case reports and 9 comments). The remaining 28 articles were retrieved for full-text review. Nineteen were excluded (14 studies did not investigate the test accuracy, 4 studies had insufficient data and 1 study only investigated PLA2R-AB in tissue). Finally, 9 articles, including 15 studies, were included in the present meta-analysis.

The characteristics of the included studies are shown in Table 1. The total population of the studies was 2212. Three articles used patients with other kidney disease as their patient controls. In total, this left 6 articles that had healthy patients and patients with other kidney disease as controls. There were 6 prospective studies and 9 retrospective studies. A more detailed description of the included studies is shown in Table S1.

Methodological quality of included studies

The methodological quality assessment for included studies is shown in Figure 2. The overall quality of the eligible studies was not robust. Although almost all studies passed quality items 1, 2, 3, 5, 6, 7, 9, 11, 13 and 14, only one study reported blinding the reference PLA2R-AB test result to the results of the biopsy test (Item 10) [18]. Four studies had not reported whether or not the time period between reference standard and index test was short enough (Item4). Two studies had not reported the execution of the biopsy test insufficient detail (Item 8). One study did not clearly state clinical data, such as when the PLA2R-AB test results were interpreted (Item 12). Two studies (Dahnrich and Zhou) did not mention their respective sponsorship sources. The rest of the seven studies were supported predominantly by grants from government and foundation sources, but Beck's financial assistance came from a pharmaceutical corporation. It should be noted that since we did not obtain the individual data from every study, we did not conduct a meta-analysis that considered individuals as a unit of analysis.

Meta-analysis

As shown in Figure3, the summary sensitivity and specificity of all studies was 78% (95% CI: 66% to 87%) and 99% (95% CI: 96% to 100%), respectively. I^2 was 93.65% for the summary

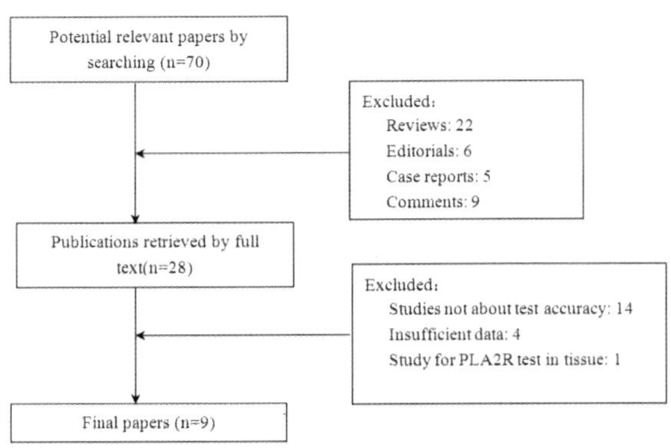

Figure 1. Flowchart for identification of studies.

Table 1. Characteristics of included eligible studies.

Year	Author	Country	Race	Case	Control1	Control2	TP no.	FP1* no.	FP2** no	FN, no.	TN1*, no.	TN2**.no	Se. %	Sp1* %	Sp2**%
2009	Beck	USA	Caucasian	12	30	30	9	0	0	3	30	30	75.0	100	100
2011	Qin	China	Asia	60	46	-	49	5	-	11	41	-	81.7	89.1	-
2011	Hoxha	Germany	Caucasian	43	107	153	21	0	0	22	107	153	48.8	100	100
2012	Murtas	Italian	Caucasian	186	92	96	111	0	0	75	92	96	59.7	100	100
2012	Hoxha	Germany	Caucasian	61	27	-	60	0	-	1	27	-	98.4	100	-
2013	Svobodova	Czech	Caucasian	28	3	-	18	2	-	10	1	-	64.3	33.3	-
2013	Dahnrich	West Europe	Caucasian	200	573	291	193	0	1	7	573	290	96.5	100	99.7
2013	Oh	Korea	Asia	100	9	14	69	2	0	31	7	14	69.0	77.8	100
2012	Zhou	China	Asia	20	26	5	15	2	0	5	24	5	75.0	92.3	100

*Other kidney disease control.
**Health control.

sensitivity and 93.83% for the summary specificity, suggesting a high heterogeneity in the sample of studies. The area under the receiver operating characteristic curve was 0.96 (95% CI: 0.94 to 0.98) and the DOR was 437 (95% CI: 74 to 2592). The SROC graph with the 95% confidence region and the 95% prediction region are shown in Figure 4. The summary positive likelihood ratio was 96.1 (95% CI: 19.5 to 472.1) and the summary negative likelihood ratio was 0.22 (95% CI: 0.14 to 0.35).

A subgroup analysis was then performed to explore potential sources of heterogeneity among studies. As shown in Table 2, the diagnostic accuracy of PLA2R-AB testing was higher in Caucasian patients than in Asian patients. Similar findings were found in subgroups with the following characteristics: larger sample sizes, healthy controls, the use of an indirect immunofluorescence method, studies have test interval between two tests and studies that were not supported by government funding. In addition, a meta-regression analysis was conducted to identify any significant sources of heterogeneity. The results suggested that testing serum PLA2R-AB after the biopsy test was significantly associated with the accuracy of PLA2R-AB testing for the detection of iMN ($P = 0.02$).

A sensitivity analysis was performed to evaluate the effect of each individual study on the pooled accuracy of PLA2R-AB testing. As shown in Table 3, a series of pooled sensitivity, specificity, DOR and area under curve (AUC) with 95% CIs were estimated after the removal of each study. The diagnostic accuracy of PLA2R-AB for iMN detection was relatively stable, with the exception of the study conducted by Dahnrich et al (2013).

The funnel plot with a superimposed regression line is shown in Figure S1. The *P* value for the slope coefficient was less than 0.001, indicating significant asymmetry. This result suggests a potential publication bias among studies.

Discussion

PLA2R is a major target antigen in autoimmune idiopathic membranous nephropathy [18–20]. Antibodies against PLA2R may serve as a new diagnostic biomarker for iMN detection. The methods for detecting PLA2R-AB, and the relationship between antibody concentration and its clinical manifestation, are not well known. Our meta-analysis suggests that the diagnostic accuracy of the serum PLA2R-AB test for iMN detection is modest, with a summary sensitivity of 78.0% and a specificity of 99%. Most of the studies included here have modest methodological quality. Moreover, the test time interval (whether or not biopsy was performed simultaneously) is a significant source of heterogeneity among studies.

To date, the etiology of iMN is not well understood. The diagnosis of iMN is still made by the exclusion of secondary causes, using the patient's medical history, physical examination, appropriate laboratory tests and renal pathological classification. Our meta-analysis suggested that PLA2R-AB may play a role in the development of iMN and might be a biomarker to help diagnose of iMN. However, the heterogeneity among studies suggested there are some potential factors that might have impact on the diagnostic accuracy of this test.

There are several possible explanations for why the testing interval is a significant source of the heterogeneity found in our meta-analysis. First, the various stages of disease may have been achieved during the testing interval. Second, the effect of immunosuppressive therapy may also be taken into account. If serum samples were collected long after the histological diagnosis, the patient may have entered an immunologically inactive stage by the time of serum collection, at which point the antibody

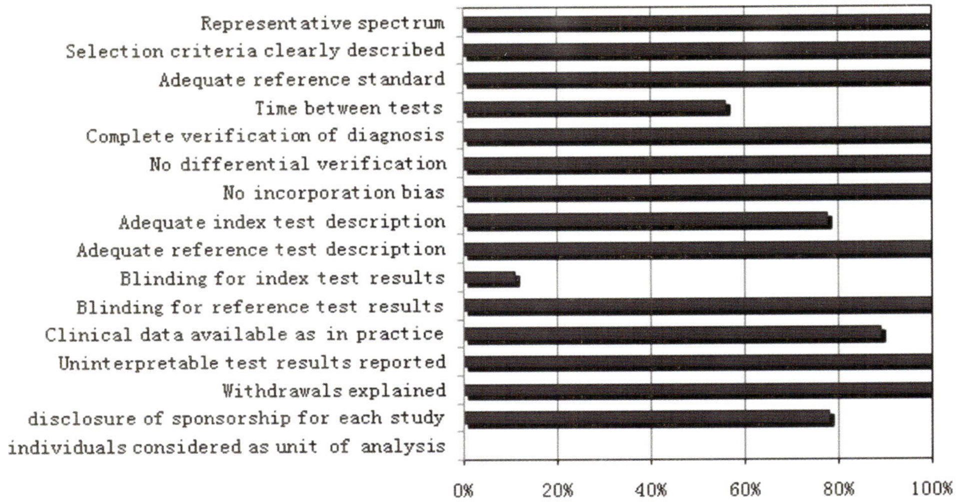

Figure 2. Proportion of all 14 quality assessment of diagnostic accuracy studies tool criteria that were fulfilled for the studies included in the meta-analysis.

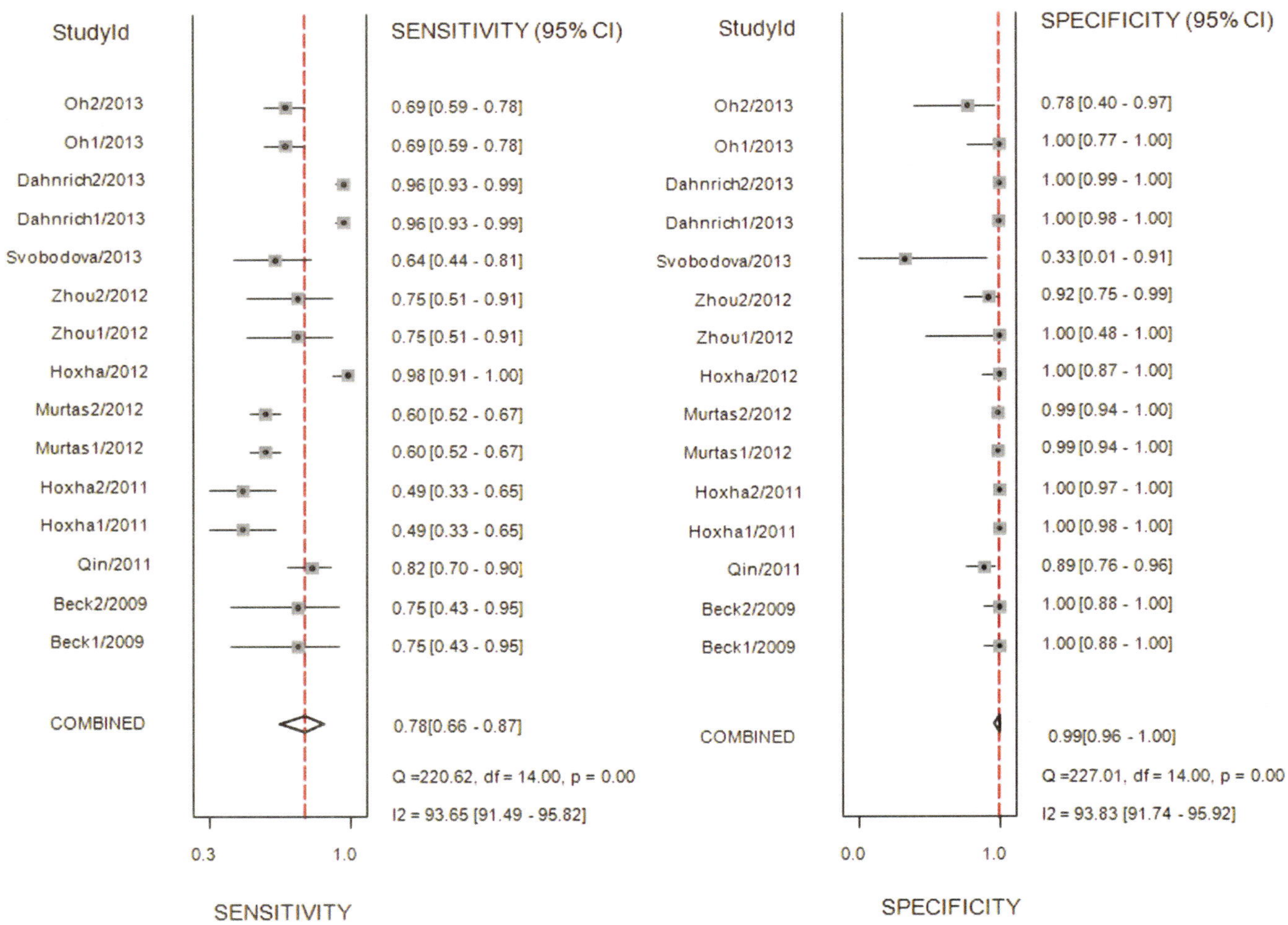

Figure 3. Forrest plots of the sensitivity and specificity of each individual study, summary sensitivity and specificity and I^2 statistic for heterogeneity.

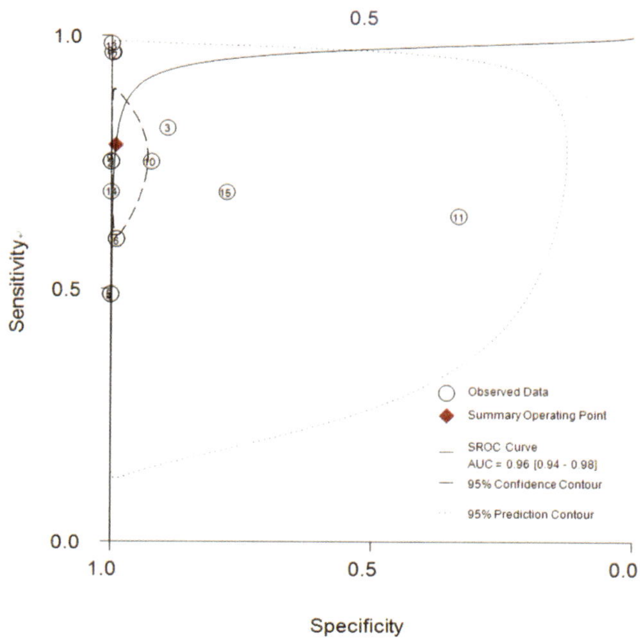

Figure 4. Summary receiver operating characteristic (SROC) graph with 95% confidence region and 95% prediction region for the diagnosis value of iMN by PLA2R-AB. Black square represents the summary estimate of sensitivity and specificity with the 95% confidence ellipse from the bivariate model. Numbers represent the reference numbers.

disappears. As previously reported in Svobodova's study (2013), circulating anti-PLA2R was measured in 37 MGN patients several months after kidney biopsy and all patients had entered spontaneous or drug-induced remission. They found that the sensitivity of anti-PLA2R was 22% (8 of 37), compared with 64% that were positive at the initial diagnosis [18]. Therefore, we suggest serological testing should be performed at the time of initial diagnosis, rather than a period of time after renal biopsy. This would thus avoid the possible confound of therapeutic intervention and disease progression.

The detection efficiency of three methods Western blotting, immunofluorescence, and ELISA is controversial in studies examining the detection of serum PLA2R-AB levels [14]. According to our findings, it seems that the immunofluorescence method has higher diagnostic accuracy than Western blotting. However, both methods have their advantages and disadvantages. Most laboratories choose to use recombinant PLA2R1 as a substrate for immunofluorescence even though it is insufficient to assess antibody concentrations [14,20,21]. On the other hand, while Western blotting uses a monoclonal antibody to confirm the location of the PLA2R band, it has relatively high laboratory demands and the assessment of a large number of clinical patients can become complicated and cumbersome [11,13]. Nevertheless, Debiec (2011) reported concordant resultsforPLA2R-AB in 42 iMN patients with both methods: Western blotting under non-reducing conditions and using glycoproteins extracted from normal human glomeruli; and immunofluorescence assay with HEK293 cells that were transfected with PLA2R1 cDNA [22,23]. More recently, ELISA has also served as a promising method for the detection of PLA2R-AB. For example, Dahnrich (2013) reported that the ELISA test for PLA2R-ABhad 96.5% sensitivity and 100% specificity [20]. However, since there were not sufficiently available studies on ELISA test evaluation, we did not include the ELISA test in our meta-analysis.

Table 2. Subgroup analysis for accuracy of PLA2R-AB for MN detection.

Subgroup	N	Sensitivity	Specificity	DOR	AUC
Race					
Caucasian	10	0.80(0.62,0.91)	1.00(0.98,1.00)	1297	0.99(0.97–0.99)
Asian	5	0.72(0.67,0.77)	0.91(0.84,0.95)	26	0.91(0.88–0.93)
Sample size					
<100 subjects	6	0.82(0.66,0.91)	0.97(0.78,1.00)	147	0.94(0.92–0.96)
>=100 subjects	9	0.76(0.59,0.88)	0.99(0.97,1.00)	465	0.97(0.96–0.99)
Control					
Patients	9	0.80(0.64,0.90)	0.98(0.89,1.00)	220	0.95(0.93–0.97)
Health	6	0.75(0.55,0.88)	1.00(0.98,1.00)	914	1.00(0.99–1.00)
Method					
Western blotting	9	0.68(0.62,0.73)	0.97(0.93,0.99)	73	0.84(0.80–0.87)
Imunofluorescence	4	0.74(0.37,0.93)	0.99(0.78,1.00)	451	0.98(0.96–0.99)
ELISA	1	-	-	-	-
Test interval					
No	8	0.68(0.62,0.73)	0.95(0.86,0.98)	39	0.78(0.74–0.81)
After biopsy test	7	0.86(0.65,0.96)	1.00(0.98,1.00)	8710	1.00(0.99–1.00)
Funding by					
Government foundation	9	0.70(0.56,0.81)	0.99(0.90,1.00)	177	0.89(0.86–0.92)
Corporation or no funding	6	0.88(0.76,0.95)	0.99(0.96,1.00)	843	0.99(0.98–1.00)

Table 3. Sensitivity analyses for the accuracy of PLA2R-AB test on iMN detection.

Study omited	Sensitivity	Specificity	DOR	AUC
Beck	0.78(0.65,0.88)	0.99(0.95,1.00)	338(54.2114)	0.96(0.94–0.98)
Qin	0.78(0.65,0.87)	0.99(0.96,1.00)	431(71,2611)	0.97(0.95–0.98)
Hoxha2011	0.82(0.70,0.89)	0.99(0.94,1.00)	298(50,1778)	0.96(0.94–0.98)
Murtas	0.81(0.68,0.89)	0.99(0.95,1.00)	592(62,5612)	0.96(0.94–0.98)
Hoxha2012	0.75(0.64,0.84)	0.99(0.96,1.00)	326(58,1840)	0.94(0.92–0.96)
Svobodova	0.79(0.66,0.88)	0.99(0.97,1.00)	581(114,2951)	0.98(0.96–0.99)
Dahnrich	0.71(0.61,0.79)	0.99(0.93,1.00)	226(34,1522)	0.89(0.86–0.92)
Oh	0.80(0.66,0.89)	0.99(0.97,1.00)	601(89,4062)	0.97(0.96–0.98)
Zhou	0.79(0.65,0.88)	0.99(0.96,1.00)	567(75,4286)	0.97(0.95,0.98)

PLA2R-AB was not found in all cases of iMN. This discrepancy could be partially due to the spontaneous remission of the disease or to the use of immunosuppressive therapy [5]. On the other hand, it is possible that iMN is not a uniform disease and might have different target antigens that have not yet been identified [24]. Our meta-analysis showed that the summary sensitivity of PLA2R-AB in all studies was only 78%. Svobodova (2013) suggested that the assessment of both circulating PLA2R antibodies and PLA2R antigen in biopsy specimens might be a better discriminator between primary and secondary MN than only assessing the levels of anti-PLA2R antibodies [18]. In some patients, MN can appear months or even years before a secondary cause is detected. Some patients who were negative for PLA2R might have been misclassified as idiopathic when they actually had a secondary form of MN [18]. This can only be examined by long-term, follow-up studies and further research on other antigens and the pathomechanism of iMN should be done in the future.

There are several limitations within this study that must be acknowledged. First, PLA2R-AB is a recently discovered biomarker, so few studies were available for our meta-analysis and our results might change as more work is done with PLA2R-AB. Second, the methodological quality of the included studies was not high. For example, the majority of studies did not report whether the serological examination results were obtained while blind to the kidney biopsy results. Such methodological limitations might have biased our final conclusions. Third, the potential publication bias among the selected studies indicates that the diagnostic value of PLA2R-AB on iMN detection may be overestimated, since studies with favorable results are more likely to be published.

In summary, the present meta-analysis suggests that there is modest diagnostic value in serum PLA2R-AB testing for the detection of iMN. Considering our limitations and the heterogeneity among our chosen studies, large and well-designed prospective studies will be needed to determine the future diagnostic value of serum PLA2R-ABtesting.

Supporting Information

Figure S1 Deeks' Funnel Plot Asymmetry Test. Funnel plot of the natural logarithm of the diagnostic odds ratio(lnDOR) against the inverse of the square root of the effective sample size (1/ESS1/2) of included studies.

Table S1 The characters detail of included studies.

Table S2 The QUADAS form for included studies.

Checklist S1 PRISMA checklist. Preferred Reporting Items for Systematic Reviews and Meta-Analyses.

Author Contributions

Conceived and designed the experiments: HG SW. Performed the experiments: YD JL. Analyzed the data: JL JH SW. Contributed reagents/materials/analysis tools: FH WL PW YD. Wrote the paper: YD SW HG YL.

References

1. Horvatic I, Galesic K (2012) [Membranous glomerulonephritis recent advances in pathogenesis and treatment]. Lijec Vjesn 134: 328 339.
2. Ponticelli C, Glassock RJ (2013) Glomerular Diseases: Membranous Nephropathy A Modern View. Clin J Am Soc Nephrol.
3. Cybulsky AV (2011) Membranous nephropathy. Contrib Nephrol 169: 107 125.
4. Ronco P, Debiec H (2010) Antigen identification in membranous nephropathy moves toward targeted monitoring and new therapy. J Am Soc Nephrol 21: 564 569.
5. Hoxha E, Kneissler U, Stege G, Zahner G, Thiele I, et al. (2012) Enhanced expression of the M-type phospholipase A2 receptor in glomeruli correlates with serum receptor antibodies in primary membranous nephropathy. Kidney Int 82: 797 804.
6. Glassock RJ (2010) The pathogenesis of idiopathic membranous nephropathy: a 50-year odyssey. Am J Kidney Dis 56: 157 167.
7. Ayalon R, Beck LH Jr (2013) Membranous nephropathy: not just a disease for adults. Pediatr Nephrol.
8. Glassock RJ (2013) Pathogenesis of membranous nephropathy: a new paradigm in evolution. Contrib Nephrol 181: 131 142.
9. Oh YJ, Yang SH, Kim DK, Kang SW, Kim YS (2013) Autoantibodies against phospholipase A2 receptor in Korean patients with membranous nephropathy. PLoS One 8: e62151.
10. Stahl R, Hoxha E, Fechner K (2010) PLA2R autoantibodies and recurrent membranous nephropathy after transplantation. N Engl J Med 363: 496 498.
11. Beck LH, Jr., Bonegio RG, Lambeau G, Beck DM, Powell DW, et al. (2009) M-type phospholipase A2 receptor as target antigen in idiopathic membranous nephropathy. N Engl J Med 361: 11 21.
12. Stanescu HC, Arcos-Burgos M, Medlar A, Bockenhauer D, Kottgen A, et al. (2011) Risk HLA-DQA1 and PLA(2)R1 alleles in idiopathic membranous nephropathy. N Engl J Med 364: 616 626.
13. Qin W, Beck LH, Jr., Zeng C, Chen Z, Li S, et al. (2011) Anti-phospholipase A2 receptor antibody in membranous nephropathy. J Am Soc Nephrol 22: 1137 1143.
14. Hoxha E, Harendza S, Zahner G, Panzer U, Steinmetz O, et al. (2011) An immunofluorescence test for phospholipase-A(2)-receptor antibodies and its clinical usefulness in patients with membranous glomerulonephritis. Nephrol Dial Transplant 26: 2526 2532.

15. Hofstra JM, Beck LH, Jr., Beck DM, Wetzels JF, Salant DJ (2011) Anti-phospholipase A(2) receptor antibodies correlate with clinical status in idiopathic membranous nephropathy. Clin J Am Soc Nephrol 6: 1286–1291.
16. Whiting P, Rutjes AW, Reitsma JB, Bossuyt PM, Kleijnen J (2003) The development of QUADAS: a tool for the quality assessment of studies of diagnostic accuracy included in systematic reviews. BMC Med Res Methodol 3: 25.
17. Deeks JJ, Macaskill P, Irwig L (2005) The performance of tests of publication bias and other sample size effects in systematic reviews of diagnostic test accuracy was assessed. J Clin Epidemiol 58: 882–893.
18. Svobodova B, Honsova E, Ronco P, Tesar V, Debiec H (2013) Kidney biopsy is a sensitive tool for retrospective diagnosis of PLA2R-related membranous nephropathy. Nephrol Dial Transplant 28: 1839–1844.
19. Khosroshahi A, Ayalon R, Beck LH Jr, Salant DJ, Bloch DB, et al. (2012) IgG4-Related Disease Is Not Associated with Antibody to the Phospholipase A2 Receptor. Int J Rheumatol 2012: 139409.
20. Dahnrich C, Komorowski L, Probst C, Seitz-Polski B, Esnault V, et al. (2013) Development of a standardized ELISA for the determination of autoantibodies against human M-type phospholipase A2 receptor in primary membranous nephropathy. Clin Chim Acta 421: 213–218.
21. Hofstra JM, Debiec H, Short CD, Pelle T, Kleta R, et al. (2012) Antiphospholipase A2 receptor antibody titer and subclass in idiopathic membranous nephropathy. J Am Soc Nephrol 23: 1735–1743.
22. Debiec H, Ronco P (2011) PLA2R autoantibodies and PLA2R glomerular deposits in membranous nephropathy. N Engl J Med 364: 689–690.
23. Debiec H, Ronco P (2011) Nephrotic syndrome: A new specific test for idiopathic membranous nephropathy. Nat Rev Nephrol 7: 496–498.
24. Murtas C, Bruschi M, Candiano G, Moroni G, Magistroni R, et al. (2012) Coexistence of different circulating anti-podocyte antibodies in membranous nephropathy. Clin J Am Soc Nephrol 7: 1394–1400.

12

The Clinical Characteristics and Pathological Patterns of Postinfectious Glomerulonephritis in HIV-Infected Patients

Christine A. Murakami[1], Doaa Attia[2], Naima Carter-Monroe[3], Gregory M. Lucas[1], Michelle M. Estrella[1], Derek M. Fine[1], Mohamed G. Atta[1]*

1 Department of Medicine, Johns Hopkins University School of Medicine, Baltimore, Maryland, United States of America, **2** Faculty of Medicine, Alexandria, Egypt, **3** Department of Pathology, Johns Hopkins University School of Medicine, Baltimore, Maryland, United States of America

Abstract

Background: Postinfectious glomerulonephritis (PIGN), a form of immune complex GN, is not well-defined in HIV-infected patients. This study characterizes PIGN in this patients' population and determine the impact of histopathological patterns on renal outcome and mortality.

Methods: HIV-infected patients with PIGN from September 1998 to July 2013 were identified. Archived slides were reviewed by a blinded renal pathologist, classified into acute, persistent and healed PIGN. Groups were compared using Wilcoxon rank-sum and Fisher's exact test. Survival analyses were performed to determine association of histopathological pattern with renal outcome and mortality.

Results: Seventy-two HIV-infected predominantly African American males were identified with PIGN. Median (interquartile range) age and creatinine at the time of renal biopsy was 48 years (41, 53) and 2.5 mg/dl (1.5, 4.9) respectively. Only 2 (3%) had acute PIGN, 42 (58%) had persistent PIGN and 28 (39%) had healed PIGN. Three patients (4%) had IgA-dominant PIGN. Only 46% of the patients had confirmed positive cultures with *Staphylococcus* the most common infectious agent. During a median follow up of 17 months, the pathological pattern had no impact on renal outcome ($P = 0.95$). Overall mortality was high occurring in 14 patients (19%); patients with healed PIGN had significantly increased mortality ($P = 0.05$).

Conclusion: In HIV-infected patients, *Staphylococcus* is the most common cause of PIGN. Renal outcome was not influenced by the histopathological pattern but those with healed PIGN had greater mortality which was potentially due to a confounder not accounted for in the study.

Editor: Antonio C. Seguro, University of São Paulo School of Medicine, Brazil

Funding: Mohamed G. Atta is supported by the National Institute of Diabetes and Digestive and Kidney Diseases grant P01DK056492. Dr. Lucas was supported by the National Institute on Drug Abuse (K24 DA035684 and R01 DA026770) and by the Johns Hopkins University Center for AIDS Research (P30 AI094189). The funders had no role in study design, data collection and analysis, decision to publish, or preparation of the manuscript.

* Email: matta1@jhmi.edu

These authors contributed equally to this work.

Introduction

Renal diseases in patients infected with HIV cover a wide array of renal pathologies [1–3]. These pathologies could be the direct effect of the HIV-1 virus, such as HIV-1 associated nephropathy (HIVAN), or the consequence of coexisting conditions such as diabetes, hypertension, intravenous drug use, or exposure to antiretroviral medications [4]. The incidence of HIVAN, the most aggressive histologic lesion in the HIV population, has substantially declined in recent years due to the introduction of highly-active antiretroviral therapy (HAART) [5,6]. However, HIV-immune complex-mediated kidney disease (HIVICK) continues to be a pervasive histologic finding [7]. HIVICK refers to a spectrum of pathological entities consisting of post-infectious glomerulonephritis (PIGN), "lupus-like' glomerulonephritis, IgA nephropathy, membranoproliferative glomerulonephritis (MPGN), and membranous nephropathy [4]. In a study by Foy *et al*, PIGN was identified as the most common immune-complex glomerulonephritis in HIV patients [4].

In recent years, the disease pattern and epidemiology of PIGN has markedly evolved [8,9]. Infections with *Staphylococcal* and gram-negative bacteria have now been identified as increasingly common antecedent of PIGN. Studies have also reported a more unfavorable prognosis than two to three decades ago; this has been attributed to changes in the disease profile as well as delayed diagnosis and treatment [8,10]. Complete remission has been reported in some studies to occur in 26% to 69% of adults with PIGN [8,11,12]. While there have been several studies describing the clinicopathologic spectrum of PIGN in the adult population, data on the prevalence and prognosis of PIGN among adults HIV patients are lacking [8,10,13]. Histologically, PIGN is characterized by diffuse endocapillary proliferative and exudative glomerulonephritis on light microscopy with granular deposits of complement 3 (C3) and immunoglobulin G (IgG) in the mesangium and glomerular basement membranes on immunofluorescence (IF). On electron microscopy, large subepithelial electron-dense deposits or "humps" are characteristic findings [14]. Although, classic cases of PIGN are diagnosed histologically without difficulty, a large number of patients have PIGN with atypical histological features [10]. In 2003, Haas reviewed 1012 renal biopsies and classified PIGN as acute or subacute glomerulonephritis (GN), persistent or progressive glomerulonephritis and healed or latent glomerulonephritis [15]. In this classification, acute or subacute GN pertains to cases with diffuse mesangial and endocapillary hypercellularity on light microscopy, multiple subepithelial humps on electron microscopy (EM), characteristic granular glomerular basement membrane staining for IgG and or C3 on IF, and clinical findings consistent with acute or subacute kidney injury. Persistent or progressive GN lacks the intense degree of diffuse mesangial and endocapillary hypercellularity seen in acute PIGN, and has variable granular mesangial C3 and or IgG deposits with some capillary wall deposits. On EM, patients with persistent PIGN have fewer subepithelial humps compared to acute PIGN. Healed or latent GN refers to cases with mild mesangial hypercellularity and immunofluorescence (IF) similar to persistent GN, with partially or markedly resorbed subepithelial deposits on EM. Although this classification may be helpful, it is not known whether it has clinical implications, particularly in HIV-infected patients.

In this study, the clinical features of PIGN in HIV-infected patients and their correlation with the different aforementioned pathological patterns are explored. In addition, the impact of these pathological findings on renal outcome and mortality is determined.

Materials and Methods

Study Design and Patient Selection

Patients with the diagnosis of PIGN on renal biopsy from September 1998 to July 2013 were identified through linkage with the institutional pathology database. Patients who met all the following criteria were included: 18 years of age and older, diagnosis of HIV-1 infection, hospital admission at Johns Hopkins University from September 1998 to July 2013. Pediatric patients, patients who received any type of organ transplantation as well as those who received care at other institutions were excluded. We initially identified 90 adult HIV-infected patients who met these criteria (Figure 1) but only 72 patients were eventually included in the study due to uncertain pathological diagnoses in 18 cases. The Institutional Review Board of Johns Hopkins University approved the study. Patient records and information were de-identified prior to analysis.

Data Collection and Definitions

The diagnosis of PIGN was established from the pathological report generated by the renal pathologist at the time of the renal biopsy. A renal pathologist, who was blinded to clinical characteristics, reviewed the slides of the 90 patients screened for this study. All renal biopsies were processed by light microscopy and EM. All but 4 slides were also examined by IF. The patients with PIGN were further subclassified into acute, persistent, or healed PIGN based on the system proposed by Haas *et al* summarized in Table 1 [15]. Demographic, clinical, laboratory and pharmaceutical data collected at the time of renal biopsy and at 2 months before and after the biopsy, were abstracted from electronic patient records. The following clinical definitions were used: HIV-1 infection based on documented diagnosis from medical records and or use of antiretroviral medications; diabetes and hypertension were defined by prescription of anti-diabetic or anti-hypertensive medications, respectively; hepatitis C virus (HCV) infection was based on presence of hepatitis C viral antibodies and/or detection of hepatitis C viral load by polymerase chain reaction. Cirrhosis was based on patient medical history and/or liver biopsy findings and end-stage renal disease (ESRD) was defined as initiation of renal replacement therapy. Nephrotic-range proteinuria was defined by >3.0 g/d (if 24 hour urine collected) or >3.0 g/g creatinine (by random urine protein-to-creatinine ratio).

Statistical Analyses

Stata statistical software version 10 (Stata Corp, College Station, TX) was used for the statistical analysis. Continuous variables were reported as median and interquartile range (IQR). Continuous and categorical variables were compared using Wilcoxon rank-sum and the Fisher's exact test, respectively. A P-value <0.05 was considered statistically significant. We used Kaplan-Meier plots and log-rank test to compare time to ESRD or death in groups with different kidney pathology features. Finally, we used Cox proportional hazards models to determine hazard ratios (HR) and 95% confidence intervals (CI).

Results

Pathological Findings

There were 1250 patients with a diagnosis of PIGN on renal biopsies performed from September 1998 to July 2013. After excluding 156 pediatric patients, 946 HIV-uninfected patients, 45 transplant recipients, 13 patients admitted at other institutions, there were 90 patients for evaluation. The blinded pathological review excluded 18 cases that were classified as immune-complex GN where there was no solid histologic evidence of PIGN. This resulted in 72 adult patients with confirmed PIGN and HIV-1 infection in the analysis (Figure 1). In the blinded pathological review of the archived renal tissues, 2 (3%) were designated as having acute PIGN, 42 (58%) persistent PIGN, and 28 (39%) healed PIGN. Three of the 72 PIGN cases (4%) were IgA-dominant PIGN. Twenty-six patients (36%) had PIGN as the sole diagnosis on their renal biopsy while 31 (43%) had PIGN with either concurrent classic FSGS or HIVAN and 15 (21%) have other pathological findings on renal biopsy.

Clinical Characteristics of Participants with Different Histological Classification of PIGN

The majority of patients were African American (89%) and male in gender (64%). The median (interquartile range [IQR]) age at the time of the renal biopsy was 48 years (41, 53). The median (IQR) CD4 count and viral load at the time of biopsy were 322 cells/mm^3 (156, 498) and 13,346 copies/mL (504, 100,566), respectively. The median (IQR) creatinine at the time of biopsy was 2.5 mg/dl (1.5, 4.9). Fifty-nine patients (82%) had hypertension and 17 (24%) had underlying diabetes mellitus. Forty out of 72 patients (56%) were coinfected with Hepatitis C. Only 12 patients (17%) exhibited a low C3 or C4. Bacterial infection was

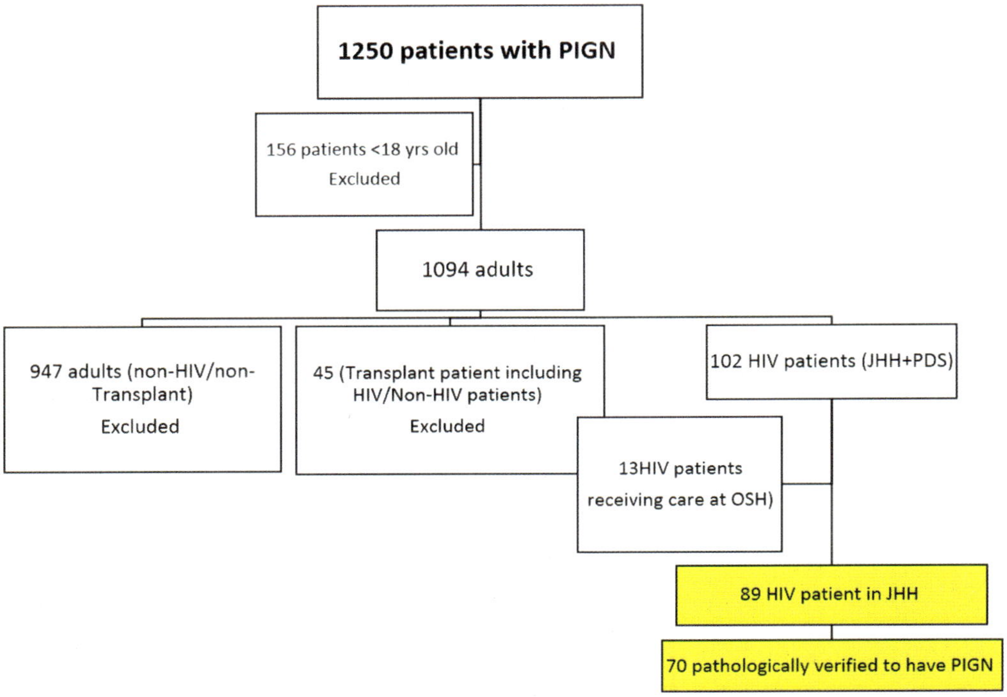

Figure 1. Screening of patients: Out of 1250 patients screened, 72 HIV infected individuals with Post infectious glomerulonephritis were included in the final analysis.

Table 1. Histopathological classification of postinfectious glomerulonephritis.

	Acute PIGN	Persistent PIGN	Healed PIGN
Light microscopy (H&E, PAS, Masson's trichrome and PAS -Methenimine silver stained slides)	• Diffuse, moderate to marked, segmental to global endocapillary hypercellularity (mostly neutrophilic)	• Focal, mild to moderate, segmental endocapillary hypercellularity (mostly mononuclear)	• Focal, absent to mild segmental endocapillary hypercellularity (mostly mononuclear)
	• ± Moderate to marked mesangial hypercellularity	• ± Mild to marked mesangial hypercellularity	• ± Absent to moderate mesangial hypercellularity
Immunofluorescence	• Granular capillary wall (GBM), with ± mesangial IgG and/or C3 deposits	• Variable granular mesangial C3± IgG with ± capillary wall (GBM) deposits	• Variable granular mesangial C3± IgG with ± capillary wall (GBM) deposits
	• Mesangial IgA in IgA -dominant PIGN	• ± IgA, IgM, C1q, kappa or lambda	• ± IgA, IgM, C1q, kappa or lambda
	• ± IgA, IgM, C1q, Kappa or lambda		
Electron microscopy	• Numerous irregularly-spaced subepithelial electron dense deposits, frequently in mesangial "notch", rare "humps", undergoing minimal to mild resorption	• Occasional to numerous subepithelial electron dense deposits, a few "humps", a few (at least 1) in mesangial "notch", undergoing variable (mild to marked) resorption	• Few subepithelial electron dense deposits, rare "humps" (up to 2), a few in mesangial "notch", undergoing moderate to marked resorption
	• ±Rare intramembranous, mesangial, subendothelial	• ± Variable numbers of subendothelial, intramembranous, mesangial	• Numerous subendothelial, intramembranous, mesangial, undergoing moderate to marked resorption

Adapted from Haas, M., Hum Pathol, 2003. 34(1): p. 3–10.

confirmed by positive blood culture in less than half of the patients (46%).

The two patients with acute PIGN were both African American males with HCV coinfection, hypertension, and history of intravenous drug use. Both presented with low C3 and normal C4 levels. At the time of renal biopsy, both were on antiretroviral therapy although one had a higher CD4 count and lower HIV-1 viral load (VL) compared to the other (CD4 657 vs. 50 and VL 400 vs. 939,000 respectively). However, the patient with better immunological status had underlying chronic kidney disease and ultimately required renal replacement therapy. The one with poor immune status had histological findings consistent with IgA-dominant PIGN. No preceding infection was identified in either patient.

The demographics and clinical characteristics of the remaining 70 patients with persistent and healed PIGN are summarized in Table 2. Hypertension and diabetes mellitus occurred in similar frequencies in the patients with persistent PIGN and healed PIGN (88% and 28% persistent PIGN vs. 79% and 23% healed, respectively). HCV coinfection was similar between the two groups, comprising 63% of patients with persistent PIGN and 56% of those with healed PIGN.

Most of the patients with persistent and healed PIGN were on antiretroviral therapy at the time of renal biopsy (66% persistent and 78% healed PIGN). The CD4 counts were also similar between the two groups. More patients with persistent PIGN (62%) exhibited statistically significant hematuria compared to those with healed PIGN ($P = 0.02$). In contrast, nephrotic-range proteinuria occurred more frequently in those with healed PIGN but these were not noted to be statistically significant ($P = 0.16$). The degree of renal dysfunction at the time of the renal biopsy was also similar between the 2 groups (median creatinine of 2.2 and 2.6 mg/dl). When identified, the heart or endocardium was the most common source of infection among patients with persistent PIGN while other infections were more frequently associated with healed PIGN (17%). However, the association between the source of infection and histopathological pattern was not statistically significant. In those with an isolated organism, *Staphylococcus* was identified as the most common infectious agent isolated in 42% of patients with persistent PIGN and 56% of those with healed PIGN.

Use of antimicrobials, angiotensin-converting enzyme inhibitor (ACE-I) and corticosteroid were similar between those with persistent PIGN and healed PIGN ($P = 0.92$, $P = 0.80$ and $P = 0.51$, respectively).

Pathological Findings

The two patients with acute PIGN have very similar pathological findings. Neither patient had crescents. Both of their renal biopsies showed subepithelial humps, subendothelial deposits and mesangial deposits. One of them had a positive C3 with trace IgM and intense IgA staining on IF while the other one was C3 negative. Both patients exhibited significant interstitial fibrosis, one with moderate interstitial fibrosis and the other with marked interstitial fibrosis. The pathological characteristics of the 70 HIV patients with persistent and healed PIGN are summarized in Table 3.

Only 3 patients out of 70 were found to have crescents on renal biopsy, all of whom had persistent PIGN. One had a fibrocellular crescent while the two others had cellular crescents. IF was positive for C3 and Ig (either IgA, IgM or IgG) on 55% of patients with persistent PIGN and 36% of patients with healed PIGN. Among the patients with positive C3 and Ig on IF, majority of the patients, both in the persistent and healed PIGN, had IgM positive deposits along with C3 (26% persistent PIGN group and 25% healed PIGN group). A small proportion of patients on both groups (19% persistent PIGN and 11% with healed PIGN) had IF that was positive for C3 only. Subepithelial humps were identified in in the majority of patients with persistent and healed PIGN. In contrast, subendothelial deposits were significantly predominant in patients with persistent PIGN compared to those with healed PIGN (57% vs 7%, $P = <0.0001$). The majority of the patients with persistent PIGN (76%) had interstitial fibrosis, mostly mild and moderate interstitial fibrosis (33% and 26% respectively). The same percentage of patients with healed PIGN (76%), had interstitial fibrosis which were mostly moderate (31%) and mild (28%). Similarly, interstitial inflammation was noted in 76% of patients with persistent PIGN and 86% of patients with healed PIGN.

Mortality and Incidence of CKD

The patients were followed up for a median (IQR) of 17 months (1–45 months). Mortality occurred in 14 out of 72 patients (19%) during the follow-up period. Among those who died, 6 patients had a sole diagnosis of PIGN, 5 with PIGN and other pathologies and 3 have PIGN with FSGS or HIVAN. Two of the patients with PIGN who died exhibited histopathological features of IgA-dominant PIGN.

Fourteen patients (19%), including one with acute PIGN, required renal replacement. None of the patients with IgA dominant PIGN required renal replacement therapy. We found no significant association between the histopathological classification of PIGN and ESRD. The cumulative progression to ESRD was similar in patients with persistent PIGN and healed PIGN (19% and 18%, respectively; $P = 0.95$ log-rank test). Individuals with healed PIGN had a similar risk of progressing to ESRD as those with persistent PIGN (HR, 0.96; 95% CI, 0.31 to 3.00). Similarly, the cumulative incidence of ESRD in patients with an exclusive diagnosis of PIGN was similar to patients with PIGN in combination with HIVAN or FSGS, and PIGN with other pathologies (15%, 25% and 14%, respectively; $P = 0.72$ log-rank test) (Table 4). Compared to those with a sole diagnosis of PIGN, the risk of progressing to ESRD was similar in those with PIGN plus HIVAN or FSGS (1.09; 95% CI 0.28–4.18) and those with PIGN plus other pathologies (0.66; 95% CI 0.11–4.06).

Mortality rates, on the other hand, showed differences based on the histopathological pattern of PIGN. The cumulative incidence of mortality in individuals with healed PIGN was higher compared to those with persistent PIGN (36% and 10%; *$P = 0.05$ log-rank test*) (Figure 2). This significant difference was eliminated in a separate analysis where cases with co-existing histopathological diagnoses were excluded. Including only those with pure PIGN, there were 15 patients with persistent PIGN and 10 patients with healed PIGN. Of these, 2 and 4 patients died respectively and the log-rank P value for this comparison was 0.41 (data not shown). However, the significant drop in the sample size may limit the interpretation of this result. Patients with IgA-dominant PIGN did not show increased mortality ($P = 0.69$) or increased need for renal replacement ($P = 0.16$).

Discussion

This is the first study to explore the clinical and pathological characteristics of PIGN in HIV- infected individuals. In this study *Staphylococcus* was the most common etiology of an identified infection prior to diagnosis of PIGN. Interestingly, renal outcome was not influenced by the histopathological pattern, but mortality was relatively high (19%) in this cohort during the follow-up period, with patients with healed PIGN having greater mortality.

Table 2. Demographics, clinical characteristics and source of Infection of 71 patients at the time of diagnosis.

	Persistent PIGN (n = 42)	Healed PIGN (n = 28)	*P*-value
Sex			
Male (%)	27 (64)	17 (61)	0.8
Female (%)	15 (36)	11 (39)	
Age (median, IQR)	45 (41, 52)	48.5 (42, 54.5)	0.47
Race - no. of patients (%)			
Black	38 (91)	24 (86)	0.41
White	2 (5)	4 (14)	
Asian	1 (2)	0 (0.00)	
Others	1 (2)	0 (0.00)	
Serum creatinine (Median, IQR)	2.2 (1.1, 4.9)	2.6 (1.9, 5.1)	0.31
CD4 count (Median, IQR)	327 (199, 506)	238 (77, 459)	0.26
Comorbidities - no. of patients (%)			
Diabetes	11 (28)	6 (23)	0.8
Hypertension	35 (88)	22 (79)	0.34
Hepatitis C	24 (63)	14 (56)	0.61
Cirrhosis	1 (3)	2 (7)	0.57
Malignancy	8 (21)	3 (11)	0.34
Other systemic diseases	5 (13)	5 (20)	0.5
Intravenous drug use	19 (50)	10 (42)	0.61
Low C3	8 (25)	2 (10)	0.28
Low C4	8 (25)	2 (10)	0.28
Site of Infection –no. of patients (%)			
Endocardium	12 (29)	4 (14)	0.59
Bone/Joint	1 (2)	2 (7)	
Pleura	1 (2)	0 (0)	
Skin	4 (10)	4 (14)	
Lung/URTI	6 (14)	5 (18)	
Others	2 (5)	0 (0.00)	
None identified	16 (38)	14 (50)	
Infectious Agent – no. of patients (%)	N = 26	N = 25	
Staphylococcus	11 (42)	14 (56)	0.31
Streptococcus	7 (27)	8 (32)	
Others	8 (31)	3 (12)	
HIV medications – no. of patients (%)			
NRTI	21 (66)	11 (78)	0.5
NNRTI	7 (22)	2 (14)	0.7
PI	19 (59)	8 (57)	1
Other medications – no. of patients (%)			
ACE Inhibitors	19 (50)	12 (46)	0.8
ARB	1 (3)	1 (4)	1
Corticosteroid	9 (23)	3 (11)	0.51
Antibiotic use	24 (62)	16 (62)	0.92
Nephrotic Proteinuria	8 (26)	11 (46)	0.16
Hematuria	23 (62)	8 (30)	0.02

PIGN has been traditionally linked to Streptococcal pharyngitis or skin infection [13]. In our HIV-infected cohort with PIGN, *Staphylococcus* was the most common causative agent identified. This supports the findings of various authors, who described a shift in the epidemiologic features of PIGN over the past decades [8,9]. Nasr *et al* described *Staphylococcus* as the most common causative

Table 3. Summary of pathological findings on 70 patients with persistent and healed PIGN.

Pathological Finding – no of patients (%)	Persistent PIGN (n = 42)	Healed (n = 28)	*p*- value
Interstitial inflammation			
Mild/Minimal	13 (31)	13 (45)	0.22
Moderate	14 (33)	8 (28)	0.80
Marked	5 (12)	3 (10)	1.00
No inflammation	10 (24)	4 (14)	0.38
Crescents			
Fibrocellular	1 (2)	0 (0)	1.00
Cellular	2 (5)	0 (0)	0.51
Subepithelial humps	31 (74)	17 (59)	0.30
Subendothelial deposits	24 (57)	2 (7)	<0.0001
Mesangial deposits	34 (81)	15 (52)	0.02
Immunofluorescence			
C3+ Ig	23 (55)	10 (34)	0.15
C3+ IgM	11 (26)	7 (24)	1.00
C3+ IgG	2 (5)	0 (0)	0.51
C3+ IgM+ IgG	10 (24)	3 (10)	0.22
C3 only	8 (19)	3 (10)	0.51
C3 negative	8 (19)	13 (45)	0.02
Interstitial fibrosis			
Mild	14 (33)	8 (28)	0.79
Moderate	11 (26)	9 (31)	0.60
Marked	7 (17)	5 (17)	1.00
No fibrosis	10 (24)	7 (24)	1.00

agent in the elderly population [16] and in IgA dominant PIGN [17]. Our study showed that this is true even in younger patients with HIV-1 infection with no pathological features of IgA-dominant PIGN.

In our HIV-infected cohort, bacterial infection was only confirmed in 46% of the patients, which is consistent with a study which revealed that in as much as 24% to 59% of patients with PIGN, the causative organism cannot be identified [13]. The low yield of bacterial culture in identifying the causative organism could be due to the diversity of organisms that can cause PIGN which include viruses and parasites. Furthermore, the role of HIV and HCV infection in the development of PIGN in this cohort is not clear although one can argue that antigens of these viruses may be playing a role in this process. Hepatitis C infection was noted in more than 50% of our HIV-infected cohort. However, the presence of HCV coinfection did not increase predisposition for a specific histological pattern of PIGN. Previous studies reported that HCV coinfection with HIV-1 increases predisposition to immune-complex glomerulonephritis [18]. HIV-1 itself may promote an increase in circulating immune complexes by promoting polyclonal hypergammaglobulinemia [19]. One study also suggested that formation of anti-HIV antibodies might play a role in forming immune complexes in some HIV patients [20] Whether HIVICK is caused by passive trapping of the circulating immune complex, or in situ deposition of antibody-antigen complex, is still not completely understood.

The lack of clinical signs of infection may explain the lower frequency of acute pattern of PIGN in our cohort. The majority of our patients with PIGN had healed and persistent PIGN on renal biopsy, and only 2 had acute PIGN. One study reported that as much as 16% of adult patients may not have any clinical manifestation of infection [13]. The absence of overt signs of acute infection is believed to be one of the reasons for delayed diagnosis [10]. Although, the patients with PIGN had comparable degrees of

Table 4. Estimated rates of mortality and ESRD 12 months following kidney biopsy, according to pathologic findings.

No. of patients (%)	PIGN only (n = 26)	PIGN+FSGS/HIVAN (n = 31)	PIGN + other* (n = 15)	*P*-value**
Mortality	6 (23)	3 (9)	5 (36)	0.09
ESRD	4 (15)	8 (25)	2 (14)	0.74

*Others: MPGN, lupus-like, membranous, diabetic glomerulosclerosis.
**Log-rank test.

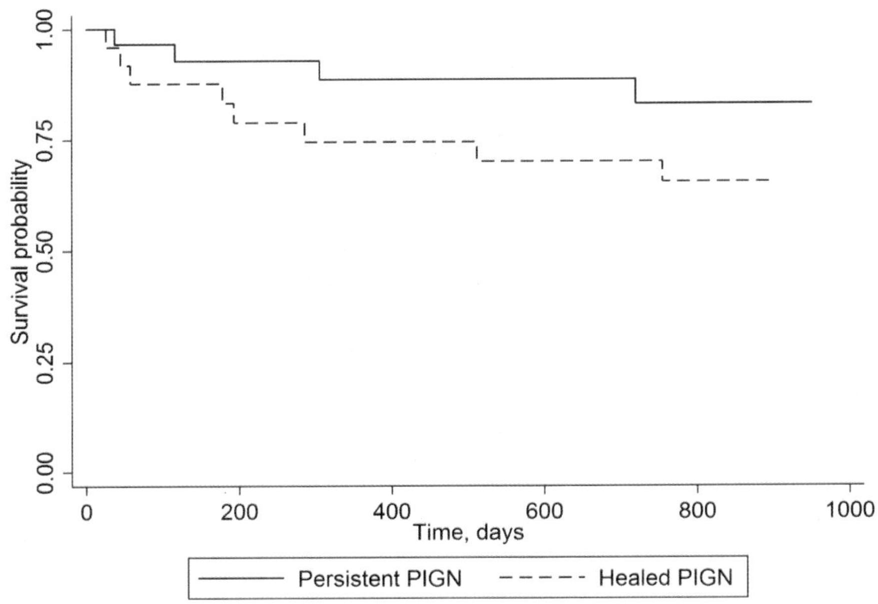

Figure 2. Mortality according to histopathological pattern of PIGN: Patients with healed PIGN had significantly worse survival compared to those of persistent PIGN, log-rank test.

renal dysfunction regardless of the histopathological pattern, early diagnosis in the HIV population may be important since patients with healed PIGN tend to have a higher mortality. Hence, PIGN should always be entertained as a differential diagnosis in HIV patients with renal dysfunction, even in the absence of a source of infection. Given the heterogeneity of renal pathologies in HIV as well as the absence of a reliable clinical indicator of PIGN in HIV patients, a timely renal biopsy is very valuable in this population.

Our study comprising of predominantly male African American HIV-infected patients, a large proportion (82%) of the patients were hypertensive. This is slightly higher than what has been previously reported [13]. However, the occurrence of hypertension did not differ between the patients with different histologic pattern of PIGN. Conversely, diabetes mellitus, which has been identified as the most frequent risk factor in a study of adults with acute PIGN [13], was only documented in 17 patients (24%) in our HIV-infected cohort. This finding may be partially explained by the demographic differences with other studies and suggests that diabetes mellitus is not a major risk factor for PIGN among young African American patients with HIV-infected patients.

Our study showed that individuals with persistent PIGN had a similar risk of progressing to ESRD as those with healed PIGN. Two prior PIGN studies identified the absence of interstitial inflammation as one of the pathological findings which correlates with renal recovery [11,13]. Interstitial fibrosis was identified by *Montseny* et al as one of the predictors of persistent renal dysfunction [8]. In our cohort of patients, the proportion of patients with interstitial inflammation and interstitial fibrosis were very similar between the persistent PIGN and healed PIGN groups. Perhaps, this explains why the mean creatinine at the time of renal biopsy and progression to ESRD during the follow-up period were similar between the two groups were similar. The association between the presence of crescents and renal outcome seems to be less straightforward in PIGN. While *Nasr* et al [13] did not find a correlation between crescents and renal outcome, another study reported poorer renal outcomes with crescentic PIGN [21]. In our patient population, only 3 patients exhibited crescents on renal biopsy. Owing to the low number of patients with crescentic GN, we cannot determine if there is a correlation between renal outcome and crescentic glomerulonephritis in HIV-infected patients. It might be worthwhile to look into this on future studies involving a larger number of HIV patients with PIGN.

Studies on HIV-infected population have suggested that HIVAN progresses more rapidly than non-HIVAN renal diseases [1,22,23]. In our study, some of the patients with PIGN had concomitant findings consistent with HIVAN. However, these patients did not show an increased progression to ESRD compared to those patients with the sole diagnosis of PIGN or with PIGN in conjunction with other pathologies. The short follow-up period of our study may not have limited our ability to distinguish differences. Perhaps and more importantly, a substantial proportion of our patients were on antiretroviral therapy at the time of diagnosis, which could have delayed the progression of HIVAN in this cohort to ESRD.

Although renal outcome did not differ between the persistent and healed PIGN groups, healed PIGN appears to correlate with higher mortality during the follow-up period. Although this may be counterintuitive and there is real possibility of a chance finding, there is evidence that at the time of biopsy more patients with healed PIGN exhibiting more nephrotic-range proteinuria which may have been associated with worse outcome in this group of patients. Alternatively, since we did not account for the timing of institution of antibiotic and HAART use, this could have played a crucial role in the different mortality between the 2 groups.

Our study has several limitations. It is a single-center study with patients mostly coming from an inner city urban hospital. Our patient population consisted mostly of African American patients; hence the results may not apply to other populations. Only patients who had renal biopsies were included, which potentially excluded the HIV patients who are coagulopathic or with severe illness. We also did not account for the duration of HIV-1 infection or timing of initiation of HAART or antibiotic therapy, which could have an impact on the renal outcome or mortality. Although the histological pattern proposed by Haas is not widely utilized in practice, our study was an attempt at using some form of standardization for the study.

In conclusion, PIGN is a common histopathologic diagnosis in HIV patients. *Staphylococcus* is the most commonly identified organism in a preceding infection in HIV-associated PIGN. The histopathological classification of PIGN has no bearing on the renal outcome but this group of patients incur overall high mortality rate. Patients with healed PIGN have the highest mortality suggesting that delayed diagnosis may have a negative impact on overall outcome.

Acknowledgments

All authors abide by the Association for Medical Ethics (AME) ethical rules of disclosure.

Author Contributions

Conceived and designed the experiments: MGA GML DMF. Performed the experiments: NCM DA CM. Analyzed the data: MGA GML. Contributed reagents/materials/analysis tools: MGA GML. Contributed to the writing of the manuscript: CM DA MGA MME.

References

1. Berliner AR, Fine DM, Lucas GM, Rahman MH, Racusen LC, et al. (2008) Observations on a cohort of HIV-infected patients undergoing native renal biopsy. Am J Nephrol 28: 478–486.
2. Nebuloni M, Barbiano di Belgiojoso G, Genderini A, Tosoni A, L N, et al. (2009) Glomerular lesions in HIV-positive patients: a 20-year biopsy experience from Northern Italy. Clin Nephrol 72: 38–45.
3. Gerntholtz TE, Goetsch SJ, Katz I (2006) HIV-related nephropathy: a South African perspective. Kidney Int 69: 1885–1891.
4. Foy MC, Estrella MM, Lucas GM, Tahir F, Fine DM, et al. (2013) Comparison of risk factors and outcomes in HIV immune complex kidney disease and HIV-associated nephropathy. Clin J Am Soc Nephrol 8: 1524–1532.
5. Lucas GM, Eustace JA, Sozio S, Mentari EK, Appiah KA, et al. (2004) Highly active antiretroviral therapy and the incidence of HIV-1-associated nephropathy: a 12-year cohort study. Aids 18: 541–546.
6. Atta MG, Gallant JE, Rahman MH, Nagajothi N, Racusen LC, et al. (2006) Antiretroviral therapy in the treatment of HIV-associated nephropathy. Nephrol Dial Transplant 21: 2809–2813.
7. Estrella MM, Fine DM, Atta MG (2010) Recent developments in HIV-related kidney disease. HIV Ther 4: 589–603.
8. Montseny JJ, Meyrier A, Kleinknecht D, Callard P (1995) The current spectrum of infectious glomerulonephritis. Experience with 76 patients and review of the literature. Medicine (Baltimore) 74: 63–73.
9. Nast CC (2012) Infection-related glomerulonephritis: changing demographics and outcomes. Adv Chronic Kidney Dis 19: 68–75.
10. Wen YK (2009) The spectrum of adult postinfectious glomerulonephritis in the new millennium. Ren Fail 31: 676–682.
11. Moroni G, Pozzi C, Quaglini S, Segagni S, Banfi G, et al. (2002) Long-term prognosis of diffuse proliferative glomerulonephritis associated with infection in adults. Nephrol Dial Transplant 17: 1204–1211.
12. Vogl W, Renke M, Mayer-Eichberger D, Schmitt H, Bohle A (1986) Long-term prognosis for endocapillary glomerulonephritis of poststreptococcal type in children and adults. Nephron 44: 58–65.
13. Nasr SH, Markowitz GS, Stokes MB, Said SM, Valeri AM, et al. (2008) Acute postinfectious glomerulonephritis in the modern era: experience with 86 adults and review of the literature. Medicine (Baltimore) 87: 21–32.
14. Haas M, Racusen LC, Bagnasco SM (2008) IgA-dominant postinfectious glomerulonephritis: a report of 13 cases with common ultrastructural features. Hum Pathol 39: 1309–1316.
15. Haas M (2003) Incidental healed postinfectious glomerulonephritis: a study of 1012 renal biopsy specimens examined by electron microscopy. Hum Pathol 34: 3–10.
16. Nasr SH, Fidler ME, Valeri AM, Cornell LD, Sethi S, et al. (2011) Postinfectious glomerulonephritis in the elderly. J Am Soc Nephrol 22: 187–195.
17. Nasr SH, D'Agati VD (2011) IgA-dominant postinfectious glomerulonephritis: a new twist on an old disease. Nephron Clin Pract 119: c18–25; discussion c26.
18. George E, Nadkarni GN, Estrella MM, Lucas GM, Sperati CJ, et al. (2011) The impact of hepatitis C coinfection on kidney disease related to human immunodeficiency virus (HIV): a biopsy study. Medicine (Baltimore) 90: 289–295.
19. Cohen SD, Kimmel PL (2008) Immune complex renal disease and human immunodeficiency virus infection. Semin Nephrol 28: 535–544.
20. Kimmel PL, Phillips TM, Ferreira-Centeno A, Farkas-Szallasi T, Abraham AA, et al. (1993) HIV-associated immune-mediated renal disease. Kidney Int 44: 1327–1340.
21. Zent R, Van Zyl Smit R, Duffield M, Cassidy MJ (1994) Crescentic nephritis at Groote Schuur Hospital, South Africa–not a benign disease. Clin Nephrol 42: 22–29.
22. Wearne N, Swanepoel CR, Boulle A, Duffield MS, Rayner BL (2012) The spectrum of renal histologies seen in HIV with outcomes, prognostic indicators and clinical correlations. Nephrol Dial Transplant 27: 4109–4118.
23. Szczech LA, Gupta SK, Habash R, Guasch A, Kalayjian R, et al. (2004) The clinical epidemiology and course of the spectrum of renal diseases associated with HIV infection. Kidney Int 66: 1145–1152.

13

IL22 Regulates Human Urothelial Cell Sensory and Innate Functions through Modulation of the Acetylcholine Response, Immunoregulatory Cytokines and Antimicrobial Peptides: Assessment of an *In Vitro* Model

Phong T. Le[1]*, Meghan M. Pearce[1], Shubin Zhang[1], Edward M. Campbell[1], Cynthia S. Fok[3], Elizabeth R. Mueller[2], Cynthia A. Brincat[2], Alan J. Wolfe[1], Linda Brubaker[2]

1 Department of Microbiology and Immunology, Stritch School of Medicine, Loyola University Chicago, Maywood, Illinois, United States of America, **2** Department of Obstetrics and Gynecology, Stritch School of Medicine, Loyola University Chicago, Maywood, Illinois, United States of America, **3** University of Minnesota, Department of Urology, Minneapolis, Minnesota, United States of America

Abstract

Human urinary disorders are generally studied in rodent models due to limitations of functional *in vitro* culture models of primary human urothelial cells (HUCs). Current HUC culture models are often derived from immortalized cancer cell lines, which likely have functional characteristics differ from healthy human urothelium. Here, we described a simple explant culture technique to generate HUCs and assessed their *in vitro* functions. Using transmission electron microscopy, we assessed morphology and heterogeneity of the generated HUCs and characterized their intercellular membrane structural proteins relative to *ex vivo* urothelium tissue. We demonstrated that our cultured HUCs are free of fibroblasts. They are also heterogeneous, containing cells characteristic of both immature basal cells and mature superficial urothelial cells. The cultured HUCs expressed muscarinic receptors (MR1 and MR2), carnitine acetyltransferase (CarAT), immunoregulatory cytokines IL7, IL15, and IL23, as well as the chemokine CCL20. HUCs also expressed epithelial cell-specific molecules essential for forming intercellular structures that maintain the functional capacity to form the physiological barrier of the human bladder urothelium. A subset of HUCs, identified by the high expression of CD44, expressed the Toll-like receptor 4 (TLR4) along with its co-receptor CD14. We demonstrated that HUCs express, at the mRNA level, both forms of the IL22 receptor, the membrane-associated (IL22RA1) and the secreted soluble (IL22RA2) forms; in turn, IL22 inhibited expression of MR1 and induced expression of CarAT and two antimicrobial peptides (S100A9 and lipocalin-2). While the cellular sources of IL22 have yet to be identified, the HUC cytokine and chemokine profiles support the concept that IL22-producing cells are present in the human bladder mucosa tissue and that IL22 plays a regulatory role in HUC functions. Thus, the described explant technique is clearly capable of generating functional HUCs suitable for the study of human urinary tract disorders, including interactions between urothelium and IL22-producing cells.

Editor: Anil Kumar, University of Missouri-Kansas City, United States of America

Funding: Funding provided by the Ralph and Marian Falk Medical Research Trust, Immunology and Infectious Disease Research Institute, Loyola University LU205650 and LU203919 (PTL), LU202567 (AJW). The funders had no role in study design, data collection and analysis, decision to publish, or preparation of the manuscript.

* Email: ple@luc.edu

Introduction

The urothelium is the layer of stratified epithelial cells that lines the lumen of the bladder and urinary tract. Whereas the urothelium forms a physical barrier, it also performs other functions [1]. For example, it responds to diverse stimuli, including mechanical, chemical and biological signals. In response, the urothelium releases mediators that contribute to the maintenance of urothelium functions and homeostasis. While most current understanding of urothelium biology and physiopathology has been gained from studying animal models, less is known about the human urothelium, mainly due to limitations in establishing a functional primary human urothelial cell (HUC) culture system.

The human urothelium is organized into three distinct cell layers: the basal, intermediate and outermost superficial layer. The superficial layer consists of terminally differentiated umbrella cells, which establish and maintain the physical barrier function through intercellular tight junctions. The apical face of the umbrella cells is covered with a unique, asymmetric unit membrane called the uroplakin plaque (Uro P), in which the four members of the uroplakin protein (UP) family are assembled into two distinct heterodimer units [2,3]. Umbrella cells also contain intracellular organelles, the discoid fusiform vesicles (DFVs); in response to mechanical stimuli, DFVs are incorporated into the cell membrane to increase bladder volume [4].

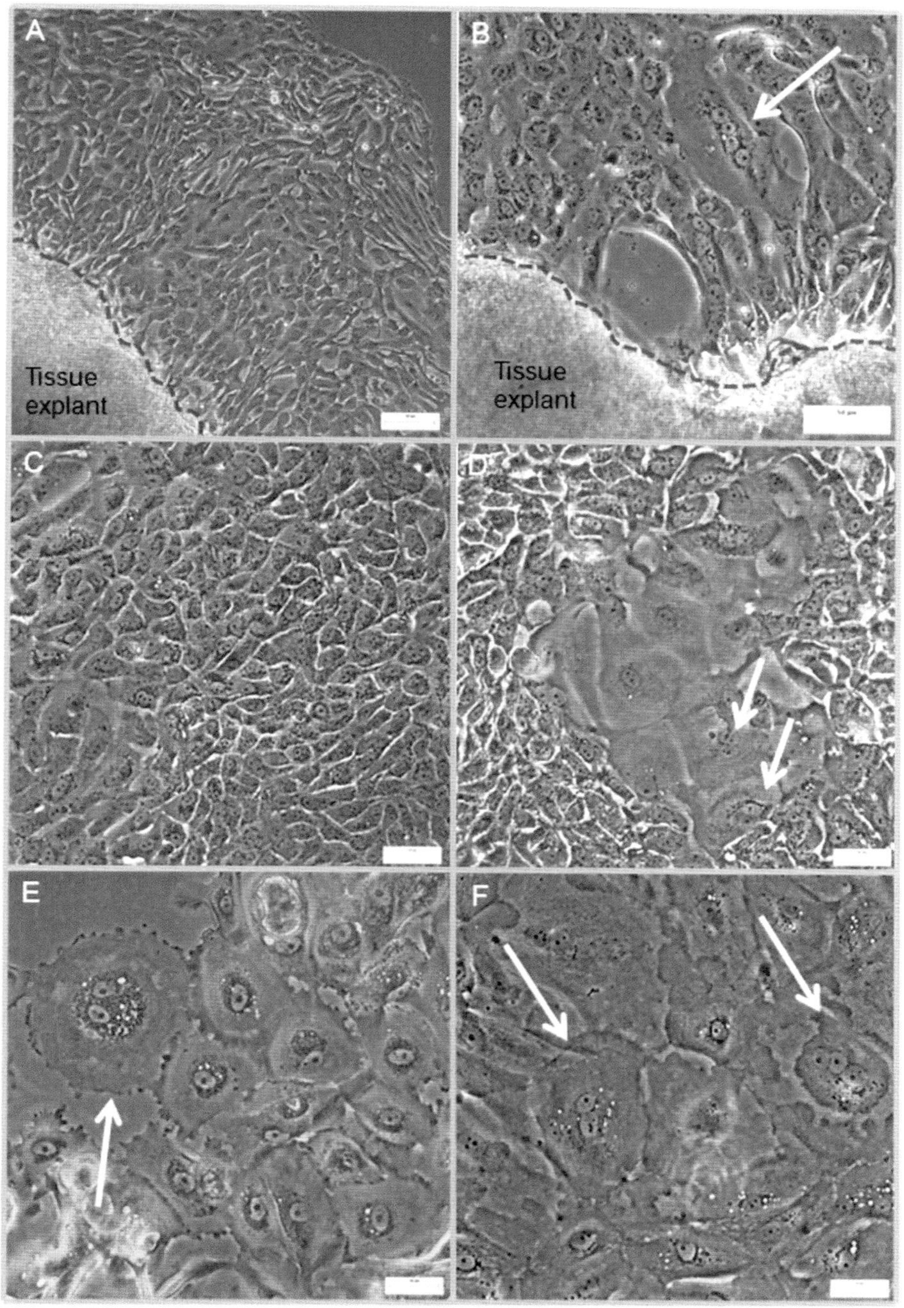

Figure 1. Cellular morphology of human urothelial cells (HUCs) generated from bladder tissue explant. (A, B) Cells growing out from the edge of two tissue explants obtained from two different biopsies; cells with typical coble-stone morphology were clearly identifiable. Arrow points to a larger cell (60–150 μm) with four nuclei and prominent nucleolus. (C, D) cells with uniform size and morphology (25–40 μm) surround a cluster of larger cells (70–100 μm); several are bi-nucleated (arrows). (E, F) clusters of larger cells (80–150 μm), many of these cells are bi-nucleated (arrows). The dotted lines demarcate the edge of the tissue explants. Scale bar = 50 μm.

The urothelium of various species has been shown to express choline acetyltransferase (ChAT) and/or carnitine acetyltransferase (CarAT), enzymes that synthesize the neurotransmitter acetylcholine (Ach) [5,6]. Urothelium also expresses cholinergic receptors, including the nicotinic and muscarinic receptors (MR) that mediate the Ach response [7,8]. Of particularly interest is the functional discovery of two main groups of MR: the MR1 (which also includes MR3 and MR5) and MR2 (which also includes MR4) [6–8]. In the urothelium, expression of MR1 is predominantly found in basal cells, while MR2 expression is restricted to umbrella cells [8]. Thus, the urothelium is a non-neuronal source of Ach, which together with expression of MR, has been implicated in the development of certain lower urinary tract disorders, via establishment of an autocrine pathway [1,9]. The modulation of this Ach response in human urothelium is not well understood.

Our recent work has convincingly demonstrated that a human urinary microbiota exists [10–12]. In other human mucosa tissues, the maintenance of organ-specific microbiota is regulated by innate and adaptive immune cells through production of various immunoregulatory cytokines and antimicrobial peptides (AMPs) that both control invasion by bacterial pathogens and potentially regulate microbial diversity [13–15]. Despite the significant disease burden of urinary tract infection, urinary incontinence, and other related urinary disorders, little is known about the immune regulation of the human bladder. Since interleukin 22 (IL22) is an important cytokine that regulates pathogen invasion in the gastrointestinal tract [16,17], it is possible that IL22 plays a similar role in maintaining the human bladder microbiota.

Human urothelial cultures currently employed are typically bladder carcinoma cell lines, whose use limits our ability to describe normal urothelial cell functions. Thus, to advance our current understanding of human urothelium biology and physiopathology, a functional *in vitro* culture system that retains key aspects of the human urothelium is needed. Such aspects would include heterogeneity of uroepithelial cell populations, as well as the expression of critical molecules that emulates their functions *in vivo*.

Here, we describe a simple explant culture technique that readily generates human urothelial cell (HUC) cultures with functional characteristics. Using, these HUC cultures, we demonstrate for the first time that IL22 plays an important role in the maintenance of human urothelium function and provide evidence that HUCs potentially interact with immune cells that contribute to the maintenance of the human bladder microbiota.

Results

Primary cultures of Human Urothelial Cells (HUCs) established from bladder biopsy

Using an explant culture technique previously established in our laboratory to generate primary cultures of human thymic epithelial cells [18], we generated HUC cultures from human bladder urothelial biopsies obtained from consenting surgical patients following human subjects institutional review board approval. The explant technique generated HUC growth from bladder biopsies in most (80–90%) of the tissue explants. Cells with epithelial cell morphology appeared at the edge of the tissue explants within 1 week in culture (**Fig. 1A, B**). Upon removal of the tissue explants (around day 10–12), clusters of the proliferating cells further expanded into growth areas of approximately 5–10 cm^2. Within this growth area, the cells appeared to be well interconnected with cobble-stone morphology, characteristic of epithelial cells in culture (**Fig. 1C, D**). Among the predominant cells with uniform size (25–40 μm in diameter), we observed clusters of larger bi-nucleated cells (70–150 μm in diameter) (**Fig. 1C–F**). Cells at this stage could be sub-cultured once; additional passages did not result in further expansion of the HUC cultures.

Phenotypes of primary cultures of HUCs

To characterize the established HUCs, we examined expression of epithelial cell-specific and other cell surface markers, using multi-color flow cytometric analysis. We first determined that HUCs uniformly express human major histocompatibility complex class I HLA-ABC, verifying that they were derived from human tissues (**Fig. 2A**). These HLA-ABC^{pos} HUCs expressed the intercellular adhesion molecule-1 (ICAM-1, CD54) (**Fig. 2A**). They also expressed the epithelial cell adhesion molecule (EpCAM, CD326) and integrin-β4 (CD104), two specific markers for epithelial cells (**Fig. 2B**). HUCs were negative for human major histocompatibility complex class II HLA-DR, suggesting that expression of HLA-DR *in vitro* requires further stimulation (**Fig. 2C**). Based on the levels of the cell surface expression of CD44, a hyaluronan binding protein, HUCs could be divided into two distinct populations (**Fig. 2C**). While both populations expressed the Toll-like receptor 4 (TLR4), only the HUC population with high expression of CD44 expressed the TLR4 co-receptor CD14 (**Fig. 2C–E**).

Ultrastructure characteristics of primary HUCs

The presence of larger, bi-nucleated cells suggested that these cells are the mature superficial umbrella cells that line the adult human bladder lumen (**Fig. 1B, D–F**). To determine if our culture system generated umbrella cells, we performed transmission electron microscopy (TEM) studies (**Fig. 3A–F**), seeking evidence of two structures that are unique to umbrella cells: the discoid fusiform vesicle (DVF) and the uroplakin plaque (Uro P). In our primary HUCs, we identified cells with numerous DVFs and Uro Ps (**Fig. 3D**); identical structures were also observed in umbrella cells that were located in the outer most layer of *ex vivo* bladder urothelium (**Fig. 4B–D**). We also observed multivesicular bodies (MVBs) with exosomes in cultured HUCs (**Fig. 3B, C**). In culture, adjacent HUCs formed lateral interdigitations (**Fig. 3E**), which increase surface connection between two cells. They also formed desmosomes (Des), which further strengthen cell-cell connections (**Fig. 3F**). These ultrastructures were similarly observed in the *ex vivo* human bladder biopsy (**Fig. 4**).

Thus, both cellular morphology and ultrastructure characteristics indicate the presence of umbrella cells in our HUC cultures. To further confirm that our culture conditions generated umbrella cells from human bladder biopsies, we performed indirect immunofluorescent staining, using anti-uroplakin and anti-keratin 20 antibodies. We detected cells positive for both uroplakins (red) and keratin 20 (green), indicative of umbrella cells (**Fig. 5**).

Since umbrella cells line the luminal surface of the bladder, they are the most likely targets for interaction with uropathogenic *Escherichia coli* (UPEC). It has been demonstrated previously that UPEC utilize type I pili to adhere to cell surface uroplakins expressed by umbrella cells [19–21]. To examine whether UPEC adhere to umbrella cells present in our primary HUCs, we incubated HUCs in the presence of the UPEC strain NU14 for 2 h, removed non-adherent bacteria through PBS washes and assessed for bacterial adherence via microscopy. NU14 adhered to HUCs (**Fig. 6A, D**). This interaction was mediated by type I pili, as the *fimH* mutant (NU14-1) exhibited decreased adherence compared to wild-type (**Fig. 6B, D**).

Functional analysis of primary HUCs

To evaluate potential functions of cultured HUCs, we assessed expression of various genes that have been implicated in urothelium physiopathology. We also assessed expression of cytokines or chemokines that potentially affect urothelium homeostasis and/or modulate immune cell functions within the human bladder mucosa tissue. By quantitative RT-PCR (qRT-PCR), we determined that primary HUCs express CarAT (**Table 1**), an enzyme that catalyzes the synthesis of acetylcholine. In contrast, expression of choline acetyltransferase (ChAT), which catalyzes acetylcholine synthesis in neurons, was not detectable in our HUC cultures (data not shown). The cultured HUCs expressed predominantly the muscarinic acetylcholine receptor group 1 (MR1); MR2 also was detectable, albeit at a very low level; perhaps, the data reflect the low percentage of umbrella cells in the cultures (**Table 1**).

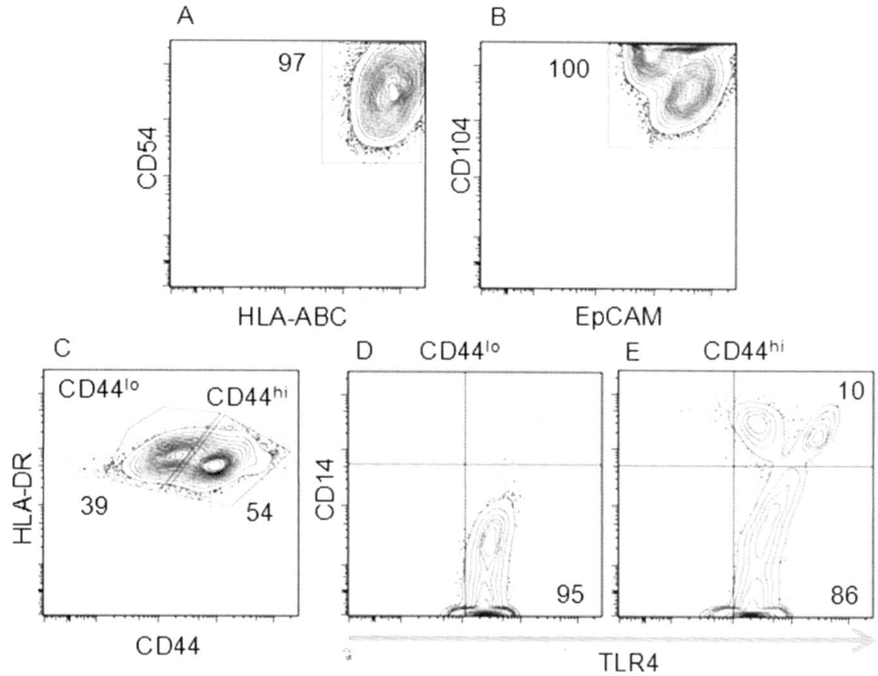

Figure 2. Flow cytometric analysis of primary HUCs. Cells were stained with eight fluorochrome-conjugated monoclonal antibodies direct against cell surface makers. Cells were analyzed for the expression of: (A) HLA-ABC and CD54 (ICAM-1); (B) CD104 and EpCAM; (C) HLA-DR, and CD44–expression of CD44 shows two distinct populations of HUCs: $CD44^{lo}$ and $CD44^{hi}$; (D, E) TLR and CD14. Representative data from 3 experiments performed with HUCs generated from 3 independent bladder biopsies.

HUCs also expressed interleukins (IL) 7, 15 and 23, and the chemokine CCL20 (**Table 1**). IL7 and IL15 play important roles in T cell functions and homeostasis [22], while CCL20 plays a role in regulating mucosa lymphoid tissue formation by attracting T cells and dendritic cells toward and into urothelium [23]. IL23 is required for regulating IL22 expression [17].

IL22 and HUC functions

IL22 has emerged as an important cytokine in the maintenance of epithelial cell homeostasis in mucosa tissues, including skin and gastrointestinal tract [16,24]. In these tissues, IL22 mediates its function through IL22RA1, the membrane form of the IL22 receptor, which is predominantly expressed in mucosa epithelial cells [16,24]. Thus, to determine if IL22 plays a regulatory role in HUC function, we first demonstrated that HUCs express IL22RA1. These cells also expressed low levels of the secreted soluble form of the IL22 receptor (IL22RA2, also known as the IL22 binding protein) (**Table 1**). To determine if HUCs could respond to IL22, we treated primary HUC cultures with a predetermined concentration of human recombinant IL22 (100 ng/mL) for 48 hours, and assessed the expression of CarAT, MR1 and two antimicrobial peptides that we found expressed in HUCs, S100A9 and lipocalin-2. Compared to untreated cultures, IL22 reduced expression of MR1 3.9-fold (or about 25% of the untreated cultures) (**Fig. 7**), while increasing S100A9 expression about 3-fold. IL22 moderately increased the expression of lipocalin-2 and CarAT (**Fig. 7**). This finding has important potential clinical significance as anti-muscarinic drugs are commonly used for treatment of certain human urinary disorders, such as urgency urinary incontinence and overactive bladder.

Discussion

Human urothelial cells (HUCs) play an important role in the normal physiology, as well as the physiopathology, of the human bladder; however, information regarding HUC function is limited by the lack of an *in vitro* culture system that generates non-malignant HUC cultures. Here, we described a simple culture explant technique that reliably generates HUC cultures from human bladder biopsies that are free of fibroblast contamination. The biopsies were obtained after IRB approval from surgical patients who consented to urothelial biopsy. A small urothelial biopsy was collected at the end of the female patients' indicated reconstructive pelvic surgery for pelvic organ prolapse and/or stress urinary incontinence. The biopsy is obtained during cystoscopy, a routine patient safety measure; clinically, the urothelium from these patients are considered grossly non-pathological, thus allowing us to interrogate normal functions of human urothelial cells. Furthermore, the generated cultures were free of fibroblasts, as verified by the high percentage of cells that co-express the epithelial cell-specific markers EpCAM and CD104. Since they consist primarily of urothelial cells, these cultures can be used to evaluate various *in vitro* functions of HUCs.

The simple explant technique described above does not require enzyme digestion of the bladder tissue, as described by others [25,26]. We found that a single step incubation of the biopsy samples in culture media at 37°C facilitates removal of the upper urothelium layer from the underlying submucosa, which is the primary cellular source for fibroblast contamination. We conclude that the HUC cultures generated from bladder explant tissues are epithelial in nature, on the basis of cell morphology and expression of epithelial cell-specific surface molecules and intermediate filament keratins. Morphologically, our HUC cultures demonstrated the cobble-stone

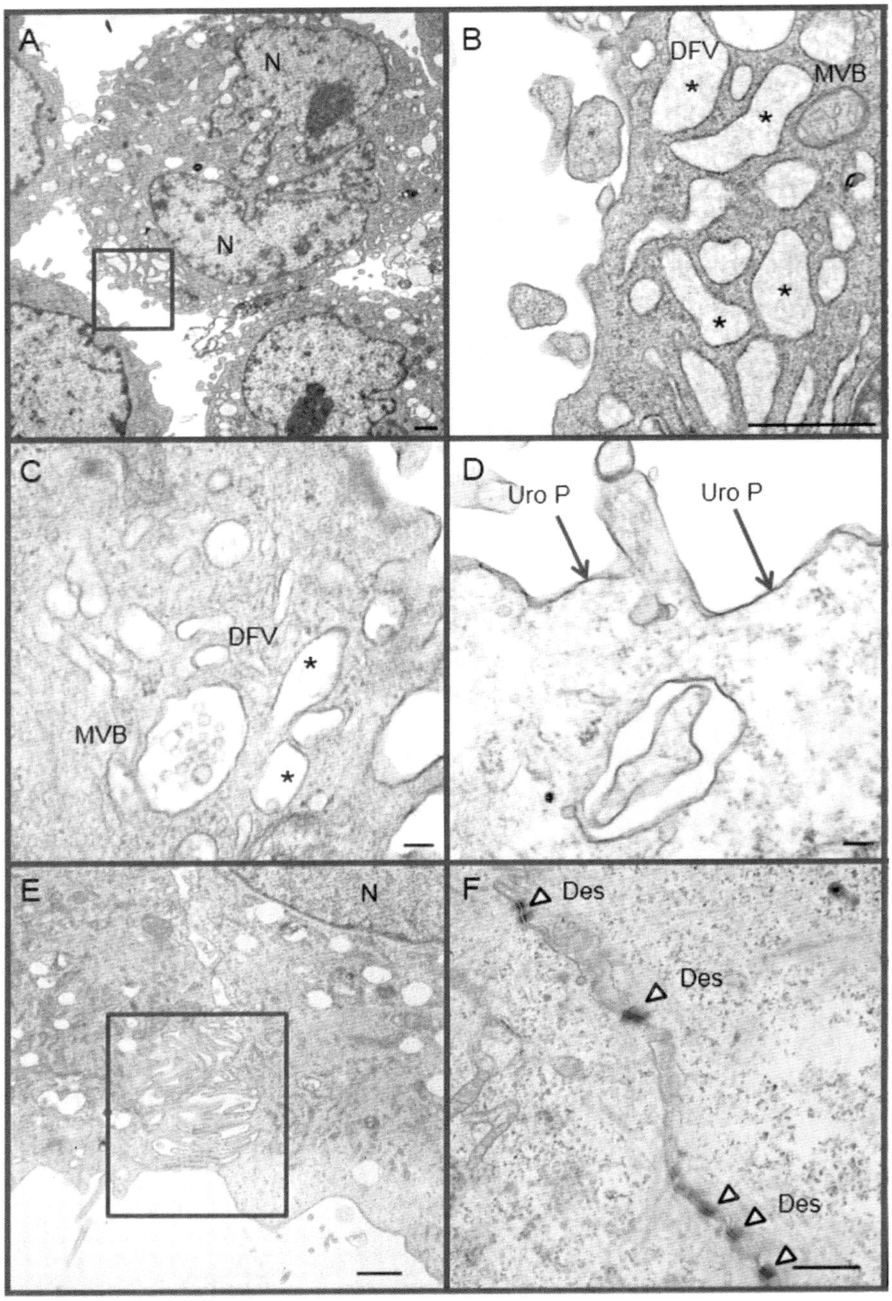

Figure 3. Ultrastructures of primary HUCs. Cultured HUCs were analyzed by TEM. (A, B) a HUC with two nuclei (N) and many discoid fusiform vesicles (DVF) - *denotes lumens of DFV; B is a higher magnification of the square area identified in A - MVB denotes multivesicular body; (C) another example of MVB and DFV in a HUC; (D) presence of uroplakins plaques (Uro P, dark line) on the cell membrane of an umbrella cell; (E) formation of lateral interdigitation between two adjacent HUCs, a higher magnification of the identified was shown in F; (F) presence of numerous desmosomes (Des, arrowheads) within a well-formed lateral interdigitation of two adjacent HUCs. Bar scale is equal to 1 μm (in A, B, E and F) and 0.1 μm (in C and D).

morphology characteristic of monolayer epithelial cell cultures. The HUCs were heterogeneous in size, comprised of islands of large cells surrounded by uniformly smaller cells. The clusters of larger cells contained many bi-nucleated cells, a cellular morphology typical of the superficial umbrella cells that line the lumen of the human bladder. We verified that the large bi-nucleated cells were umbrella cells by demonstrating that they express specific markers for umbrella cells: uroplakins (UPs) and cytokeratin 20 [4,27]. Furthermore, TEM revealed that the bi-nucleated cells displayed uroplakin plaques (Uro Ps) and discoid fusiform vesicles (DFVs), both unique ultrastructures of umbrella cells [4].

Uro Ps are characteristic membrane structures composed of four UP types (Ia, Ib, II and III). UPIa is only expressed on the cell surface when it forms heterodimers with UPII [2]. When this

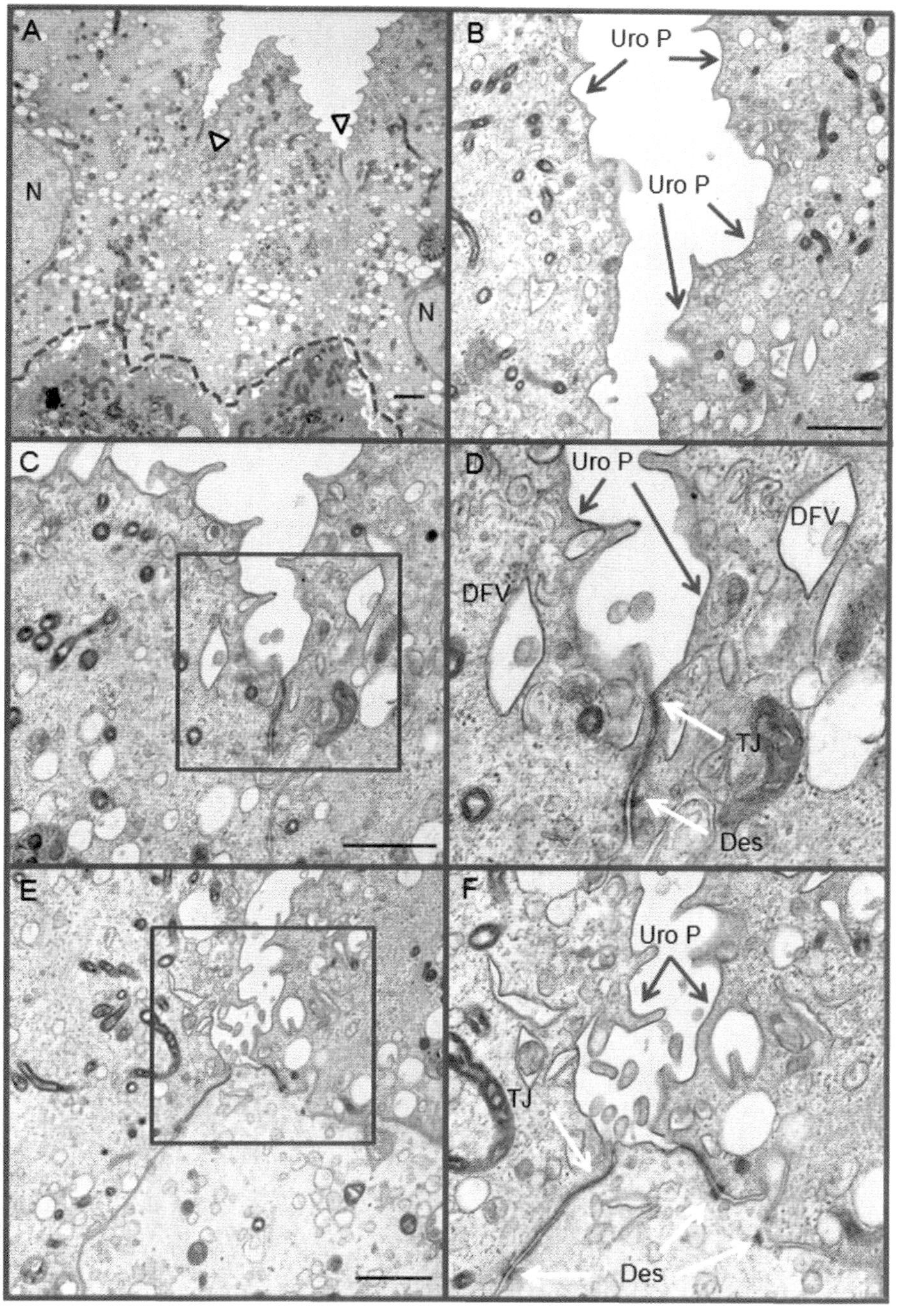

Figure 4. Ultrastructures of *ex vivo* human bladder urothelium. Bladder tissue biopsy was immediately processed for TEM study. (A) Surface umbrella cells with numerous DFVs. Arrowheads point to tight junctions (TJ) between two adjacent umbrella cells; dotted line demarcates junction between the upper umbrella cells and the underlying urothelial cells. (B) A higher magnification photograph of umbrella cells showing DVFs and uroplakins plaques (Uro P), which appear as darker lines associated with the cell membrane. (C, E) Higher magnification of TJ structures shown in A. (E, F) enlargement of areas shown in C and E (square boxes) showing DFVs, Uro P, TJ and desmosomes (Des). Bar scale = 1 μm.

complex is properly assembled, it is expressed on the cell surface where it serves as a receptor for UPEC via the adhesive FimH tip of UPEC's type I pili, which selectively binds UPIa [19–21]. We demonstrated that UPEC adhered to HUCs in a FimH-dependent manner, indicating that UPs are functionally assembled and expressed on the HUC cell surface. We propose that these HUC cultures may be a useful tool to investigate the interactions between the human urothelium and UPEC, as well as the newly discovered urinary microbiota [11,12].

That these cultures were indeed epithelial and free of fibroblast contamination was shown by their homogeneous co-expression of two epithelial cell-specific cell adhesion molecules: EpCAM and integrin-β4 (CD104). Expression of both cell surface markers also showed that cultured HUCs maintain expression of molecules that are critical for cell-cell interaction and intercellular structures.

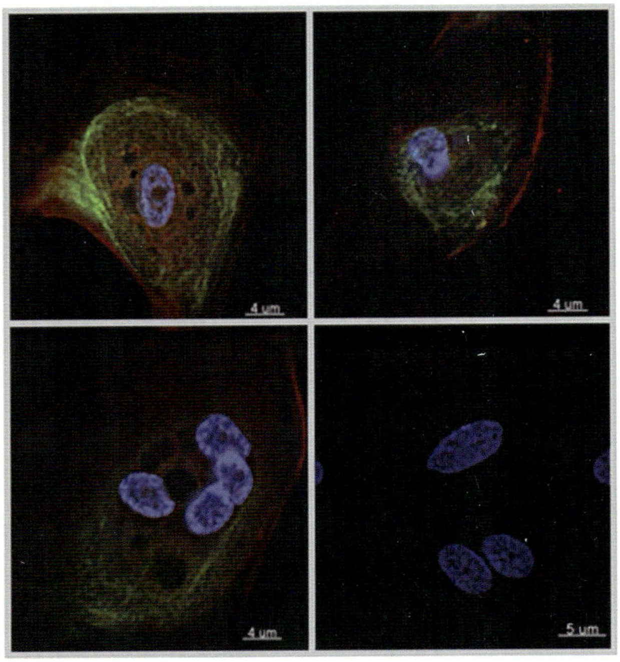

Figure 5. Immunofluorescent staining of cultured HUCs. HUCs were fixed and double stained with anti-uroplakins (PE, Red) and keratin-20 (FITC, green). DAPI (blue) was used to stain the nucleus. Lower right panel is a negative control stained with mouse and rabbit IgG. Representative images from 3 experiments from 3 independent biopsies.

CD104 is important for forming hemi-desmosomes in urothelial cells of the basal layer, allowing them to anchor to the basal lamina [28]. EpCAM mediates homotypic cell adhesion through homodimerization, contributing to the formation of tight junctions through interaction with claudin 7 [29,30]. We determined that cultured HUCs expressed claudin 7 (data not shown), indicating that they maintain their ability to form tight junctions. These cell-cell interactions at the monolayer cell level were revealed by TEM, which demonstrated that adjacent HUCs form lateral interdigitations with desmosomes. The expression of adhesion molecules, coupled to the existence of intercellular structures, indicates that the cultured HUCs maintain their ability to recapitulate the physical barrier function of urothelium *in vitro*. The HUCs generated from our explant technique are thus a potential source of cells to generate stratified human urothelium *in vitro*.

The cultured HUCs also uniformly express ICAM-1 (also known as CD54). It has been shown that expression of ICAM-1 is increased in bladder biopsies from patients with interstitial cystitis (IC), but undetectable in non-pathological bladder biopsies [31]. However, urothelial cells from IC patients express HLA-DR, while our cultured HUCs are HLA-DR negative. Whether the constitutive expression ICAM-1 is a unique feature of cultured HUCs remains to be determined.

In addition to the heterogeneity in cell size, cultured HUCs are also segregated into two distinct populations based on the expression of cell surface CD44. Expression of CD44 has been shown as a marker for basal urothelial cells; its expression is reduced in the intermediate layer and undetectable in the superficial umbrella cells [32,33]. The two levels of CD44 expression suggest that HUCs in culture undergo differentiation from the less mature basal cells into the more differentiated and mature umbrella cells. The two populations of CD44-expressing

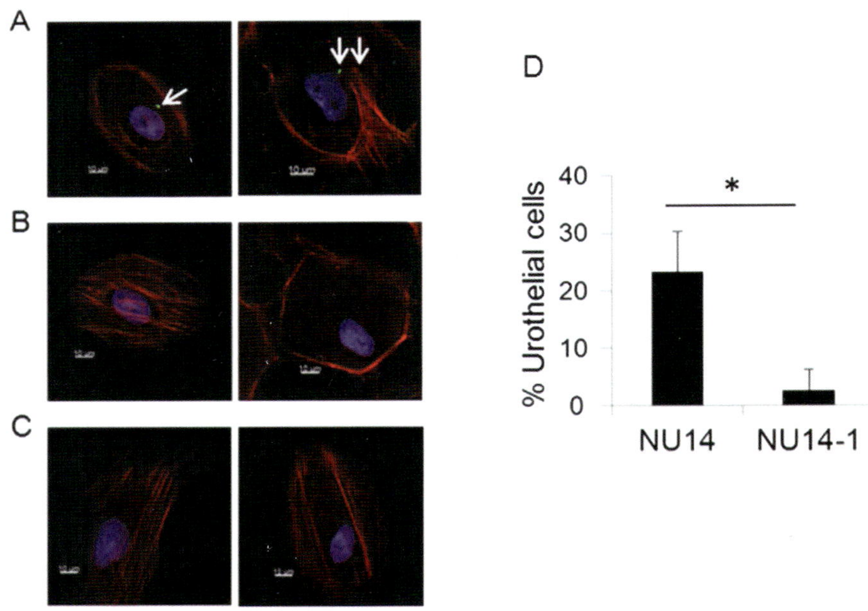

Figure 6. Uropathogenic *E. coli* strain NU14 adheres to HUCs. HUCs were exposed to NU14 (A), the isogenic *fimH* mutant NU14-1 (B) or media alone (C). After 2 h, the HUCs were washed and stained for the presence of adherent bacteria (green). Host cell actin (red) and nuclei (blue) were counterstained. Merged images show NU14 (A, arrows) adhering to urothelial cells. The percentage of urothelial cells with adherent bacteria was quantified (D) by scoring at least 200 urothelial cells from random fields of view for the presence of adherent bacteria. The percentage represents the number of urothelial cells with adherent bacteria divided by the total number of urothelial cells examined. Data are representative of at least three (A–C) or two (D) independent experiments performed with cells derived from independent biopsies. Between experiments, the average percentage of urothelial cells with adherent NU14 ranged from 8 to 23%. The errors bars represent the standard deviation of two coverslips per strain per experiment. Scale bars, 10 μm. *Indicates $p<0.05$, Student's t-test.

Table 1. Expression of cytokines, cytokine receptors, chemokines in primary HUCs (#Number of copies/μg total RNA).

Genes	Experiment 1	Experiment 2	Experiment 3
MR1	2.7×10^5 (2×10^4)#	1.3×10^4 (6.8×10^3)	8.4×10^4 (1.8×10^4)
MR2	2.3×10^3 (2×10^2)	1.7×10^3 (2.4×10^2)	0.3×10^3 (3)
CarAT	8.1×10^5 (1×10^5)	2.9×10^5 (1.6×10^4)	1.6×10^5 (1.0×10^4)
IL7	1.2×10^6 (1.7×10^5)	4.1×10^6 (2.0×10^5)	3.1×10^5 (4.8×10^4)
IL15	1.2×10^4 (3.2×10^3)	2.6×10^5 (4.0×10^4)	6.4×10^3 (1.3×10^3)
IL23	6.4×10^3 (1.3×10^3)	1.2×10^4 (9.2×10^2)	7.1×10^3 (1.1×10^3)
CCL20	6.4×10^5 (1.7×10^5)	4.5×10^6 (1.2×10^5)	1.5×10^6 (7.8×10^5)
IL22RA1	4.2×10^5 (2.1×10^4)	1.3×10^6 (1.4×10^5)	1.1×10^5 (1×10^4)
IL22RA2	8.1×10^2 (2.4×10^2)	5.4×10^3 (9.0×10^2)	0.6×10^3 (50)

Data were from three independent cultures of HUCs established from three different human bladder biopsies. Transcript levels were determined by qRT-PCR. #Values represent the average of triplicates; numbers in parentheses are standard errors of the mean.

HUCs also showed distinct patterns of expression of the Toll-like receptor 4 (TLR4) and its co-receptor CD14. While both $CD44^{lo}$ and $CD44^{hi}$ subpopulations expressed TLR4, only the $CD44^{hi}$ HUCs expressed the CD14 co-receptor, suggesting that HUCs control signaling through TLR4 by regulating the expression of CD14.

The defense function of HUCs may be partially due to the co-expression of CD44 (which binds hyaluronic acid or HA) and TLR4/CD14 receptor complex (which responds to lipopolysaccharide of Gram-negative bacteria). Since CD44 facilitates the interaction of UPEC and urothelial cells in a murine model [34], the binding of HA to CD44 could function as a natural blocking ligand. Indeed, small case series report that intravesical HA treatment may have a role in reducing cystitis recurrence and mean UTI-recurrence time in humans [35,36]. Thus, CD44/HA and TLR4/CD14 could collaborate to diminish bacterial infection. In addition to its regulatory role in the expression of S100A9 and lipocalin-2 as we reported here, whether IL22 also contributes to urothelium defense mechanisms against bacterial infection by regulating HUC production of HA or HUC expression of TLR4/CD14 remains to be elucidated.

The establishment of HUC cultures free of fibroblast contamination allows us to interrogate the potential functions that HUCs play in maintaining mucosa immunity of the human bladder. This clinically important aspect will advance our current knowledge deficit regarding the immune function of the human bladder, especially in the face of the emerging knowledge regarding the urinary microbiota [10–12]. For example, in the gastrointestinal tract, IL22 has emerged as an important regulatory cytokine. It maintains homeostasis in enterocytes and controls colonization of gut pathogens by modulating expression of antimicrobial peptides (AMPs), such as RegIIIγ, calprotectin, and lipocalin-2 [37,38]. First, we showed that cultured HUCs express the membrane from of IL22R (IL22RA1). We then showed that IL22 increases expression of lipocalin-2 and the S100A9 subunit of calprotectin, but not the second subunit of calprotectin (S100A8) or RegIIIγ (data not shown). Selective expression of AMPs by HUCs may reflect the unique composition of tissue-specific microbiota, as well as a specific mechanism for controlling infections of tissue-specific

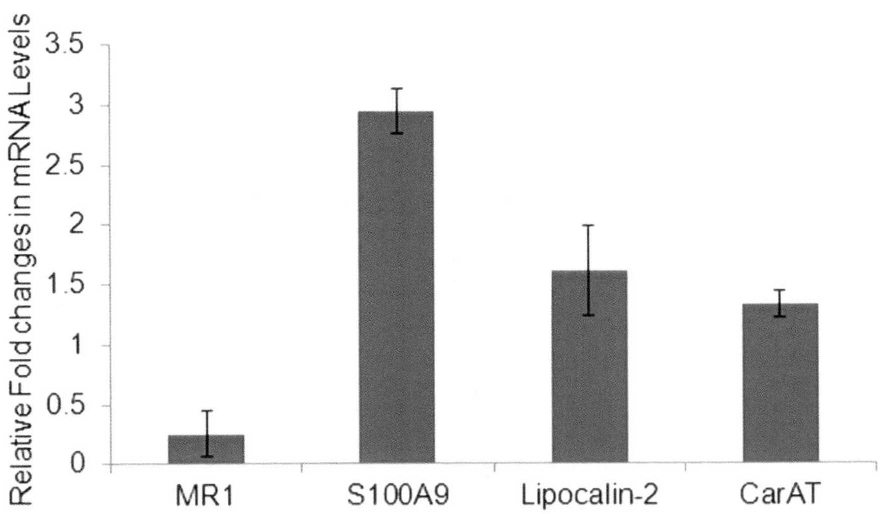

Figure 7. Effect of IL22 on the expression of MR1, S100A9, lipocalin-2, and CarAT by primary HUCs. Transcript levels were measured by qRT-PCR and expressed as fold change of treated versus untreated HUC cultures. Values represent the average of two independent experiments performed with two different HUC cultures. Errors bars are standard deviations.

pathogens. For example, RegIIIγ expression in enterocytes is induced by IL22 and is important for preventing *Candida albicans* infection in the gastrointestinal tract; UTI due to *C. albicans* has been described, but is a very uncommon lower urinary tract disorder [37,39].

Lipocalin-2 has been shown to bind to a subset of iron chelators (siderophores) secreted by bacteria to obtain iron from the host [40]. The ability of siderophores to salvage host iron permits UPEC to grow in urine [41]. Sequestration of iron by siderophores is also required for UPEC to establish intracellular bacterial communities (IBC) in bladder urothelial cells. These IBCs have been associated with recurrent UTIs [42]. An IL22-mediated increase in lipocalin-2 expression would be expected to oppose bacterial salvage of host iron and thus inhibit UPEC growth in urine, UPEC invasion of HUCs, establishment of IBCs within HUCs, and recurrent UTIs.

In the absence of its subunit S100A8, S100A9 forms homodimers that can bind calcium. By sequestering calcium, S100A9 could control host-bacterial interactions that depend on calcium. S100A9 homodimers also interact with TLR4 to mediate an inflammatory response [43]. It is possible that, by modulating the expression of S100A9, IL22 could mediate an anti-inflammatory response through TLR4 in the HUC population that does not express the TLR4 co-receptor CD14.

Normal human bladder tissue is known to express both S100A9 and lipocalin-2; in bladder cancer, expression of both increases [44]. However, how their expression is regulated in health and diseases is not well understood; we provided the first direct evidence showing that IL22 regulates the expression of lipocalin-2 and S100A9 in primary HUCs express.

We also evaluated possible functions of IL22 in the physiopathology of lower urinary tract disorders. Bladder urothelium has recently been identified as a contributing factor in the development of overactive bladder. Increased release of acetylcholine by urothelium coupled with expression of muscarinic receptors by urothelial cells establishes a potential autocrine pathway [9]. It has been reported that human urothelial cells express CarAT, but not ChAT [6–8]. Indeed, our cultured HUCs expressed CarAT, but not ChAT. Furthermore, our cultured HUCs predominantly expressed MR1. We showed that IL22 potently inhibits MR1 expression, while only moderately increasing CarAT expression. IL22 could serve as a regulatory cytokine that contributes to the physiopathology of overactive bladder by modulating the acetylcholine response through inhibition MR1 expression. Whether IL22 also mediates a similar response in detrusor muscle cells remains to be determined.

While the cellular sources of IL22 in the human bladder have yet to be identified, it is known in other tissues that T cells and various innate cell types produce IL22 [24]. It is possible that HUCs can recruit these cells into the bladder submucosa and into urothelium itself. The high level of expression of the chemokine CCL20 by HUCs supports this notion. Indeed, we have preliminary TEM data showing that cells with lymphocyte morphology are present within the basal layer of urothelium (unpublished observation). Furthermore, HUCs also express IL7, IL15 and IL23, cytokines required for IL22-producing cell survival and expression of IL22.

Materials and Methods

Human Urothelial Cell Culture

The project was fully reviewed and approved by the Institutional review Board (RRB) for the protection of human subjects (Loyola University Health Science Division). Following IRB approval, and after written informed consent, a cystoscopically-directed biopsy was taken at the completion of reconstructive surgery in consenting adult women. The tissue was placed in saline and immediately transported to the laboratory. Bladder biopsy was transferred into culture media and incubated at 37°C for 2 hours to loosen the lamina propria. The culture media consists of a 3:1 DMEM:Ham's F12 medium with 5% FCS, 5.5 μg/mL (Life Technology), bovine insulin (Sigma-Aldrich), 0.4 μg/mL hydrocortisone (Invitrogen), 9.0 ng/mL cholera toxin (Sigma-Aldrich), 0.3% adenine hydrochloride, 1 mM sodium pyruvate, 10 ng/ml epidermal growth factor, 2.5 μg/ml amphotericin B, and 55 ng/ml gentamicin sulfate (Invitrogen). The urothelium layer was then separated from the lamina propria under dissecting microscope, cut into 1×1 cm^2 fragments; the fragments were then anchored under coverslips to propagate HUCs. Tissue explants were removed after 1–2 weeks in culture and the proliferating cells were allowed to expand. The cells were then used or passage once and then used for experiments.

Flow Cytometric Analysis

Harvested cells were washed once in RPMI-1640 media containing 2% FBS and $2–3\times10^5$ cells were stained with a cocktail of fluorochrome-conjugated monoclonal antibodies for flow cytometric analysis using BD LSRFostessa; flow cytometric data were analyzed using Flowjo 7.5.5 (Treestar). All antibodies and their optimal dilutions were listed in Table 2.

Transmission Electron Microscopy

Culture cells or bladder tissues were fixed in 4% glutaraldehyde in 0.1 M cacodylate buffer and then stained with 1% osmium in 0.1 M cacodylate buffer. Prepared cells or tissues were embedded in resin block, sectioned and analyzed using Hitachi- H600, 75 KV transmission electron microscope.

Immunofluorescence assay

Briefly, 10^4 primary HUCs in cultured medium were seeded into 24 well plates containing glass coverslips pre-treated with bovine plasma fibronectin (Sigma-Aldrich) and incubated at 37°C and 5% CO^2 overnight. HUCs were then fixed in 3.7% formaldehyde in 0.1 M piperazine-N, N'bis (2-ethanesulfonic acid) PIPES buffer, pH 6.8 for 20 minutes at 4°C. Cells were then blocked and permeabilized with a blocking solution (10% normal goat serum, 0.1% triton X-100 in PBS) for 1 hour at room temperature and then stained with a mouse anti-human cytokeratin 20 (Abcam) and rabbit anti-bovine uroplakins (a gift from Dr. Tung-Tien Sun, NYU). After washing, cells were stained with a cocktail of goat anti-mouse IgG-FITC and donkey and donkey anti-rabbit IgG-PE (InVitrogen). To label actin, cells were stained with Cy5-labeled phalloidin at 1:300 dilution in PBS for 30 minutes. Coverslips were then mounted onto glass slides with ProLong Gold Antifade containing DAPI (Invitrogen). Cells were examined using an epifluorescent DeltaVision microscope (Applied Precision) with a 60X objective lens and images were deconvolved with SoftWoRx software (Applied Precision).

Quantitative RT-PCR

Total RNA was isolated using Trizol reagent (Sigma, Aldrich) according to manufacturer's protocol. Isolated RNA was then treated with DNase using Ambion DNA-free kit and 0.5–2 μg of RNA was used for cDNA synthesis using the Invitrogen's SuperScript II synthesis kit. Quantitative RT-PCR was performed on an Applied Biosystems 7100 as we have previously described [45]. Sequences for the primers are presented in Table 3; all are

Table 2. Antibodies Used in the Study.

Monoclonal antibodies	Clone	Sources	Dilutions
Anti-HLA ABC-PE	W6/32	eBioscience/Affymatrix	1:5#
Anti-HLA DR-eF450	LN3	eBioscience/Affymatrix	1:10
Anti-CD14-AF700	M5E2	Biolegends	1:5
Anti-CD44-APC-eF780	IM7	eBioscience/Affymatrix	1:40
Anti-CD54-FITC	HCD54	Biolegends	1:5
Anti-CD284 (TLR4)-PE-Cy7	HTA125	eBioscience/Affymatrix	1:5
Anti-CD104-eF660	439-98	eBioscience/Affymatrix	1:10
Anti-CD326 (EpCam)-PerCp-eF710	1B7	eBioscience/Affymatrix	1:10

#A volume of 5 μL of the indicated dilution was used.

selected using Primer Express software (Aplied Biosystems). Samples were normalized to the housekeeping gene *Gapdh*. Levels of transcript were extrapolated from a standard curve constructed with five known concentrations ranging from 10 copies/μl to 100,000 copies/μl. Data were expressed as number of copies/μg RNA.

UPEC growth conditions

E. coli cystitis isolate NU14 and its isogenic *fimH* mutant NU14-1 [46] were grown under conditions known to induce type 1 piliation, namely serial subculture in static Luria Bertani broth for a total of 48 h at 37°C [47,48]. Expression of type I pili by NU14, but not NU14-1, was confirmed by mannose-sensitive agglutination of 1% yeast in PBS [49].

UPEC adherence assay

Bacterial adherence assays were performed, as previously described with modification [19]. Briefly, 10^4 primary urothelial cells in TE medium were seeded into 24 well plates containing glass coverslips pre-treated with bovine plasma fibronectin (Sigma-Aldrich) and incubated at 37°C and 5% CO^2 overnight. Prior to infection, the culture media was replaced with a medium consisting of RPMI, 5% FBS and Ham's F-12. In duplicate wells, 10^5 bacteria (NU14 or NU14-1) were added per well and the plate was centrifuged at 1400 rpm for 5 min to initiate bacteria contact with host cells. After 2 h of incubation at 37°C, the wells were washed five times with PBS to remove non-adherent bacteria and fixed in 3.7% formaldehyde in 0.1 M piperazine-N, N'bis (2-ethanesulfonic acid) PIPES buffer, pH 6.8 for 20 minutes at 4°C. Cells were blocked and permeabilized with block solution (10% normal goat serum, 0.1% triton X-100 in PBS) for 1 hour. The bacteria were stained with rabbit anti-*E. coli* antibodies (AbCam) followed by goat anti-rabbit Alexa Fluor 546 (Invitrogen) both diluted 1:200 in block solution and incubated at 4°C for 1 h each. To label host actin, cells were stained with Cy5-labeled phalloidin at 1:300 dilution in PBS for 30 minutes. Coverslips were then mounted onto glass slides with ProLong Gold Antifade containing DAPI (Invitrogen). Cells were examined using a DeltaVision microscope (Applied Precision) with a 60X objective lens and images were deconvolved with SoftWoRx software (Applied

Table 3. Primer Sequences.

Genes	Forward	Reverse	Reference
GAPDH	GCACCGTCAAGGCTGAGAAC	CTTGTCATCAATGGAAATCCCATCACCATC	NM_008238.1
CarAT	GGACACAGTCAGCAACTTCAGC	CGGTTCACCTTGTCTTTGATGA	NM_000755.3
MR1	CGAAGTGGTGATCAAGATGCC	TGTTGTACGGTGTCCAGGTGA	NM_000738
MR2	CGACAGGTTGTTAGCGACATGA	TGTTCCCGATAATGGTCACCA	NM_000739
IL7	CAGACCAAGCGCAAAGTAGAAA	CGTAGTCATGATGACCGCAACT	GI:186363
IL15	CTTGCCATAGCCAGCTCTTCTT	CTGCACAAATCTATGGTTCCCA	GI:71680273
IL23p19	AGCTGTAATGCTGCTGTTGCTG	GGATCCTTTGCAAGCAGAACTG	GI:45768274
CCL20	TGTCAGTGCTGCTACTCCACCT	TCCATTCCAGAAAAGCCACAG	GI:18088856
IL22RA1	GCATGGAAGGTTCTGGCAA	AGGTACTGTGGTGTCCCTTCCT	NM_021258.3
IL22RA2	CAGTCAACGCATGAGTCTCTGA	CCTCCCGTAATAAGGTTCCTGT	NM_181309.1
S100A8	GGCCAAGCCTAACCGCTATAA	GACGTCTGCACCCTTTTTCCT	NM_002964.4
S100A9	GTGCAAGACGATGACTTGCAA	CAGCATGATGAACTCCTCGAAG	NM_002965.3
Lipocalin-2	CTGGATCAGGACTTTTGTTCCA	GGAAGACGATGTGGTTTTCAGG	NM_005564.3
RegIIIγ	CCTCCTCAAGTCGCAGACACTA	GCACAGACACCAGTTTTCCAGA	NM_001008387.2

Precision). To quantify the number of urothelial cells with adherent bacteria, at least 200 urothelial cells were scored for the presence or absence of adherent bacteria. The percentage of urothelial cells with adherent UPEC was calculated by dividing the number of urothelial cells with bacteria by the total number of urothelial cells examined.

Acknowledgments

We would like to thank Pat Simms at the FACS Core for her excellent technical skill in performing flow cytometric analysis, Linda Fox at Image Core for the TEM study and Mary Tulke RN for all her hard work in facilitating the recruitment of patients for bladder biopsy samples. We also like to thank Dr. David Klumpp at Northwestern University for the UPEC NU 14 and NU 14-1 and Dr. Tun-Tien Sun at NYU for the anti-uroplakin antibody.

Author Contributions

Conceived and designed the experiments: PTL SZ MMP EMC AJW. Performed the experiments: SZ MMP. Analyzed the data: SZ MMP EMC PTL. Contributed reagents/materials/analysis tools: CSF ERM LB CAB EMC. Contributed to the writing of the manuscript: PTL MMP AJW LB.

References

1. Birder LA (2005) More than just a barrier: Urothelium as a drug target for urinary bladder pain. Am J Physiol Renal Physiol 289: F489–95.
2. Tu L, Sun T-T, Kreibich G (2000) Specific heterodimer formation is a prerequisite for uroplakins to exit from the endoplasmic reticulum. Mol Biol Cell: 13: 4221–30.
3. Wu X, Kong XP, Pellicer A, Kreibich G, Sun T-T (2009) Uroplakins in urothelial biology, function, and disease. Kidney Int.: 75: 1153–65.
4. Truschel ST, Ruiz WG, Shulman T, Pilewski J, Sun TT, et al. (1999) Primary uroepithelial cultures. A model system to analyze umbrella cell barrier function. J Biol Chem 274: 15020–15029.
5. Yoshida M, Inadome A, Maeda Y, Satoji Y, Masunaga K, et al. (2006) Non-neuronal cholinergic system in human bladder urothelium. Urology 67: 425–430.
6. Lips KS, Wunsch J, Zarghooni S, Bschleipfer T, Schukowski K, et al. (2007) Acetylcholine and molecular components of its synthesis and release machinery in the urothelium. Eur Urol 51: 1042–1053.
7. Ishii M, Kurachi Y (2006) Muscarinic acetylcholine receptors. Curr Pharm Des 12: 3573–3581.
8. Bschleipfer T, Schukowski K, Weidner W, Grando SA, Schwantes U, et al. (2007) Expression and distribution of cholinergic receptors in the human urothelium. Life Sci 80: 2303–2307.
9. de Groat WC (2006) Integrative control of the lower urinary tract: Preclinical perspective. Br J Pharmacol 147: S25–40.
10. Wolfe AJ, Toh E, Shibata N, Rong R, Kenton K, et al. (2012) Evidence of uncultivated bacteria in the adult female bladder. J Clin Microbiol 50: 1376–1383.
11. Hilt EE, McKinley K, Pearce MM, Rosenfeld AB, Zilliox MJ, et al. (2014) Urine is not sterile: Use of enhanced urine culture techniques to detect resident bacterial flora in the adult female bladder. J Clin Microbiol 52: 871–876.
12. Pearce MM, Hilt EE, Rosenfeld AB, Zilliox MJ, Thomas-White K, et al. (2014) The female urinary microbiome: A comparison of women with and without urgency urinary Incontinence. mBio: 5(4): e01283–14.
13. Edwards LA, Nistala K, Mills DC, Stephenson HN, Zilbauer M, et al. (2010) Delineation of the innate and adaptive T-cell immune outcome in the human host in response to campylobacter jejuni infection. PLoS One 5: e15398.
14. Rahman A, Fahlgren A, Sundstedt C, Hammarstrom S, Danielsson A, et al. (2011) Chronic colitis induces expression of beta-defensins in murine intestinal epithelial cells. Clin Exp Immunol 163: 123–130.
15. Fahlgren A, Hammarstrom S, Danielsson A, Hammarstrom ML (2004) Beta-defensin-3 and -4 in intestinal epithelial cells display increased mRNA expression in ulcerative colitis. Clin Exp Immunol 137: 379–385.
16. Sanos SL, Vonarbourg C, Mortha A, Diefenbach A (2011) Control of epithelial cell function by interleukin-22-producing RORgammat+ innate lymphoid cells. Immunology 132: 453–465.
17. Sanos SL, Bui VL, Mortha A, Oberle K, Heners C, et al. (2009) RORgammat and commensal microflora are required for the differentiation of mucosal interleukin 22-producing NKp46+ cells. Nat Immunol 10: 83–91.
18. Beaudette-Zlatanova BC, Knight KL, Zhang S, Stiff PJ, Zuniga-Pflucker JC, et al. (2011) A human thymic epithelial cell culture system for the promotion of lymphopoiesis from hematopoietic stem cells. Exp Hematol 39: 570–579.
19. Martinez JJ, Mulvey MA, Schilling JD, Pinkner JS, Hultgren SJ (2000) Type 1 pilus-mediated bacterial invasion of bladder epithelial cells. EMBO J 19: 2803–2812.
20. Zhou G, Mo WJ, Sebbel P, Min G, Neubert TA, et al. (2001) Uroplakin ia is the urothelial receptor for uropathogenic escherichia coli: Evidence from in vitro FimH binding. J Cell Sci 114: 4095–4103.
21. Xie B, Zhou G, Chan S, Shapiro E, Kong XP, et al. (2006) Distinct glycan structures of uroplakins Ia and Ib: Structural basis for the selective binding of FimH adhesin to uroplakin Ia. J Biol Chem.: 281(21): 14644–53.
22. Guimond M, Fry TJ, Mackall CL (2005) Cytokine signals in T-cell homeostasis. J Immunother 28: 289–294.
23. Schutyser E, Struyf S, Van Damme J (2003) The CC chemokine CCL20 and its receptor CCR6. Cytokine Growth Factor Rev 14: 409–426.
24. Wolk K, Witte E, Witte K, Warszawska K, Sabat R (2010) Biology of interleukin-22. Semin Immunopathol 32: 17–31.
25. Hutton KA, Trejdosiewicz LK, Thomas DF, Southgate J (1993) Urothelial tissue culture for bladder reconstruction: An experimental study. J Urol 150: 721–725.
26. Southgate J, Hutton KA, Thomas DF, Trejdosiewicz LK (1994) Normal human urothelial cells in vitro: Proliferation and induction of stratification. Lab Invest 71: 583–594.
27. Veranic P, Romih R, Jezernik K (2004) What determines differentiation of urothelial umbrella cells? Eur J Cell Biol 83: 27–34.
28. Spinardi L, Rietdorf J, Nitsch L, Bono M, Tacchetti C, et al. (2004) A dynamic podosome-like structure of epithelial cells. Exp Cell Res 295: 360–374.
29. Trzpis M, McLaughlin PM, Popa ER, Terpstra P, van Kooten TG, et al. (2008) EpCAM homologues exhibit epithelial-specific but different expression patterns in the kidney. Transgenic Res 17: 229–238.
30. Trzpis M, McLaughlin PM, de Leij LM, Harmsen MC (2007) Epithelial cell adhesion molecule: More than a carcinoma marker and adhesion molecule. Am J Pathol 171: 386–395.
31. Green M, Filippou A, Sant G, Theoharides TC (2004) Expression of intercellular adhesion molecules in the bladder of patients with interstitial cystitis. Urology 63: 688–693.
32. Liu AY, Vencio RZ, Page LS, Ho ME, Loprieno MA, et al. (2012) Bladder expression of CD cell surface antigens and cell-type-specific transcriptomes. Cell Tissue Res 348: 589–600.
33. Southgate J, Trejdosiewicz LK, Smith B, Selby PJ (1995) Patterns of splice variant CD44 expression by normal human urothelium in situ and in vitro and by bladder-carcinoma cell lines. Int J Cancer 62: 449–456.
34. Rouschop KM, Sylva M, Teske GJ, Hoedemaeker I, Pals ST, et al. (2006) Urothelial CD44 facilitates escherichia coli infection of the murine urinary tract. J Immunol 177: 7225–7232.
35. De Vita D, Giordano S (2012) Effectiveness of intravesical hyaluronic acid/ chondroitin sulfate in recurrent bacterial cystitis: A randomized study. Int Urogynecol J Pelvic Floor Dysfunct. 23: 1707–1713.
36. De Vita D, Antell H, Giordano S (2013) Effectiveness of intravesical hyaluronic acid with or without chondroitin sulfate for recurrent bacterial cystitis in adult women: A meta-analysis. Int Urogynecol J Pelvic Floor Dysfunct 24: 545–552. via the Internet. 20130325.
37. Zelante T, Iannitti RG, Cunha C, De Luca A, Giovannini G, et al. (2013) Tryptophan catabolites from microbiota engage aryl hydrocarbon receptor and balance mucosal reactivity via interleukin-22. Immunity 39: 372–385.
38. Liu JZ, Pezeshki M, Raffatellu M (2009) Th17 cytokines and host-pathogen interactions at the mucosa: Dichotomies of help and harm. Cytokine 48: 156–160.
39. Fisher JF, Kavanagh K, Sobel JD, Kauffman CA, Newman CA (2011) Candida urinary tract infection: Pathogenesis. Clin Infect Dis 52 Suppl 6: S437–51.
40. Flo TH, Smith KD, Sato S, Rodriguez DJ, Holmes MA, et al. (2004) Lipocalin 2 mediates an innate immune response to bacterial infection by sequestrating iron. Nature 432: 917–921.
41. Zhang JP, Normark S (1996) Induction of gene expression in escherichia coli after pilus-mediated adherence. Science 273: 1234–1236.
42. Reigstad CS, Hultgren SJ, Gordon JI (2007) Functional genomic studies of uropathogenic escherichia coli and host urothelial cells when intracellular bacterial communities are assembled. J Biol Chem 282: 21259–21267.
43. Tsai SY, Segovia JA, Chang TH, Morris IR, Berton MT, et al. (2014) DAMP molecule S100A9 acts as a molecular pattern to enhance inflammation during influenza A virus infection: Role of DDX21-TRIF-TLR4-MyD88 pathway. PLoS Pathog 10: e1003848.
44. Dokun OY, Florl AR, Seifert HH, Wolff I, Schulz WA (2008) Relationship of SNCG, S100A4, S100A9 and LCN2 gene expression and DNA methylation in bladder cancer. Int J Cancer 123: 2798–2807.

45. Zook EC, Zhang S, Gerstein RM, Witte PL, Le PT (2013) Enhancing T lineage production in aged mice: A novel function of Foxn1 in the bone marrow niche. J. of Immunol 191: 5583–5589.
46. Langermann S, Palaszynski S, Barnhart M, Auguste G, Pinkner JS, et al. (1997) Prevention of mucosal escherichia coli infection by FimH-adhesin-based systemic vaccination. Science 276: 607–611.
47. Berry RE, Klumpp DJ, Schaeffer AJ (2009) Urothelial cultures support intracellular bacterial community formation by uropathogenic escherichia coli. Infect Immun 77: 2762–2772.
48. Hultgren SJ, Schwan WR, Schaeffer AJ, Duncan JL (1986) Regulation of production of type 1 pili among urinary tract isolates of escherichia coli. Infect Immun 54: 613–620.
49. Eshdat Y, Speth V, Jann K (1981) Participation of pili and cell wall adhesion in the yeast agglutination activity of escherichia coli. Infect Immun 34: 980–986.

14

A Non-Invasive Laboratory Panel as a Diagnostic and Prognostic Biomarker for Thrombotic Microangiopathy: Development and Application in a Chinese Cohort Study

Tao Zhang[1], Huimei Chen[1,2]*, Shaoshan Liang[1], Dacheng Chen[1], Chunxia Zheng[1], Caihong Zeng[1], Haitao Zhang[1], Zhihong Liu[1]*

1 National Clinical Research Center of Kidney Diseases, Jinling Hospital, Nanjing University School of Medicine, Nanjing 210002, P. R. China, **2** Jiangsu Key Laboratory of Molecular Medicine, Nanjing University School of Medicine, Nanjing, 210093, P. R. China

Abstract

Background: Thrombotic microangiopathy (TMA) in the kidney is a histopathologic lesion that occurs in a number of clinical settings and is often associated with poor renal prognosis. The standard test for the diagnosis of TMA is the renal biopsy; noninvasive parameters such as potential biomarkers have not been developed.

Methods: We analyzed routine parameters in a cohort of 220 patients with suspected TMA and developed a diagnostic laboratory panel by logistic regression. The levels of candidate markers were validated using an independent cohort (n = 46), a cohort of systemic lupus erythematosus (SLE) (n = 157) and an expanded cohort (n = 113), as well as 9 patients with repeat biopsies.

Results: Of the 220 patients in the derivation cohort, 51 patients with biopsy-proven TMA presented with a worse renal prognosis than those with no TMA (P = 0.002). Platelet and L-lactate dehydrogenase (LDH) levels showed an acceptable diagnostic value of TMA (AUC = 0.739 and 0.756, respectively). A panel of 4 variables - creatinine, platelets, ADAMTS13 (a disintegrin and metalloprotease with thrombospondin type 1 repeats 13) activity and LDH - can effectively discriminate patients with TMA (AUC = 0.800). In the validation cohort, the platelet and LDH levels and the 4-variable panel signature robustly distinguished patients with TMA. The discrimination effects of these three markers were confirmed in patients with SLE. Moreover, LDH levels and the 4-variable panel signature also showed discrimination values in an expanded set. Among patients undergoing repeat biopsy, increased LDH levels and panel signatures were associated with TMA status when paired evaluations were performed. Importantly, only the 4-variable panel was an independent prognostic marker for renal outcome (hazard ratio = 3.549; P<0.001).

Conclusions: The noninvasive laboratory diagnostic panel is better for the early detection and prognosis of TMA compared with a single parameter, and may provide a promising biomarker for clinical application.

Editor: Nancy Lan Guo, West Virginia University, United States of America

Funding: This work was supported in part by National Basic Research Program of China 973 Program No.2012CB517600 (No.2012CB517606) (to Z.L.)(http://www.973.gov.cn/AreaMana.aspx), National Natural Science Foundation (NSF) Grant 81370788 (to H.C.) (http://www.nsfc.gov.cn/), The National Key Technology R&D Program (2011BAI10B04) (to Z.L.) (http://kjzc.jhgl.org/) and Six Talent Peaks Project of Jiangsu Province (2012-WSN-071) (to H.C.) (http://archives.nuist.edu.cn/rcgf/). The funders had no role in study design, data collection and analysis, decision to publish, or preparation of the manuscript.

* Email: chenhuimei@nju.edu.cn (HC); liuzhihong@nju.edu.cn (ZL)

Introduction

Thrombotic microangiopathy (TMA) is a pathological lesion that results in thrombosis in capillaries and arterioles, due to an endothelial injury [1–3]. TMA lesions in the kidney usually present in two different forms with considerable overlap: (1) glomerular involvement with capillary thrombi, capillary loops with double contours and mesangiolysis with microhemorrhage, that is most frequently seen in patients with hemolytic uremic syndrome; or (2) predominant arteriolar involvement with thrombi and fibrinoid necrosis, particularly in thrombotic thrombocytopenic purpura and malignant hypertension [4,5].

TMA lesions occur in a number of other kidney diseases as well, including IgA nephropathy, systemic lupus erythematosus (SLE), antiphospholipid antibody syndrome, systemic sclerosis, pre-eclampsia, infections, medications and post transplantation [2,6,7]. The presence of TMA in the kidney has been proven to be associated with poor renal prognosis [8,9]. Nephrologists often face a typical situation in which patients are suspected of having TMA lesions on the basis of renal disorders. In such cases, it is difficult to decide on an early therapy before the results of a renal biopsy are obtained [10]. While the interpretation of the renal biopsy has become more standardized and the invasive procedure safer over time, bleeding and subsequent functional impairment nevertheless still occur, especially in the patients with coagulopathy [11].

Heterogeneous disorders with TMA are usually characterized by microangiopathic hemolytic anemia (MAHA) [12], thrombocytopenia and/or ischemic organ failure. It is questionable as to whether these abnormalities can predict TMA, since they are also observed in patients without TMA, and studies have been inconsistent [13,14]. Hence, we enrolled cohorts of patients with renal damage and MAHA and/or thrombocytopenia to determine whether a single parameter or a diagnostic panel could predict the histological TMA. In addition, the association between the noninvasive prediction and a poor renal outcome was further investigated.

Methods

Ethics statement

The study was approved by the Ethics Committee of Jinling Hospital. Because this study was retrospective, the Ethics Committee agreed to waive the requirement for the informed consent, and the data were analyzed anonymously.

Patient selection and study design

We enrolled a cohort of suspected patients from the Research Institute of Nephrology, Jinling Hospital, Nanjing University School of Medicine, PR China during July 2011 to July 2012 (n = 266). The enrollment criteria were: renal damage (proteinuria, hematuria or renal dysfunction) and microangiopathic hemolytic anemia (hemoglobin level below 120 g/L for males, 110 g/L for females, at least 5 schistocytes per high power field in a peripheral blood smear, elevated LDH above 240 u/L [normal 60–240 u/L]) or thrombocytopenia (platelet counts below 100×10^9/L of blood at any time in the course of the disease) [15]. Patients were randomly divided into two cohorts: (1) derivation cohort (n = 220) and (2) validation cohort (n = 46).

In addition, 157 patients diagnosed with SLE were selected from the suspected patients, and 113 patients were enrolled in an expanded group for external validation. SLE was defined according to the 1997 American College of Rheumatology revised criteria for SLE [16]. The independent patients were enrolled in the expanded group according to the criteria: (1) renal damage (proteinuria, hematuria or renal dysfunction) and (2) fever (temperature of >38°C, no infection), elevated LDH (more than 240 u/L) or non-renal anemia. The information and profiles of patients during the follow-up sessions were also reviewed through October 2013.

Definitions

TMA in the kidney was defined by the histologic feature of occlusive fibrin-platelet thrombi in at least one glomerulus or one arteriole, with one or more of the following: (1) glomerular endothelial swelling and detachment, capillary wall thickening and double contour formation, mesangial lysis with microhemorrhage, and erythrocytolysis, and/or (2) obliterative arteriolopathy defined as luminal occlusion with mural myxoid or fibrinoid change, thickening of the vessel wall, with or without erythrocytolysis, luminal thrombosis and concentric spindle cell proliferation or hypercellularity [2,5].

All patients accepted adjunctive treatments, including protecting the organ function, symptomatic and immunosuppressive treatment. Glomerularfiltration rate was estimated (eGFR) using the simplified MDRD (Modification of Diet in Renal Disease) formula. End stage renal disease (ESRD) was defined as eGFR< 15 mL/min/1.73 m^2 or a need for permanent dialysis therapy. During follow-up, the combined event defined as ESRD or a doubling of the serum creatinine level and death. The renal survival rate was defined as the percentage of patients who had preservation of renal function independent of ESRD and death, while the survival rate was defined as the percentage of live patients.

Laboratory features

Physical exams and routine laboratory tests were performed on the suspected patients. Serum ADAMTS13 activity was measured by the Fluorescence Resonance Energy Transfer (FRET) assay (United States Patent No.7270976) [17]. Serum anti-ADAMTS13 IgG antibodies (Sekisui Diagnostics, USA), vWF (von Willebrand factor) (Sunbiote, Shanghai, China), thrombomodulin (Diaclone Research, Besancon, France), E-selectin (R&D Systems, Minneapolis, Minnesota, USA) and soluble vascular cellular adhesion molecule-1 (sVCAM-1, VCAM) (R&D Systems, Minneapolis, Minnesota, USA) were measured using enzyme linked immunosorbent assays. The concentrations of endothelial cells in the circulation were sorted using a magnetic microbead sorting system (MACS, Miltenyi Biotec, Germany), according to the manufacturer's instructions [18].

Statistical analysis

All data were given a numerical code and statistical analysis was performed using SPSS software, version 19.0 or RMS software, version 2.12.2. Comparisons of proportions or mean values between patients with or without TMA in the kidney were calculated by the Mann-Whitney test or chi-square ($\chi2$) test.

Logistic regression was used to identify 6 parameters - hemoglobin, platelets, serum creatinine, LDH, ADAMTS13 activity and THBD - that discriminated between patients with and without TMA in the kidney. Regression estimated from this panel defined a diagnostic signature or individual predictors, and the greatest area under the receiver-operating-characteristic (ROC) curve as the best-fitting model was used. The area under the curve (AUC) was calculated, and sensitivity and specificity were used to evaluate the ability of these to discriminate TMA in the kidney. The best sub-set panel was then fit to 1000 additional bootstrap samples. Cross-validated measures of discrimination (i.e., the AUC), model fit (i.e., calibration-curve intercept and slope) and a locally estimated scatterplot-smoothed (loess) calibration plot were obtained [19].

Cumulative incidence of poor renal outcome was calculated using Kaplan-Meier survival probabilities (1- survival probabilities) and comparisons were made using the log-rank test. Cox regression was performed to test the association of the pathologic findings and the 4-variable panel signature with the renal outcome. A two-tailed P value less than 0.05 is considered to be statistically significant.

Results

In the derivation cohort of 220 patients, 51 (23.2%) patients were histologically proven to have TMA by renal biopsy. Compared with patients without TMA, the patients with TMA presented a worse renal outcome (P = 0.002, log-rank test; Figure 1) at the 12-month follow-up, with a renal survival rate of 54.9% (P = 0.015; Table 1).

Correlation between laboratory parameters and TMA lesions

The levels of serum creatinine, LDH and thrombomodulin (THBD) were significantly higher in patients with TMA than those

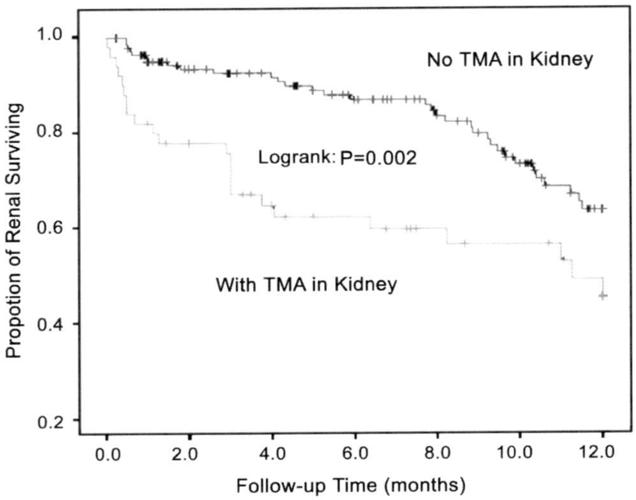

Figure 1. Comparison of renal outcome in suspected patients. After 12 months of follow-up, the patients with TMA had a worse outcome of renal survival than those without TMA (Log rank: P = 0.002).

without TMA, while levels of hemoglobin, platelets and ADAMTS13 activity were remarkably lower (all $P<0.05$; Table 1). With a cutoff of 0.05 (P value, in Table 1), 6 laboratory parameters were included in the next binary logistic regression analysis. The ROC curve showed that these 6 parameters individually can distinguish patients with TMA in the derivation set (all $P<0.05$; Figure 2A). Only the platelet and LDH levels showed acceptable discrimination values ($0.7 \leq AUC < 0.8$), while levels of hemoglobin, serum creatinine, ADAMSTS13 activity and THBD had low discrimination accuracy ($0.5 \leq AUC < 0.7$). With the use of the cutoff point of $97.5 \times 10^9/L$, platelets had 82.4% sensitivity and 60.9% specificity, and with the cutoff point of 289 u/L, LDH had 67.3% sensitivity and 74.1% specificity (Table S1 in File S1).

In an independent validation cohort, platelet and LDH levels also could discriminate patients with TMA from those without TMA (Figure 2B; Table S2 in File S1). Thus, the levels of platelets and LDH showed acceptable predictive probabilities of patients with TMA in the kidney.

Correlation between the 4-variable panel and TMA lesions

Furthermore, multiple logistic regression analysis in the derivation set indicated that levels of serum creatinine (SCr), platelets (PLT), LDH and ADAMTS13 activity were valid predictors of renal TMA lesions (all $P<0.05$; Table 2), with the final panel signature:

$$-0.371 - 0.002 \times \text{ADAMTS13activity}$$
$$+ 0.140 \times \text{SCr} + 0.004 \times \text{LDH} - 0.010 \times \text{PLT}$$

The units of measurement are as listed in Table 1. In the equation, −0.371 was the intercept, and −0.002, 0.140, 0.004 and −0.010 were the slopes (coefficients), respectively, for the ADAMTS13 activity, SCr (mg/dL), LDH and PLT values in the best-fitting logistic-regression model. The intercept and slopes have no intrinsic units of measurement.

The ROC curve showed that this 4-variable model yielded an AUC of 0.800 (95% confidence interval [CI], 0.723 to 0.877; $P< 0.001$), suggesting a good discrimination between patients with TMA in the kidney and those without TMA (Figure 3A). With the use of the cutoff point of 0.248, this diagnostic panel has 81.6% sensitivity and 66.9% specificity. The diagnostic panel for the prediction of TMA was validated in the independent cohort, with an AUC of 0.815 ($P<0.001$; Figure 3B). The use of the cut-off of 0.248 predicted the presence of TMA with 80.0% sensitivity and 61.5% specificity.

Bootstrap validation of this 4-variable panel yielded a cross-validated estimate of the AUC of 0.777, which is an estimate of the expected value of the AUC in the combined derivation and validation cohorts. The calibration-curve intercept and slope were 0.07 and 0.64, respectively. It was revealed that the predicted probabilities of a biopsy showing TMA in the kidney tended to be relatively higher than the actual probabilities (Figure 3C). The loess-smoothed estimates of the unadjusted and cross-validated calibration curves were overlaid on a diagonal reference line representing good model calibration ($P = 0.489$). The close correspondence of the two curves to the reference line shows good fit and reflects the above interpretation of the intercept and slope estimates of the calibration curve (Figure 3C).

Evaluation of LDH, platelet and the 4- variable panel in extra cohorts

Since renal TMA lesions occur in a number of kidney diseases, we focused on a specific condition and 157 renal patients diagnosed with SLE were selected in extra validation (Table S3 in File S1). All levels of platelets, LDH and the 4-variable panel could discriminate patients with TMA in SLE. The ability of discrimination in the 4-variable panel was higher than the levels of platelets and LDH, with an AUC of 0.872 (Figure 4A). With the use of the cutoff point of 0.248, the diagnostic panel has 74.1% sensitivity and 83.6% specificity.

To further enhance the application of these markers, we enrolled another independent group of 113 patients and determined the association between the levels of LDH, platelets and the 4-variable panel and TMA lesions (Table S4 in File S1). ROC curve analysis showed that the levels of LDH and the 4-variable panel yielded an AUC of 0.843 and 0.825, showing a good discrimination of TMA (both $P<0.001$; Figure 4B). However, platelet levels could not predict patients with TMA lesions in this cohort ($P = 0.068$).

Evaluation of LDH and the 4-variable panel in patients with repeat biopsy

We then analyzed, in a subset of 9 patients who underwent repeat renal biopsy, levels of LDH and the 4-variable panel in paired blood samples taken at the time of the first and second biopsy (Table S5 in File S1). It is interesting to note that the 4-variable panel signature plummeted from 0.248 or higher in the same subset of patients when they presented with TMA at the first biopsy, but with no TMA at second biopsy (Figure 5A). On the contrary, for the only patient who had no TMA at first biopsy but exhibited TMA at the second biopsy, the 4-variable panel dramatically increased to greater than 0.248. For the other 5 patients, the 4-variable signature was significantly decreased after treatment ($P = 0.030$), although they each presented without TMA at the two biopsies and the signature was 0.248 or less.

A similar pattern of LDH changes were observed in the patients with repeat biopsy, and increased LDH levels were associated with TMA status (Figure 5B). However, an LDH value of 289 u/L was

Table 1. Clinical laboratory data for suspected patients in derivation cohort (n = 220).

	TMA	No TMA	P Value
Number of patients	**51**	**169**	
Age (year)	26 (963)	28 (1370)	0.450
Male (n, %)	10 (19.6)	45 (26.6)	0.310
Clinical diagnosis			
HUS/TTP (n, %)	15 (29.4)	0 (0)	<0.001
Primary glomerulonephritis & acute interstitial nephritis (n, %)	0 (0)	22 (13.0)	0.003
Autoimmune diseases (n, %)	29 (56.9)	144 (85.2)	<0.001
SLE (n, %)	27/29 (93.1)	130/144 (90.3)	1.000
Pregnancy/postpartum (n, %)	5 (9.8)	1 (0.6)	0.003
Malignant hypertension (n, %)	1 (2.0)	0 (0)	0.232
Post-transplantation (n, %)	1 (2.0)	2 (1.2)	0.549
Laboratory profiles			
Urine protein (g/24 h)	1.5 (0.310.6)	2.5 (0.29.8)	0.073
Erythrocyturia ($\times 10^4$/mL)	18 (110000)	24 (19000)	0.364
Hemoglobin (g/L)	74.2±16.1	87.1±21.6	<0.001
Platelets ($\times 10^9$/L)	73 (10275)	108 (34441)	<0.001
Serum creatinine (umol/L)	347.2 (52.21697.5)	162.7 (33.61556.0)	<0.001
Globulin (g/L)	22.0±5.7	23.3±6.6	0.289
C3 (g/L)	0.62±0.29	0.57±0.30	0.219
C4 (g/L)	0.16±0.10	0.14±0.10	0.098
L-lactate dehydrogenase (u/L)	418 (1292920)	267 (64878)	<0.001
ADAMTS13 antibody (Au/mL)	16.6 (2.184.9)	16.6 (1.681.3)	0.862
ADAMTS13 activity (ng/mL)	616±331	772±255	0.001
NEC (/ml)	19.7±6.8	20.7±8.9	0.654
E-selectin (ng/mL)	65.2±37.3	73.1±72.8	0.636
VCAM (ng/mL)	2011±1070	2460±1340	0.073
Thrombomodulin (ng/mL)	6.3±4.3	4.4±2.8	<0.001
vWF (%)	184±127	215±120	0.080
After 12-months of follow up			
Renal survival rate (%)	54.9 (28/51)	74.6 (126/169)	0.015
Survival rate (%)	94.1 (48/51)	98.2 (166/169)	0.138

Values are expressed as medians (range), means ± standard deviation or percentages. *P* values were calculated by Mann-Whitney U test, Fisher's exact test or chi-square test as appropriate. HUS: hemolytic uremic syndrome; TTP: thrombotic thrombocytopenic purpura; SLE: systemic lupus erythematosus; C3: Complement component 3; C4: Complement component 4; ADAMTS13: A Disintegrin and Metalloprotease with ThromboSpondin type 1 repeats 13; NEC: normal endothelial cells; VCAM: vascular cell adhesion molecule; vWF: von Willebrand factor.

not a good cut-off level to discriminate TMA status in this group of patients.

Association of LDH levels and the 4-variable panel with renal survival

To further evaluate whether LDH levels and the 4-variable panel can serve as a predictor of renal survival in patients with suspected TMA, we performed a Kaplan-Meier survival analysis. As suspected, patients with a higher 4-variable panel signature had a statistically significant worse renal outcome ($P<0.001$, log-rank test; Figure 6A). However, the pattern of increased LDH concentrations was not associated with a poorer renal outcome ($P = 0.183$, log-rank test; Figure 6B).

Furthermore, the renal survival was only 53.9% in patients with a panel signature of more than 0.248, but was 79.5% in patients with a panel signature of less than 0.248. The Cox proportional hazard survival regression model revealed that TMA lesions increased the risk for a poor renal outcome, with a hazard ratio of 2.235 (95% CI 1.306 to 3.826, $P = 0.003$), while a panel signature 0.248 or greater had a hazard ratio of 3.549 (95% CI 2.034 to 3.549, $P<0.001$). These two diagnostic factors showed a similar predictive effect on renal outcome ($P = 0.964$).

Discussion

Histological TMA in the kidney has been frequently described in association with a large number of underlying diseases [20–22]. Although the causes of TMA in the kidney are unclear, it has been reported that there is a significantly worse renal outcome among patients with TMA [16,22]. Kaplan et al. [23] reported that death rates were as high as 25% and progression to ESRD occurred in half of the patients with TMA within 10 years after diagnosis. In agreement with published studies [24], we confirmed that patients

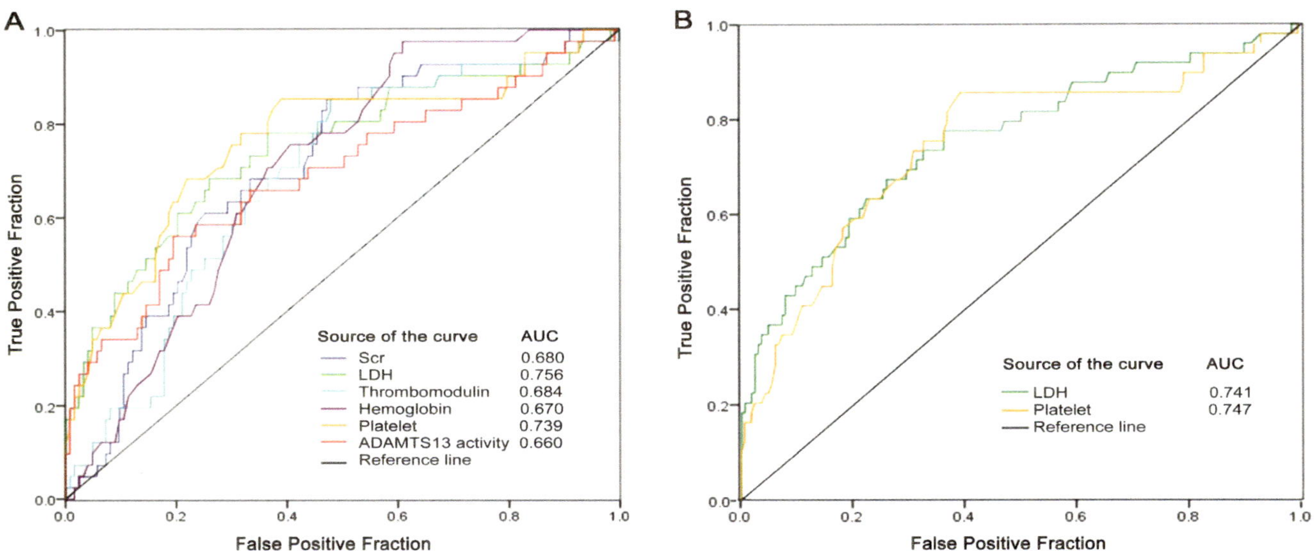

Figure 2. Receiver operating characteristic curves of laboratory parameters. (A) The fraction of true positive results (sensitivity) and the fraction of false positive results (1-specificity) for LDH, HGB, SCr, PLT, THBD and ADAMTS13 activity were developed in 220 patients (all $P \leq 0.001$), and the levels of platelet and LDH showed acceptable discrimination, with AUC 0.739 and 0.756, respectively. (B) The levels of platelet and LDH could discriminate patients with TMA from those with no TMA in the validation cohort (n = 46), with AUC 0.747 and 0.741, respectively.

with renal biopsy-proven TMA presented with a poor outcome in the kidney and the patients with TMA had a 2.24-fold higher risk of renal failure than those without TMA.

The renal biopsy represents the gold standard in the management of patients with TMA, but a noninvasive diagnostic method for detection of TMA would be a valuable clinical application. Few studies have focused on the prediction of the histopathologic lesions, although abnormalities in the urinalysis and an increase in serum creatinine have been observed in patients with TMA lesions [25]. In addition, reports have demonstrated that laboratory variables were involved in clinical conditions associated with TMA [26–28], including hemolytic uremic syndrome and thrombotic thrombocytopenic purpura. Increased levels of LDH are associated with the severity of hemolysis and tissue ischemia, which might increase the risk of tissue lesions [29]. A deficiency of ADAMTS13 was related to thrombus formation and was subsequently noted in patients with thrombocytopenic purpura, who often suffered from TMA lesions in the kidney [30,31].

This study is the first to demonstrate the potential of routine laboratory parameters to be used in the detection of TMA without renal biopsy. Six parameters - serum creatinine, platelets, hemoglobin, THBD, ADAMTS13 activity and LDH - had moderate diagnostic value for TMA. The strengths of this study are that we developed a diagnostic panel based on 4 laboratory variables (levels of serum creatinine, LDH, platelets and ADAMTS13 activity). This panel can noninvasively and accurately predict histological TMA. This is supported by the high AUC values of 0.800 derived from patients with and without TMA (sensitivity 81.6%; specificity 66.9%). Similar effects were noted when the predictive panel was validated using an independent population. The cross-validation further revealed that the 4-variable model tended to have high sensitivity, but a relatively low specificity. To the best of our knowledge, this is the first noninvasive biomarker that can detect TMA in the kidney. In addition, each individual parameter of the 5 or 6 variable model could not reach statistical significance ($P < 0.05$, data not shown). The model of fewer variables could discriminate patients with TMA in derivation cohort, including the levels of LDH and platelets, but this effect was not proven by all different validation cohorts.

The 3 markers, LDH, platelets and the 4-variable panel, were further evaluated in a group of patients with SLE and expanded sets of patients. SLE is often reported with TMA lesions in the kidney [6,22], and there were 157 patients diagnosed with SLE

Table 2. Results of logistic regression analysis (n = 220).

Variable	B	S.E	Sig.	Exp (B)	95% CI
					Lower-Upper
Serum creatinine	0.140	0.060	0.020	1.150	1.022–1.295
LDH	0.004	0.001	0.002	1.004	1.001–1.006
Platelet	−0.010	0.004	0.021	0.990	0.981–0.998
ADAMTS 13 Activity	−0.002	0.001	0.014	0.998	0.996–1.000

Abbreviations: B: coefficient of regression; S.E.: Standard Error; Sig: P value; Exp (B): odds ratio; CI: confidence interval. LDH: L-lactate dehydrogenase; ADAMTS 13: a disintegrin and metalloprotease with thrombospondin type 1 repeats 13.

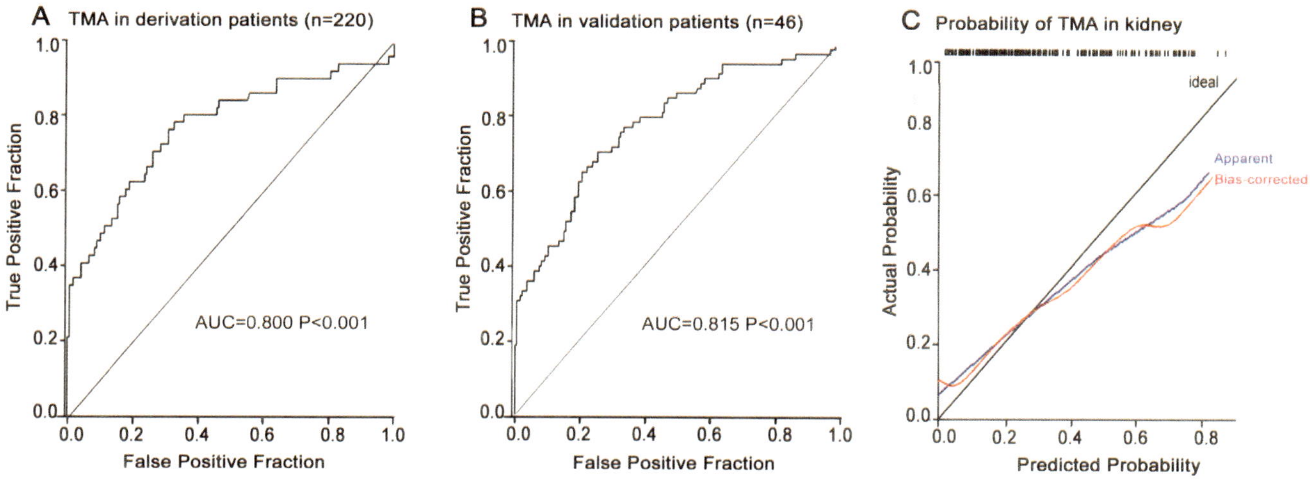

Figure 3. Receiver operating characteristic curves and calibration curve for a diagnostic panel. (A) The diagnostic panel was developed in the derivation group of 220 suspected patients, with AUC 0.800, P<0.001. (B) This marker was validated in 46 independent patients, with AUC 0.815, P<0.001. (C) Bootstrap validation shows the calibration curve of the diagnostic panel. Cross-validated estimates of the AUC, calibration-curve intercept and slope were 0.777, 0.07 and 0.64, respectively. The loess-smoothed estimates of the cross-validated and unadjusted calibration curves are overlaid on a diagonal reference line representing good model calibration.

among the suspected patients investigated. Focusing on one particular disease, all 3 markers showed discrimination values for patients with TMA. Because some patients with TMA exhibit little or no signs of clinical manifestations [31–33], we expanded the application of these markers. LDH levels and the 4-variable panel still demonstrated good discrimination, while platelets did not. Thus, LDH levels and the 4-variable panel might have wide usage in different cohorts of patients. In addition, data from patients with a repeat biopsy confirmed the association of increased LDH levels and the 4-variable signature with TMA status.

Another important finding of our study was that the 4-variable panel also serves as a prognostic biomarker for renal patients. The increased signature of the 4-variable panel was an independent prognostic parameter. The prognostic value of the 4-variable panel was similar with the histological diagnosis of TMA. As a noninvasive biomarker, the 4-variable panel showed an advantage in clinical application. However, LDH levels did not exhibit a prognostic value for renal outcome. Therefore, the 4-variable panel might not only diagnose TMA but also help predict renal

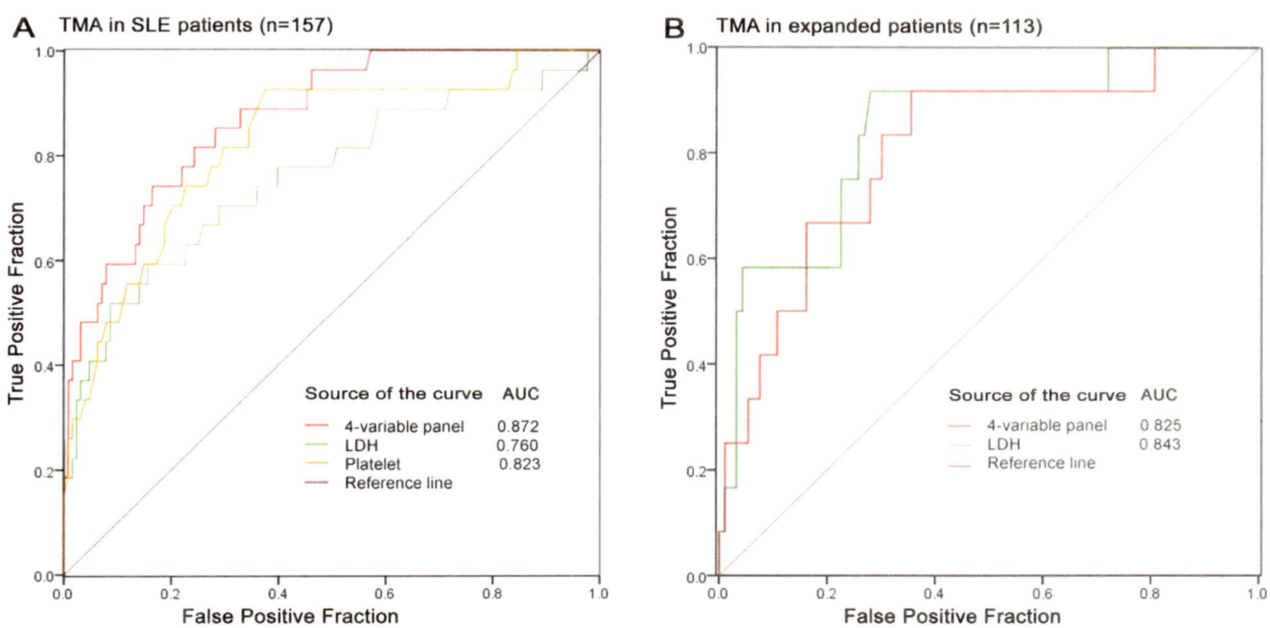

Figure 4. Evaluation of LDH, platelet and 4-variable panel in extra cohorts. (A) All levels of platelet, LDH and the 4-variable panel were evaluated in 157 suspected patients diagnosed with SLE and could discriminate patients with TMA, with an AUC of 0.823, 0.76 and 0.872, respectively. (B) To further validate in another independent group of 113 patients and ROC curve analysis showed that the levels of LDH and the 4-variable panel yielded an AUC of 0.843 and 0.825, showing an good discrimination of TMA (both P<0.001).

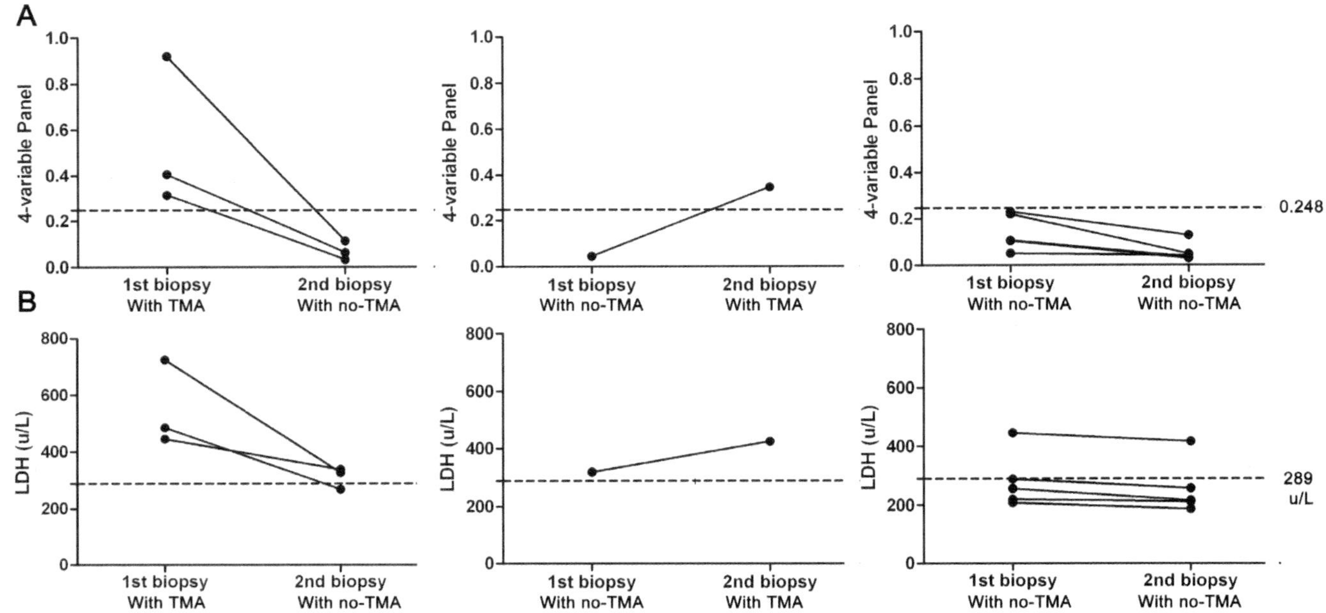

Figure 5. Evaluation of LDH and 4-variable panel in patients with repeat biopsy. (A)We analyzed paired first and second levels of LDH and 4-variable panel in a subset of 9 patients, who underwent repeat renal biopsy. The first figure shows 4-variable panel signature plummeted from 0.248 or greater in the same subset of patients, when three patients presented TMA at first biopsy but no TMA at second biopsy. In the second figure, only one patient had no TMA at first biopsy and TMA at second biopsy and 4-variable panel dramatically increased to 0.348. For other 5 patients, 4-variable signature was significantly decreased after treatment, although they consistently presented without TMA at two biopsies and the signature was 0.248 or less. (B) Similar pattern of LDH changes was observed in the patients with repeat biopsy, and increased LDH levels were associated with TMA status.

outcome with a higher accuracy than other single laboratory parameter.

Although our current assay may become a promising diagnostic tool for TMA, we acknowledge three potential limitations of this study. It is retrospective and will need to be validated with a prospective cohort of patients. Furthermore, the evaluation of prognosis was rendered difficult because of the variable nature of the treatments received. In addition, the number of patients with certain diseases was small and some validations were calculated using non-independent data, which prevented an in-depth

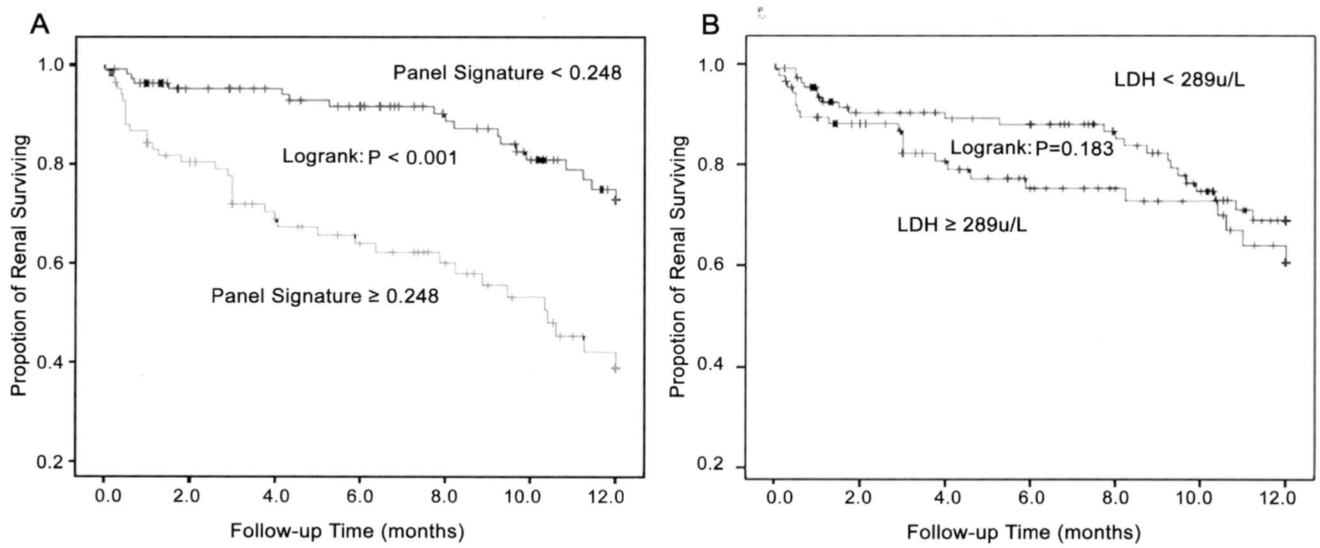

Figure 6. Association of LDH levels and 4-variable panel with renal survival. (A) Using the cutoff value of 0.248, suspected patients were divided into two groups by more or less than the value and the renal survival of two groups followed up 12 months was significantly different ($P < 0.001$). (B) The pattern of increased LDH concentrations (more than the cutoff point of 289 u/L) associated statistically poorer renal outcome was not observed ($P = 0.183$).

evaluation of the usefulness of the diagnostic panel for specifically predicting TMA in the kidney.

Conclusions

In conclusion, our results provide compelling evidence for the potential use of laboratory parameters as a noninvasive diagnostic and prognostic tool for TMA in the kidney. The 4-variable panel showed an advantage for the early detection of renal TMA lesions without renal biopsy and in directly predicting renal prognosis. In order for this concept to be incorporated into routine clinical practice in the near-future, validation is needed in large-scale prospective trials.

Supporting Information

File S1 Includes table S1–S5. **Table S1,** Diagnosis of TMA in kidney among patients (n = 220). **Table S2,** Laboratory variables in the validation group of internal patients (n = 46). **Table S3,** Clinical laboratory data for suspected patients with SLE (n = 157). **Table S4,** Clinical laboratory data for patients in expanded group (n = 113). **Table S5,** The laboratory feature of patients with/without TMA in the kidney at first renal biopsy and repeat biopsy.

Acknowledgments

We thank all the patients and their families who participated in this study.

Author Contributions

Conceived and designed the experiments: TZ HC ZL. Performed the experiments: TZ HC DC CZ SL CZ. Analyzed the data: TZ HC ZL. Contributed reagents/materials/analysis tools: DC SL HZ. Contributed to the writing of the manuscript: TZ HC ZL.

References

1. Moake JL (2002) Thrombotic microangiopathies. N Engl J Med 347: 589–600.
2. El Karoui K, Hill GS, Karras A, Jacquot C, Moulonguet L, et al. (2012) A clinicopathologic study of thrombotic microangiopathy in IgA nephropathy. J Am Soc Nephrol 23: 137–148.
3. Goldberg RJ, Nakagawa T, Johnson RJ, Thurman JM (2010) The role of endothelial cell injury in thrombotic microangiopathy. Am J Kidney Dis 56: 1168–1174.
4. van den Born BJ, van der Hoeven NV, Groot E, Lenting PJ, Meijers JC, et al. (2008) Association between thrombotic microangiopathy and reduced ADAMTS13 activity in malignant hypertension. Hypertension 51: 862–866.
5. Laurence J (2000) Pathological and therapeutic distinctions in HUS/TTP. Lancet 355: 497; author reply 497–498.
6. Hughson MD, Nadasdy T, McCarty GA, Sholer C, Min KW, et al. (1992) Renal thrombotic microangiopathy in patients with systemic lupus erythematosus and the antiphospholipid syndrome. Am J Kidney Dis 20: 150–158.
7. Eremina V, Jefferson JA, Kowalewska J, Hochster H, Haas M, et al. (2008) VEGF inhibition and renal thrombotic microangiopathy. N Engl J Med 358: 1129–1136.
8. Garg AX, Suri RS, Barrowman N, Rehman F, Matsell D, et al. (2003) Long-term renal prognosis of diarrhea-associated hemolytic uremic syndrome: a systematic review, meta-analysis, and meta-regression. JAMA 290: 1360–1370.
9. Reynolds JC, Agodoa LY, Yuan CM, Abbott KC (2003) Thrombotic microangiopathy after renal transplantation in the United States. Am J Kidney Dis 42: 1058–1068.
10. Clark WF (2012) Thrombotic microangiopathy: current knowledge and outcomes with plasma exchange. Semin Dial 25: 214–219.
11. Stiles KP, Yuan CM, Chung EM, Lyon RD, Lane JD, et al. (2000) Renal biopsy in high-risk patients with medical diseases of the kidney. Am J Kidney Dis 36: 419–433.
12. Symmers WS (1952) Thrombotic microangiopathic haemolytic anaemia (thrombotic microangiopathy). Br Med J 2: 897–903.
13. George JN, Vesely SK, James JA (2007) Overlapping features of thrombotic thrombocytopenic purpura and systemic lupus erythematosus. South Med J 100: 512–514.
14. D'Angelo WA, Fries JF, Masi AT, Shulman LE (1969) Pathologic observations in systemic sclerosis (scleroderma). A study of fifty-eight autopsy cases and fifty-eight matched controls. Am J Med 46: 428–440.
15. Cataland SR, Yang SB, Witkoff L, Kraut EH, Lin S, et al. (2009) Demographic and ADAMTS13 biomarker data as predictors of early recurrences of idiopathic thrombotic thrombocytopenic purpura. Eur J Haematol 83: 559–564.
16. Hochberg MC (1997) Updating the American College of Rheumatology revised criteria for the classification of systemic lupus erythematosus. Arthritis Rheum 40: 1725.
17. Peng J, Gong L, Si K, Bai X, Du G (2011) Fluorescence resonance energy transfer assay for high-throughput screening of ADAMTS1 inhibitors. Molecules 16: 10709–10721.
18. White LE, Cui Y, Shelak CM, Lie ML, Hassoun HT (2012) Lung endothelial cell apoptosis during ischemic acute kidney injury. Shock 38: 320–327.
19. Austin PC, Tu JV (2004) Bootstrap methods for developing predictive models. Am Stat 58: 131–137.
20. Baliga RS, Wingo CS (2003) Quinine induced HUS-TTP: an unusual presentation. Am J Med Sci 326: 378–380.
21. Noris M, Remuzzi G (2010) Thrombotic microangiopathy after kidney transplantation. Am J Transplant 10: 1517–1523.
22. Hu WX, Liu ZZ, Chen HP, Zhang HT, Li LS, et al. (2010) Clinical characteristics and prognosis of diffuse proliferative lupus nephritis with thrombotic microangiopathy. Lupus 19: 1591–1598.
23. Kaplan B, Meier-Kriesche HU (2002) Death after graft loss: an important late study endpoint in kidney transplantation. Am J Transplant 2: 970–974.
24. Michael M, Elliott EJ, Craig JC, Ridley G, Hodson EM (2009) Interventions for hemolytic uremic syndrome and thrombotic thrombocytopenic purpura: a systematic review of randomized controlled trials. Am J Kidney Dis 53: 259–272.
25. Droz D, Nochy D, Noel LH, Heudes D, Nabarra B, et al. (2000) Thrombotic microangiopathies: renal and extrarenal lesions. Adv Nephrol Necker Hosp 30: 235–259.
26. Vesely SK, George JN, Lammle B, Studt JD, Alberio L, et al. (2003) ADAMTS13 activity in thrombotic thrombocytopenic purpura-hemolytic uremic syndrome: relation to presenting features and clinical outcomes in a prospective cohort of 142 patients. Blood 102: 60–68.
27. Park YA, Waldrum MR, Marques MB (2010) Platelet count and prothrombin time help distinguish thrombotic thrombocytopenic purpura-hemolytic uremic syndrome from disseminated intravascular coagulation in adults. Am J Clin Pathol 133: 460–465.
28. Cataland SR, Yang S, Wu HM (2012) The use of ADAMTS13 activity, platelet count, and serum creatinine to differentiate acquired thrombotic thrombocytopenic purpura from other thrombotic microangiopathies. Br J Haematol 157: 501–503.
29. Cohen JA, Brecher ME, Bandarenko N (1998) Cellular source of serum lactate dehydrogenase elevation in patients with thrombotic thrombocytopenic purpura. J Clin Apher 13: 16–19.
30. Furlan M, Robles R, Solenthaler M, Wassmer M, Sandoz P, et al. (1997) Deficient activity of von Willebrand factor-cleaving protease in chronic relapsing thrombotic thrombocytopenic purpura. Blood 89: 3097–3103.
31. Galbusera M, Noris M, Rossi C, Orisio S, Caprioli J, et al. (1999) Increased fragmentation of von Willebrand factor, due to abnormal cleavage of the subunit, parallels disease activity in recurrent hemolytic uremic syndrome and thrombotic thrombocytopenic purpura and discloses predisposition in families. The Italian Registry of Familial and Recurrent HUS/TTP. Blood 94: 610–620.
32. George JN (2006) Clinical practice. Thrombotic thrombocytopenic purpura. N Engl J Med 354: 1927–1935.
33. Hastings MC, Wyatt RJ, Ault BH, Jones DP, Lau KK, et al. (2007) Diagnosis of de novo localized thrombotic microangiopathy by surveillance biopsy. Pediatr Nephrol 22: 742–746.

15

Mosaicism of Podocyte Involvement Is Related to Podocyte Injury in Females with Fabry Disease

Michael Mauer[1,2], Emily Glynn[3], Einar Svarstad[4,5], Camilla Tøndel[5,6], Marie-Claire Gubler[7], Michael West[8], Alexey Sokolovskiy[3], Chester Whitley[1], Behzad Najafian[3]*

1 Department of Pediatrics, University of Minnesota, Minneapolis, United States of America, **2** Department of Medicine, University of Minnesota, Minneapolis, United States of America, **3** Department of Pathology, University of Washington, Seattle, United States of America, **4** Department of Medicine, Haukeland University Hospital, Bergen, Norway, **5** Department of Clinical Medicine, University of Bergen, Bergen, Norway, **6** Department of Pediatrics, Haukeland University Hospital, Bergen, Norway, **7** U983, Université René Descartes, Hôpital Necker-Enfants Malades AP-HP, Paris, France, **8** Division of Nephrology, Department of Medicine, Dalhousie University, Halifax, Nova Scotia, Canada

Abstract

Background: Fabry disease. an X-linked deficiency of α-galactosidase A coded by the GLA gene, leads to intracellular globotriaosylceramide (GL-3) accumulation. Although less common than in males, chronic kidney disease, occurs in ~15% of females. Recent studies highlight the importance of podocyte injury in Fabry nephropathy development and progression. We hypothesized that the greater the % of podocytes with active wild-type GLA gene (due to X-inactivation of the mutant copy) the less is the overall podocyte injury.

Methods: Kidney biopsies from 12 treatment-naive females with Fabry disease, ages 15 (8–63), median [range], years were studied by electron microscopy and compared with 4 treatment-naive male patients.

Results: In females, 51 (13–100)% of podocytes (PC) per glomerulus had no GL-3 inclusions, this consistent with a non-Fabry podocyte phenotype (NFPC). In PC with GL-3 inclusions [Fabry podocyte phenotype (FPC)], GL-3 volume density per podocyte was virtually identical in females and males, consistent with little or no cross-correction between FPC and NFPC. %NFPC per glomerulus (%NFPC/glom) correlated with age in females ($r = 0.65$, $p = 0.02$), suggesting a survival disadvantage for FPC over time. Age-adjusted %NFPC/glom was inversely related to foot process width (FPW) ($r = -0.75$, $p = 0.007$), an indicator of PC injury. GL-3 volume density in FPC in females correlated directly with FPW.

Conclusions: These findings support important relationships between podocyte mosaicism and podocyte injury in female Fabry patients. Kidney biopsy, by providing information about podocyte mosaicism, may help to stratify females with Fabry disease for kidney disease risk and to guide treatment decisions.

Editor: Stuart E. Dryer, University of Houston, United States of America

Funding: This work was supported by an NIH RDCRN U54 grant (5U54NS065768-04) and an investigator initiated grant from Genzyme, a Sanofi Company. The funder provided support in the form of research grants for authors [BN, MM, and MLW], and travel support and honoraria for authors [BN, MM, CT, and MLW] but did not have any additional role in the study design, data collection and analysis, decision to publish, or preparation of the manuscript. The specific roles of these authors are articulated in the 'author contributions' section.

* Email: najafian@u.washington.edu

Introduction

Fabry disease is a storage disease caused by deficiency of the α-galactosidase A (αGal A) enzyme that hydrolyzes the terminal α-galactosyl moieties from glycolipids and glycoproteins. This leads to the accumulation of its substrates, predominately globotriaosylceramide (GL-3) in various cell types and organs, causing a constellation of complications including skin lesions, strokes, cardiac arrhythmias and cardiomyopathy, neuropathies and renal failure. [1] αGal A is encoded by the GLA gene located on the X chromosome locus Xq21.3-q22. Similar to other X-linked diseases, the complications are typically less frequent and more variable in severity in females, [2,3,4] although they can be as severe as in male patients. [5,6] A significant proportion of female patients suffer from important complications, including 40% with clinical renal disease (mainly proteinuria) [7] and about 15% with serious renal events. [2] Fabry disease is associated with significant life expectancy reductions in both sexes. [8] It is of great importance to understand the factors associated with disease severity in females. Currently, there are no reliable tests to identify females at greater risk to develop kidney failure, thus justifying earlier treatment with enzyme replacement therapy (ERT). Podocytes are terminally differentiated cells with pivotal role in preserving glomerular structure and function. [9] Recent studies suggest that GL-3 accumulation in podocytes plays an important role in the pathophysiology of Fabry nephropathy. [10] These cells are also much more resistant to ERT than most other kidney cell types. [11,12] Similar to other "terminally differentiated cells" podocytes do not easily regenerate following injury [13]. Continuous podocyte loss leads to progressive reduction of these cells in the glomeruli, this eventually reaching critical levels causing irreversible glomerular scarring [14]. Despite recent evidence that higher doses of ERT during childhood may result in partial to almost complete clearance of podocytes from GL-3 inclusions, [15] there is no consensus as to when to initiate ERT, especially in females, and the relative clinical effectiveness of the different licensed ERT doses remain unsettled. [16,17,18] We hypothesized that podocytes, due to random X-inactivation, are heterogeneously involved by Fabry disease in female patients and that this heterogeneity could influence podocyte injury. Herein we describe a method to quantify the % of podocytes with the Fabry phenotype and report an inverse relationship in females between age-adjusted % podocytes with no GL-3 inclusions in glomeruli and foot process width, a sensitive indicator of podocyte injury [19], supporting a relationship between X-inactivation and podocyte injury in females with Fabry disease. We also found no evidence of cross-correction between podocytes without and with the Fabry phenotype in females with Fabry disease.

Methods

These studies were performed in accordance with principles of the Declaration of Helsinki and were reviewed and approved by the Institutional Review Board of the University of Minnesota, Comité. de Protection des Personnes "Ile-De-France II." and the Regional Ethics Committee of Western Norway. Informed consents approved by the institutional board review committees were obtained prior to these studies.

Subjects and Clinical Parameters

Kidney biopsies from 12 ERT-naive females with Fabry disease, age 15 (8–63) years were studied by electron microscopy for distribution of podocyte involvement by the Fabry phenotype. Biopsies were obtained for assessment of the severity of the lesions of Fabry nephropathy in order to aid clinical decision-making regarding ERT initiation and/or as a baseline biopsy prior to ERT initiation. Biopsies from 4 ERT-naive males with Fabry disease, age 14 (7–18), were studied for comparison; 7/16 patients presented here were included in our previous publications. [10,15] The demographic and clinical data of all patients are presented in Table 1.

9/12 female and 3/4 male patients had results of GLA mutation analysis in their medical records confirming the diagnosis of Fabry disease (Table 1). The diagnosis of Fabry disease in the other patients was based on family history or clinical findings with or without reduced leukocyte αGal A activity and confirmed by the kidney biopsy findings. Protein excretion per gram creatinine (UPCR) was based on urine samples obtained close to the date of biopsy. GFR was estimated by the plasma clearance of iohexol where available or by creatinine clearance. Except for one of the patients where we were not able to find information about the use of renin-angiotensin system blockers, none of the patients were receiving these drugs.

Biopsies from 6 healthy living kidney donors, age 37 (16–52) were used to estimate normal control values for podocyte foot process with (FPW), as described below.

Biopsy Tissue Preparation and Electron Microscopy

Electron microscopy specimens were fixed in 2.5% glutaraldehyde, and embedded in PolyBed. Random glomerular sections were prepared as previously described. [20] Thin sections were mounted on formvar coated copper slot grids. Overlapping digital low magnification (~10,000 x) images of the entire glomerular profiles were obtained using a JEOL CX100 electron microscope for the podocyte mosaicism studies. High magnification (~30,000 x) images were obtained according a systematic uniform random sampling protocol for estimation of fraction of the volume (Vv) of PC cytoplasm occupied by GL-3 inclusions [Vv(Inc/PC)], Vv of inclusions/glomerular mesangial cell [Vv(Inc/Mes)], Vv of inclusions/glomerular endothelial cell [Vv(Inc/Endo)], and podocyte average FPW as previously described [10,20].

Identification of Podocytes with and without the Fabry Phenotype

Observers were masked to any of the patient characteristics. Montages of complete glomerular profiles were prepared from the above images in Adobe Photoshop software (Adobe Photoshop CS5 Extended, version 12.0×32). Twice digital magnification was applied to the images. Podocyte nuclei were identified and glomerular profiles with less than 10 podocyte nuclei (n = 3) were excluded from these studies. The cytoplasmic profiles surrounding each podocyte nucleus were carefully examined for presence of GL-3 inclusions. Podocyte nuclear profiles with cytoplasmic GL-3 inclusions, consistent with Fabry phenotype podocytes (FPC) or without cytoplasmic GL-3 inclusions, consistent with non-Fabry phnotype podocytes (NFPC) cytoplasmic GL-3 inclusions were counted in each glomerulus and %NFPC/glom was calculated. The maximum number of immediately adjacent podocytes, including podocytes on the other side of the same capillary loop, which were NFPC was recorded as an estimate of the size of podocyte mosaic patches on the section.

Electron Microscopy Stereology

Based on the best quality of tissue preservation and images, one glomerulus per biopsy was arbitrarily selected for detailed GL-3 volume density measurement in podocytes with visible nuclei on the section. Boundaries of nuclei and cell membranes, excluding the tertiary foot processes were traced using the magnetic lasso tool in separate layers in Adobe Photoshop (Figure 1). Similarly, the most convex points of cytoplasmic GL-3 inclusions were connected using the magnetic lasso tool to draw a polygon around the GL-3 inclusion aggregates in a separate layer. The tracings were colored differentially for nuclei, cytoplasm and inclusions (Figure 1). The observed magnification was calculated from the average of 10 horizontal and 10 vertical random measurements performed on images from a SPI grating carbon replica #02902-AB (Structure Probe, Inc., West Chester, PA, USA) with horizontal and vertical lines 0.463 μm apart obtained at the same magnification as for the montage images. Subsequently, the measurement tool of the software was calibrated. The area of cell, nucleus and inclusion aggregate profiles were obtained separately for each podocyte profile with a visible nucleus from the Adobe Photoshop measurement log. The fractional volume of GL-3 inclusions per each nucleated podocyte profile with GL-3 inclusions [Vv(Inc/

Table 1. Clinical characteristics of subjects.

Case	Sex	Age (year)	UPCR (mg/g)	UACR (mg/g)	GFR (ml/min/1.73 m^2)	GLA Mutation	Mutation Type	Aangiokeratoma	Corneal Opacity
1	F	8	40	NA	NA*	NA	NA	+	+
2	F	11	0.02	53	105	c.800T>G (p.M267R)	Missense	+	+
3	F	12	29	NA	109	W236X	Nonsense	−	−
4	F	13	0	NA	97	Y216D	Missense	−	+
5	F	13	60	5	100	NA	NA	+	−
6	F	14	62	11	90	c.800T>G (p.M267R)	Missense	NA	NA
7	F	16	30	12	127	NA	NA	−	−
8	F	34	150	NA	118	R301Q	Missense	+	−
9	F	34	100	5	99	R112C	Missense	−	+
10	F	39	100	NA	78	1270T	Missense	+	+
11	F	39	40	ND	99	N215S	Missense	+	−
12	F	63	1150	NA	46	C.427G>C p.Ala143Pro	Missense	+	−
13	M	7	0	NA	183	Y216D	Missense	+	+
14	M	16	92	12	112	c.1212_1214delAAG	Deletion	+	+
15	M	18	251	135	96	c.800T>G(p. M267R)	Missense	+	+
16	M	23	102	NA	111	NA	NA	NA	NA

Abbreviations: UPCR = urine protein/creatinine ratio; UACR = urine albumin/creatinine ratio; GFR = glomerular filtration rate; NA = data not available; *Serum creatinine within the normal range; F = female; M = male; ND = Not detectable.

FPC)] was estimated as follows: $V_V(Inc/FPC) = \frac{A_{inclusions} \times 100}{A_{cell} - A_{nucleus}}$. The overall average glomerular volume fraction of GL-3 inclusions per podocytes [Vv(Inc/PC)], endothelial cells [Vv(Inc/Endo)] and mesangial cells [Vv(Inc/Mes)] were estimated using unbiased stereology methods as previously detailed. [10] For clarity, we emphasize that Vv(Inc/FPC) is an estimate of GL-3 inclusion density in nucleated podocyte profiles with GL-3 inclusions, while Vv(Inc/PC) is an estimate of the same parameter in all visible podocyte profiles regardless of GL-3 content and including the podocytes with and without visible nuclei over 3 (1–3), median (range), glomeruli per biopsy. Average foot process width (FPW) was also estimated using unbiased stereology methods as detailed elsewhere. [10,20,21] In order to compare podocyte injury in FPC *vs.* NFPC in female patients with Fabry disease, FPW was separately estimated in systematically and uniformly obtained electron micrographs with and without FPC.

Statistical Analyses

Statistica 8.0 (Statsoft, Inc.) was used for statistical analysis. Comparison between groups was made by student t-test after confirming homogeneity of variances. Relationships between variables were evaluated using Pearson correlation. Partial correlations were performed to control for confounding variables. Random effects model variance component analysis was performed to estimate % contribution of biopsies (inter-subject) and glomeruli (intra-subject) variations to total variance of %NFPC per glomerulus (%NFPC/glom). $p<0.05$ was considered statistically significant.

Results

Electron Microscopy Examination of Kidney Biopsies

Examination of electron micrographs from all biopsies allowed easy and reliable distinction between male and female patients by the identification in females of podocytes with visible nuclei without GL-3 cytoplasmic inclusions, termed non-Fabry podocytes (NFPC) (Figure 1) in contrast with podocytes containing GL-3 inclusions, termed Fabry phenotype podocytes (FPC). However, mosaicism of the Fabry phenotype was not easily identifiable in the other glomerular or extra-glomerular cells, perhaps, at least in part, due to uncertainty about cellular boundaries (*e.g.*, mesangial or endothelial cells). In 4 female patient biopsies, no GL-3 inclusions were identified in endothelial and/or mesangial cells, thus, comments about mosaicism could not be made in those cell types. In 7/12 female patient biopsies, parietal epithelial cell profiles with no GL-3 inclusions were identified while occasional parietal epithelial cells with enlarged cytoplasm had abundant GL-3 inclusions. Characteristic lamellar GL-3 inclusions were not easily identified in proximal tubular epithelial cells. Distal tubular epithelial cells showed variable GL-3 inclusions in both males and females. Thus, this variability could not be accounted for X-inactivation mosaicism in those cells.

Distribution of GL3 Inclusions among Podocytes in Males and Females

54 (27–87) podocytes per biopsy were examined for presence of GL-3 inclusions in female patients. 51 (13–100)% of podocyte profiles per biopsy with visible nuclei and no GL-3 inclusions, were classified as NFPC in these females. NFPC were distributed as

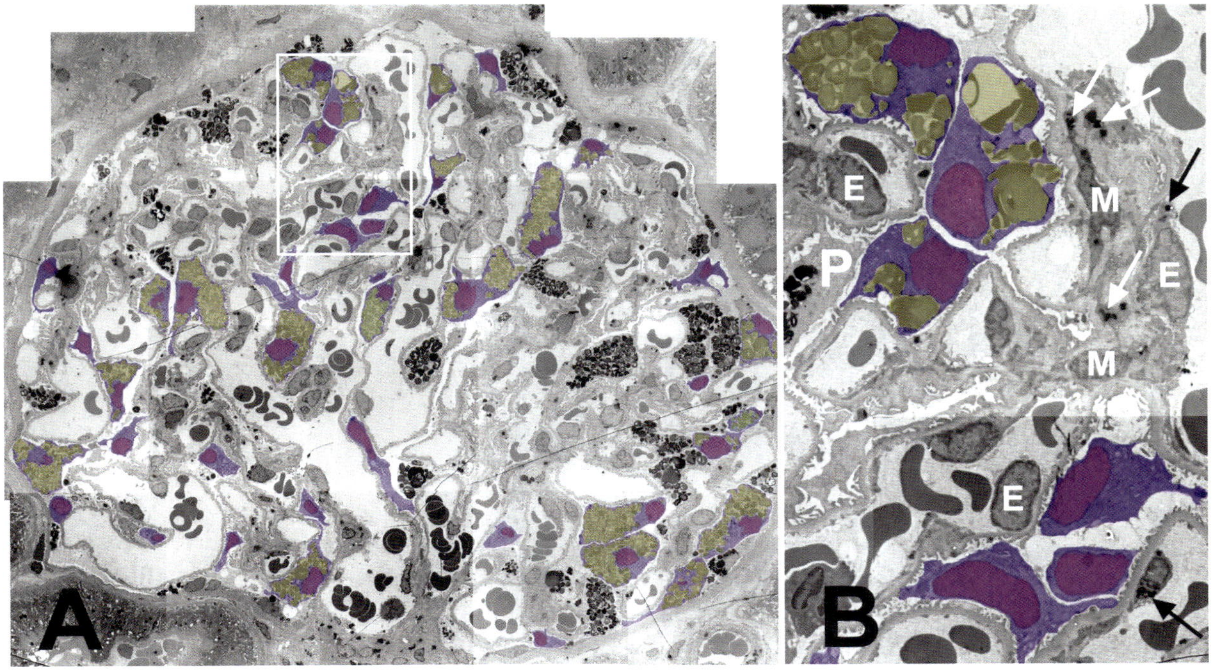

Figure 1. Mosaicism of podocyte Fabry phenotype in a glomerulus from a female patient with Fabry disease. (**A**) Montage image of a glomerulus (~3,000×). Podocyte bodies with visible nuclei are colored blue, podocyte nuclei purple, and GL-3 inclusions yellow. The white rectangle is magnified in B. (**B**) Magnified view of three podocyte profiles without (at the bottom) and three other podocyte profiles with GL-3 inclusions (on the top). Arrows show GL-3 inclusions in mesangial (M) cells (black) and endothelial (E) cells. P is a podocyte profile with no visible nucleus on this section.

single cells among FPC or in patches composed of 2–6 podocytes (Figure 1).

Two biopsies from female patients (one with 3 and another with 2 glomeruli) had no GL-3 inclusions in podocytes with visible nuclei (cases #9 and #11, Table 1). Case #9 showed rare podocyte profiles that were filled with GL-3. However, because these GL-3 containing podocytes had no visible nuclei they were not included in calculation of %NFPC per glomerulus. This case had a missense mutation (R112C) with GFR, UPCR and UACR values all within the normal range (Table 1). Clinical examination revealed corneal opacities, but no angiokeratoma. Echocardiograms showed normal left ventricular size and function with an estimated ejection fraction of 55–60% and normal right ventricular size and systolic function. Case #11 had distal tubular cells with GL-3 inclusions. This case had a cardiac variant mutation (N215S) with normal GFR and UPCR values and no detectable albumin in the urine (Table 1). The diagnosis of Fabry disease was made based on known family history. Clinical examination revealed angiokeratoma, but no corneal opacities. Clinically, she was asymptomatic. No echocardiograms were available from this case. None of these two subjects had a history of stroke. In order to determine whether random sectioning through podocytes may have obscured the observation of GL-3 inclusions in podocyte profiles 4 male patients with Fabry disease were similarly studied, 1–3 (median 2.5) glomeruli, containing 18–36 (median 22) podocyte profiles per glomerulus with visible nuclei were examined (Table 1). All podocyte profiles from these glomeruli contained abundant GL-3 inclusions, consistent with FPC, except for two very small profiles in a 7-year-old boy. The volume fraction of GL-3 inclusions per FPC [Vv(Inc/FPC)] was nearly identical in males (0.56±0.11) and females (0.53±0.13; $p=0.54$).

Inter- and Intra-subject Variations of Podocyte Phenotype Mosaicism

Biopsies from 9 female patients with more than one glomerulus (3 (2–5), median (range)) available for electron microscopy were used to compare inter- and intra- subject variability of podocytes with the Fabry the phenotype. The %NFPC/glom in 2–4 glomeruli per biopsy in female patients is shown in Figure 2. Variance component analysis showed that only 9.6% of total variance in podocyte Fabry phenotype mosaicism originated from inter-glomerular (intra-subject) variation, while the vast majority of variance lay in differences in this parameter among the subjects.

Relationships Between % Podocytes with no GL-3 Inclusions and Female Patient Characteristics, Renal Function and Other Glomerular Structural Parameters

Values of %NFPC/glom, Vv(Inc/PC), volume fraction of GL-3 inclusions per mesangial cells [Vv(Inc/Mes)], volume fraction of inclusions per endothelial cells [Vv(Inc/Endo)], and foot process width (FPW) are provided in Table 2. The average %NFPC/glom was calculated in biopsies from female patients with more than one available glomerulus. There was a direct relationship between age and %NFPC/glom ($r=0.65$; $p=0.02$, Figure 3). No statistically significant relationship was found between %NFPC/glom and urine albumin/creatinine ratio (UACR) (available in 6/12 patients), urine protein creatinine ratio (UPCR) or glomerular filtration rate (GFR). As expected, %NFPC/glom was inversely related to Vv(Inc/PC) ($r=-0.70$, $p=0.02$) for all podocytes. Simple linear regression analysis revealed no statistically significant relationships between %NFPC/glom and foot process width, Vv(Inc/Endo), Vv(Inc/Mes). However, adjusted for age, significant inverse relationships were found between %NFPC/glom and FPW ($r=-0.75$, $p=0.007$), and Vv(Inc/Mes) ($r=0.70$, $p=0.02$), but not with Vv(Inc/Endo).

To better visualize the relationships between %NFPC/glom and FPW and UPCR, 10 female patients were grouped into 5 age-matched pairs, 3 pairs with identical ages and the 2 other pairs with ages no more than 2 years apart. Except for one pair, in each pair, the subject with lower %NFPC/glom had greater FPW value, suggestive of an inverse relationship between the extent of podocyte injury and the number of NFPC in age-matched Fabry females (Figure 4). Even an 8 year old female with 20% NFPC/glom (case #1) had greater FPW than an 11 year old (case #2) with 50% NFPC/glom. The one exception was a pair with greater FPW in a 14 year old girl with 22% NFPC/glom (case #6) compared to a 16 years old with 13% %NFPC/glom (case #7) (Figure 4). The relationships between %NFPC/glom and UPCR among the above pairs paralleled the relationships between %NFPC/glom and FPW, except for cases #2 and #3 with almost identical %NFPC/glom (50 and 52%, respectively) and slightly (~15%) greater UPCR for case#2 (Figure 4). However, the relationship between %NFPC and UPCR remained not statistically significant after age adjustment. Also, when adjusted for age, Vv(Inc/FPC) in females correlated with FPW ($r=0.64$, $p=0.03$). In females with Fabry disease, FPW in electron micrographs where glomerular basement membranes were covered by FPC (562±160 nm) was not statistically different from those where glomerular basement membranes were covered by NFPC (663±283 nm). On the other hand, FPW in either of these areas were greater than FPW in normal control biopsies (406±34 nm, $p=0.037$ for FPC and $p=0.048$ for NFPC).

Discussion

We recently demonstrated that the fraction of the volume of podocytes occupied by GL-3 [Vv(Inc/PC)] increases with age in children with Fabry disease and is directly correlated with FPW and to proteinuria,[9] the latter a strong predictor of renal disease risk among Fabry disease patients.[23] Increased FPW is a common concomitant of injury in podocytes and is seen in a variety of conditions known to be associated with injury in these cells. [21,22], [23] Thus careful examination of this cell in Fabry disease is important. This is the first study to provide unbiased electron microscopic morphometric measures of the heterogeneity of podocyte involvement in females with Fabry disease, almost certainly as a result of X-inactivation. Gubler *et al* first described the heterogeneous distribution of GL-3 inclusions in podocytes in 3 females with Fabry disease. [24] Valbuena *et al* also described variable podocyte GL-3 accumulation in 4 females with Fabry disease. [25] However, no quantitative assessment of podocyte GL-3 or statistical analyses was provided in these reports. Similar to these studies, [24,25] we found that a distinction between Fabry and non-Fabry phenotype, consistent with cells carrying active mutant or wild-type GLA, respectively, could be easily made in podocytes but not in other renal cells of female patients. This could be due to distinct borders of podocyte cell bodies from their neighbor cells, or because podocytes are apparently very long lived [26] and may thus retain GL-3 inclusions for years while other cell types are more frequently replaced.

Importantly, we documented, through unbiased morphometric measurements, that the average fraction of podocyte cytoplasm occupied by GL-3 was virtually identical in male and female patients, suggesting that FPC do not benefit from the enzymatic activity of the adjacent NFPC or from the generally higher residual plasma αGal A in females than on males. [27] [28,29].

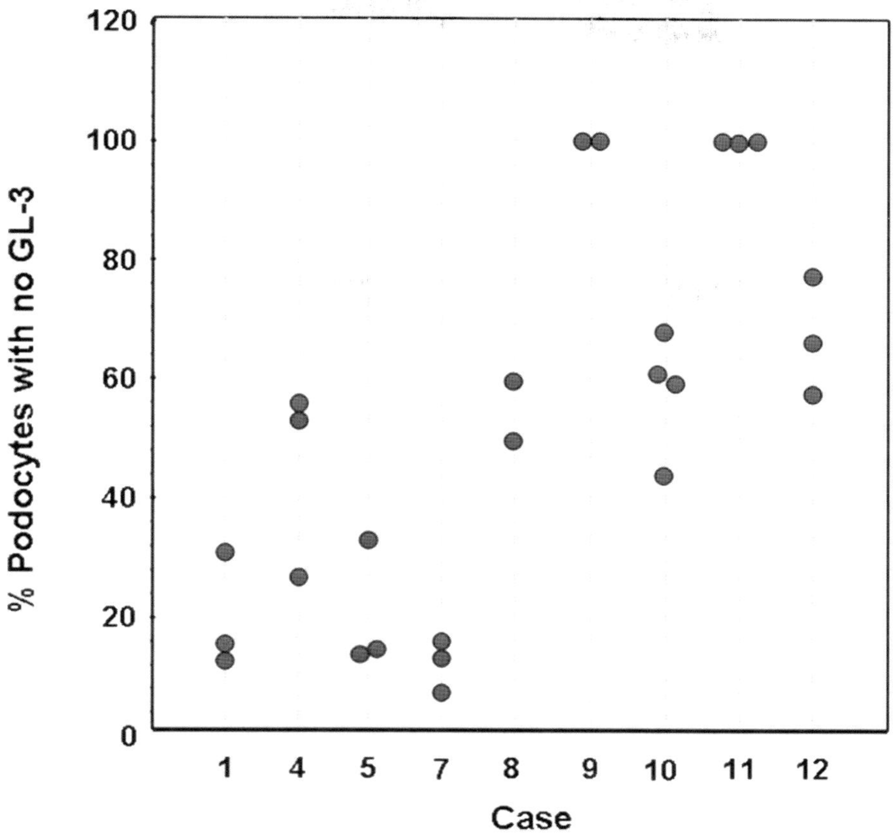

Figure 2. Intra- and inter-subject variability of podocyte mosaicism for Fabry phenotype in females. X axis shows case numbers (see Table 1). Each vertical dashed line represents a biopsy and each circle represents % podocytes with no GL-3 inclusions in one glomerulus.

Also important, we found that inter-glomerular variation in podocyte phenotype mosaicism in a given female Fabry patient's renal biopsy is much smaller than inter-patient variation. This suggests that estimation of podocyte phenotypic mosaicism even in a single glomerulus is representative of this phenomenon in the biopsy and validates the study of podocyte phenotype mosaicism in a few glomeruli. It also suggests that podocyte mosaciasm in females is established relatively early in embryogenesis. It should be noted that in these studies we used random profiles of glomeruli. Although we observed NFPC in patches of up to 5 cells in these two-dimensional glomerular cross-sections, these patches are likely larger in three dimensions. Nonetheless we posit that these patches are not very large, otherwise we might have expected greater inter-glomerular variability as a result of random sectioning through glomeruli.

This study is the first to show a quantitative relationship in females with Fabry disease between the X-inactivation phenomenon and podocyte injury manifest as increased FPW. Although X-inactivation may play a role in the clinical phenotypic expression of X-linked diseases, a direct link between skewed X-inactivation and severity of the Fabry phenotype has been controversial. Dobrovolny *et al.* reported that the trend line between the age and the Mainz severity score index (MSSI) [30] was steeper in 10 Fabry females with *vs.* 28 without unfavorably skewed X-inactivation in leukocytes, urinary and salivary cells. This suggested that random X-inactivation could influence the severity of the Fabry phenotype in female patients. [31] In contrast, Maier *et al.* found that in 46% of the 28 Fabry females studied, skewed X-inactivation did not correlate with phenotype severity. [4] Similarly, in a more recent study, while confirming random X-inactivation in leukocytes in ~82% of 77 female Fabry patients, there was no relationship between X-inactivation ratios and age, αGal A activity, MSSI scores, cardiac involvement, neuropathic pain or proteinuria. [32] We did not find a statistically significant relationship between % NFPC/glom and UPCR. However, in regression models including UPCR among the predictor variables, UPCR accounted for much less of the variance for rates of GFR decline in women than in men with Fabry disease. [33] Also, increased UPCR can reflect parameters other than podocyte injury, such as impaired tubular reabsorption reabsorption of filtered protein. However, after adjusting for age, we documented a significant inverse relationship between %NFPC/glom and FPW, a widely accepted indicator of podocyte injury. Thus, having more NFPC in glomeruli was associated with less podocyte injury. However, having a greater proportion of NFPC in older females with Fabry disease is not necessarily indicative of less podocyte injury. In fact, the observed increase in the %NFPC/glom with age in female patients in the current study is suggestive of progressive FPC loss with aging due to a survival disadvantage caused by the Fabry phenotype. Thus, glomeruli of older female patients may have fewer total podocytes than those of younger females with lesser %NFPC/glom, a hypothesis that remains to be tested in future studies. On the other hand, our side-by-side comparisons of age-matched female pairs revealed a robust inverse relationship between %NFPC/glom and FPW. However, given that Fabry disease is genetically heterogeneous, with more

Table 2. Glomerular Structural Parameters.

Case	Sex	Age (year)	%NFPC/glom	Vv(Inc/PC)	Vv(Inc/Mes)	Vv(Inc/Endo)	Vv(Inc/FPC)	FPW* (nm)
1	F	8	20	0.28	0.03	0.08	0.50	524
2	F	11	50	0.43	0.02	0	0.62	426
3	F	12	52	0.21	0	0	0.42	372
4	F	13	45	0.20	0	0.03	0.42	464
5	F	13	21	0.26	0.03	0.03	0.68	663
6	F	14	22	0.38	0.07	0.02	0.53	602
7	F	16	13	0.51	0.03	0.02	0.67	461
8	F	34	55	0.43	0.01	0.01	0.70	620
9	F	34	100	0	0	0.01	0	427
10	F	39	58	0.21	0.01	0	0.35	654
11	F	39	100	0.02	0.01	0	0	441
12	F	63	68	0.16	0.04	0.06	0.48	673
13	M	7	8**	0.21	0.01	0.09	0.58	369
14	M	16	0	0.44	0.10	0.37	0.56	551
15	M	18	0	0.50	0.16	0.21	0.61	823
16	M	23	0	0.34	0.56	0.27	0.65	714

Abbreviations: %NFPC/glom = % non-Fabry podocytes per glomerulus; Vv(Inc/PC) = volume fraction of GL3 inclusions per podocyte; Vv(Inc/Mes) = volume fraction of GL3 inclusions per mesangial cell; Vv(Inc/Endo) = volume fraction of GL3 inclusions per endothelial cell; Vv(Inc/FPC) = volume fraction of GL3 inclusions per Fabry podocytes; FPW = foot process width; F = female; M = male; *Normal values for FPW obtained from biopsies from 6 healthy living donors was 406±34 nm. **The biopsy contained two very small podocyte profiles with no GL3 inclusions, most likely due to random sectioning.

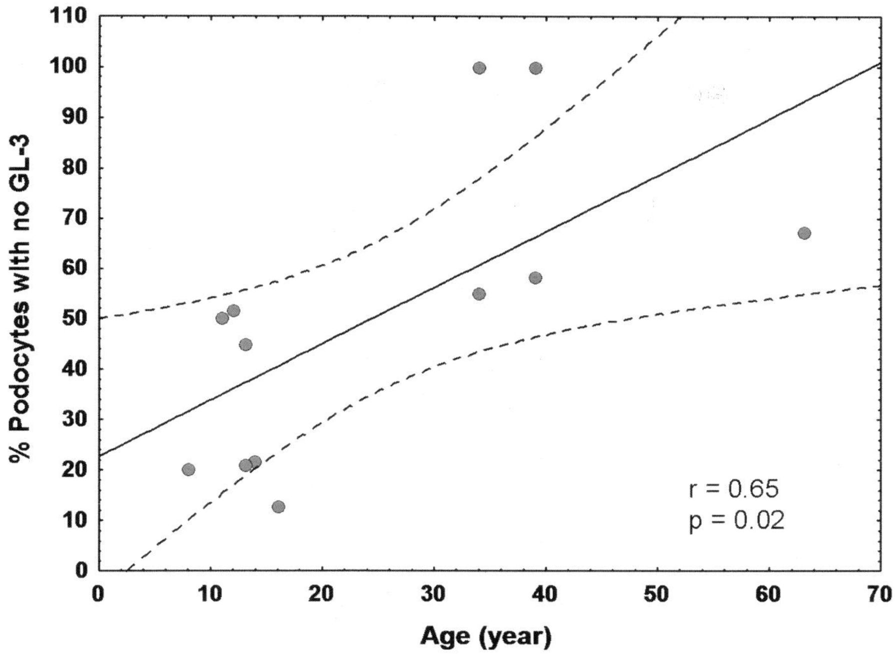

Figure 3. Relationship between age and % podocytes with no GL-3 in females. Dashed lines represent 0.95 confidence interval.

than registered 600 mutations, [34] it should be expected that attempts to explain all phenotype variation by a single parameter such as mosaicism will necessarily be overambitious. [35,36] Nevertheless, it will be interesting to examine if a relationship can be found between podocyte mosaicism status in the kidney and skewed X-inactivation in other organs or cell types, especially that of leukocytes. However, some of the cases presented in this study were from historical archived material and no simultaneous blood samples or skin biopsies had been obtained for x-inactivation studies at the time other biopsies were performed.

The relationship between podocyte mosaicism and podocyte injury in female Fabry patients suggests that the status of podocyte

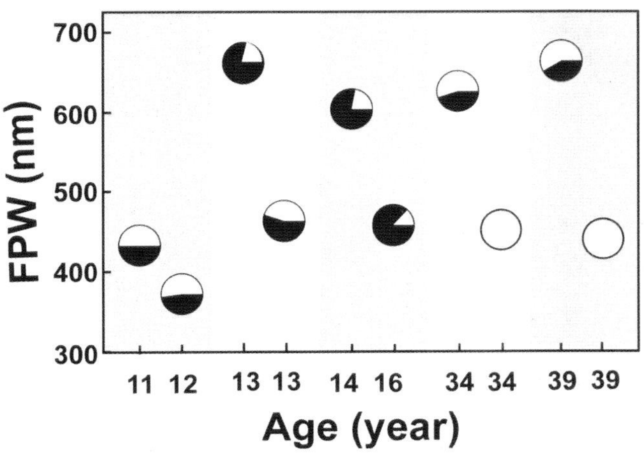

Figure 4. Relationships between podocyte mosaicism and foot process width in age-matched paired females. Each vertical grey or white band represents an age-matched pair. Each pie chart represents %NFPC/glom as white and %FPC/glom as black area. Abbreviation: FPW: foot process width.

X-inactivation, after making adjustment for the age of the patient, could help to identify females with greater risk of progression of Fabry nephropathy. Although it would be desirable to use less invasive methods to obtain information about the proportion of cells with active mutant GLA, the status of mosaicism may be cell type and organ specific. Moreover, as outlined above, studies attempting to link X-inactivation in peripheral blood leukocytes and clinical manifestations of Fabry females have produced contradictory results. [4,31] Thus far, renal biopsy may be the only reliable way to obtain information about podocyte mosaicism in these patients.

Importantly, the present study showed that not only podocyte mosaicism for Fabry phenotype and podocyte injury are linked in female patients, but also podocyte injury in these patients is not limited to FPC and extends to NFPC, evidenced by increased FPW in GBM areas covered by NFPC compared with normal control biopsies. This is consistent with experimental studies performed by Matsusaka et al. where following administration of the immunotoxin LMB2 to the mice chimeric for hCD25 (LMB2 receptor), not only hCD25+ podocytes, but also hCD25- podocytes were injured and showed foot process widening, suggesting that specific injury to some podocytes can induce non-specific injury to other podocytes, [14] a phenomenon that if severe enough could lead to a vicious cycle of podocyte loss and glomerulosclerosis.

To our knowledge, this is the first report of the finding of rare cells with GL-3 inclusions in kidney biopsies from female Fabry patients. We encountered two females, ages 34 (case #9) and 39 years (case #11), with known Fabry disease by mutation analysis with very rare kidney cells with GL-3 inclusions. One (case #11), had a cardiac variant GLA mutation (N215S) [37] and the other (case #9) had a missense mutation (R112C). Thus, in contrast to males, the finding of even rare cells with GL3 inclusions in kidney biopsies from females should raise strong suspicion for Fabry disease. Notably, both of these subjects had very mild phenotypes, raising suspicion that the favorable skewed X-inactivation (predominantly affecting the mutant copy of GLA) observed in kidney biopsies may have also been present in other organs, especially since R112C mutation has been associated with classical Fabry disease causing ESRD [38], while case #9 in the present study had normal renal function and no history of cardiac disease or strokes. We did not have access to blood samples or other biopsies from these subjects to do correlative studies with our findings in kidney biopsies.

This study has some limitations. Although, it is the largest kidney biopsy study of females with Fabry disease, given the heterogeneity of Fabry mutations and clinical manifestations, additional studies are needed to confirm our results. We did not examine the status of X-inactivation in podocytes directly, rather we studied their apparent phenotype as to presence/absence of GL-3 inclusions in cell body profiles as a surrogate for X-inactivation. However, the easy discrimination between males and females on biopsies based on podocyte mosaicism supports validity of this surrogate. We cannot exclude the possibility of overestimation of %NFPC/glom in this study due to missing GL-3 inclusions in a single section through podocyte cell bodies. However, among 4 biopsies examined from male patients, only 2 of 98 podocyte nucleated profiles, both of very small size, had no GL-3 inclusions. Thus, we believe the extent of %NFPC/glom overestimation due to random sectioning is trivial.

In summary, this is the first study showing that mosaicism of podocytes in females with Fabry disease is related to podocyte injury. The extent of podocyte mosaicism for the Fabry phenotype is quite uniform among the glomeruli. The fraction of the cell body occupied by GL-3 in affected podocytes in females is the same as in males, indicating the absence of significant cross-correction. The relative number of podocytes without the Fabry phenotype increases with age in female patients, suggesting either a disproportionate loss of Fabry-affected podocytes over time and/or selection bias. Information about podocyte mosaicism in kidney biopsies may be useful to identify females with Fabry disease with increased risk of developing progressive podocyte and nephron loss. The methodology we introduced is applicable to future longitudinal biopsy studies to test this hypothesis.

Acknowledgments

Special thanks to Frieda Maiers, Ann Palmer and Paul Murry for their help with electron microscopy images and histologic measurements, Cathy Bagne for clinical coordinator assistance, and Kristina Chayet for secretarial assistance.

Author Contributions

Conceived and designed the experiments: MM BN. Performed the experiments: MM EG AS BN. Analyzed the data: AS BN. Contributed reagents/materials/analysis tools: MM ES CT MG MW CW. Contributed to the writing of the manuscript: MM BN EG ES CT MG AS MW CW.

References

1. Zarate YA, Hopkin RJ (2008) Fabry's disease. Lancet 372: 1427–1435.
2. Wilcox WR, Oliveira JP, Hopkin RJ, Ortiz A, Banikazemi M, et al. (2008) Females with Fabry disease frequently have major organ involvement: lessons from the Fabry Registry. Mol Genet Metab 93: 112–128.
3. MacDermot KD, Holmes A, Miners AH (2001) Anderson-Fabry disease: clinical manifestations and impact of disease in a cohort of 60 obligate carrier females. J Med Genet 38: 769–775.
4. Maier EM, Osterrieder S, Whybra C, Ries M, Gal A, et al. (2006) Disease manifestations and X inactivation in heterozygous females with Fabry disease. Acta Paediatr Suppl 95: 30–38.
5. Wang RY, Lelis A, Mirocha J, Wilcox WR (2007) Heterozygous Fabry women are not just carriers, but have a significant burden of disease and impaired quality of life. Genet Med 9: 34–45.
6. Gibas AL, Klatt R, Johnson J, Clarke JT, Katz J (2008) Disease rarity, carrier status, and gender: a triple disadvantage for women with Fabry disease. J Genet Couns 17: 528–537.
7. Deegan PB, Baehner AF, Barba Romero MA, Hughes DA, Kampmann C, et al. (2006) Natural history of Fabry disease in females in the Fabry Outcome Survey. J Med Genet 43: 347–352.
8. Mehta A, Ricci R, Widmer U, Dehout F, Garcia de Lorenzo A, et al. (2004) Fabry disease defined: baseline clinical manifestations of 366 patients in the Fabry Outcome Survey. Eur J Clin Invest 34: 236–242.
9. Reiser J, Sever S (2013) Podocyte biology and pathogenesis of kidney disease. Annu Rev Med 64: 357–366.
10. Najafian B, Svarstad E, Bostad L, Gubler MC, Tondel C, et al. (2011) Progressive podocyte injury and globotriaosylceramide (GL-3) accumulation in young patients with Fabry disease. Kidney Int 79: 663–670.
11. Thurberg BL, Rennke H, Colvin RB, Dikman S, Gordon RE, et al. (2002) Globotriaosylceramide accumulation in the Fabry kidney is cleared from multiple cell types after enzyme replacement therapy. Kidney Int 62: 1933–1946.
12. Germain DP, Waldek S, Banikazemi M, Bushinsky DA, Charrow J, et al. (2007) Sustained, long-term renal stabilization after 54 months of agalsidase beta therapy in patients with Fabry disease. J Am Soc Nephrol 18: 1547–1557.
13. Kriz W, LeHir M (2005) Pathways to nephron loss starting from glomerular diseases-insights from animal models. Kidney Int 67: 404–419.
14. Matsusaka T, Sandgren E, Shintani A, Kon V, Pastan I, et al. (2011) Podocyte injury damages other podocytes. J Am Soc Nephrol 22: 1275–1285.
15. Tondel C, Bostad L, Larsen KK, Hirth A, Vikse BE, et al. (2013) Agalsidase benefits renal histology in young patients with Fabry disease. J Am Soc Nephrol 24: 137–148.
16. Terryn W, Cochat P, Froissart R, Ortiz A, Pirson Y, et al. (2013) Fabry nephropathy: indications for screening and guidance for diagnosis and treatment by the European Renal Best Practice. Nephrol Dial Transplant 28: 505–517.
17. Najafian B, Mauer M, Hopkin RJ, Svarstad E (2013) Renal complications of Fabry disease in children. Pediatr Nephrol 28: 679–687.
18. Warnock DG, Mauer M (2014) Fabry Disease: Dose Matters. J Am Soc Nephrol.
19. Kriz W, Shirato I, Nagata M, LeHir M, Lemley KV (2013) The podocyte's response to stress: the enigma of foot process effacement. Am J Physiol Renal Physiol 304: F333–347.
20. Najafian B, Mauer M (2011) Quantitating glomerular endothelial fenestration: an unbiased stereological approach. Am J Nephrol 33 Suppl 1: 34–39.
21. Toyoda M, Najafian B, Kim Y, Caramori ML, Mauer M (2007) Podocyte detachment and reduced glomerular capillary endothelial fenestration in human type 1 diabetic nephropathy. Diabetes 56: 2155–2160.
22. Deegens JK, Dijkman HB, Borm GF, Steenbergen EJ, van den Berg JG, et al. (2008) Podocyte foot process effacement as a diagnostic tool in focal segmental glomerulosclerosis. Kidney Int 74: 1568–1576.
23. Topham PS, Haydar SA, Kuphal R, Lightfoot JD, Salant DJ (1999) Complement-mediated injury reversibly disrupts glomerular epithelial cell actin microfilaments and focal adhesions. Kidney Int 55: 1763–1775.
24. Gubler MC, Lenoir G, Grunfeld JP, Ulmann A, Droz D, et al. (1978) Early renal changes in hemizygous and heterozygous patients with Fabry's disease. Kidney Int 13: 223–235.
25. Valbuena C, Carvalho E, Bustorff M, Ganhao M, Relvas S, et al. (2008) Kidney biopsy findings in heterozygous Fabry disease females with early nephropathy. Virchows Arch 453: 329–338.
26. Wolf G, Chen S, Ziyadeh FN (2005) From the periphery of the glomerular capillary wall toward the center of disease: podocyte injury comes of age in diabetic nephropathy. Diabetes 54: 1626–1634.
27. Pinto LL, Vieira TA, Giugliani R, Schwartz IV (2010) Expression of the disease on female carriers of X-linked lysosomal disorders: a brief review. Orphanet J - Rare Dis 5: 14.
28. Migeon BR (2006) The role of X inactivation and cellular mosaicism in women's health and sex-specific diseases. JAMA 295: 1428–1433.
29. Aerts JM, Groener JE, Kuiper S, Donker-Koopman WE, Strijland A, et al. (2008) Elevated globotriaosylsphingosine is a hallmark of Fabry disease. Proc Natl Acad Sci U S A 105: 2812–2817.
30. Whybra C, Kampmann C, Krummenauer F, Ries M, Mengel E, et al. (2004) The Mainz Severity Score Index: a new instrument for quantifying the Anderson-Fabry disease phenotype, and the response of patients to enzyme replacement therapy. Clin Genet 65: 299–307.
31. Dobrovolny R, Dvorakova L, Ledvinova J, Magage S, Bultas J, et al. (2005) Relationship between X-inactivation and clinical involvement in Fabry heterozygotes. Eleven novel mutations in the alpha-galactosidase A gene in the Czech and Slovak population. J Mol Med (Berl) 83: 647–654.
32. Elstein D, Schachamorov E, Beeri R, Altarescu G (2012) X-inactivation in Fabry disease. Gene 505: 266–268.
33. Warnock DG, Ortiz A, Mauer M, Linthorst GE, Oliveira JP, et al. (2012) Renal outcomes of agalsidase beta treatment for Fabry disease: role of proteinuria and timing of treatment initiation. Nephrol Dial Transplant 27: 1042–1049.

34. (2013) The Human Gene Mutation Database at the Institute of Medical Genetics in Cardiff.
35. Ashton-Prolla P, Tong B, Shabbeer J, Astrin KH, Eng CM, et al. (2000) Fabry disease: twenty-two novel mutations in the alpha-galactosidase A gene and genotype/phenotype correlations in severely and mildly affected hemizygotes and heterozygotes. J Investig Med 48: 227–235.
36. Eng CM, Ashley GA, Burgert TS, Enriquez AL, D'Souza M, et al. (1997) Fabry disease: thirty-five mutations in the alpha-galactosidase A gene in patients with classic and variant phenotypes. Mol Med 3: 174–182.
37. Bekri S, Enica A, Ghafari T, Plaza G, Champenois I, et al. (2005) Fabry disease in patients with end-stage renal failure: the potential benefits of screening. Nephron Clin Pract 101: c33–38.
38. Wang C, Wang Y, Zhu F, Xiong J (2013) A Missense Mutation of the alpha-Galactosidase A Gene in a Chinese Family of Fabry Disease with Renal Failure. Kidney Blood Press Res 37: 221–228.

Urinary Calprotectin and Posttransplant Renal Allograft Injury

Martin Tepel[1] ❡, Christoffer Borst[1] ❡, Claus Bistrup[1], Niels Marcussen[2], Nikolaos Pagonas[3,4], Felix S. Seibert[3,4], Robert Arndt[3], Walter Zidek[3], Timm H. Westhoff[3,4]*

1 Department of Nephrology, Odense University Hospital, and University of Southern Denmark, Institute of Molecular Medicine, Cardiovascular and Renal Research, Institute of Clinical Research, Odense, Denmark, **2** Department of Pathology, Odense University Hospital, and University of Southern Denmark, Odense, Denmark, **3** Department of Nephrology, Charité, Campus Benjamin Franklin, Berlin, Germany, **4** Medizinische Klinik I, Univ.-Klinik Marienhospital Herne, Ruhr-University Bochum, Bochum, Germany

Abstract

Objective: Current methods do not predict the acute renal allograft injury immediately after kidney transplantation. We evaluated the diagnostic performance of urinary calprotectin for predicting immediate posttransplant allograft injury.

Methods: In a multicenter, prospective-cohort study of 144 incipient renal transplant recipients, we postoperatively measured urinary calprotectin using an enzyme-linked immunosorbent assay and estimated glomerular filtration rate (eGFR) after 4 weeks, 6 months, and 12 months.

Results: We observed a significant inverse association of urinary calprotectin concentrations and eGFR 4 weeks after transplantation (Spearman $r = -0.33$; $P<0.001$). Compared to the lowest quartile, patients in the highest quartile of urinary calprotectin had an increased risk for an eGFR less than 30 mL/min/1.73 m^2 four weeks after transplantation (relative risk, 4.3; $P<0.001$; sensitivity, 0.92; 95% CI, 0.77 to 0.98; specificity, 0.48; 95% CI, 0.31 to 0.66). Higher urinary calprotectin concentrations predicted impaired kidney function 4 weeks after transplantation, as well as 6 months and 12 months after transplantation. When data were analyzed using the urinary calprotectin/creatinine-ratio similar results were obtained. Urinary calprotectin was superior to current use of absolute change of plasma creatinine to predict allograft function 12 months after transplantation. Urinary calprotectin predicted an increased risk both in transplants from living and deceased donors. Multivariate linear regression showed that higher urinary calprotectin concentrations and older donor age predicted lower eGFR four weeks, 6 months, and 12 months after transplantation.

Conclusions: Urinary calprotectin is an early, noninvasive predictor of immediate renal allograft injury after kidney transplantation.

Editor: Stanislaw Stepkowski, University of Toledo, United States of America

Funding: This work was supported by Deutsche Forschungsgemeinschaft (German Research Foundation, Research Unit FOR 1368) and the European Union (Interreg 4A, grant number 62-1.2-10). The funders had no role in study design, data collection and analysis, decision to publish, or preparation of the manuscript.

* Email: timm.westhoff@marienhospital-herne.de

❡ These authors contributed equally to this work.

Introduction

The immediate function of a renal allograft within the first weeks after kidney transplantation may vary considerably. The renal allograft may immediately start urine production. In contrast, the renal allograft may be damaged. An impaired renal allograft function within the first weeks or within the first year is detrimental to the longevity of the allograft and accounts for a 40% decrease in long-term graft survival [1–5]. A major role of ischemia-reperfusion injury for impaired renal allograft function has been confirmed in the literature [6].

Current methods do not predict the acute renal allograft injury immediately after kidney transplantation [7]. Recently, urinary calprotectin concentrations have been identified as a marker of acute kidney injury in the non-transplant population [8,9]. Calprotectin is a calcium-binding complex of two proteins of the so-called S100 group. It serves as a mediator protein of the innate immune system. Calprotectin is derived predominantly from neutrophils and mononuclear cells and activates Toll-like receptor 4 thereby amplifying inflammatory activity [10]. The innate immune system plays a crucial role in the pathophysiology of ischemia-reperfusion injury in the kidney. Neutrophils and macrophages migrate into the transplant within 6 h of reperfusion and release proinflammatory cytokines and other soluble inflammatory mediators [11]. After ischemia-reperfusion injury of the tubular epithelial cells, Toll-like receptor 4 maintains and amplifies the inflammatory response [12]. In the present study we tested the hypothesis that urinary calprotectin at the first postoperative days predicts acute renal allograft injury and allograft function, i.e. estimated glomerular filtration rate (eGFR) 4 weeks, 6 months, and 12 months after transplantation.

Materials and Methods

Approval

The study protocol was in accordance with the ethical standards of the Declarations of Helsinki and Istanbul. The study was approved by the local ethics committees (Den Videnskabsetiske Komite for Region Syddanmark, Projekt-ID: 8-20100098 and Ethik-Komitee Charité Universitätsmedizin Berlin).

Study population

We performed a multicenter prospective-cohort study of 144 patients receiving kidney transplants. Patients who were at least 18 years old and who were scheduled to receive living donor kidney transplants or deceased donor kidney transplants were recruited. Written informed consent was obtained from all patients before entry into the study. Baseline characteristics of donors and recipients and information on organ procurement were prospectively obtained from medical records. Induction therapy, immunosuppressive therapy, concomitant medications, and transplant biopsy were all made by the clinicians at each institution according to their local protocols. Delayed graft function was defined by at least one dialysis session within 7 days of transplantation [13]. Hemodialysis within 1 week after transplantation was performed because of uremic symptoms (29% of cases), hypervolemia causing dyspnoe (50% of cases), hyperkalemia (21% of cases). The treating physicians were unaware of the calprotectin concentrations. During follow up, one recipient died during the first year posttransplant due to a cardiovascular event. Six recipients lost graft function during the first year posttransplant. eGFR was available after 12 months in 123 patients.

Enzyme-linked immunosorbent assay for urinary calprotectin and urinary kidney injury molecule-1

We collected one urine sample postoperatively. We aliquoted urine supernatants into cryovials, labeled each with a random barcode, and stored samples at −20°C. The enzyme-linked immunosorbent assay (ELISA) for urinary calprotectin was performed as previously published by our group using the PhiCal-Calprotectin assay kit (Immundiagnostik AG, Bensheim, Germany) according to the manufacturer's protocol [8,9]. Calprotectin concentrations were measured by personnel blinded to patient information. The coefficient of variation was less than 6% Urinary kidney injury molecule-1 (KIM-1) concentrations was measured using ELISA kits according to the manufacturer's protocol (dianova, Hamburg, Germany). The coefficient of variation was less than 10%.

Assessment of allograft function

Plasma creatinine was routinely measured. The absolute change in plasma creatinine was calculated as plasma creatinine preoperatively minus the first postoperative day. Four weeks, 6 months, and 12 months after transplantation we determined estimated glomerular filtration rate (eGFR) in kidney recipients according to the Chronic Kidney Disease Epidemiology Collaboration (CKD-EPI) equation [14].

$$eGFR = 141 \times \min(Cr/\kappa,1)^{\alpha} \times \max(Cr/\kappa,1)^{-1.209} \times 0.993^{Age} \times 1.018$$

[if female] × 1.159 [if black], where Cr is plasma creatinine in mg/dL, κ is 0.7 for females and 0.9 for males, α is −0.329 for females and −0.411 for males, min indicates the minimum of Cr/κ or 1, and max indicates the maximum of Cr/κ or 1.

CKD-EPI equation is recommended in transplanted patients because it more accurately gives true glomerular filtration rate measured by plasma clearance of (99 m)Tc-diethylenetriamine pentaacetic acid [15].

Histological findings

In 98 patients a baseline biopsy was performed at transplantation as benchmark for comparison of post-transplantation histology in case a post-transplant indication biopsy was necessary. Median number of glomeruli in the baseline biopsy was 7 (IQR, 3 to 11). The severity of lesions (arteriolar hyalinosis, arteriolosclerosis, interstitial fibrosis) was scored semiquantitatively as published [16,17].

Statistics

Continuous data are presented as median and interquartile range (IQR). Non-parametric Mann-Whitney test or Kruskal-Wallis test with Dunn's Multiple Comparison Test were used as appropriate to detect differences between the groups. Frequency counts were calculated for categorical data. Differences in these categorical variables between the groups were analyzed by Chi-square test or Fisher's exact text as appropriate. Associations between variables were determined using non-parametric Spearman correlation. We performed receiver operating characteristic (ROC) curve analysis to detect the accuracy of urinary calprotectin, urinary KIM-1, and absolute change in plasma creatinine for predicting eGFR after transplantation.

We performed linear regression for associations between urinary calprotectin and eGFR four weeks after kidney transplantation while adjusting for donor age, donor gender, living-donor vs. deceased-donor status, recipient age, recipient gender, delayed graft function, recipient months on dialysis before transplantation, and use of prednisolone. For regression analyses urinary calprotectin concentrations were log-transformed to obtain normal distributed data to obtain normal distributed data as tested by Kolmogoroff-Smirnov-test. Multivariate models were constructed with backward variable selection, using $P<0.05$ for variable retention.

Data were analyzed using GraphPad prism software (version 5.0, GraphPad Software, San Diego, CA, USA) and SPSS for windows (version 15.0; SPSS, Chicago, IL, USA). All statistical tests were two-sided. Two-sided p-values less than 0.05 were considered to indicate statistical significance.

Results

Characteristics of cohort at baseline

Urinary calprotectin concentrations were measured in 144 patients after renal allograft transplantation. 85 transplant recipients were male (59%), and 59 were female (41%). Median age of recipients was 52 years (IQR, 45 to 59 years). The cause of chronic kidney disease was diabetic nephropathy in 14 cases (10%), hypertensive nephropathy in 19 cases (13%), chronic glomerulonephritis in 53 cases (37%), polycystic kidney disease in 22 cases (15%), and other/unknown in 36 cases (25%). The number of patients with second or more transplants was 17 (12%). Median time on dialysis before transplantation was 26 months (IQR, 4 to 71 months). 31 patients (22%) were smokers, 125 patients (87%) had hypertension, and 15 patients (10%) had a history of cardiovascular events. There was no association of calprotectin and cardiac events (Spearman r = 0.08; 95% CI, 0.08 to 0.25; P = 0.31). 68 patients (47%) received kidneys from living

Table 1. Clinical characteristics of 144 patients with renal allograft.

Characteristic	All patients	Q1	Q2	Q3	Q4	P-value
Age of the donor	52	51	56	51	52	0.13
(years)	(45–59)	(45–57)	(49–66)	(46–57)	(43–67)	
Deceased kidney	76	11	19	16	30	<0.001
(number (%))	(53%)	(31%)	(53%)	(44%)	(83%)	
Cold-ischemia time	600	398	754	415	607	0.26
(min)	(290–840)	(163–840)	(293–914)	(166–664)	(447–798)	
HLA mismatches	3	3	3	3	3	0.37
(range, 0 to 6)	(2–4)	(2–4)	(3–4)	(2–4)	(2–4)	
Age of recipient	52	52	53	50	53	0.18
(years)	(45–59)	(40–61)	(39–61)	(42–58)	(48–65)	
Gender male, n (%)	85 (59)	22 (61)	22 (61)	19 (53)	22 (61)	0.86
Duration of dialysis	26	5	29	22	72	<0.001
(months)	(4–71)	(0–32)	(5–68)	(7–59)	(25–90)	
Body weight (kg)	79 (66–89)	74 (64–89)	82 (69–91)	79 (68–97)	77 (65–89)	0.36
Body mass-index	26	24	25	26	26	0.10
(kg/m^2)	(23–29)	(23–27)	(24–28)	(24–30)	(23–29)	
Systolic blood	148	150	152	145	144	0.19
pressure (mmHg)	(130–161)	(135–166)	(136–170)	(124–154)	(128–169)	
Diastolic blood	84	85	87	80	80	0.75
pressure (mmHg)	(76–94)	(76–97)	(78–92)	(75–97)	(71–94)	

Continuous data are presented as median (interquartile range). Data are shown for all patients and according to quartiles (Q) of urinary calprotectin concentrations (with Q1, less than 286 ng/mL; Q2, 286 to 576 ng/mL; Q3, 577 to 1694 ng/mL; Q4, more than 1694 ng/mL). Categorical data are presented as numbers (percent). Groups containing continuous data were compared using Kruskal-Wallis test, whereas groups containing categorical data were compared using Chi-squared test.

donors, and 76 patients (53%) from deceased donors. 101 patients (70%) received tacrolimus, 43 patients (30%) cyclosporine A, 144 patients (100%) mycophenolate acid, and 75 patients (52%) prednisolone, respectively. The clinical characteristics of patients and their allograft are shown in **Table 1**.

Urinary calprotectin concentrations predict allograft function

The median urinary calprotectin concentration was 576 ng/mL (IQR, 286 to 1694 ng/mL). In the lowest calprotectin quartile eGFR was 51 mL/min/1.73 m^2 (IQR, 42 to 63 mL/min/1.73 m^2), then eGFRs were 46 mL/min/1.73 m^2 (IQR, 37 to 56 mL/min/1.73 m^2) and 40 mL/min/1.73 m^2 (IQR, 30 to 49 mL/min/1.73 m^2), and finally in the highest calprotectin quartile eGFR was 33 mL/min/1.73 m^2 (IQR, 21 to 58 mL/min/1.73 m^2) ($P = 0.004$; **Figure 1A**). 6 months after transplantation eGFRs were 52 mL/min/1.73 m^2 (IQR, 41 to 72 mL/min/1.73 m^2) and 40 mL/min/1.73 m^2 (IQR, 26 to 58 mL/min/1.73 m^2) in the lowest and highest calprotectin quartile, respectively ($P<0.05$; **Figure 1B**). 12 months after transplantation eGFRs were 59 mL/min/1.73 m^2 (IQR, 43 to 68 mL/min/1.73 m^2) and 44 mL/min/1.73 m^2 (IQR, 27 to 62 mL/min/1.73 m^2) in the lowest and highest calprotectin quartile, respectively ($P<0.05$; **Figure 1C**).

We observed a significant association of urinary calprotectin levels with eGFR 4 weeks after transplantation (Spearman $r = -0.33$; 95% CI, -0.47 to -0.17; $P<0.001$; **Figure 2A**), 6 months after transplantation (Spearman $r = -0.20$; 95% CI, -0.36 to -0.03; $P = 0.018$), and 12 months after transplantation (Spearman $r = -0.22$; 95% CI, -0.39 to -0.04; $P = 0.015$).

Figure 2B indicates that 48.6% of patients with urinary calprotectin concentrations in the highest quartile (i.e., more than 1694 ng/mL) showed an eGFR in the lowest quartile (i.e., less than 30 mL/min/1.73 m^2) 4 weeks after renal transplantation. On the other hand, only 8.3% of patients with urinary calprotectin concentrations in the lowest quartile (i.e., less than 286 ng/mL) showed an eGFR in the lowest quartile (relative risk, 4.3; $P<0.001$; sensitivity, 0.92; 95% CI, 0.77 to 0.98; specificity, 0.48; 95% CI, 0.31 to 0.66). As the likelihood ratio equals 1.78, patients with higher urinary calprotectin concentrations more likely showed worse renal function.

The predictive effect of urinary calprotectin could be observed both in transplants from living donors and deceased donors. In transplants from living donors the relative risk was 4.9 ($P = 0.039$; sensitivity, 0.94; 95% CI, 0.71 to 1.00; specificity, 0.41; 95% CI, 0.18 to 0.67; likelihood ratio, 1.60). In transplants from deceased donors the relative risk was 3.5 ($P = 0.030$; sensitivity, 0.89; 95% CI, 0.67 to 0.99; specificity, 0.47; 95% CI, 0.24 to 0.71; likelihood ratio, 1.70).

Receiver-operating characteristic (ROC) curves showed that urinary calprotectin was able to predict the eGFR in the lowest quartile (i.e., less than 30 mL/min/1.73 m^2) 4 weeks after renal transplantation. Urinary calprotectin resulted in an area under curve (AUC) of 0.75 (95% CI, 0.66 to 0.84; $P<0.001$).

Figure 3A shows ROC curves and summary data for the AUC according to eGFR 4 weeks after transplantation. Higher values for area under curve were observed with lower eGFR 4 weeks after transplantation, ranging from 0.89 (95% CI, 0.80 to 0.99; $P<0.001$) with eGFR less than 15 mL/min/1.73 m^2 ($n = 7$) to 0.69

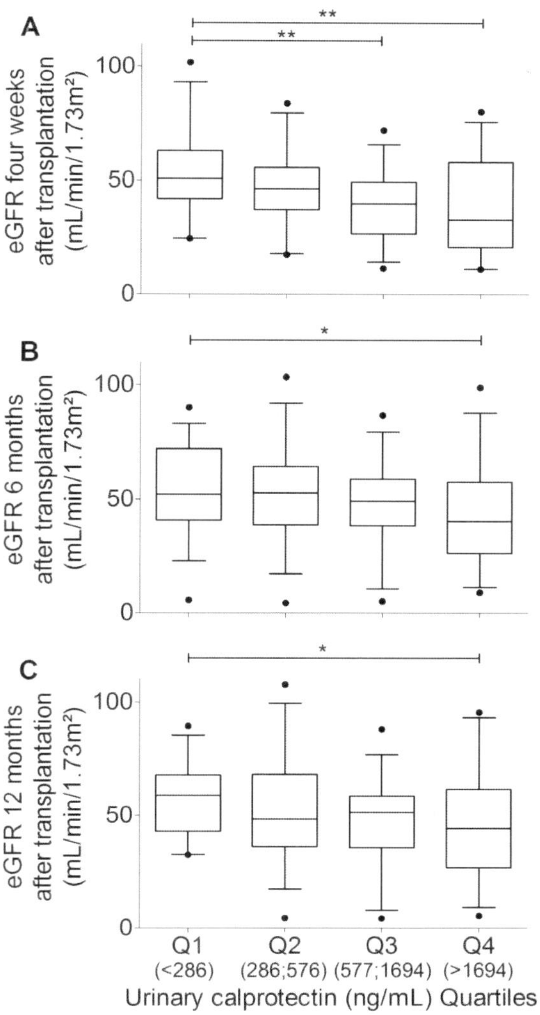

Figure 1. Urinary calprotectin concentrations predict renal allograft function. Box-and-whiskers-plots showing the reduction of estimated glomerular filtration rate (eGFR) four weeks (**A**), 6 months (**B;** n = 135), and 12 months (**C;** n = 123) after transplantation with increasing quartiles (Q) of urinary calprotectin concentrations. Boxes indicate median and interquartile ranges, whiskers indicate 5 to 95 percentile. Significant differences between the shown groups were **P<0.01 and *P<0.05 by Kruskal-Wallis test and Dunn's multiple comparison test.

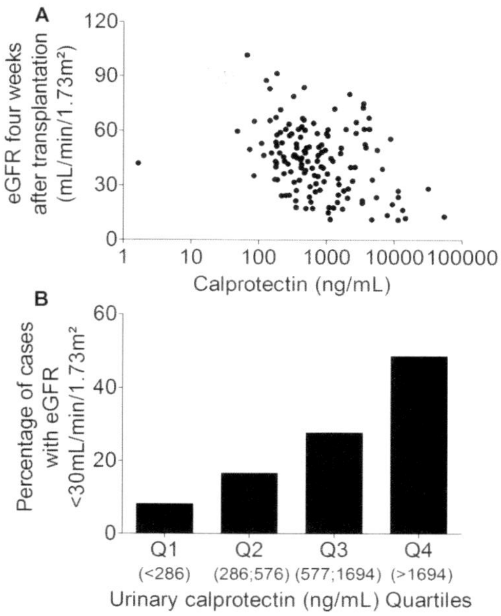

Figure 2. Association of urinary calprotectin with estimated glomerular filtration rate. A. Dot plot depicting the significant association of urinary calprotectin levels (log scale) with estimated glomerular filtration rate (eGFR) four weeks after transplantation. Spearman r = −0.33; P<0.001. **B.** Percentage of cases with estimated glomerular filtration rate (eGFR) after 4 weeks in the lowest quartile (i.e., less than 30 mL/min/1.73 m^2) is shown. Bar graph shows percentages of cases from the contingency table, therefore there are no error bars. Chi-square derived from the contingency table was 17.10; P<0.001.

(95% CI, 0.60 to 0.77; P<0.001) with eGFR less than 40 mL/min/1.73 m^2 (n = 58).

When data were analyzed using the urinary calprotectin/creatinine-ratio similar results were obtained: The median urinary calprotectin/creatinine-ratio was 1.15 ng/g (IQR 0.67 to 3.00 ng/g). In the lowest calprotectin/creatinine quartile eGFR 4 weeks after renal transplantation was 46 mL/min/1.73 m^2 (IQR, 34 to 64 mL/min/1.73 m^2) whereas the highest quartile showed an eGFR of 36 mL/min/1.73 m^2 (IQR, 21 to 55 mL/min/1.73 m^2; P = 0.041). Receiver-operating characteristic (ROC) curves showed that urinary calprotectin/creatinine ratio was able to predict the eGFR in the lowest quartile (i.e., less than 30 mL/min/1.73 m2) 4 weeks after renal transplantation (AUC, 0.66; 95% CI, 0.55 to 0.77; P = 0.004).

For comparison, data were obtained using urinary kidney injury molecule-1 (KIM-1). The median urinary KIM-1 was 0.56 ng/mL (IQR, 0.29 to 1.14 ng/mL). In the lowest KIM-1 quartile eGFR was 48 mL/min/1.73 m^2 (IQR, 28 to 60 mL/min/1.73 m^2), then eGFRs were 34 mL/min/1.73 m^2 (IQR, 24 to 45 mL/min/1.73 m^2) and 40 mL/min/1.73 m^2 (IQR, 33 to 51 mL/min/1.73 m^2), and finally in the highest KIM-1 quartile eGFR was 28 mL/min/1.73 m^2 (IQR, 18 to 44 mL/min/1.73 m^2) (P = 0.06). 6 months after transplantation eGFRs were 54 mL/min/1.73 m^2 (IQR, 38 to 62 mL/min/1.73 m^2) and 34 mL/min/1.73 m^2 (IQR, 25 to 58 mL/min/1.73 m^2) in the lowest and highest KIM-1 quartile, respectively (P = 0.17). 12 months after transplantation eGFRs were 51 mL/min/1.73 m^2 (IQR, 40 to 60 mL/min/1.73 m^2) and 32 mL/min/1.73 m^2 (IQR, 27 to 57 mL/min/1.73 m^2) in the lowest and highest KIM-1 quartile, respectively (P = 0.25). Urinary KIM-1 levels were associated with eGFR 4 weeks after transplantation (Spearman r = −0.23; P = 0.034). We observed that 55.0% of patients with urinary KIM-1 in the highest quartile (i.e., more than 1.14 ng/mL) showed an eGFR in the lowest quartile (i.e., less than 30 mL/min/1.73 m^2) 4 weeks after renal transplantation, and 25.0% of patients with urinary KIM-1 in the lowest quartile (i.e., less than 0.29 ng/mL) showed an eGFR in the lowest quartile (relative risk, 2.0; P = 0.11). As depicted in **Figure 3B** KIM-1 resulted in an AUC of 0.61 (95% CI, 0.48 to 0.75; P = 0.09), indicating that calprotectin, but not KIM-1 predicted the eGFR in the lowest quartile (i.e., less than 30 mL/min/1.73 m^2).

We observed that urinary calprotectin was superior to current use of absolute change of plasma creatinine to predict allograft function. Urinary calprotectin resulted in an AUC of 0.76 (95% CI, 0.65 to 0.88; P<0.001) to predict eGFR less than 30 mL/min/1.73 m^2 12 months after transplantation, whereas the

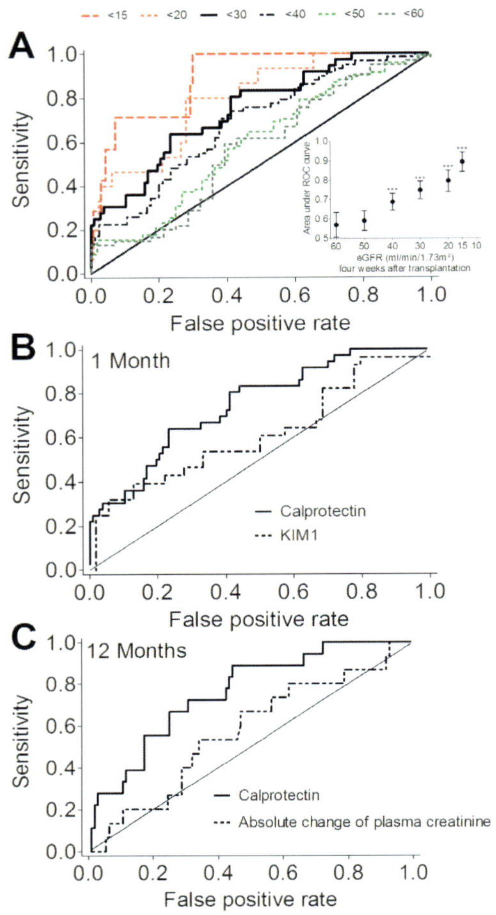

Figure 3. Calprotectin predicts kidney function. A. Receiver-operating characteristic (ROC) curves and summary data (**Inset**) for area under curve showing that urinary calprotectin concentrations predicted impaired kidney function 4 weeks after transplantation. All analyses were performed in the entire population. eGFR after 4 weeks in mL/min/1.73 m^2 are indicated in the legend above the curves. The inset indicates each area under curve per eGFR curve. ***P<0.001. **B.** Receiver-operating characteristic (ROC) curves for urinary calprotectin and urinary kidney injury molecule-1 (KIM-1) concentrations for predicting the eGFR in the lowest quartile (i.e., less than 30 mL/min/1.73 m^2) 1 month after renal transplantation. **C.** Receiver-operating characteristic (ROC) curves for urinary calprotectin and absolute change of plasma creatinine for predicting the eGFR in the lowest quartile (i.e., less than 30 mL/min/1.73 m^2) 12 months after renal transplantation.

absolute change of plasma creatinine resulted in an AUC of 0.57 (95% CI, 0.42 to 0.72; P = 0.38) (**Figure 3C**).

Univariate and multivariate linear regression analyses are shown in **Tables 2 and 3**. Multivariate linear regression showed that higher urinary calprotectin concentrations (P<0.001), older donor age (P<0.001), and delayed graft function (P = 0.039) predicted lower eGFR four weeks after transplantation, but not donor gender, living-donor vs. deceased-donor status, recipient age, recipient gender, recipient months on dialysis before transplantation, or prednisolone. As shown in **Table S1** using mixed model analyses for estimated glomerular filtration rate 4 weeks after kidney transplantation confirmed these results. We also found that that higher urinary calprotectin concentrations and older donor age predicted lower eGFR 6 months as well as 12 months after transplantation.

Median eGFR 4 weeks after transplantation were not significantly different between the subgroups without or with prednisolone (46 mL/min/1.73 m^2; IQR, 33 to 53 mL/min/1.73 m^2; vs. 43 mL/min/1.73 m^2; IQR, 25 to 59 mL/min/1.73 m^2; P = 0.66). Furthermore, median urinary calprotectin concentrations were not significantly different between the subgroups without or with prednisolone (552 ng/mL; IQR, 262 to 1260 ng/mL; vs. 638 ng/mL; IQR 302 to 2239 ng/mL; P = 0.29).

Patients with delayed graft function showed higher urinary calprotectin levels, however that difference was only marginally significant (819 ng/mL; IQR 346 to 2627 ng/mL; vs. 522 ng/mL; IQR, 262 to 1308 ng/mL; P = 0.09). Multivariate logistic regression showed that living-donor vs. deceased-donor status (P = 0.003) predicted delayed graft function. In contrast urinary calprotectin (P = 0.51), donor age (P = 0.54), donor gender (P = 0.68), recipient age (P = 0.57) as well as recipient gender (P = 0.19) did not show significant effects. For delayed graft function urinary calprotectin resulted in an AUC of 0.59 (95% CI, 0.49 to 0.69; P = 0.09). For delayed graft function urinary KIM-1 resulted in an AUC of 0.52 (95% CI, 0.39 to 0.65; P = 0.74).

We also analyzed urinary calprotectin levels in a subgroup of 38 patients who were anuric before renal transplantation. We would like to emphasize that that subgroup of 38 patients were anuric before renal transplantation, but not after transplantation. 5 out of 10 previously anuric patients (50.0%) with urinary calprotectin concentrations in the highest quartile showed a creatinine clearance in the lowest quartile. On the other hand, none out of 10 previously anuric patients (0.0%) with urinary calprotectin concentrations in the lowest quartile showed a creatinine clearance in the lowest quartile (P = 0.03).

Histological findings

Histological evaluation could be performed in 98 baseline biopsies obtained at the time of transplantation. Urinary calprotectin concentrations were similar in patients receiving a graft without or with arteriolar hyalinosis (grade 0, median, 426 ng/mL (IQR, 233 to 1643 ng/mL); vs. grade >0, median, 659 ng/mL (IQR, 357 to 1260 ng/mL; P = 0.29)). Urinary calprotectin concentrations were also similar in patients receiving a graft without or with arteriolosclerosis (grade 0, median, 463 ng/mL (IQR, 238 to 1204 ng/mL) vs. grade 1, median, 616 ng/mL (IQR, 355 to 1191 ng/mL; P = 0.52)) and receiving a graft without or with interstitial fibrosis (grade 0, median, 478 ng/mL (IQR, 241 to 1476 ng/mL) vs. grade 1, median, 724 ng/mL (IQR, 390 to 1024 ng/mL; P = 0.59)). Only 13 patients had suspected rejection during the first 4 postoperative weeks, only 1 patient showed BANFF grade 1A rejection. These data may indicate that preexisting renal lesions per se may not affect postoperative urinary calprotectin concentrations.

Discussion

In the present study we showed that postoperative urinary calprotectin predicts kidney allograft function after transplantation. We observed that use of urinary calprotectin was superior to current use of absolute change of plasma creatinine to predict allograft function after transplantation. It is noteworthy to acknowledge the biologically plausible role of calprotectin in the mechanisms of ischemic reperfusion injury after kidney transplantation. The tubular damage leads to a secondary activation of the innate immune system with immigration of granulocytes and monocytes. Moreover it leads to an amplification and activation of toll-like receptors [18]. Calprotectin is a ligand of toll-like receptors, which is constitutively expressed in both proximal and

Table 2. Univariate linear regression analyses for estimated glomerular filtration rate 4 weeks after kidney transplantation.

Variable	B	SE of B	P	95% CI of B
Urinary calprotectin	−8.391	2.432	0.001	−13.201 to −3.580
Donor age	−0.577	0.120	<0.001	−0.814 to −0.339
Donor gender (0 = female; 1 = male)	5.168	2.755	0.063	−0.283 to 10.619
Donor status (0 = LD; 1 = DD)	−3.308	3.493	0.345	−10.219 to 3.603
Recipient age	−0.040	0.117	0.735	−0.271 to 0.192
Recipient gender (0 = female; 1 = male)	1.212	2.801	0.666	−4.329 to 6.753
Delayed graft function (0 = no DGF; 1 = DGF)	−5.638	3.409	0.101	−12.382 to 1.106
Duration of dialysis before transplantation (months)	−0.005	0.040	0.897	−0.084 to 0.074
Prednisolone (0 = no; 1 = yes)	2.002	3.223	0.536	−4.374 to 8.379

B indicates regression coefficient; SE indicates standard error; CI indicates confidence interval. Calprotectin was analyzed as a continuous variable. Regression analyses were performed after logarithmic transformation of urinary calprotectin concentrations.
LD indicates living donor; DD indicates deceased donor. DGF indicates delayed graft function.

distal tubules [19]. Hall et al. [20] reported that neutrophil gelatinase-associated lipocalin predicted dialysis within one week after kidney transplantation. They reported that 34 out of 91 patients (37%) had delayed graft function, defined by at least one dialysis session within the first postoperative week [20]. However, it is well-known that the clinical decision to perform postoperative hemodialysis may be influenced by several factors beyond renal allograft function, for example fluid overload and clinical uremic status of the patient.

Looking at the results for urinary calprotectin and urinary KIM-1 it may be speculated that an increased neutrophil and macrophage response to ischemia-reperfusion injury may cause increased calprotectin levels. This may be supported by the finding that urinary calprotectin but not urinary KIM-1 was significantly associated with renal allograft function.

A study by Szeto et al. in 63 kidney transplant recipients investigated urinary mRNA of neutrophil gelatinase-associated lipocalin, kidney injury molecule-1, interleukin-18, surfactant protein-C, and S100 calcium-binding proteins A8 and A9 according to histologic groups observed in biopsies from biopsy because of progressive worsening of allograft function. They showed that urinary mRNA of KIM-1 may provide prognostic information about renal function decline, irrespective of the kidney pathology [21]. No data are available for urinary calprotectin protein and pathology because of progressive worsening of allograft function.

The present study confirms previous reports that donor age has a large impact on allograft function. However, there is no treatment to adjust for the fact of using allografts from older subjects. It should be noted that urinary calprotectin predicted allograft function even after adjustment for donor age. Hence, measurements of urinary calprotectin may add to the diagnostic procedures.

Beside the use of urinary calprotectin for prediction of immediate renal allograft injury, its determination immediately after kidney transplantation may be helpful and a necessary step for the implementation of future strategies to improve outcome after kidney transplantation. In summary, urinary calprotectin is an early, noninvasive predictor of acute renal allograft injury after kidney transplantation.

Table 3. Multivariate linear regression analyses for estimated glomerular filtration rate 4 weeks, 6 months and 12 months after kidney transplantation.

Variable	B	SE of B	P	95% CI of B
4 weeks after transplantation				
Urinary calprotectin	−9.636	2.199	<0.001	−13.985 to −5.287
Donor age	−0.571	0.115	<0.001	−0.797 to −0.344
Delayed graft function	−5.925	2.839	0.039	−11.539 to −0.312
6 months after transplantation				
Urinary calprotectin	−5.516	2.416	0.024	−10.295 to −0.737
Donor age	−0.808	0.127	<0.001	−1.058 to −0.557
12 months after transplantation				
Urinary calprotectin	−5.895	2.816	0.038	−11.470 to −0.318
Donor age	−0.735	0.148	<0.001	−1.027 to −0.443

B indicates regression coefficient; SE indicates standard error; CI indicates confidence interval. Calprotectin was analyzed as a continuous variable. Regression analyses were performed after logarithmic transformation of urinary calprotectin concentrations.
LD indicates living donor; DD indicates deceased donor. DGF indicates delayed graft function.

Acknowledgments

Supported by Deutsche Forschungsgemeinschaft (German Research Foundation, Research Unit FOR 1368) and the European Union (Interreg 4A, grant number 62-1.2-10).

Author Contributions

Conceived and designed the experiments: MT THW. Performed the experiments: MT C. Borst C. Bistrup NM NP FS RA WZ THW. Analyzed the data: MT C. Borst C. Bistrup NM NP FS RA WZ THW. Contributed reagents/materials/analysis tools: MT C. Borst C. Bistrup NM NP FS RA WZ THW. Contributed to the writing of the manuscript: MT C. Borst C. Bistrup NM NP FS RA WZ THW.

References

1. Siedlecki A, Irish W, Brennan DC (2011) Delayed graft function in the kidney transplant. Am J Transplant 11: 2279–2296.
2. Yarlagadda SG, Coca SG, Formica RN, Poggio ED, Parikh CR (2009) Association between delayed graft function and allograft and patient survival: a systematic review and meta-analysis. Nephrol Dial Transplant 24: 1039–1047.
3. Hariharan S, McBride MA, Cherikh WS, Tolleris CB, Bresnahan BA, et al. (2002) Post-transplant renal function in the first year predicts long-term kidney transplant survival. Kidney Int 62: 311–318.
4. Resende L, Guerra J, Santana A, Mil-Homens C, Abreu F, et al. (2009) First year renal function as a predictor of kidney allograft outcome. Transplant Proc 41: 846–848.
5. Raimundo M, Guerra J, Teixeira C, Santana A, Silva S, et al. (2013) Intermediate early graft function is associated with increased incidence of graft loss and worse long-term graft function in kidney transplantation. Transplant Proc 45: 1070–1072.
6. Terasaki PI, Cecka JM, Gjertson DW, Takemoto S (1995) High survival rates of kidney transplants from spousal and living unrelated donors. N Engl J Med 333: 333–336.
7. Knoll GA (2009) Predicting the ideal serum creatinine level following kidney transplantation. Nat Clin Pract Nephrology 5: 72–73.
8. Heller F, Frischmann S, Grünbaum M, Zidek W, Westhoff TH (2011) Urinary calprotectin and the distinction between prerenal and intrinsic acute kidney injury. Clin J Am Soc Nephrol 6: 2347–2355.
9. Seibert FS, Pagonas N, Arndt R, Heller F, Dragun D, et al. (2013) Calprotectin and neutrophil gelatinase-associated lipocalin in the differentiation of pre-renal and intrinsic acute kidney injury. Acta Physiol 207: 700–708.
10. Vogl T, Tenbrock K, Ludwig S, Leukert N, Ehrhardt C, et al. (2007) Mrp8 and Mrp14 are endogenous activators of Toll-like receptor 4, promoting lethal, endotoxin-induced shock. Nat Med 13: 1042–1049.
11. Li L, Okusa MD (2010) Macrophages, dendritic cells, and kidney ischemia-reperfusion injury. Semin Nephrol 30: 268–277.
12. Anders HJ (2010) Toll-like receptors and danger signaling in kidney injury. J Am Soc Nephrol 21: 1270–1274.
13. Daly PJ, Power RE, Healy DA, Hickey DP, Fitzpatrick JM, et al. (2005) Delayed graft function: a dilemma in renal transplantation. BJU Int 96: 498–501.
14. Levey AS, Stevens LA, Schmid CH, Zhang YL, Castro AF, et al. (2009) A new equation to estimate glomerular filtration rate. Ann Intern Med 150: 604–612.
15. White CA, Akbari A, Doucette S, Fergusson D, Knoll GA (2010) Estimating glomerular filtration rate in kidney transplantation: is the new chronic kidney disease epidemiology collaboration equation any better? Clin Chem 56: 474–477.
16. Sis B, Mengel M, Haas M, Colvin RB, Halloran PF, et al. (2010) Banff '09 meeting report: antibody mediated graft deterioration and implementation of Banff working groups. Am J Transplant 10: 464–471.
17. De Vusser K, Lerut E, Kuypers D, Vanrenterghem Y, Jochmans I, et al. (2013) The predictive value of kidney allograft baseline biopsies for long-term graft survival. J Am Soc Nephrol 24: 1913–1923.
18. Wen X, Murugan R, Peng Z, Kellum JA (2010) Pathophysiology of acute kidney injury: a new perspective. Contrib Nephrol 165: 39–45.
19. Fujiu K, Manabe I, Nagai R (2011) Renal collecting duct epithelial cells regulate inflammation in tubulointerstitial damage in mice. J Clin Invest 121: 3425–3441.
20. Hall IE, Yarlagadda SG, Coca SG, Wang Z, Doshi M, et al. (2010) IL-18 and urinary NGAL predict dialysis and graft recovery after kidney transplantation. J Am Soc Nephrol 21: 189–197.
21. Szeto CC, Kwan BC, Lai KB, Lai FM, Chow KM, et al. (2010) Urinary expression of kidney injury markers in renal transplant recipients. Clin J Am Soc Nephrol 5: 2329–2337.

17

Outcome of Patients with Primary Immune-Complex Type Mesangiocapillary Glomerulonephritis (MCGN) in Cape Town South Africa

Ikechi G. Okpechi[1]*, Thandiwe A. L. Dlamini[1], Maureen Duffield[2], Brian L. Rayner[1], George Moturi[3], Charles R. Swanepoel[1]

1 Division of Nephrology and Hypertension, Groote Schuur Hospital and University of Cape Town, South Africa, **2** Division of Anatomical Pathology, National Health and Laboratory Services (NHLS), University of Cape Town, South Africa, **3** Department of Medicine, Aga Khan University Hospital, Nairobi, Kenya

Abstract

Background and Aim: Mesangiocapillary glomerulonephritis (MCGN) is a common cause of chronic kidney disease in developing countries. Data on the renal outcome of patients with idiopathic MCGN is limited. The aim of this study is to investigate the outcome of patients with idiopathic MCGN presenting to the Groote Schuur Hospital (GSH) Renal Unit in Cape Town.

Materials and Methods: A retrospective study of patients with idiopathic MCGN followed up at our clinic. Seventy-nine patients with no identifiable cause of MCGN were included for analysis. A composite renal outcome of persistent doubling of serum creatinine or end stage renal disease (ESRD) was used. Kaplan Meier survival and Cox regression analysis were used to assess survival and identify factors predicting the outcome.

Results: The mean age at biopsy was 33.9±13.6 years and 41.8% were black. Mean duration of follow up was 13.5±18.8 months. Twenty-three patients (34.2%) reached the composite endpoint. Overall, median renal survival was 38.7±11.7 months (95% CI 15.7–61.8) with 2-year and 5-year renal survival of 61% and 40.3% respectively. No significant difference was found for renal survival between males and females, treatment or non-treatment with immunosuppression, presence or absence of crescents or histological type of MCGN ($p>0.05$). On univariate Cox-regression analysis, factors found to be associated with the outcome were the estimated glomerular filtration rate at biopsy (OR 0.97 [95%CI: 0.95–0.99], $p<0.0001$), black race (OR 3.03 [95%CI: 1.27–7.21], $p=0.012$) and presence of interstitial fibrosis in the biopsy (OR 2.64 [95%CI: 1.07–6.48], $p=0.034$). Age, systolic blood pressure and attaining complete or partial remission approached significant values with the endpoint.

Conclusions: The outcome of idiopathic MCGN in Cape Town is poor and requires further prospective studies to improve our understanding of this common disease.

Editor: Giuseppe Remuzzi, Mario Negri Institute for Pharmacological Research and Azienda Ospedaliera Ospedali Riuniti di Bergamo, Italy

Funding: The authors have no support or funding to report.

* Email: Ikechi.Okpechi@uct.ac.za

Introduction

Mesangiocapillary glomerulonephritis (MCGN; also known as membranoproliferative GN [MPGN]) is a histological pattern of glomerular injury characterized by mesangial hypercellularity, increased mesangial matrix and thickening of glomerular capillary walls secondary to subendothelial deposition of immune complexes and/or complement factors, cellular entrapment, and new basement membrane formation [1,2]. MCGN has traditionally been divided into three distinct morphological types: type I (classical MCGN), is characterized by the presence of subendothelial deposits of immune complexes; type II MCGN (dense deposit disease), characterized by the presence of dense deposits in the basement membrane and type III MCGN, (considered as a variant of type I) and characterized by the presence of additional subepithelial deposits.

MCGN is a common cause of glomerulonephritis and the nephrotic syndrome in many low to middle income countries but especially in Africa [3–8]. In Romania, MCGN was the most frequent primary glomerulonephritis (GN) and was responsible for 29.4% of all primary glomerulonephritides reported from 1995 to 2004 [3]. In a previous study from our centre, we reported MCGN to account for 20.4% of all primary GN with 90.4% of cases being type I MCGN [6]. However, IgA nephropathy remains the most common primary glomerular disease reported from many developed countries where the occurrence of primary MCGN has steadily declined in recent decades [9–12]. Although the "hygiene hypothesis" [13,14] may explain some of the differences in prevalence of glomerular diseases seen in emerging and developed countries, results from recent research in this field has now made some authors to question the existence of idiopathic MCGN [15]. Their doubt is predominantly borne out of advances in methods of analysis of biopsy specimens and a more thorough and detailed evaluation of patients to identify possible causes of so-called idiopathic MCGN [15]. However, these studies have been published from high income countries where IgAN is still predominant. Sethi et al have therefore proposed a new classification for MCGN based on immune complex deposition (with or without complement) and sole complement deposition in the glomerulus denoting dysregulation of the alternative pathway of complement [16] (see Figure S1 and Figure 2).

The treatment recommendation of the KDIGO on the use of immunotherapies in idiopathic MCGN is only limited to cases in which crescents are present [17] and treatment of adults with the disease is often unrewarding as approximately 60% of patients will progress to end-stage renal disease (ESRD) within 10 years [18–20]. Given that so-called idiopathic MCGN is the most frequent primary GN seen in our population, the aim of this study is to report on the outcome of patients in Cape Town with idiopathic MCGN and to identify the factors that predict renal outcomes in such patients who are longitudinally followed up in our centre.

Materials and Methods

Ethics Statement

The study received approval from the Human Research Ethics Committee (HREC REF: 227/2012) of the University of Cape Town. All patient records/information was anonymized and de-identified prior to analysis.

Study population

Hospital records of patients who had a kidney biopsy performed between January 2000 to December 2011 and who were diagnosed with idiopathic MCGN and followed up at the renal clinic at Groote Schuur Hospital Cape Town were retrieved for retrospective collection of data. The written records and the electronic records of these patients were rigorously assessed in order to exclude patients with MCGN with possible secondary cause. All selected patients were proven to have tested negative for common viral infections (HIV, Hepatitis B and C), other commonly encountered infections (such as mycobacterium tuberculosis, syphilis) and autoimmune diseases (lupus and rheumatoid arthritis). As these patients were not acutely ill at presentation or showing evidence for any chronic infections, tests for malaria, schistosomiasis, leprosy among other possible infections that have been reported to be associated with MCGN were not performed; and although these infections are unusual in Cape Town, the patients never manifested any features of them during follow up. Serum protein electrophoresis, urine protein electrophoresis and bone marrow biopsy were not clinically indicated and were thus not performed in our patients. We identified 85 patients with complete records and with no known secondary causes of MCGN but excluded 6 patients whose biopsies only had C3 complement deposits alone.

Data Collection

Demographic, clinical and biochemical records of patients included in the study were obtained at the time of biopsy and during follow-up visits to the renal clinic. Data collected therefore included age at time of biopsy, gender, indication for biopsy, duration of follow up, serial recorded blood pressures (systolic and diastolic) and various laboratory measurements (serum albumin, creatinine, cholesterol, complements (C3 and C4 – expressed as normal or low) and proteinuria [g/24 hrs]. The racial grouping of our patient population was categorized as Black Africans and non-Black Africans (to include patients of mixed ancestry and Whites). The estimated glomerular filtration rate was calculated using the Modification of Diet in Renal Disease (MDRD) formula [21]. Treatment received by the patients was also recorded.

Histology

Light microscopic and immunohistochemical features of the renal biopsies were noted and recorded. Histological data collected included number of glomeruli per biopsy, percentage of sclerosed glomeruli reported, degree of interstitial fibrosis (none, mild, moderate or severe), presence of crescentic lesions and type of deposit present on immunohistochemical analysis (IgA, IgG, IgM or C3). All patients included had immune complex type MCGN (immune complex deposits were present with or without complement deposit) according to the newly proposed classification of Sethi et al [16]. Those with only C3 deposits were excluded in the analysis. Electron microscopic examination of all biopsy specimens was performed. All the histological specimens were reviewed by one pathologist (M.D.).

Definitions used in this study

Blood pressure. Hypertension was defined as systolic BP (SBP) persistently ≥140 mmHg and/or diastolic BP (DBP) ≥ 90 mmHg or if on treatment with anti-hypertensive medications [22]. Blood pressure at biopsy and average BP during follow up visits were recorded.

Remission. As there is no guideline for defining remission in MCGN, we used the following criteria and categorized patients into 3 groups: complete remission (CR), partial remission (PR) or no remission (NR) [23]:

- CR was defined as proteinuria of <0.2 g/day with stable eGFR if normal at baseline or increase in eGFR by 25% if abnormal at baseline.
- PR was defined as reduction in proteinuria (for proteinuria between 0.2 and 2.9 g) and stable eGFR if normal at baseline or increase in eGFR by 25% if abnormal at baseline.
- NR was defined as persistent proteinuria of ≥3 g/day or progressive or worsening renal impairment.

Study end-point

The composite end point of this study was persistent doubling of the serum creatinine over the baseline value or end-stage renal disease (ESRD). For patients who reached the end point, the period of follow-up was the interval between first renal biopsy and the time the end point was reached.

Statistics

The data were analyzed using IBM SPSS Statistics 21 software (SPSS, Chicago, IL). Categorical variables were presented as percentages and continuous variables as means ± SD. Comparison was made between those reaching the end-point and those not reaching the end-point using the Student's t-test, chi-square test or Fisher's exact test. Estimate of survival was done using the Kaplan–Meier survival method. Renal survival with time to ESRD was assessed using Kaplan–Meier estimates and log-rank test for comparison of survival estimates between groups. Univariate analysis was performed using Cox regression analysis to assess the association between relapse-free survival and explanatory variables. Significant P-value was taken as $P<0.05$.

Results

Baseline characteristics of the patients

There were a total of 79 patients eligible for inclusion in the study with renal biopsy diagnosis of MCGN and with no clinical or biochemical evidence for a secondary cause of MCGN. The mean age of all the patients was 33.9±13.6 years with 74.7% of the patients being males. Racial distribution of the subjects was 41.8%, 54.4% and 3.8% for blacks, patients of mixed ancestry and whites respectively. We observed that 20.3% of the patients were either actively abusing substance (predominantly methamphetamines – called "*Tik*" in Cape Town) or were referred to us from a correctional services department for treatment. Nephrotic syndrome was by far the most frequent indication for renal biopsy in 77.9%. Other features at time of biopsy are shown in Table 1.

Histological characteristics of the renal biopsies

Table 2 summarizes the histological features of the biopsies. The average number of glomeruli per biopsy was 16.5±10.5 with an average of 6.2% glomeruli reported as sclerosed. In 63.5% the interstitium was completely normal with no evidence of fibrosis at the time of biopsy; severe interstitial fibrosis was present in 4.1%. IgM deposits (59.4%) and C3 deposits (69.8%) were more frequently seen.

Comparison of the features of patients reaching or not reaching end-point

Twenty-three of 79 patients (34.2%) reached the end-point. There were more black African patients reaching end-point than non-black patients (60.9% vs 33.9%; p = 0.044). Average of all systolic and diastolic blood pressures during follow up visits were significantly higher in those who reached the end-point than in those who did not reach the end-point ($p<0.05$) (Table 3). However, SBP and DBP at initial presentation, although higher in those reaching the end-point were not significantly different. A significantly higher proportion of patients had attained a complete or partial remission at six months after diagnosis in those not reaching end-point than in those who did (36.2% vs 4.8%; p = 0.007).

The frequencies of immune (IgA, IgG and IgM) or complement (C3) deposits observed in the biopsies were not significantly different in both groups. Presence of any interstitial fibrosis (mild, moderate or severe) was significantly higher in the group reaching end-point (56.5% vs 30.4%; p = 0.041); although there were more patients in the group that reached end-point with crescentic lesion present on biopsy, this was not significantly different between the 2 groups. Of all the biochemical features, only serum creatinine (and estimated GFR) at presentation were significantly different between the 2 groups (Table 4). Those who reached the end-point had a significantly higher value of serum creatinine (p = 0.001) at the time of renal biopsy (which was usually the first presentation of the patient). There were more patients in the end-

Table 1. Demographic, clinical and biochemical features of all the patients.

Baseline characteristics (n = 79)	Value
Mean age (years)	33.9±13.6
Gender (Male) (%)	74.7
Ethnicity (%):	
- Blacks	41.8
- Mixed ancestry	54.4
- Whites	3.8
Mean duration of follow-up (months)	13.5±18.8
Hypertension at biopsy (%)	65.8
Oedema present at biopsy (%)	84.8
History of substance abuse or incarceration (%)	20.3
History of schizophrenia (%)	5.1
SBP at biopsy (mmHg)	159.9±30.1
DBP at biopsy (mmHg)	95.8±17.8
Indication for renal biopsy (%):	
- Nephrotic syndrome	77.9
- Nephrotic-nephritic syndrome	10.3
- AKI	5.9
Serum albumin at biopsy (g/L)	25.9±7.3
Serum cholesterol at biopsy (mmol/L)	6.7±2.3
Serum creatinine at biopsy (μmol/L)	180.6±166.8
Estimated MDRD GFR at biopsy (ml/min/1.73 m^2)	65.1±35.2
Proteinuria at biopsy (g/24 hrs)	8.2±6.4
Low complement C3 at biopsy (%)	15.2
Low complement C4 at biopsy (%)	-

SBP – Systolic blood pressure, DBP – Diastolic blood pressure, AKI – Acute kidney injury, MDRD – Modification of diet in renal failure, GFR – Glomerular filtration rate.

Table 2. Histological features of the renal biopsies (n = 79).

Variable	Value
Number of glomeruli	16.5±10.5
Interstitial fibrosis (%):	
- No fibrosis	63.5
- Mild fibrosis	24.3
- Moderate fibrosis	8.1
- Severe fibrosis	4.1
Mean percentage of sclerosed glomeruli (%)	6.2
Crescentic lesions present (%)	17.1
Immunohistochemical features (%):	
- IgA deposit present	18.8
- IgG deposit present	43.8
- IgM deposit present	59.4
- C3 deposit present	69.8

Ig – Immunoglobulin, C3 – Complement 3.

point group with low serum complement; however, this was not significantly different from those not reaching the end-point.

As treatment often followed a conservative care approach, use of an angiotensin converting enzyme inhibitor (ACE-i) or angiotensin receptor blocker (ARB) was common but was not significantly different between the 2 groups (87.0% vs 92.9%; p = 0.409). There were more patients who reached endpoint that received immunosuppression therapy: prednisone: 52.2% vs 25.0%; p = 0.034, pulse cyclophosphamide: 26.1% vs 8.9%; p = 0.071, Azathioprine: 8.7% vs 3.6%; p = 0.635).

Survival Analysis

The cumulative renal survival curve is shown in Figure 1. Overall, the median renal survival was 38.7±11.7 months (95% confidence interval [95%CI]: 15.7–61.8) with 2-year and 5-year renal survival being 61.0% and 40.3% respectively. Kaplan-Meier

Table 3. Comparison of clinical and histological factors associated with outcome.

Factors	End-point		p
	NO (n = 56)	YES (n = 23)	
Age at biopsy (years)	33.0±12.6	36.1±16.0	0.364
Duration of follow-up (Months)	11.6±17.1	17.9±22.1	0.178
Gender (Male) (%)	71.4	82.6	0.398
Race (%):			**0.044**
- Blacks	33.9	60.9	
- Non-Blacks	66.1	39.1	
Hypertension at biopsy (%)	64.3	69.6	0.796
SBP at initial presentation (mmHg)	155.3±29.4	167.9±30.6	0.198
Average SBP at follow-up (mmHg)	141.7±19.8	168.1±30.1	**0.003**
DBP at initial presentation (mmHg)	93.4±18.5	100.0±16.3	0.257
Average DBP at follow-up (mmHg)	88.4±13.8	99.2±19.2	**0.018**
Complete or partial remission at 6 months:	36.2	4.8	**0.007**
Histological features (%):			
- IgA deposits present	22.7	21.1	1.000
- IgG deposits present	47.7	57.9	0.585
- IgM deposits present	68.2	68.4	1.000
- C3 deposits present	62.8	78.9	0.252
- Any interstitial fibrosis present (%)	30.4	56.5	**0.041**
- Any crescentic lesion present (%)	14.3	26.1	0.330

SBP – Systolic blood pressure, DBP – Diastolic blood pressure, Ig – Immunoglobulin, C3 – Complement 3.

Table 4. Comparison of biochemical and treatment factors associated with outcome.

Factors	End-point		p
	NO (n = 56)	YES (n = 23)	
Complement C3 at biopsy	1.05±0.41	1.23±0.62	0.311
Low complement C3 at biopsy (%)	14.3	17.4	0.706
Complement C4 at biopsy	0.36±0.33	0.37±0.19	0.891
Low complement C4 at biopsy (%)	-	-	-
Serum cholesterol (mmol/L)	6.1±1.4	7.9±3.2	0.079
Serum albumin at biopsy (g/L)	26.1±6.9	25.2±8.2	0.667
Serum creatinine at biopsy (μmol/L)	124.7±86.9	315.2±229.0	**0.001**
Estimated MDRD GFR at biopsy (ml/min)	75.3±30.6	40.5±34.0	**<0.0001**
Proteinuria at biopsy (g/day)	8.1±6.9	8.3±5.2	0.872
Treatment with ACE-i/ARB (%)	92.9	87.0	0.409
Treatment with prednisone (%)	25.0	52.2	**0.034**
Treatment with cyclophosphamide (%)	8.9	26.1	0.071
Treatment with Azathioprine (%)	3.6	8.7	0.635

MDRD – Modification of Diet in Renal Disease; GFR – Glomerular filtration rate; ACE-I – Angiotensin converting enzyme inhibitors; ARB – Angiotensin receptor blockers.

renal survival curves for differences in outcome based on race (log rank p = 0.009), gender (log rank p = 0.995), treatment with I/V cyclophosphamide (log rank p = 0.440) and presence or absence of interstitial fibrosis (log rank p = 0.028) are shown in figure 2. *Cox univariate regression analysis for predictors of end-point.*

Factors associated with the end-point, identified through Cox-regression analysis are shown in Table 5. Estimated GFR at biopsy (OR 0.97 [95%CI 0.95–0.99], p<0.0001), being of black African descent (OR 3.03 [95%CI 1.27–7.21], p = 0.012) and presence of interstitial fibrosis at biopsy (OR 2.64 [95%CI 1.07–6.48], p = 0.034) were the factors identified to be associated with the end-point. Early complete or partial remission (at six months after renal biopsy) did not influence the renal outcome in these patients (OR: 0.17 [95%CI: 0.02–1.27]; p = 0.084).

Discussion

The analysis of our data of patients with idiopathic MCGN in Cape Town shows that a number of important demographic,

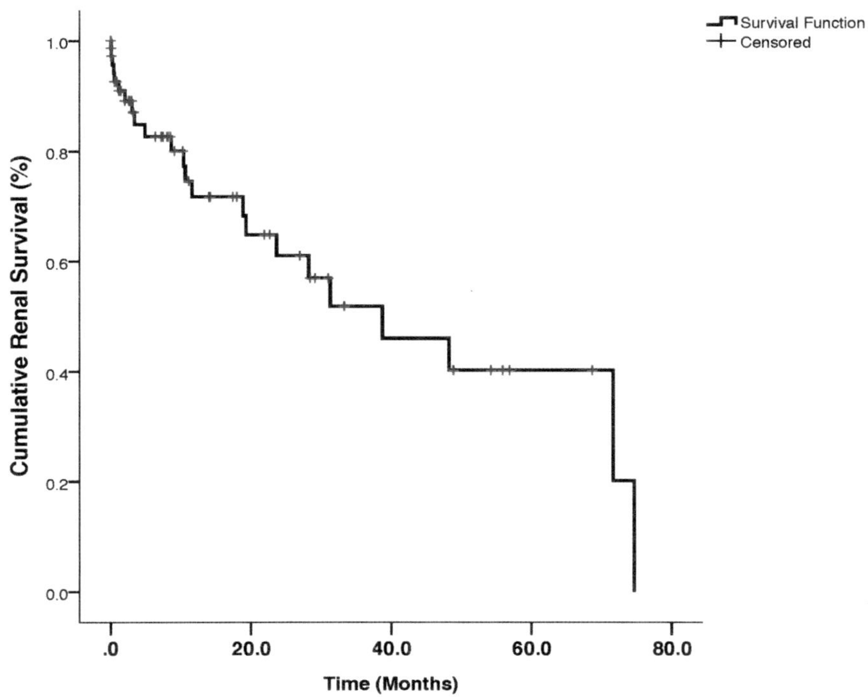

Figure 1. Kaplan-Meier curve for overall renal survival in the study population.

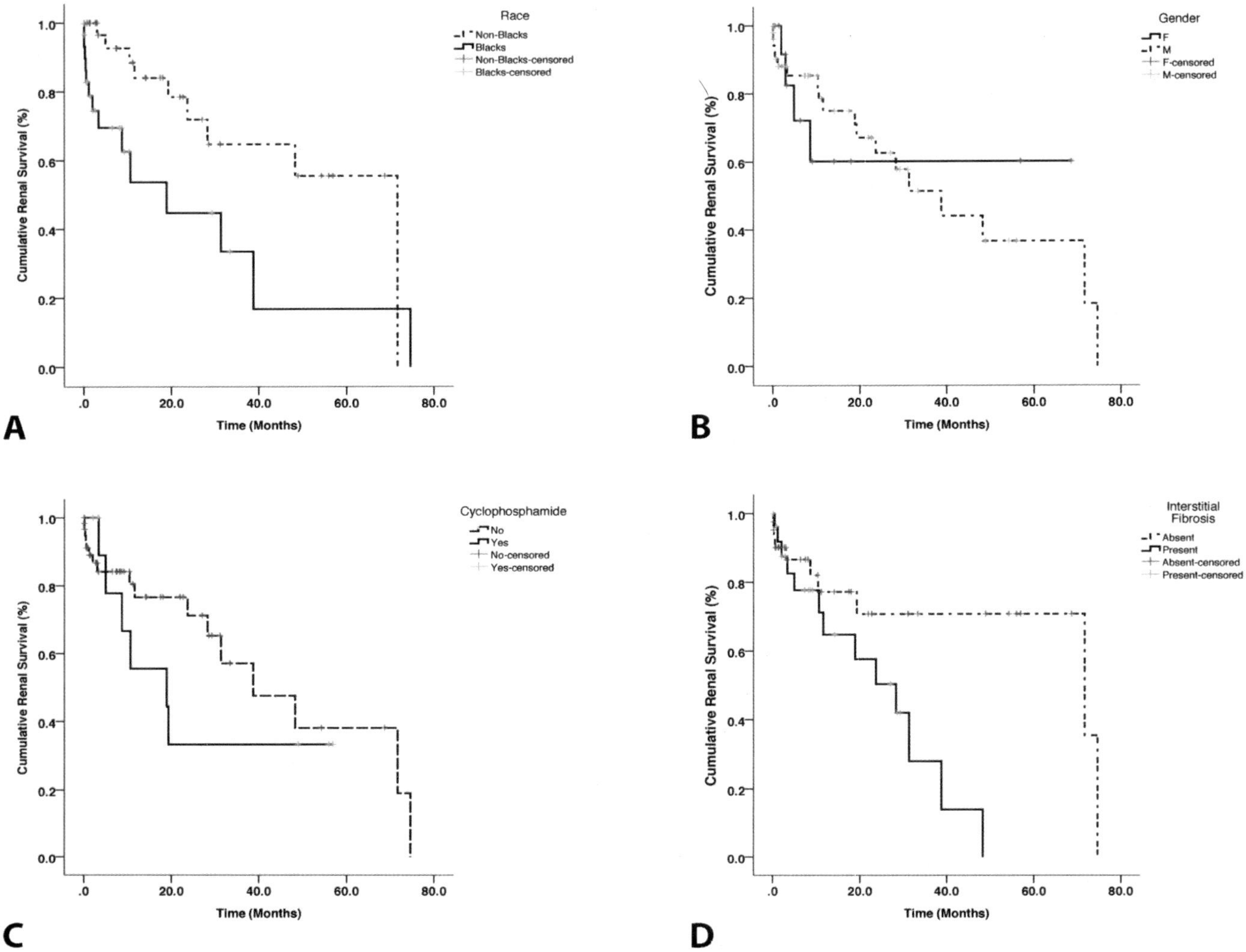

Figure 2. Kaplan-Meier curve for renal survival based on histological features of MCGN. (A) shows differences in outcome between Black Africans and non-Black Africans (log rank $p = 0.009$); (B) shows gender differences in outcome (log rank $p = 0.995$); (C) differences between patients who received treatment with cyclophosphamide and those who didn't receive treatment (log rank $p = 0.440$) and (D) shows differences in outcomes based on the presence of interstitial fibrosis in the biopsy (log rank $p = 0.028$).

Table 5. Cox univariate regression analysis for predictors of the end-point.

Variable	OR (95% CI)	P value
Age	1.03 (0.99–1.06)	0.089
Gender (Female)	0.99 (0.33–2.99)	0.995
Estimated GFR at biopsy	0.97 (0.95–0.99)	**<0.0001**
Average SBP during follow-up	1.01 (0.99–1.03)	0.082
Average DBP during follow-up	1.00 (0.98–1.03)	0.982
Remission status at 6 months (CR/PR)	0.17 (0.02–1.27)	0.084
Race (Blacks)	3.03 (1.27–7.21)	**0.012**
Interstitial fibrosis (Present)	2.64 (1.07–6.48)	**0.034**
Crescent (Present)	1.66 (0.64–4.29)	0.295
Cyclophosphamide (Yes)	1.45 (0.56–3.78)	0.443

GFR – Glomerular filtration rate; SBP – systolic blood pressure; DBP – diastolic blood pressure; CR – complete remission, PR – partial remission.

clinical and histological features may adversely predict the renal outcome in these patients. Given that there are no published recent outcome studies on idiopathic MCGN, this study has shown that in comparison with previous studies, the renal outcome of patients with idiopathic MCGN remains dismally low in comparison to outcomes in previously published studies (Table 6) [18–20,24–28]. Importantly, we have observed that lower estimated GFR at presentation (often a surrogate of late presentation), being of black African ethnicity and presence of interstitial fibrosis in the renal histology were the predicting factors of renal outcome in our patients. The 2-year and 5-year renal survival was found to be low in this study.

Late presentation of patients is common in many centres in Africa and is thought to be an important factor responsible for disease outcome [7,29,30]. Many late presenters will have markedly elevated serum creatinine (low eGFR) and may have features of ureamia or be in need of dialysis at first presentation. Late presenters may account for 36.5% of our patients having significant interstitial fibrosis on histology (Table 2). Reasons for late presentation are often tied to poverty (lack of transportation, long distances to health care facility, lack of health insurance, low level of education), cultural beliefs (visits to the traditional healer) or due to late referral. Although in this study we did not evaluate the duration of symptoms in our patients, many patients often report having been ill for many weeks and in some instances many months before presenting to hospital. In one study, late evaluation of patients with chronic kidney disease (CKD) was reported to be associated with greater burden and severity of comorbid disease, black ethnicity, lack of health insurance, and shorter duration of survival [31]. However, late presentation alone may not explain the elevated serum creatinine as the pathogenesis of MCGN itself (involving complement activation, capillary wall damage and reduction in filtration at the glomerulus) may have accounted for this. We did not exclude the possible effects of genetic factors relative to outcome in this study; hence our finding of the black race being associated with outcome may be put down to socio-economic factors rather than genetic as many of the black patients who use the public health care system in South Africa are indigent.

Although SBP and DBP during follow-up were not predictors of the endpoint on regression analysis, they were significantly higher in those patients reaching endpoint than those who didn't. Uncontrolled hypertension combined with impaired sieving function with consequent protein overload play a pathogenic role in the progression of CKD. The utility of adequate BP control to reduce progression of kidney disease in diabetic and non-diabetic CKD has been shown from various studies and is recommended by various guidelines [21,22,32,33]. One systematic review and meta-analysis of randomized controlled trials on the effects of intensive BP lowering on the progression of CKD has reported that in 5 trials that involved 1703 patients, intensive BP lowering reduced the risk of progressive kidney failure by 27% in people with proteinuria at baseline [34]. In one large population based study, the odds ratios to develop progression of urine albumin excretion during follow-up was 1.91 (95% CI 1.72 to 2.12) per 10-mmHg increase in BP during follow-up and this was independent of baseline BP and other biochemical and patient factors during follow-up [35]. In our study, several patients were receiving treatment with an agent that blocked the renin angiotensin aldosterone pathway. Previous studies from our centre have also highlighted inadequate control of BP as a factor for poor outcomes in patients with proliferative and non-proliferative glomerulonephritis [36,37]. Poor BP control may be related to the disease process or in some instances to poor adherence to therapy. Emphasis on BP control in patients with MCGN may therefore be useful in improving renal outcomes since, unlike in many other glomerular diseases, immunosuppression has a limited role in the treatment of patients.

Renal survival in MCGN has often been reported to be low and with probably worse outcomes in comparison with other glomerular diseases, probably due to lack of specific therapy for MCGN. Recommendations from the KDIGO guideline for treatment of MCGN are limited to cases with abnormal renal function and are drawn mainly from small observational studies [17]. It was interesting that treatment with immunosuppression did not make any difference with regards to the outcome even though there were more patients in our study who reached endpoint that received immunosuppression (Table 4). Renal survival in this study was found to be 61% at 2 years and 40.3% at 5 years, much lower than for studies reported from developed countries. Although some older studies have found type of MCGN to predict outcome, we did not apply this to our study given the new approach to classifying patients with MCGN [16]. However, like some previous studies have reported, we found that any degree of interstitial fibrosis present at time of biopsy (mild/moderate/severe) is a poor prognostic factor for renal outcome.

Given recent publications on this subject, a major question that this study needed to address is whether everything was done to exclude all known secondary causes of MCGN before a labeling of the "idiopathic" diagnosis. The answer to that question is "yes – as far as was possible" given the clinical features of the patients at time of presentation and during follow up. All the patients included in this study had the immune-complex type of MCGN hence, secondary causes will include various chronic bacterial and viral infections, autoimmune diseases and monoclonal gammopathy (dysproteinaemia). All the patients included in this study tested negative for HIV, hepatitis B and C, syphilis and did not demonstrate serological or histological features of post-infectious glomerulonephritis. Our patients also tested negative for cryoglobulins and commonly occurring autoimmune diseases like SLE and rheumatoid arthritis. As it was not clinically indicated, no patient was tested for a dysproteinaemia and there were no features to suggest the disease being present at time of presentation or during the period of follow-up. Our patients typically present at a younger age (mean age in this study is 33.9±13.9 years) compared to other studies where dysproteinaemias have been reported [38,39]. The lack of evidence for a secondary cause of MCGN is supported by the absence of clinical manifestation of any chronic infection or systemic disease during the period of follow up in our patients. However, the high frequency of patients with IgM deposits (59.4%) in their biopsy may be suggestive of a recent (maybe sub-clinical infection) at time of biopsy.

There still remains on our part a persistent and a renewed concern that there is a huge gap in our understanding of this common disease in Cape Town even though we continue to see many "healthy" patients presenting with nephrotic syndrome in whom renal histology show MCGN that is labeled as idiopathic after a detailed and thorough assessment. It could be that we have continued to miss a yet to be identified sub-clinical chronic antigenaemic process possibly resulting from an environmental exposure to drugs (substance abuse), tattoo ink or previous incarceration from one of the correctional services department in Cape Town all of which we have observed to be quite common amongst these patients. Further prospective studies are required to reprove this.

There were a number of limitations for this study. Firstly is our inability to assess for the monoclonality of the Ig deposits at time of biopsy. However, as our patients were young and never exhibited clinical features to suggest monoclonal gammopathy at any time

Table 6. Summary of some selected studies reporting outcomes in idiopathic MCGN.

Author (Year publication) [REF]	Sample size	Country of study	Study design	Mean duration of follow-up (years)	Study population	Renal survival	Predictors of outcome
Habib R (1973) [18]	105	France	Retrospective	5.75	Paediatric	Type I: 66% Type II: 45%	Crescents, Type II disease, nephrotic syndrome, macroscopic haematuria, impaired renal function at presentation
Swainson et al (1983) [24]	40	UK	Observational	5–22	Adult and Paediatric	5-year: 58% 10-year: 48%	Low complements, crescents, impaired renal function at presentation
Cameron et al (1983) [20]	104	UK	Observational	8	Adult and paediatric	Type I: 62% Type II: 51%	Glomerulosclerosis, crescents, nephrotic syndrome, Type II disease
McEnery (1990) [25]	76	USA	Retrospective	10.6	Paediatric	10-year: 82% 20-year: 56%	Not analyzed
Orlowski et al (1988) [26]	50	Poland	Observational	10	Adult	5-year: 90% 10-year: 82%	Hypertension
Schmitt et al (1990) [19]	220	Germany	Retrospective	5	Adult and Paediatric	5-year: 51% 10-year: 36%	Hypertension, crescents, interstitial fibrosis
Perdersen (1995) [27]	37	Denmark	Observational	2.7	Adult and Paediatric	5-year: 35% 10-year: 16%	Older age, hypertension
Little et al (2006) [28]	70	UK	Retrospective	13.8	Adult and paediatric	8.3-20 years: 30%*	Nephrotic range proteinuria, crescents, mesangial proliferation
This study	79	South Africa	Retrospective	1.1	Adult	2-year: 61.0% 5-year: 40.3%	Abnormal serum creatinine at presentation, black race, interstitial fibrosis, hypertension

UK – United Kingdom; USA – United States of America.
*Median time to ESRD.

during follow-up, this diagnosis was clinically excluded. Secondly, given the high number of patients with intravenous drug abuse and the common finding of IgM deposition in glomeruli, our study is also limited by the absence of routine testing for IgG/IgM mixed cryoglobulins. However, given that cryoprecipitates which can occasionally be observed as hyaline-like globules were not observed in the histological materials of these patients further makes this unlikely. Finally, the retrospective design of this study limited the type of data that can be collected and analyzed. This therefore warrants a prospective study of patients with "idiopathic" MCGN with emphasis on a more rigorous evaluation to exclude or identify possible secondary causes. For now however, patients identified with MCGN in whom we are unable to find a cause, efforts to reduce proteinuria and treat BP to target will be our major aim.

Conclusions

The outcome of idiopathic MCGN in Cape Town is poor and is related to socio-demographic as well as to some clinical and histological features at time of presentation. Being the most frequent primary glomerular disease reported in Cape Town, there is need for a prospectively designed study of idiopathic MCGN in order to increase our understanding of its pathogenesis and maybe find ways to its treatment.

Supporting Information

Figure S1 Glomerular features of one of our study patients identified with immune complex type MCGN. A – The H&E stain showing increased lobulation of the displayed glomerulus and increased mesangial matrix; B – silver stain showing double contours/splitting of the glomerular basement membrane; C – F shows positive immunohistochemical stains for C3, IgG, IgA and IgM respectively; G–I are the electron micrographs (x 30,000) showing sub-endothelial and intramembranous deposits. (Courtesy Dr M Duffield and Mr. D. Rademeyer – National Health and Laboratory Services [NHLS] Cape Town).

Acknowledgments

None

Author Contributions

Conceived and designed the experiments: IGO TALD MD BLR GM CRS. Performed the experiments: IGO TALD MD BLR GM CRS. Analyzed the data: IGO TALD MD BLR GM CRS. Contributed reagents/materials/analysis tools: IGO TALD MD BLR GM CRS. Wrote the paper: IGO TALD MD BLR GM CRS.

References

1. D'Amico G, Ferrario F (1992) Mesangiocapillary glomerulonephritis. J Am Soc Nephrol. 2 (10 Suppl): S159–166.
2. Sethi S, Nester CM, Smith RJ (2012) Membranoproliferative glomerulonephritis and C3 glomerulopathy: resolving the confusion. Kidney Int. 81: 434–441.
3. Covic A, Schiller A, Volovat C, et al (2006) Epidemiology of renal disease in Romania: a 10 year review of two regional renal biopsy databases. Nephrol Dial Transplant 21: 419–424.
4. Barsoum RS, Francis MR (2000) Spectrum of glomerulonephritis in Egypt. Saudi J Kidney Dis Transpl 11: 421–429.
5. Khalifa EH, Kaballo BG, Suleiman SM, Khalil EA, El-Hassan AM (2004) Pattern of glomerulonephritis in Sudan: histopathological and immunofluorescence study. Saudi J Kidney Dis Transpl 15: 176–179.
6. Okpechi I, Swanepoel C, Duffield M, Mahala B, Wearne N, et al (2011) Patterns of renal disease in Cape Town South Africa: a 10-year review of a single-centre renal biopsy database. Nephrol Dial Transplant 26: 1853–1861.
7. Okpechi IG, Rayner BL, Swanepoel CR (2010) Nephrotic syndrome in adult black South Africans: HIV-associated nephropathy as the main culprit. J Natl Med Assoc. 102: 1193–1197.
8. Asinobi AO, Gbadegesin RA, Adeyemo AA, Akang EE, Arowolo FA, et al (1999) The predominance of membranoproliferative glomerulonephritis in childhood nephrotic syndrome in Ibadan, Nigeria. West Afr J Med. 18: 203–206.
9. Kawamura T, Usui J, Kaseda K, Takada K, Ebihara I, et al (2013) Primary membranoproliferative glomerulonephritis on the decline: decreased rate from the 1970s to the 2000s in Japan. Clin Exp Nephrol. 17: 248–254.
10. Hanko JB, Mullan RN, O'Rourke DM, McNamee PT, Maxwell AP, et al (2009) The changing pattern of adult primary glomerular disease. Nephrol Dial Transplant 24: 3050–3054.
11. Schena FP (1997) Survey of the Italian Registry of Renal Biopsies. Frequency of the renal diseases for 7 consecutive years. The Italian Group of Renal Immunopathology. Nephrol Dial Transplant 12: 418–426.
12. Rychlík I, Jancová E, Tesar V, Kolsky A, Lácha J, et al (2004) The Czech registry of renal biopsies. Occurrence of renal diseases in the years 1994–2000. Nephrol Dial Transplant 19: 3040–3049.
13. Strachan DP (1989) Hay fever, hygiene, and household size. BMJ 299: 1259–1260.
14. Johnson RJ, Hurtado A, Merszei J, Rodriguez-Iturbe B, Feng L (2003) Hypothesis: dysregulation of immunologic balance resulting from hygiene and socioeconomic factors may influence the epidemiology and cause of glomerulonephritis worldwide. Am J Kidney Dis 42: 575–581.
15. Fervenza FC, Sethi S, Glassock RJ (2012) Idiopathic membranoproliferative glomerulonephritis: does it exist? Nephrol Dial Transplant. 27: 4288–4294.
16. Sethi S, Fervenza FC (2011) Membranoproliferative Glomerulonephritis: Pathogenetic Heterogeneity and Proposal for a New Classification. Semin Nephrol 31: 341–348.
17. Kidney Disease: Improving Global Outcomes (KDIGO) Glomerulonephritis Work Group. KDIGO Clinical Practice Guideline for Glomerulonephritis (2012) Kidney int. 2(suppl): 139–274.
18. Habib R, Kleinknecht C, Gubler MC, Maiz HB (1973) Idiopathic membranoproliferative glomerulonephritis. Morphology and natural history. Perspect Nephrol Hypertens 1: 491–514.
19. Schmitt H, Bohle A, Reineke T, Mayer-Eichberger D, Vogl W (1990) Long-term prognosis of membranoproliferative glomerulonephritis type I. Significance of clinical and morphological parameters: an investigation of 220 cases. Nephron 55: 242–250.
20. Cameron JS, Turner DR, Heaton J, Williams DG, Ogg CS, et al (1983) Idiopathic mesangiocapillary glomerulonephritis. Comparison of types I and II in children and adults and long-term prognosis. Am J Med. 74: 175–192.
21. National Kidney Foundation K/DOQI clinical practice guidelines for chronic kidney disease; evaluation, classification and stratification (2002) Am J Kidney Dis 39(2 Suppl 1): S1–S266.
22. Mancia G, De Backer G, Dominiczak A, Cifkova R, Fagard R, et al (2007) 2007 Guidelines for the Management of Arterial Hypertension: The Task Force for the Management of Arterial Hypertension of the European Society of Hypertension (ESH) and of the European Society of Cardiology (ESC). J Hypertens 25: 1105–1187.
23. Renal Disease Subcommittee of the American College of Rheumatology Ad Hoc Committee on Systemic Lupus Erythematosus Response Criteria (2006) The American college of rheumatology response criteria for proliferative and membranous renal disease in systemic lupus erythematosus clinical trials. Arthritis Rheum 54: 421–432.
24. Swainson CP, Robson JS, Thomson D, MacDonald MK (1983) Mesangiocapillary glomerulonephritis: a long-term study of 40 cases. J Pathol 141: 449–468.
25. McEnery PT (1990) Membranoproliferative glomerulonephritis: the Cincinnati experience – cumulative renal survival from 1957 to 1989. J Pediatr 116: S109–S114.
26. Orlowski T, Rancewicz Z, Lao M, Juskowa J, Klepacka J, et al (1988) Long-term immunosuppressive therapy of idiopathic membranoproliferative glomerulonephritis. Klin Wochenschr 66: 1019–1023.
27. Pedersen RS (1995) Long-term prognosis in idiopathic membranoproliferative glomerulonephritis. Scand J Urol Nephrol 29: 265–272.
28. Little MA, Dorman A, Gill D, Walshe JJ (2000) Mesangioproliferative glomerulonephritis with IgM deposition: clinical characteristics and outcome. Ren Fail 22: 445–457.
29. Naicker S, Aboud O, Gharbi MB (2008) Epidemiology of acute kidney injury in Africa. Semin Nephrol. 28: 348–353.
30. Olowu WA (2003) Renal failure in Nigerian children: factors limiting access to dialysis. Pediatr Nephrol. 18: 1249–1254.
31. Kinchen KS, Sadler J, Fink N, Brookmeyer R, Klag MJ, et al (2002) The timing of specialist evaluation in chronic kidney disease and mortality. Ann Intern Med. 137: 479–486.
32. Jafar TH, Stark PC, Schmid CH, Landa M, Maschio G, et al (2003) Progression of chronic kidney disease: the role of blood pressure control, proteinuria, and angiotensin-converting enzyme inhibition: a patient-level meta-analysis. Ann Intern Med 139: 244–252.

33. Chobanian AV, Bakris GL, Black HR, Cushman WC, Green LA, et al (2003) The seventh report of the Joint National Committee on Prevention, Detection, Evaluation, and Treatment of High Blood Pressure: the JNC7 report. JAMA 289: 2560–2572.
34. Lv J, Ehteshami P, Sarnak MJ, Tighiouart H, Jun M, et al (2013) Effects of intensive blood pressure lowering on the progression of chronic kidney disease: a systematic review and meta-analysis. CMAJ. 185: 949–957.
35. Brantsma AH, Atthobari J, Bakker SJ, de Zeeuw D, de Jong PE, et al (2007) What predicts progression and regression of urinary albumin excretion in the nondiabetic population? J Am Soc Nephrol. 18: 637–645.
36. Ayodele OE, Okpechi IG, Swanepoel CR (2013) Long-term renal outcome and complications in South Africans with proliferative lupus nephritis. Int Urol Nephrol. 45: 1289–1300.
37. Okpechi IG, Ayodele OE, Jones ES, Duffield M, Swanepoel CR (2012) Outcome of patients with membranous lupus nephritis in Cape Town South Africa. Nephrol Dial Transplant. 27: 3509–3515.
38. Zand L, Kattah A, Fervenza FC, Smith RJ, Nasr SH, et al (2013) C3 glomerulonephritis associated with monoclonal gammopathy: a case series. Am J Kidney Dis. 62: 506–514.
39. Sethi S, Zand L, Leung N, Smith RJ, Jevremonic D, et al (2010) Membranoproliferative glomerulonephritis secondary to monoclonal gammopathy. Clin J Am Soc Nephrol. 5: 770–782.

18

Role of WNT10A-Expressing Kidney Fibroblasts in Acute Interstitial Nephritis

Akihiro Kuma[1,2], Sohsuke Yamada[3], Ke-Yong Wang[4], Noriaki Kitamura[1], Takahiro Yamaguchi[1], Yoshiko Iwai[1], Hiroto Izumi[5], Masahito Tamura[2], Yutaka Otsuji[2], Kimitoshi Kohno[6]*

1 Department of Molecular Biology, School of Medicine, University of Occupational and Environmental Health, Kitakyushu, Japan, **2** Second Department of Internal Medicine, Cardiology and Nephrology, School of Medicine, University of Occupational and Environmental Health, Kitakyushu, Japan, **3** Department of Pathology and Cell Biology, School of Medicine, University of Occupational and Environmental Health, Kitakyushu, Japan, **4** Bio-information Research Center, University of Occupational and Environmental Health, Kitakyushu, Japan, **5** Department of Occupational Pneumology, Institute of Industrial Ecological Science, University of Occupational and Environmental Health, Kitakyushu, Japan, **6** The President Laboratory, University of Occupational and Environmental Health, Kitakyushu, Japan

Abstract

WNT signaling mediates various physiological and pathological processes. We previously showed that WNT10A is a novel angio/stromagenic factor involved in such processes as tumor growth, wound healing and tissue fibrosis. In this study, we investigated the role of WNT10A in promoting the fibrosis that is central to the pathology of acute interstitial nephritis (AIN). We initially asked whether there is an association between kidney function (estimated glomerular filtration rate; eGFR) and WNT10A expression using kidney biopsies from 20 patients with AIN. Interestingly, patients with WNT10A expression had significantly lower eGFR than WNT10A-negative patients. However, changes in kidney function were not related to the level of expression of other WNT family members. Furthermore, there was positive correlation between WNT10A and α-SMA expression. We next investigated the involvement of WNT10A in kidney fibrosis processes using COS1 cells, a kidney fibroblast cell line. WNT10A overexpression increased the level of expression of fibronectin and peroxiredoxin 5. Furthermore, WNT10A overexpression renders cells resistant to apoptosis induced by hydrogen peroxide and high glucose. Collectively, WNT10A may induce kidney fibrosis and associate with kidney dysfunction in AIN.

Editor: Robert Dettman, Northwestern University, United States of America

Funding: This work was supported by JSPS KAKENHI (Grant Number 22249025) and an UOEH grant for advanced research to Ke-Yong Wang. The funders had no role in study design, data collection and analysis, decision to publish, or preparation of the manuscript.

* Email: k-kohno@med.uoeh-u.ac.jp

Introduction

Acute interstitial nephritis (AIN) is a general cause of acute kidney injury (AKI). Patients with AIN can either completely recover or progress to chronic kidney disease (CKD) or end-stage renal disease (ESRD) [1]. Although several antifibrotic strategies have been proposed, there are no effective treatments for kidney fibrosis. Kidney fibrosis is generally considered to result from tissue inflammation and the tissue repair/wound healing responses [2]. Wound healing is a complex process involving several signal transduction systems, and ultimately can result in scar formation. The first phase begins with tissue damage caused by anti-inflammatory cytokines [3]. The next phase is defined by deposition of granulation tissue and new extracellular matrix (ECM) proteins. Acute inflammatory reactions are considered to be a part of early wound healing and play a key role in triggering fibrosis. Since prevention of the initial fibrotic process in AIN may lead to retention of kidney function, we investigated what kinds of signaling systems mediate kidney fibrosis associated with AIN.

There are two major WNT signaling pathways, the canonical (involving β-catenin) [4] and the non-canonical pathways (independent of β-catenin) [5,6]. WNT is a family of highly conserved glycoproteins, and 19 WNT members have been identified so far in humans [7]. The WNT/Frizzled signal transduction system is a highly complex cascade that is fundamental for a wide variety of physiological processes, as well as pathological states. Some WNT proteins were previously investigated in kidney interstitial fibrosis [8,9], but the relation between WNT10A and kidney fibrosis has not been determined. We asked whether WNT10A promotes kidney fibrosis. We previously reported that WNT10A is expressed in dermal fibroblasts, and that α-SMA-positive cells are involved in wound healing [10]. Myofibroblasts, or activated fibroblasts with α-SMA expression, differentiate from diverse sources including local interstitial fibroblasts, vascular pericytes, and endothelial cells [11]. Furthermore, they produce ECM (collagen and fibronectin). Therefore, we hypothesized that WNT10A expression in myofibroblasts may also play an important role in tissue repair and the fibrotic processes associated with AIN.

Here, we discovered that WNT10A is expressed in kidney fibroblasts expressing α-SMA. Patients with WNT10A expression had a significantly lower estimated glomerular filtration rate (eGFR) than WNT10-negative patients. We investigated mechanism of fibroblasts (COS1) behavior with WNT10A expression.

Materials and Methods

Cell culture and conditioned media

COS1 cells (kidney fibroblasts of African green monkey) were purchased from ATCC (VA, USA) and cultured in Dulbecco's

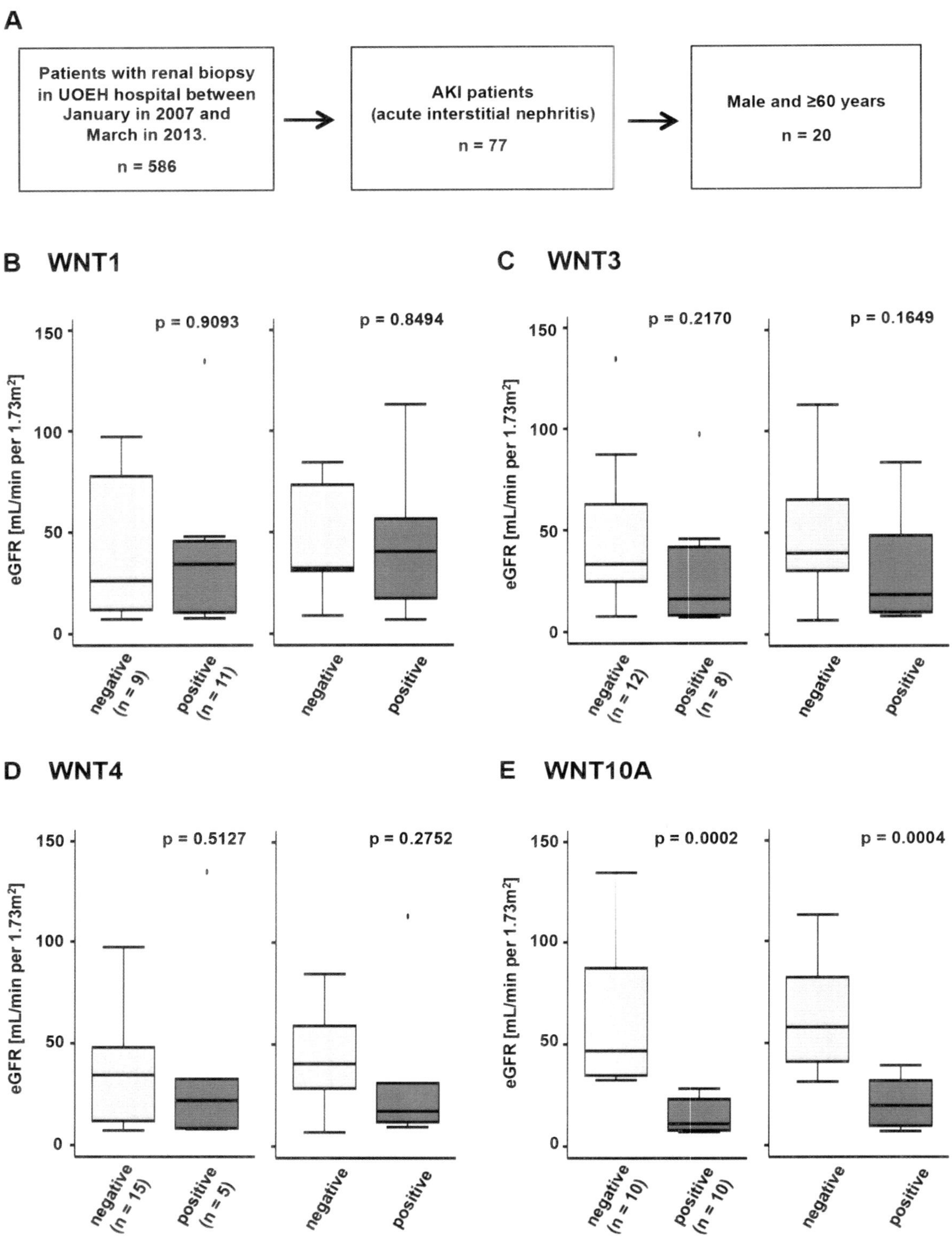

Figure 1. The relationship between WNT family gene expression and kidney function. (A) Patient selection method to evaluate eGFR among AIN patients. eGFR (mL/min per 1.73 m^2) of AIN patients with (B) WNT1, (C) WNT3, (D) WNT4, and (E) WNT10A. (B) WNT1 negative-expression; n = 9, positive-expression; n = 11 (C) WNT3 negative-expression; n = 12, positive-expression; n = 8 (D) WNT4 negative-expression; n = 15, positive-expression; n = 5 (E) WNT10A negative expression; n = 10, positive-expression; n = 10. Light gray box indicates eGFR of patients without WNT protein expression, and dark gray box indicates eGFR of patients with WNT protein expression. The left panels show kidney function on kidney biopsy, and right panels show kidney function on discharge. Data of each category is shown in Table 2.

modified Eagle's medium (Nissui Seiyaku, Tokyo, Japan) containing 10% fetal bovine serum and 5.5 mM glucose. Low glucose medium (LM) contained 5.5 mM glucose, moderate-high glucose medium (MM) contained 11 mM glucose, and high glucose medium (HM) contained 22 mM glucose. Cell lines were maintained in a 5% CO_2 atmosphere at 37°C.

Plasmid construction and transfectants

The WNT10A cDNA expression plasmid was constructed by PCR as described previously [10]. The PCR product was cloned into the pGEM-T easy vector (Promega, WI, USA). The full-length cDNA fragment was recloned into the pEB-Multi vector (Wako). COS1 cells were transfected with either vector (control cells) or pEB-WNT10A (WNT10A-overexpressing cells; COS1-10A) using the X-tremeGENE 9 (Roche, Basel, Switzerland) and cultured with normal medium for three days. After that, medium was changed to 300 μg/ml hygromycin contining medium and cultured for 21 days. The resulting colonies were isolated and the cellular expression levels of WNT10A were confirmed by Western blotting with an anti-WNT10A antibody.

Preparation of human kidney samples

Patients (Japanese) who were hospitalized with AKI in the Department of Nephrology of University of Occupational and Environmental Health (UOEH) hospital in Kitakyushu, Japan, received kidney biopsy to diagnose the cause of AKI between January 2007 and March 2013. Human kidney tissue samples were examined in the department of nephrology and pathology at UOEH. The diagnosis was re-evaluated and confirmed by at least three board-certified nephrologists and one board-certified surgical pathologist. All the intended procedures of the present study, including use of specimens from human subjects, were approved by the Ethics Committee of UOEH in Kitakyushu, Japan. Especially, written consent of next of kin for research use of the materials was obtained according to the guidelines of the Japanese Society of Pathology and also approved by the Ethics Committee of UOEH, where the biopsy was performed.

Histology and Immunohistochemical staining

Deparaffinized and rehydrated 3-μm sequential sections from kidney samples were stained with hematoxylin and eosin (HE) or Masson's trichrome stain, or underwent immunohistochemistry (IHC) preparations. IHC was performed as previously described [12]. For IHC performed by the antibody-linked dextran polymer method (EnVision; DAKO, Glostrup, Denmark), samples were incubated in 10% H_2O_2 for 5 min to block endogenous peroxidase activity. Then, these sections were rinsed and incubated with the indicated antibodies for 30 min, respectively. The second antibody-peroxidase-linked polymers were then applied, and the sections were incubated with a solution consisting of 20 mg of 3.3′-diaminobenzidine tetrahydrochloride, 65 mg of sodium azide, and 20 ml of 30% H_2O_2 in 100 ml of Tris-HCl (50 mM, pH 7.6). After counterstaining with Mayer's haematoxylin, sections were observed under a light microscope. The immune-reactivity with WNT proteins and α-SMA in each case were assessed semi-quantitatively by evaluating the proportion of positive cells over total stromal cells. For WNT proteins or α-SMA expression, positive areas that were equal to or more than 10% or 50% were considered positively stained respectively, in accord with the performance of receiver operating characteristic (ROC) curve analyses. Finally, to assess the co-localization of both proteins in the same or at least in adjacent fibrogenic cells (i.e., myofibroblasts), we stained tissues in consecutive sections with rabbit polyclonal anti-WNT10A antibodies and mouse monoclonal anti-human α-SMA, respectively, as previously described [13]. For fibronectin expression, positive areas that were equal to or more 30% were considered positively stained. All histological and immunohistochemical staining was evaluated by two independent observers (a certified surgical pathologist and a nephrology doctor) using a blind protocol design (observers were blinded to the clinicopathological data).

Immunofluorescence staining

Control and WNT10A-overexpressing cells was cultured on 6 well-plate for 72 hours and fixed with 15% formalin for 10 minutes after washing with PBS. Cells were incubated with 0.2% (v/v) Triton X-100 with PBS for 10 minutes at room temperature. Cells were treated with 4% (w/v) skimmed milk (DS Pharma Biomedical Co., Ltd., Osaka, Japan) in PBS and incubated for 30 minutes at room temperature, washed with PBS, and incubated for 1 hour at room temperature with each primary antibody (anti-WNT10A and anti-fibronectin antibody). Primary antibodies were used at a 1:100 dilution. Cells were reacted with Alexa 488 conjugated anti-rabbit IgG for 45 minutes at room temperature. After washed with PBS containing DAPI, specimens were observed.

Table 1. Patient characteristics.

Characteristics	All	WNT10A(−)	WNT10A(+)	p-value
Number (n)	20	10	10	
Age (years, mean±S.D)	70.6±7.1	71.2±6.5	70.0±8.0	0.717
α-SMA positive (n, %)	10 (50)	1 (5)	9 (45)	0.0005
Fibronectin positive (n, %)	12 (60)	3 (15)	9 (45)	0.0062
Strongly interstitial fibrosis (n, %)	7 (35)	1 (5)	6 (30)	0.0191
Drug induced AIN (n, %)	4 (20)	1 (5)	3 (15)	0.264
Unknown AIN (n, %)	6 (30)	3 (15)	3 (15)	1.000
Crescentic nephritis (n, %)	9 (45)	5 (25)	4 (20)	0.653
MPA (n, %)	1 (5)	1 (5)	0 (0)	0.305
Administer maintenance HD (n, %)	3 (15)	0 (0)	3 (15)	0.060

AIN; acute interstitial nephritis, MPA; microscopic polyangiitis, HD; hemodialysis.
S.D; standard deviation.

Table 2. eGFR according to WNT proteins.

WNT protein	negative	positive	p-value
WNT1	26.06 [11.79–77.82]	34.28 [16.05–41.68]	0.9093
	32.31 [30.90–73.46]	40.40 [19.27–55.58]	0.8494
WNT3	33.29 [25.32–55.43]	16.05 [8.08–39.69]	0.2170
	39.91 [31.31–62.76]	19.27 [11.28–44.44]	0.1649
WNT4	34.28 [17.45–46.81]	21.66 [8.16–32.30]	0.5127
	40.40 [29.82–57.87]	17.14 [11.89–30.90]	0.2752
WNT10A	46.81 [35.45–84.91]	11.12 [7.93–22.74]	0.0002
	57.87 [44.25–79.96]	19.27 [10.05–30.64]	0.0004

eGFR; median [interquartile range] mL/min per 1.73 m^2 above (on biopsy), below (on discharge).

Western blotting analysis

Whole-cell lysates were prepared as previously described [14]. The 50 μg of protein from whole-cell lysates were separated by sodium dodecyl sulfate-polyacrylamide gel electrophoresis and transferred to polyvinylidene difluoride microporous membranes (Millipore, MA, USA). The blotted membranes were treated with 5% (w/v) skimmed milk in 10 mM Tris, 150 mM NaCl and 0.2% (v/v) Tween 20, and incubated for 1 h at room temperature with the primary antibody. anti-β-actin (Santa Cruz, CA, USA) antibody was used as an internal control at a 1:5,000 dilution. The membranes were then incubated for 45 minutes at room temperature with a peroxidase-conjugated secondary antibody, and visualized using an ECL kit (GE Healthcare Bio-Science, Buckinghamshire, UK). The detection was performed with an LAS-4000 mini (Fujifilm, Tokyo, Japan).

Antibodies

For western blotting and IHC, the following antibodies were used: anti-WNT10A (SAB3500393) was purchased from Sigma-Aldrich (MO, USA), anti-WNT1 (PAB11850) and anti-WNT3 (PAB7032) were purchased from Abnova (Taipei, Taiwan), and anti-WNT4 (sc-13962), anti-fibronectin (sc-9068), anti-COL1A1 (sc-25974), anti-COL3A1 (sc-28888), anti-PRDX2 (sc-23967), anti-PRDX4 (sc-23974) and anti-caspase9 (sc-56076) were purchased from Santa Cruz, and anti-caspase-3 (9662), anti-cleaved caspase-3 (9664), and anti-PARP (9532) were purchased from Cell Signaling Technology (MA, USA), anti-αSMA (M851) was purchased from Dako, and anti-PRDX3 (ab16751) was purchased from Abcam (MA, USA). To generate anti-PRDX1 and anti-PRDX5 antibodies, the synthetic peptides PDVQKSKEYFSKQK and GLTCSLAPNIISQL were used as immunogens, respectively, and the antisera obtained from immunized rabbits were affinity purified using the synthetic peptide antigens [15].

PRDX5 siRNA knockdown

Double-stranded RNA oligonucleotides 25 base pairs long were commercially generated (Life technologies, CA, USA): 5′-GGAUGGCAUAGUGAAGGCCCUGAAU-3′ and 5′-AUUCAGGGCCUUCACUAUGCCAUCC-3′ for PRDX5#1; 5′-CCUGAGACGCUCAGCGGGCUAUAUA-3′ and 5′-UAUAUAGCCCGCUGAGCGUCUCAGG-3′ for PRDX5#3. siRNA transfections were performed as previously described [16,17]. A sample of 5 μL of Lipofectamine 2000 (Qiagen, Hilden, Germany) was diluted in 250 μL Opti-MEM medium (Invitrogen, CA, USA) and incubated for 5 minutes at room temperature. Next, 250 pmol of siRNA and Lipofectamine 2000, serving as the control siRNA, were gently mixed in 250 μL Opti-MEM and incubated for 20 minutes at room temperature. Oligomer-Lipofectamine complexes and aliquots of 2×10^5 WNT10A-overexpressing cells in 500 μL culture medium were combined and incubated for 48 hr. Whole cell extracts (50 μg) were prepared from cells after siRNA transfection, and western blotting was performed.

Cytotoxicity analysis

Cytotoxicity analysis (water-soluble tetrazolium salt: WST-8 assay) was performed as described previously [18,19]. Briefly, 2.5×10^3 cells were seeded into 96-well plates. After 24 hours, to induce oxidative stress, cells were incubated with the indicated concentrations of H_2O_2 in the serum-free medium for 4 hours. After 48 hours, surviving cells were analyzed using a Cell Counting Kit −8 (Dojindo, Kumamoto, Japan) for 2 hours at 37°C. The absorbance was then measured at 450 nm.

Cell proliferation assay

Cell lines were seeded into 12-well plates (2×10^4 cells per well). For the purposes of analysis, the 0 hour was taken to be 24 hours after seeding. The cells were harvested with trypsin and counted every 24 hours.

Statistical analysis

Statistical analyses of the data were carried out using STATA SE12 (Stata Co., TX, USA). Comparison between the two groups was performed by Mann-Whitney U-test or Student's t-test. The X^2 test was used for dichotomous variables. A p-value <0.05 was considered significant.

Results

Patients with WNT10A expression had a lower estimated eGFR

A total of 586 patients received kidney biopsy in the hospital of UOEH during a 75-month period starting in 2007. Of these patients, 77 were AKI and diagnosed with AIN. We investigated the relationship between eGFR and the expression of WNT proteins (WNT1, 3, 4, and 10A) in kidney tissue of 20 patients (Fig. 1A). We selected 20 male patients over 60 years of age because patient background was statistically matched. Primary causes of AIN were rapidly progressive glomerulonephritis (50%), drug-induced AIN (20%), and unknown AIN (30%) (Table 1). Interestingly, 10 patients with WNT10A expression had significantly lower eGFR (median; 11.12 mL/min per 1.73 m^2, [interquartile range; 7.93–22.74 mL/min per 1.73 m^2]) than that

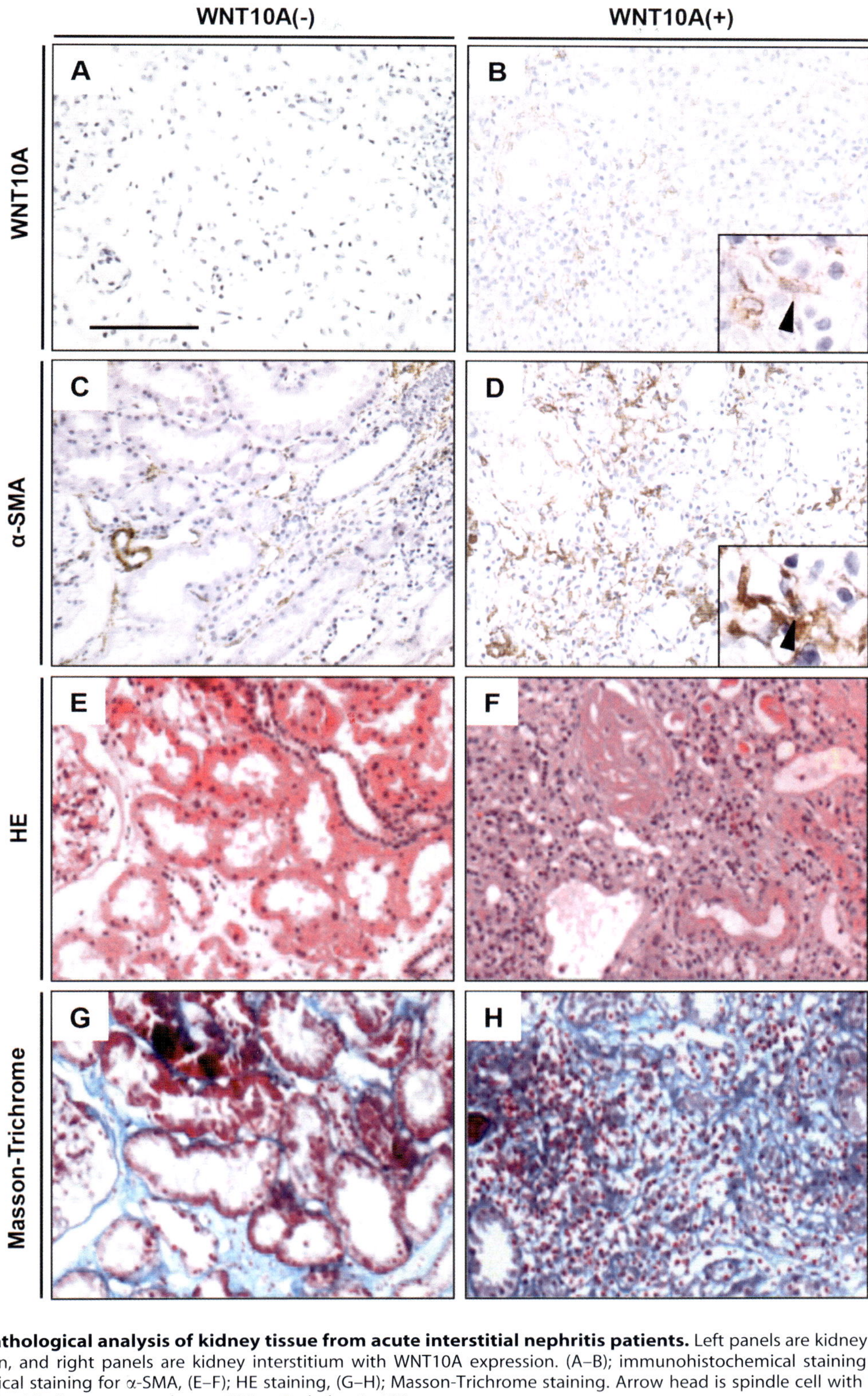

Figure 2. Histopathological analysis of kidney tissue from acute interstitial nephritis patients. Left panels are kidney interstitium without WNT10A expression, and right panels are kidney interstitium with WNT10A expression. (A–B); immunohistochemical staining for WNT10A, (C–D); immunohistochemical staining for α-SMA, (E–F); HE staining, (G–H); Masson-Trichrome staining. Arrow head is spindle cell with WNT10A and α-SMA positive respectively. All photos were taken at 200×. Scale bar is 100 μm.

(46.81 [35.45–84.91]) of the 10 patients without WNT10A expression on kidney biopsy (Fig. 1E left panel). Concerning eGFR on discharge, patients with WNT10A expression also had significantly lower eGFR (19.27 [10.05–30.64] vs 57.87 [44.25–79.96]) (Fig. 1E right panel). However, expression of other WNT proteins (WNT1, 3, and 4) was not correlated with altered kidney function both on biopsy and discharge (Fig. 1B, C and D, Table 2). There was not statistical correlation between high WNT10A

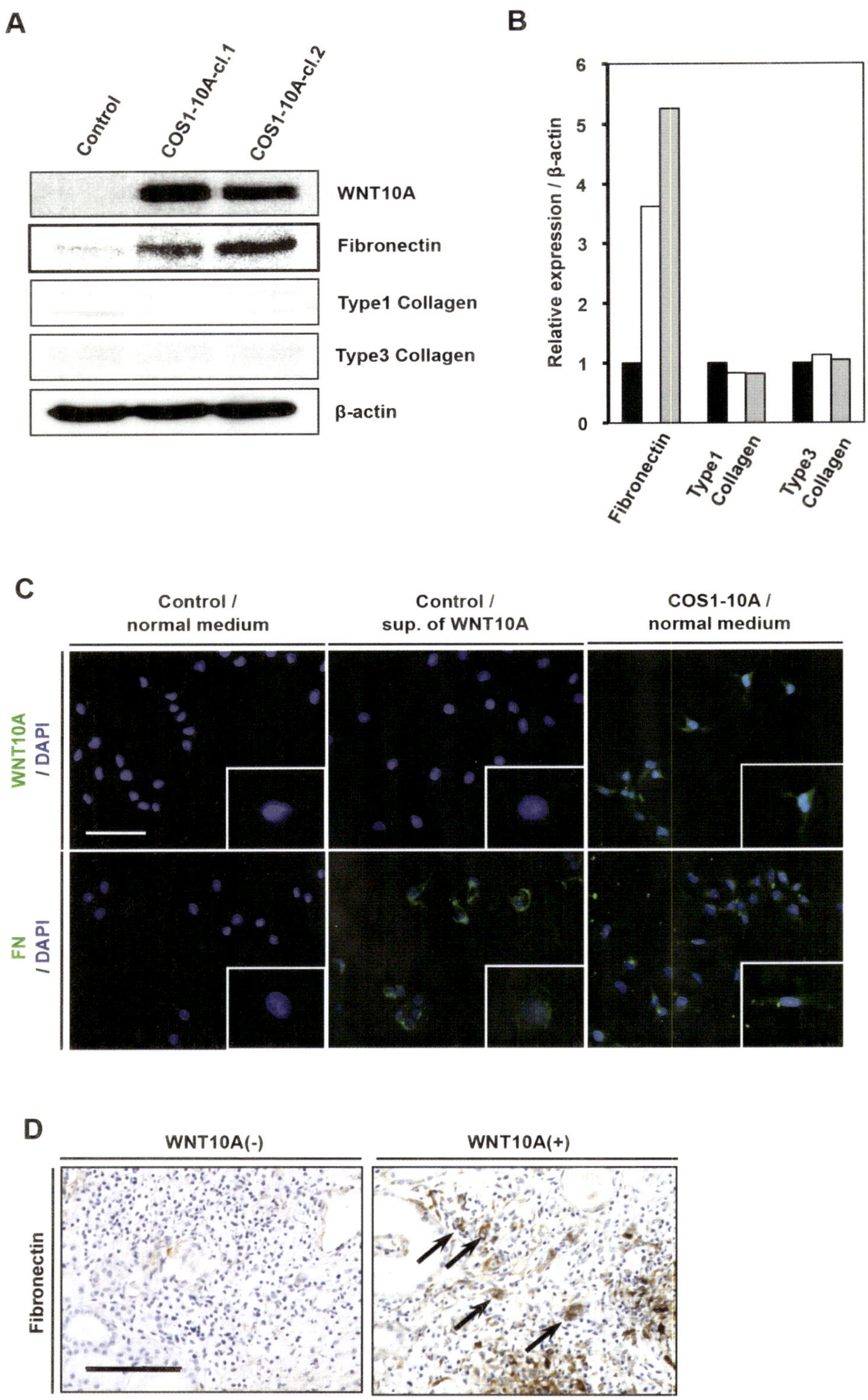

Figure 3. WNT10A overexpression enhances fibronectin expression in COS1 cells. (A) The expression of ECM components in WNT10A-overexpressing cells. Western analysis was performed using whole lysates obtained from control and WNT10A-overexpressing cells (COS1-10A). (B) Relative expression of fibronectin, type 1 collagen, and type 3 collagen, which were normalized to β-actin expression. The black bar shows control cells, white and gray bars showed COS1-10A-cl.1 and COS1-10A-cl.2 respectively. (C) Immunofluorescence staining for WNT10A (green), fibronectin (FN) (green), and DAPI (blue). Control cells treated with normal medium (left panel), control cells treated with supernatant (sup.) of WNT10A-overexpressing cells (middle panel), and COS1-10A cells treated with normal medium (right panel). Each cell was cultured for 72 hours. All photos were taken at 200×. Scale bar is 100 μm. (D) Immunohistochemical staining for fibronectin (brown) in AIN tissues. Kidney tissues from WNT10A-negative (left panel) or -positive (right panel) patients are shown. Arrows indicate fibronectin-positive cells. All photos were taken at 200×. Scale bar is 100 μm.

expression in kidney tissue and low eGFR (data not shown). Furthermore, three patients with WNT10A-positive tissue progressed to ESRD and were administered hemodialysis therapy (Table 1). No patient whose biopsied tissue was negative for WNT10A expression received renal replacement therapy. Thus, WNT10A expression may be correlated with poor prognosis of kidney function.

WNT10A and α-SMA expression in kidney fibroblasts associated with AIN

WNT10A expression in kidney tissues obtained from AIN patient biopsies was much higher than that of samples from chronic kidney disease patients (Fig. 2B and Fig. S1). Inflammatory cells (primarily lymphocytes) were found associated with uriniferous tubules in tissues from patients with AIN (Fig. 2F). Fibroblasts that are α-SMA positive are thought to be myofibroblasts or activated fibroblasts that produce ECM components, such as type 1 collagen, type 3 collagen, and fibronectin. Some α-SMA-expressing cells were present at the interstitium of uriniferous tubules in kidneys without AIN (Fig. S2). Many more α-SMA-positive cells were identified in WNT10A-positive AIN cases (Fig. 2B and D) compared with WNT10A-negetive AIN cases (Fig. 2A and C). The consecutive IHC sections also demonstrated co-localization of both WNT10A and α-SMA in the same or at least in adjacent myofibroblasts/fibroblasts (Fig. 2B and D). Moreover, there was a significantly close positive correlation to the IHC WNT10A-positive and α-SMA-positive expression pattern ($p = 0.0005$) (Table 1). Finally, Masson-Trichrome staining showed that more ECM was found in WNT10A-positive AIN (Fig. 2H) than in WNT10A-negetive AIN (Fig. 2G). WNT10A expression in kidney tissue had significantly strong kidney fibrosis (fibrosis area is equal or more than 20%) compared with WNT10A-negative expression ($p = 0.0191$) (Table 1). However, there was not statistical correlation between high WNT10A expression (positive area is equal or more than 30%) and strong kidney fibrosis ($p = 0.7782$) (data not shown). Thus, WNT10A protein expression in α-SMA-expressing fibroblasts may contribute to the kidney interstitial fibrotic process characteristic of AIN.

Fibroblasts with WNT10A expression produce fibronectin

We investigated the involvement of WNT10A in the kidney fibrosis processes of AIN using COS1 cells, a cell line derived from kidney fibroblasts of the African green monkey. Two WNT10A-overexpressing COS1 cells (COS1-10A) were established (Fig. 3A). Interestingly, WNT10A overexpression enhances the expression of fibronectin (an ECM component) about three to five fold but does not alter the expression of type 1 and type 3 collagen (Fig. 3B). WNT10A is a secreted protein. In contrast to normal medium, supernatant from WNT10A-overexpressin COS1 cells induced fibronectin expression in untransfected COS1 cells (Fig. 3C). As expected, kidney tissues with WNT10A expression also expressed fibronectin (Fig. 3D). Furthermore, there was statistical positive correlation to the IHC WNT10A-positive and fibronectin-positive expression ($p = 0.0062$) in kidney tissues (Table 1). This indicates that WNT10A signaling plays a role in fibronectin synthesis and in activating stromagenic factors to induce fibrosis.

WNT10A protects fibroblasts from oxidative stress

We previously reported that WNT10A expression is induced by treatment with hydrogen peroxide [10], suggesting that WNT10A signaling might induce the expression of antioxidant protein genes to protect cells. In this study, we found that WNT10A overexpression enhanced the expression of peroxiredoxin (PRDX) 5, but not PRDX 1, 2, 3 and 4 (Fig. 4A). COS1-10A cells expressed PRDX5 at approximately twice the level of control cells (Fig. 4B). PRDXs are a ubiquitous family of multifunctional antioxdant thioredoxin-dependent peroxidase that scavenge reactive oxygen species (ROS), suggesting that WNT10A overexpressing cells may be resistant against oxidative stress. As we expected, COS1-10A cells may be resistant to oxidative stress because WNT10A overexpression renders cells resistant to hydrogen peroxide (Fig. 4C). Down regulation of PRDX5 expression by siRNA sensitizes cells to hydrogen peroxide (Fig. 4D and E). COS1-10A cells expressed weakly active caspase-3 than control cells under hydrogen peroxide (Fig. 4F). WNT10A prevented apoptosis from oxidative stress via PRDX5 expression.

WNT10A prevented apoptosis of fibroblasts from high-glucose stress

High glucose triggers cell apoptosis, the generation of free radicals, and oxidative stress [20]. The control COS1 cells demonstrated poor survival following treatment with moderate- and high-glucose (MM and HM) compared with treatment with low-glucose medium (LM). However, COS1-10A cells survived even when treated with MM and HM, indicating that WNT10A overexpression protected fibroblasts from high glucose stress (Fig. 5A). Thus, high glucose stress leads to apoptosis of COS1 cells. As shown in Fig. 5B, control COS1 cells expressed caspase-3, cleaved caspase-3, PARP (poly ADP ribose polymerase), and cleavage-PARP compared with COS1-10A (Fig. 5B). WNT10A also prevented apoptosis from high glucose stress.

Discussion

The kidney is exposed to several kinds of stresses including oxidative stress, high glucose stress, hypoxic stress, and uremic stress. Oxidative stress in the kidney is considered a major cause of kidney injury and inflammation [21]. The pathogenesis and recovery processes of AKI is regulated by a wide variety of pathways in various inflammatory cells that produce cytokines/chemokines and ROS. Tissue-specific fibrosis is differentially regulated by intrinsic and extrinsic mechanisms that involve organ-specific autocrine and paracrine systems. The molecular mechanisms that determine progressive CKD after AKI are largely unknown. A previous report showed that persistently high profibrotic signaling activity induces paracrine signaling that drives fibroblasts proliferation and inflammation [22]. WNT signaling is persistently active in areas exposed to stress. However, following AKI, WNT signaling becomes widely activated in kidney [23]. Since WNT10A induces angio/stromagenesis [10], we considered the possibility that there may be a relationship between WNT10A, tissue fibrosis, and inflammation. In contrast to AIN tissue, WNT10A hardly expressed in kidney of chronic kidney disease (Fig. S1). Therefore, we hypothesized that WNT10A-positive cells are found in proximity to areas of severe tissue injury, and that secreted WNT10A might be involved in fibrotic synthesis on AIN.

Tissue repair and fibrosis from injury involves multiple evolutionarily-conserved processes. Hydrogen peroxide can function as a chemoattractant following injury to transmit an immediate damage signal. After the initial response, angio/stromagenesis occurs leading to formation of new blood vessels, the appearance of (myo) fibroblasts, and the ECM gradually forming granulation tissue. The tissue remodeling after granulation is regulated by contractile fibroblasts called myofibroblasts [24]. The sources of renal myofibroblasts are local resident fibroblasts that arise from proliferation (50%), and nonproliferat-

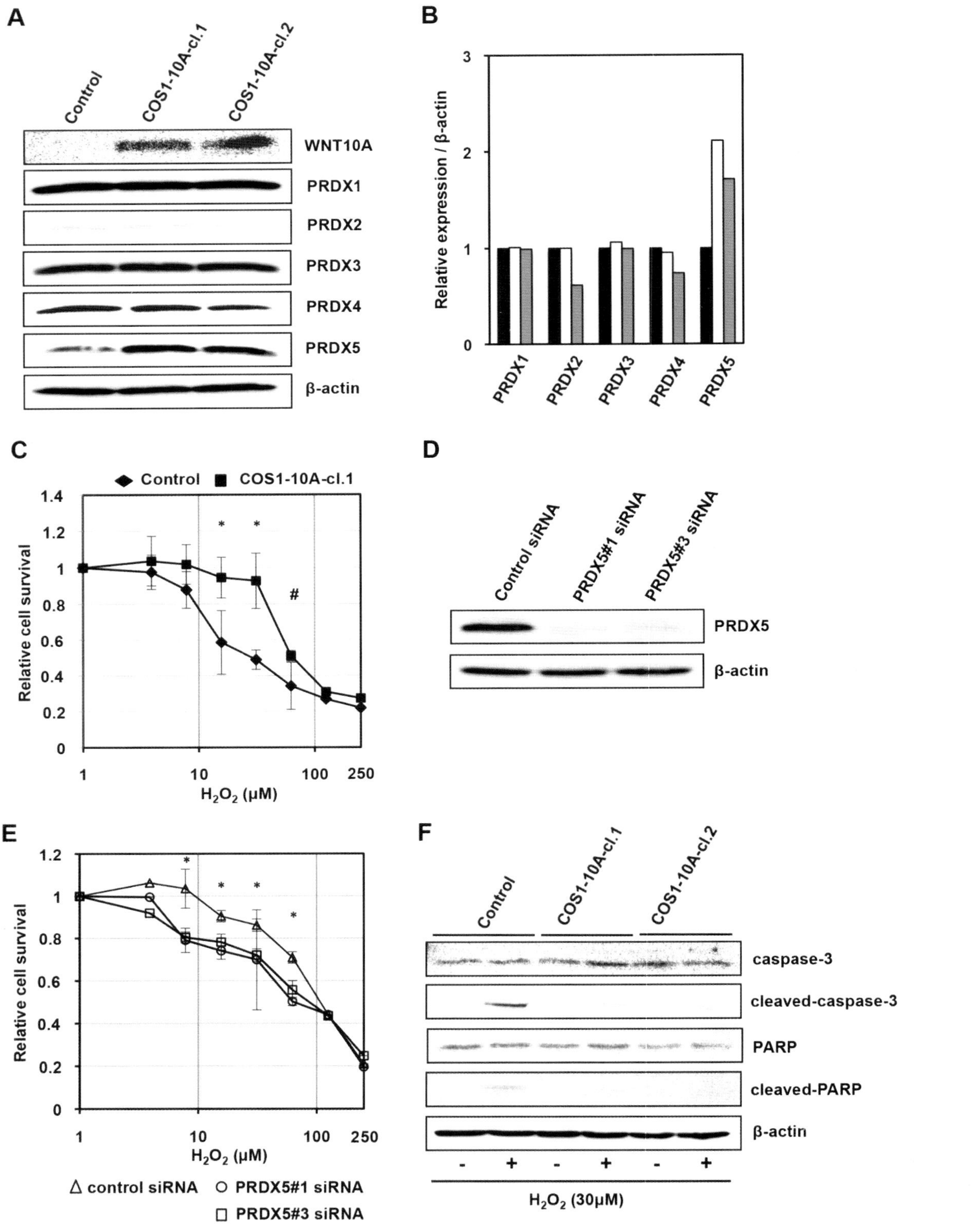

Figure 4. WNT10A protected fibroblasts against oxidative stress. (A) Western blot analysis of peroxiredoxin (PRDX)1, 2, 3, 4, and 5. Western blot analysis was performed using whole lysates obtained from COS1-vector (control) and COS1-10A cells. Only PRDX5 was increased with expression of WNT10A. (B) Relative expression of PRDX1, 2, 3, 4, and 5 normalized to β-actin expression. The black bar shows control cells, white and gray bars show COS1-10A-cl.1 and COS1-10A-cl.2 respectively. (C) The sensitivity of control and WNT10A-overexpressing cells (COS1-10A-cl.1) to H_2O_2. All values are the means of at least three independent experiments. Bars indicate standard deviation. *$p<0.01$ vs control. #$p<0.05$ vs control. (D) Downregulation of PRDX5 in WNT10A-overexpressing cells (COS1-10A-cl.1) by two kinds of siRNA. (E) The sensitivity of siRNA transfected cells to H_2O_2. All values are the means of at least three independent experiments. Bars indicate standard deviation. *$p<0.05$ vs PRDX5#1 and #3 siRNA. (F) Western blot analysis of caspase-3 and PARP expression. Western blot analysis was performed using whole lysates obtained from COS1-vector (control) and COS1-10A. Each cells were cultured in normal medium or medium containing hydrogen peroxide (30 μM) for 4 hours.

ing myofibroblasts derived from bone marrow (35%) [25]. It has been proposed that the remaining progenitor population is derived from circulating fibrocytes, local pericytes, and resident epithelial cells, although this remains to be fully characterized [26,27]. α-SMA expression induces fibroblasts into myofibroblasts [28]. Persistent myofibroblasts activation results in hypertrophic scars including keloid tissue or tissue fibrosis. Local activating fibroblasts express α-SMA and become fibrotic tissue [29]. Activation of WNT-β-catenin signaling has been reported in kidney and skin fibrosis [30,31]. WNT10A expression in kidney tissue associated with α-SMA and fibronectin expression, and interstitial fibrosis (Table 1). The patients with WNT10A expression showed significantly lower eGFR than patients without WNT10A expression on kidney biopsy (Fig. 1 and 2), suggesting that WNT10A may induce persistent myofibroblasts activation leading to tissue fibrosis.

TGF-β and connective tissue growth factor are cytokines that up-regulate fibronectin expression during fibrogenesis [32]. As shown in Fig. 3, WNT10A overexpression enhances the expression of one of the ECM components, fibronectin. This data supports relation between WNT10A and fibronectin expression in AIN kidney tissue (Fig. 3D and Table 1). Consequently, WNT10A increases synthesis of interstitial fibrosis. Fibronectin has two different forms, cellular and plasma fibronectin. Cellular fibronectin is expressed by fibroblasts and is deposited locally into the ECM [33]. In general, locally-produced cellular fibronectin

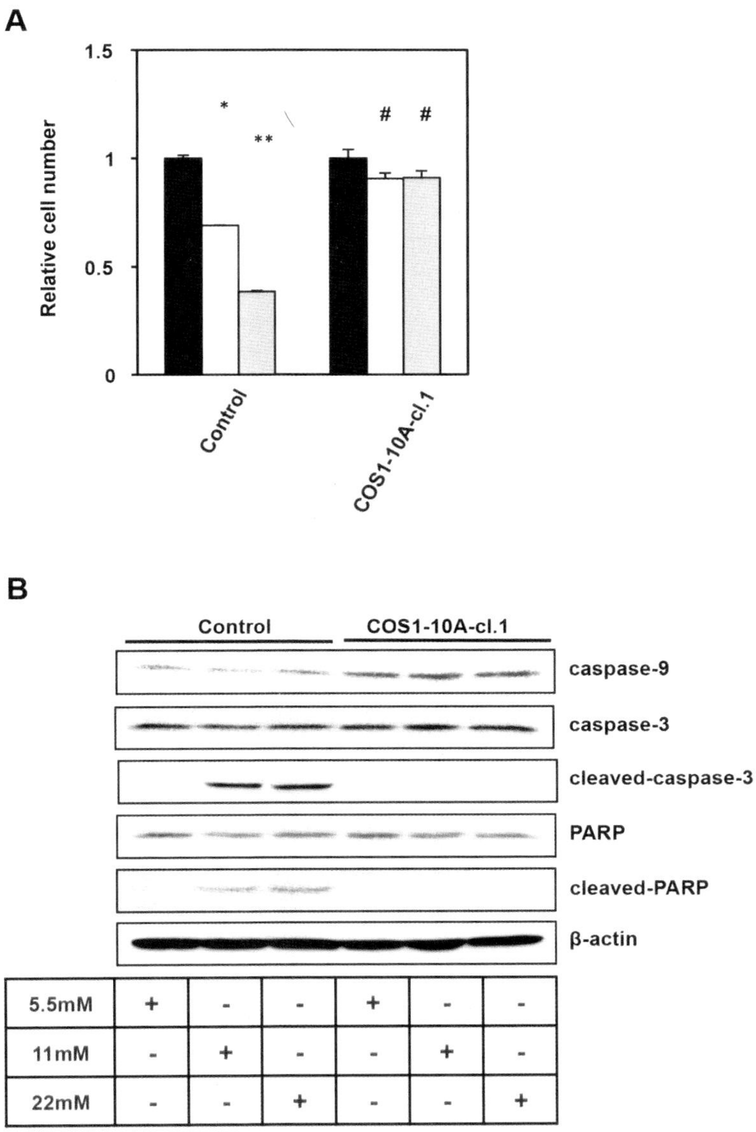

Figure 5. WNT10A protected fibroblasts against high glucose stress. (A) Proliferation assay. Control and WNT10A-overexpressing cells (COS1-10A-cl.1) (2×10^4 cells/well) were seeded into a 12-well plate, and incubated in normal DMEM. After 24 hours, cells (0hr) were harvested, and other cells were cultured in each medium (5.5 mM, 11 mM, and 22 mM of glucose concentration) for 72 hours. Proliferative rates for 72 hours were compared. Black bar (5.5 mM), white bar (11 mM), gray bar (22 mM). All values are the means of at least three independent experiments. Bars indicate standard deviation. *p<0.001 vs 5.5 mM, **p<0.001 vs 5.5 mM and 11 mM, #p<0.05 vs 5.5 mM (B) Caspase and PARP expression. Whole lysates obtained from control and WNT10A-overexpressing cells treated with each medium (5.5 mM, 11 mM, and 22 mM of glucose concentration) were analyzed by western blotting.

appears at the injury site within the early phase after tissue injury [34]. Plasma fibronectin is synthesized by hepatocytes and secreted into the blood plasma. Plasma fibronectin levels have been shown to increase after major trauma resulting in vascular tissue damage and inflammation such as atherosclerosis and ischemic diseases [35,36]. Previous studies suggested that mechanical stress contributes to injury and fibrosis by inducing epithelial-mesenchymal transition (EMT) via a mechanism driven by TGF-β1 and WNT signaling [37,38].

PRDXs are a ubiquitous family of multifunctional antioxidant thioredoxin-dependent peroxidases that scavenge reactive oxygen species (ROS). There are six distinct members located in various subcellular compartments. PRDX1, PRDX2, and PRDX6 are in the cytoplasm, and PRDX3 is in mitochondria. And PRDX4 is in endoplasmic reticulum and secreted. PRDX5 is expressed in mitochondria, the peroxisome, and the cytosol [39]. ROS are involved in initiation and implementation of apoptosis. PRDXs can efficiently eliminate hydrogen peroxide and participate in physiological processes such as apoptosis [40]. WNT10A promotes PRDX5 expression, and protects COS1 cells from oxidative stress (Fig. 4). Our study showed that WNT10A prevented COS1 cells from apoptosis by hydrogen peroxide. So, WNT10A may be helpful of fibroblasts to synthesize ECM under oxidative stress. As mentioned above, AKI is exposed several kinds of stresses including oxidative stress. WNT10A in kidney fibroblasts might play an important role in AKI/AIN.

We also investigated the relation between high glucose and WNT10A in COS1 cells. High glucose induces caspase-3-dependent apoptosis in fibroblasts, and activation of caspase caused by high glucose stress is independent of Fas/FasL signaling pathways system [41]. Activation of caspase-3 requires proteolytic cleavage of its inactive zymogen into active subunits. Cleaved caspase-3 causes apoptosis by degrading PARP. Our results show that WNT10A overexpression COS1 cells weaker expressed cleaved caspase-3 and PARP than control cells (Fig. 5B). WNT10A protected cells from apoptosis caused by high glucose stress. Consequently, a proliferation of WNT10A-overexpressing COS1 cells was small reduction than control cells (Fig. 5A).

3-hydroxy-3-methylglutaryl-coenzyme A (HMG-CoA) reductase inhibitors (statins) are used as therapy for hyperlipidemia. Statins inhibit kidney fibrosis and inflammation in rats [42,43], and inhibits fibronectin expression in human airway fibroblasts [44]. Several studies have reported that statins are anti-inflammatory and block proliferation by G1 arrest of the cell cycle [45,46,47]. Our investigation also indicated that simvastatin suppressed proliferation of COS1 via inducing apoptosis regardless of WNT10A expression (data not shown). Our work suggests that it will be important to study the effects of statins during kidney fibrosis in a clinical setting.

In conclusion, we should point out that WNT10A expression leads to loss of kidney function due to excess tissue fibrosis. WNT10A enhances the synthesis of fibronectin. Furthermore, WNT10A expression in kidney is thought to promote kidney fibrosis following severe kidney dysfunction. COS1 cells with WNT10A expression are not induced to apoptosis against for hydrogen peroxide and high glucose. Thus, these findings might imply kidney fibroblasts with WNT10A-expression maintain their viability and cause kidney fibrosis under several kinds of stresses in AKI. We expect that WNT10A expression in kidney tissue may be a bio-maker of prognosis for AKI. Further studies to validate our conclusions in other model systems such as animal model and 3-D culture system will be critical for understanding the role of WNT10A in kidney fibrosis.

Supporting Information

Figure S1 Expression of WNT10A in the kidney tissues of a chronic kidney disease (CKD) patient (left panel) and AIN patient (right panel). Immunohistochemical staining for WNT10A (brown). CKD patient had taken therapy for IgA nephropathy for a few decades. All photos were taken at 200×. Scale bar is 100 μm.

Figure S2 Expression of α-SMA in the kidney tissues. Each tissue is minor glomerular abnormalities (left panel) and AIN with WNT10A expression (right panel). Few myofibroblasts with α-SMA expression can be seen in the circumference of uriniferous tubule in minor glomerular abnormalities. Immunohistochemical staining for α-SMA (brown). All photos were taken at 200×. Scale bar is 100 μm.

Acknowledgments

We thank Naoko Une, Akiko Matsumura and Michiko Kurihara for their technical assistance.

Author Contributions

Conceived and designed the experiments: AK KK. Performed the experiments: AK SY KYW NK TY YI HI MT YO KK. Analyzed the data: AK SY KYW MT YO KK. Contributed reagents/materials/analysis tools: AK SY KYW HI KK. Wrote the paper: AK KK.

References

1. Eddy AA (2000) Molecular basis of renal fibrosis. Pediatr Nephrol 15: 290–301.
2. Liu Y (2006) Renal fibrosis: new insights into the pathogenesis and therapeutics. Kidney Int 69: 213–217.
3. Wynn TA, Ramalingam TR (2012) Mechanisms of fibrosis: therapeutic translation for fibrotic disease. Nat Med 18: 1028–1040.
4. Moon RT, Kohn AD, De Ferrari GV, Kaykas A (2004) WNT and beta-catenin signalling: diseases and therapies. Nat Rev Genet 5: 691–701.
5. Kohn AD, Moon RT (2005) Wnt and calcium signaling: beta-catenin-independent pathways. Cell Calcium 38: 439–446.
6. Carroll TJ, Das A (2011) Planar cell polarity in kidney development and disease. Organogenesis 7: 180–190.
7. Nusse R (2005) Wnt signaling in disease and in development. Cell Res 15: 28–32.
8. He W, Dai C, Li Y, Zeng G, Monga SP, et al. (2009) Wnt/beta-catenin signaling promotes renal interstitial fibrosis. J Am Soc Nephrol 20: 765–776.
9. Dai C, Stolz DB, Kiss LP, Monga SP, Holzman LB, et al. (2009) Wnt/beta-catenin signaling promotes podocyte dysfunction and albuminuria. J Am Soc Nephrol 20: 1997–2008.
10. Yasuniwa Y, Izumi H, Wang KY, Shimajiri S, Sasaguri Y, et al. (2010) Circadian disruption accelerates tumor growth and angio/stromagenesis through a Wnt signaling pathway. PLoS One 5: e15330.
11. Grande MT, López-Novoa JM (2009) Fibroblast activation and myofibroblast generation in obstructive nephropathy. Nat Rev Nephrol 5: 319–328.
12. Kitada S, Yamada S, Kuma A, Ouchi S, Tasaki T, et al. (2013) Polypeptide N-acetylgalactosaminyl transferase 3 independently predicts high-grade tumors and poor prognosis in patients with renal cell carcinomas. Br J Cancer 109: 472–481.
13. Noguchi H, Yamada S, Nabeshima A, Guo X, Tanimoto A, et al. (2014) Depletion of apoptosis signal-regulating kinase 1 prevents bile duct ligation-induced necroinflammation and subsequent peribiliary fibrosis. Am J Pathol 184: 644–661.
14. Igarashi T, Izumi H, Uchiumi T, Nishio K, Arao T, et al. (2007) Clock and ATF4 transcription system regulates drug resistance in human cancer cell lines. Oncogene 26: 4749–4760.
15. Shiota M, Izumi H, Miyamoto N, Onitsuka T, Kashiwagi E, et al. (2008) Ets regulates peroxiredoxin1 and 5 expressions through their interaction with the high-mobility group protein B1. Cancer Sci 99: 1950–1959.

16. Miyamoto N, Izumi H, Noguchi T, Nakajima Y, Ohmiya Y, et al. (2008) Tip60 is regulated by circadian transcription factor clock and is involved in cisplatin resistance. J Biol Chem 283: 18218–18226.
17. Izumi H, Takahashi M, Uramoto H, Nakayama Y, Oyama T, et al. (2011) Monocarboxylate transporters 1 and 4 are involved in the invasion activity of human lung cancer cells. Cancer Sci 102: 1007–1013.
18. Wakasugi T, Izumi H, Uchiumi T, Suzuki H, Arao T, et al. (2007) ZNF143 interacts with p73 and is involved in cisplatin resistance through the transcriptional regulation of DNA repair genes. Oncogene 26: 5194–5203.
19. Miyamoto N, Izumi H, Miyamoto R, Kubota T, Tawara A, et al. (2009) Nipradilol and timolol induce Foxo3a and peroxiredoxin 2 expression and protect trabecular meshwork cells from oxidative stress. Invest Ophthalmol Vis Sci 50: 2777–2784.
20. Sedeek M, Callera G, Montezano A, Gutsol A, Heitz F, et al. (2010) Critical role of Nox4-based NADPH oxidase in glucose-induced oxidative stress in the kidney: implications in type 2 diabetic nephropathy. Am J Physiol Renal Physiol 299: F1348–1358.
21. Joshi S, Peck AB, Khan SR (2013) NADPH oxidase as a therapeutic target for oxalate induced injury in kidneys. Oxid Med Cell Longev 2013: 462361.
22. Hinz B, Phan SH, Thannickal VJ, Prunotto M, Desmoulière A, et al. (2012) Recent developments in myofibroblast biology: paradigms for connective tissue remodeling. Am J Pathol 180: 1340–1355.
23. Kawakami T, Ren S, Duffield JS (2013) Wnt signalling in kidney diseases: dual roles in renal injury and repair. J Pathol 229: 221–231.
24. Tomasek JJ, Gabbiani G, Hinz B, Chaponnier C, Brown RA (2002) Myofibroblasts and mechano-regulation of connective tissue remodelling. Nat Rev Mol Cell Biol 3: 349–363.
25. LeBleu VS, Taduri G, O'Connell J, Teng Y, Cooke VG, et al. (2013) Origin and function of myofibroblasts in kidney fibrosis. Nat Med 19: 1047–1053.
26. Humphreys BD, Lin SL, Kobayashi A, Hudson TE, Nowlin BT, et al. (2010) Fate tracing reveals the pericyte and not epithelial origin of myofibroblasts in kidney fibrosis. Am J Pathol 176: 85–97.
27. Zeisberg M, Kalluri R (2004) The role of epithelial-to-mesenchymal transition in renal fibrosis. J Mol Med (Berl) 82: 175–181.
28. El Kahi CG, Atiyeh BS, Abdallah Hajj Hussein I, Jurjus R, Dibo SA, et al. (2009) Modulation of wound contracture alpha-smooth muscle actin and multispecific vitronectin receptor integrin alphavbeta3 in the rabbit's experimental model. Int Wound J 6: 214–224.
29. Hinz B, Celetta G, Tomasek JJ, Gabbiani G, Chaponnier C (2001) Alpha-smooth muscle actin expression upregulates fibroblast contractile activity. Mol Biol Cell 12: 2730–2741.
30. Wei J, Melichian D, Komura K, Hinchcliff M, Lam AP, et al. (2011) Canonical Wnt signaling induces skin fibrosis and subcutaneous lipotrophy: a novel mouse model for scleroderma? Arthritis Rheum 63: 1707–1717.
31. Surendran K, Schiavi S, Hruska KA (2005) Wnt-dependent β-catenin signaling is activated after unilateral ureteral obstruction, and recombinant secreted fizzled-related protein 4 alters the progression of renal fibrosis. J Am Soc Nephrol 16: 2373–2384.
32. Leask A, Abraham DJ (2004) TGF-beta signaling and the fibrotic response. FASEB J 18: 816–827.
33. Mao Y, Schwarzbauer JE (2005) Fibronectin fibrillogenesis, a cell-mediated matrix assembly process. Matrix Biol 24: 389–399.
34. Gabbiani G (2003) The myofibroblast in wound healing and fibrocontractive diseases. J Pathol 200: 500–503.
35. Song KS, Kim HK, Shim W, Jee SH (2001) Plasma fibronectin levels in ischemic heart disease. Atherosclerosis 154: 449–453.
36. Claudepierre P, Allanore Y, Belec L, Larget-Piet B, Zardi L, et al. (1999) Increased Ed-B fibronectin plasma levels in spondyloarthropathies: comparison with rheumatoid arthritis patients and a healthy population. Rheumatology (Oxford) 38: 1099–1103.
37. Heise RL, Stober V, Cheluvaraju C, Hollingsworth JW, Garantziotis S (2011) Mechanical stretch induces epithelial-mesenchymal transition in alveolar epithelia via hyaluronan activation of innate immunity. J Biol Chem 286: 17435–17444.
38. Chen JH, Chen WL, Sider KL, Yip CY, Simmons CA (2011) β-catenin mediates mechanically regulated, transforming growth factor-β1-induced myofibroblast differentiation of aortic valve interstitial cells. Arterioscler Thromb Vasc Biol 31: 590–597.
39. Wood ZA, Schröder E, Robin Harris J, Poole LB (2003) Structure, mechanism and regulation of peroxiredoxins. Trends Biochem Sci 28: 32–40.
40. Oláhová M, Taylor SR, Khazaipoul S, Wang J, Morgan BA, et al. (2008) A redox-sensitive peroxiredoxin that is important for longevity has tissue- and stress-specific roles in stress resistance. Proc Natl Acad Sci U S A 105: 19839–19844.
41. Liu J, Jiang Y, Mao J, Gu B, Liu H, et al. (2013) High levels of glucose induces a dose-dependent apoptosis in human periodontal ligament fibroblasts by activating caspase-3 signaling pathway. Appl Biochem Biotechnol 170: 1458–1471.
42. Gianella A, Nobili E, Abbate M, Zoja C, Gelosa P, et al. (2007) Rosuvastatin treatment prevents progressive kidney inflammation and fibrosis in stroke-prone rats. Am J Pathol 170: 1165–1177.
43. Vieira JM Jr, Mantovani E, Rodrigues LT, Dellê H, Noronha IL, et al. (2005) Simvastatin attenuates renal inflammation, tubular transdifferentiation and interstitial fibrosis in rats with unilateral ureteral obstruction. Nephrol Dial Transplant 20: 1582–1591.
44. Schaafsma D, McNeill KD, Mutawe MM, Mutawe MM, Ghavami S, et al. (2011) Simvastatin inhibits TGFβ1-induced fibronectins in human airway fibroblasts. Respir Res 12: 113.
45. Bereswill S, Muñoz M, Fischer A, Plickert R, Haag LM, et al. (2010) Anti-inflammatory effects of resveratrol, curcumin and simvastatin in acute small intestinal inflammation. PLoS One 5: e15099.
46. Yagi H, Kato T, Nagata T, Habu T, Nozaki M, et al. (1995) Regulation of the mouse histone H2A.X gene promoter by the transcription factor E2F and CCAAT binding protein. J Biol Chem 270: 18759–18765.
47. Javanmoghadam-Kamrani S, Keyomarsi K (2008) Synchronization of the cell cycle using lovastatin. Cell Cycle 7: 2434–2440.

19

Renal Involvement in Non-Hodgkin Lymphoma: Proven by Renal Biopsy

Shi-Jun Li, Hui-Ping Chen, Ying-Hua Chen, Li-hua Zhang, Yuan-Mao Tu, Zhi-hong Liu*

National Clinical Research Center of Kidney Diseases, Jinling Hospital, Nanjing University of Medcine, Nanjing, China

Abstract

Aims: To determine the spectrum of renal lesions in patients with kidney involvement in non-Hodgkin's lymphoma (NHL) by renal biopsy.

Methods: The clinical features and histological findings at the time of the renal biopsy were assessed for each patient.

Results: We identified 20 patients with NHL and renal involvement, and the diagnosis of NHL was established following the kidney biopsy in 18 (90%) patients. The types of NHL include the following: chronic lymphocytic leukemia/small lymphocytic lymphoma (n = 8), diffuse large B-cell lymphoma (n = 4), T/NK cell lymphoma (n = 3), lymphoplasmacytic lymphoma (n = 2), cutaneous T-cell lymphoma (n = 1), mucosa-associated lymphoid tissue lymphoma (n = 1) and mantle cell lymphoma (n = 1). All presented with proteinuria, and 15 patients had impaired renal function. The pathological findings included (1) membranoproliferative glomerulonephritis-like pattern in seven patients; (2) crescent glomerulonephritis in four; (3) minimal-change disease in three, and glomeruli without specific pathological abnormalities in three; (4) intraglomerular large B-cell lymphoma in one; (5) intracapillary monoclonal IgM deposits in one; (6) primary diffuse large B-cell lymphoma of the kidneys in one; and (7) lymphoma infiltration of the kidney in eight patients.

Conclusion: A wide spectrum of renal lesions can be observed in patients with NHL, and NHL may be first proven by renal biopsies for evaluation of kidney injury or proteinuria. Renal biopsy is necessary to establish the underlying cause of renal involvement in NHL.

Editor: Maria Pia Rastaldi, Fondazione IRCCS Ospedale Maggiore Policlinico & Fondazione D'Amico per la Ricerca sulle Malattie Renali, Italy

Funding: The authors have no support or funding to report.

* E-mail: zhihong—liu@hotmail.com

Introduction

Renal involvement in non-Hodgkin lymphoma (NHL) has been reported previously, including glomerulonephritis, acute kidney injury (AKI), and lymphoma infiltrating the kidney parenchyma [1–4]. Previous studies have shown that up to 10% of patients with NHL and lymphocytic leukemia may have kidney injury [5]. However, a limited number of cases of GN have been described in patients with NHL demonstrated by renal biopsy in the literature to date [6–8]. Considering that the morphology of glomerular injury in patients with lymphoma are often heterogeneous, the myriad of etiologies of renal injury due to NHL often present a diagnostic challenge to clinician. Here, we retrospectively analyzed the spectrum of renal lesions proven by renal biopsy in patients with NHL in single center, to better establish the relationship between renal injury and NHL.

Materials and Methods

Patient selection

We reviewed the renal pathology archives of the Research Institute of Nephrology at Nanjing University of Medicine from 2001 through 2012 and identified 20 patients with NHL and renal dysfunction of sufficient severity and/or proteinuria that a renal biopsy was obtained. The diagnosis of NHL was based on the 2008 WHO classification system [9]. This study was approved by the Ethical Committee of Nanjing University. According to the ethics committee recommendation, written consent was not required for this non interventional study. Patients or surrogates provided verbal informed consent prior to study inclusion. Verbal consent was obtained through a session of patient or family information explaining the study, its aims and the non interventional design. The consent was recorded in the medical chart of each patient. Patients or relatives had the opportunity to decline study participation at any time.

Data collection

Baseline data at the time of renal biopsy were obtained from the medical records for all cases. The following data were collected: sex, age, clinical presentation, ultrasound of kidneys, extra renal presentations and relevant clinical history.

Clinical and laboratory data at the time of kidney biopsy were assessed for each patient. Cryoglobulinemia was detected by cold precipitation of serum samples from blood that had been collected and processed at 37°C. Proteinuria was defined as a urine protein level >0.4 g/24 h, and hematuria, assessed using light microscopy, was defined as a red blood cell count >10,000/ml in the urinary sediment. Nephrotic syndrome was defined as a urinary protein excretion >3.5 g/d and a serum albumin level <30 g/L. Impaired renal function was defined as a GFR<60 ml/min per 1.73 m^2according to the Modification of Diet in Renal Disease (MDRD) formula. Acute kidney injury was defined according to the KIDIGO criteria.

Renal biopsy studies

All patients underwent a percutaneous renal biopsy. No symptom perirenal haematoma and macroscopic haematuria have been observed in these patients. Each renal sample contained more than 10 glomeruli. The renal biopsy procedure was as follows: the samples were embedded in paraffin and sectioned at 2 μm, followed by hematoxylin-eosin, Masson, periodic acid-Schiff or periodic acid-silver methenamine (PASM) staining. For immunofluorescence (IF), the samples were sectioned at 3 μm using a cryostat, followed by use of a panel of FITC-conjugated rabbit anti-human antibodies to IgG, IgM, IgA, C3, C1q, and κ and λ light chains (polyclonal, Dako Corporation). These samples were also stained with Congo red. The intensity of the immunofluorescence staining was semiquantitatively scored on a scale of 0 to 2+. Immunophenotyping of the lymphomas was performed on frozen sections using the immunoperoxidase and avidin-biotin techniques. The phenotype of the cellular infiltrate was studied using biotinylated anti-CD4, -CD8, -CD20 and -CD68 antibodies (Dako) and visualized using a peroxidase-streptavidin conjugate. Electron microscopy was performed using a Hitachi 7500 electron microscope after routine sections were prepared from renal tissues, followed by double staining with uranyl acetate and lead citrate. Renal biopsies from all patients were reviewed by two renal pathologists.

Results

Clinical findings

The clinical characteristics of all 20 patients are summarized in Table 1. There were 17 men and 3 women aged 16 to 68 years at the time of renal biopsy (mean age 53 years). At the time of the renal biopsy, only 2 (10%) of 20 patients had an established diagnosis of NHL, the remaining 18 patients had renal biopsies performed before the diagnosis of the lymphoma. Six patients (30%) presented with recurring fever of unknown origin. Enlargement of the inguinal, axillary, submaxillary or supraclavicular lymph nodes were found in eight patients (40%). Computed tomography (CT) scans revealed numerous intumesced lymph nodes in the neck, mediastinal septum and retroperitoneal space in five patients (25%). CT revealed markedly enlarged kidneys bilaterally in nine (45%) patients, enlargement of the spleen in three patients. (See Table 1). The anatomic sites of sampling used for the primary diagnosis of the lymphoid neoplasm were the lymph nodes (n = 7), bone marrow (n = 6), gastrointestinal tract (n = 2), nasal cavity/sinus (n = 2), kidney (n = 2) and skin (n = 1).

Of the 20 patients with NHL, 16 (80%) had B-cell neoplasms, including chronic lymphocytic leukemia/small lymphocytic lymphoma (CLL/SLL, n = 8), diffuse large B-cell lymphoma (DLBCL, n = 4), lymphoplasmacytic lymphoma (LPL, n = 2), mucosa-associated lymphoid tissue lymphoma (MALT, n = 1) and mantle cell lymphoma (MCL, n = 1). Four patients (20%) had mature T/NK-cell neoplasms, including extra nodal NK/T-cell lymphoma, nasal type T/NK cell lymphoma (n = 2), cutaneous T-cell lymphoma (n = 1) and adult T-cell lymphoma (n = 1).

All patients presented with proteinuria, and 15 patients (75%) had impaired renal function(eGFR<60 ml/min). The mean serum creatinine level was 228±181 μmol/l (range 50 to 752 μmol/L). Microscopic hematuria was found in 15 patients (75%), and gross hematuria in 4 patients (20%). Renal symptoms included nephrotic syndrome in 6 patients, while accompanied by AKI in 4 patients; rapidly progressive glomerulonephritis (RPGN) in 5 patients; AKI in 5 patients and mild proteinuria/microscopic hematuria in the remaining 4 patients (see Table 2).

Eighteen patients (90%) had anemia (5.9 to 11.3 g/dl), five had leukocytosis, three had leucopenia and three had thrombopenia. Two patients were positive for ANA, two were positive for cytoplasmic antineutrophil cytoplasmic antibodies (C-ANCA) and anti-proteinase 3 ANCA (PR3-ANCA) and one was positive for anti-glomerular basement membrane antibody (anti-GBM). IgM (kappa) monoclonal protein was detected in five patients by immunofixation electrophoresis. Cryoglobulinemia was also identified in three patients (see Table 2).

Histological findings

The histological findings of 20 patients are summarized in Table 3. Membranoproliferative glomerulonephritis -like patterns was found in seven patients with B-cell lymphoma. Light microscopy showed increased cellularity in all glomeruli and accentuation of the lobular architecture (Fig. 1 A). Silver staining showed double contours within the capillary loops. Capillary loops contained infiltrating leucocytes (more than 10 cells). Immunofluorescence studies revealed granular staining in a lobular pattern for IgG, IgM or C3 in five patients (Fig. 1 B). IgG was undetectable, and only IgM and C3 were present in mesangial area in case 6 and 18. The interstitium was diffusely or focally infiltrated by mononuclear cells. Electron microscopy showed fine subendothelial and mesangial electron-dense deposits together with frequent double-contoured appearance (Fig. 1 C).

Crescent glomerulonephritis was demonstrated in 4 patients, two patients had T/NK cell lymphoma, and the remaining two had CLL/SLL. No evidence of immune complex deposition was found in case1, 2; and serum PR3-ANCA was positive in case 2. IgG line deposits along the GBM and anti-GBM antibody was positive in case 7. Cellular crescents and focal necrotizing capillary by LM and IgG, IgM, IgA and C3 deposits in the mesangial and capillary were confirmed in case 8. In addition to the glomerular lesions, mononuclear cell infiltration was observed in the peritubular capillaries (PTCs) in all 4 patients.

Three patients (case 4,10,11) had minimal change in the glomeruli observed by light microscopy and no immune complex deposition by IF assay, but ultrastructural examination of these glomeruli revealed extensive effacement of the foot processes characteristic of minimal-change disease (MCD). The other three patients(case 3,5,17) revealed glomeruli without specific pathological abnormalities, ultrastructural examination revealed only segmental effacement of the foot processes, and the IF assay showed staining for IgG and IgM deposits in the glomeruli in two patients(case 3,5). Mononuclear cell infiltration was also observed in the PTCs in five patients (Fig. 1 E, F).

Primary diffuse large B-cell lymphoma of the kidney was found in case 13. Severe cell infiltration throughout the cortex and marked destruction of both the glomeruli and the tubular structure, with only two ruined glomeruli were observed. The accumulation of large atypical lymphoid cells with hyperchromatic nuclei was observed in renal specimens under high-power magnification (Fig. 2A). IF did not reveal any glomerular immune deposits. The lymphoid cell were positive for CD20 (+++) (Fig. 2B) and CD79a (+) but negative for CD3, CD43 and CD138.

Intraglomerular large B-cell lymphoma was identified in case 14. Lymphoid cells were present only within the lumina of the

Table 1. Clinical features of patients with NHL and renal involvement

Patient	Sex	Age	Type of lymphoma	Biopsy site	Clinical symptoms of lymphoma	Renal symptoms	Treatment	Patient outcome	Renal Outcome (Scr μmol/l)
1	M	16	T/NK	Nasal mucosa	Anemia, fever, nasal discharge	RPGN	EPOCH	Died (1 yr)	NA
2	F	38	T/NK	Nasal mucosa	Fever, nasal discharge	NS	Steroids	Died (2 mo)	NA
3	F	39	TCL	Lymph node	Fever, lymphadenectasis	proteinuria	CHOP	Died (2 mo)	NA
4	M	40	TCL	Skin	Skin rash	NS	Steroids	NA	NA
5	M	61	CLL/SLL	Bone marrow	Anemia, weakness	AKI	Chlorambucil	Died (2 mo)	NA
6	F	57	CLL/SLL	Lymph node	Anemia, lymphadenectasis	RPGN	Chlorambucil	NA	NA
7	M	64	CLL/SLL	Lymph node	Lymphadenectasis	RPGN	FC	Died (3 mo)	NA
8	M	55	CLL/SLL	Lymph node	Lymphadenectasis	RPGN	FC	Alive (3 yr)	dialysis
9	M	59	CLL/SLL	Bone marrow	Leucocytosis	RPGN	Steroids	Alive (6 yr)	126
10	M	61	CLL/SLL	Bone marrow	Anemia, weakness	NS+AKI	FC	Alive (3 yr)	137
11	M	68	CLL/SLL	Bone marrow	Anemia, lymphadenectasis	NS+AKI	Steroids	Died (4 mo)	NA
12	M	62	CLL/SLL	Bone marrow	Anemia, leucopenia	AKI	CTX	Alive (1 yr)	350
13	M	47	DLBCL	Kidney	Fever, weakness	AKI	CHOP	Alive (1 yr)	109
14	M	56	DLBCL	Kidney	Anemia	AKI	CHOP	Died (2 yr)	NA
15	M	62	DLBCL	Lymph node	Anemia, lymphadenectasis	AKI	Steroids	Alive (8 yr)	156
16	M	37	DLBCL	Ileum	Fever, diarrhea	proteinuria	CHOP	Died (2 yr)	NA
17	M	53	LPL	Lymph node	Anemia, lymphadenectasis	proteinuria	Steroids	Alive (2 yr)	89
18	M	68	LPL	Bone marrow	Fever, Anemia, skin rash	proteinuria	CTX	Died (1 yr)	NA
19	M	65	MCL	Lymph node	Anemia, lymphadenectasis	NS+AKI	CHOP	Alive (1 yr)	101
20	M	52	MALT	Stoma mucosa	Anemia, stomachache	NS+AKI	R+Steroids	Alive (1 yr)	249

CLL/SLL: chronic lymphocytic leukemia/small lymphocytic lymphoma, DLBCL: diffuse larger B-cell lymphoma, T/NK:T/NK cell lymphoma, TCL: T-cell lymphoma, MALT: mucosa-associated lymphoid tissue lymphoma, MCL: mantle cell lymphoma, LPL: lymphoplasmacytic lymphoma, NS: nephritic syndrome,
AKI: acute kidney injury, RPGN: rapidly progressive glomerulonephritis, R: radiotherapy, NA: not available.
CHOP: cyclophosphamide, hydroxydaunomycin, oncovin, prednisone. CTX: cyclophosphamide.
EPOCH:Etoposide, prednisone, oncovin, cyclophosphamide, hydroxydaunomycin, FC: fludarabine, cyclophosphamide

glomerular capillaries and not within the interstitium (Fig 2C). Large pleomorphic lymphoid cells often occluded the glomerular capillaries. The lymphoid cells had large vesicular nuclei. In the IF analysis of frozen sections, the lymphoid cells were $CD45^+$, $CD3^-$ and $CD20^{3+}$ (Fig 2D).

Intracapillary monoclonal IgM deposits (ICMDD) was observed in case 12. The most striking glomerular lesions consisted of periodic acid Schiff-positive intracapillary deposits that were variable in size and distribution (Fig. 3A). In the IF assay, all of the deposits were strongly stained for IgM and the κ light chain (Fig. 3B, C). EM revealed large intracapillary deposits that dilated the capillary lumen. No organized structure was observed (Fig. 3D).

The monomorphic lymphocytes infiltrates were patchy in 7 cases, diffuse in case 13 (Table 3), renal tubules were separated and atrophic or destroyed as a result of interstitial infiltrates. Staining with various immunohistochemical markers revealed that the infiltrating lymphocyte cells were positive for predominance of CD20, while $CD68^+$ cells within the infiltration (Table 3), which is consistent with B-cell lymphoma.

Outcome

During follow-up, two patients were lost, nine patients died. Among those who died, three patients with T/NK cell lymphoma died of infection after they received specific chemotherapy; the remaining six patients died as a direct or indirect result of the lymphoma during the first 2 years after NHL diagnosis. In these nine patients, four patients had AKI, four patients had CKD in last record. At the end of the follow-up period (6-96 months, average 35 months), three patients had normal serum creatinine, five patients had renal function stable or improved after chemotherapy, and one patient required permanent hemodialysis. (See Table 1).

Discussion

In this study, we confirmed that a wide spectrum of NHL is associated with renal injury, particularly with B-cell lymphocytic type NHL. CLL/SLL was the most common type of lymphoma associated with renal involvement (40%), followed by DLBCL and NK/T-cell lymphoma (20%). The profile of the NHL reported in the literature is similar to that observed our study. Kowalewska et al. [6] found a similar pattern of distribution; among 18 patients with neoplasms and kidney injury, the most common type of lymphoma was CLL/SLL, followed by DLBCL. However, Sun et al. [10] showed that the most common subtype of lymphoma was DLBCL (36.2%) in China, followed by extranodal NK/T-cell lymphoma, nasal type (11.0%); CLL/SLL accounted for only 3.7% of all lymphoid neoplasm. This finding suggests that renal involvement may be commonly associated with CLL/SLL. The pathogenesis of CLL/SLL-associated glomerulonephritis is not well understood. Notably, four of eight patients with CLL/SLL had serum positive for ANA or ANCA, three had M-component and two had cryoglobulinemia in their sera. Therefore, glomerulonephritis may also be related to the production of cryoglobulins

Table 2. Summary of clinical data in patients with NHL and renal involvement

Patient	Hb (g/L)	WBC (*10^9/L)	Scr (μmol/l)	eGFR (ml/min)	albumin (g/L)	globulin (g/L)	Urine protein (g/d)	Urine RBC (10^4/ml)	Urine NAG (U/g·cr)	Urine RBP (mg/L)	Renal size (mm/mm)	Antibody or Cryo	SIFE
1	70	6.6	187	44.8	33	31.3	2.72	2500	40.7	65.5	115/109	N	N
2	90	4.1	61	105	28.2	35.3	3.5	95	31.2	1.51	103/101	ANA PR3-ANCA	N
3	65	4.5	100	52.7	32.6	28.8	1.58	N	47.6	1.32	104/100	N	N
4	147	5.2	95	85.9	20.4	16.4	5.37	15	39.4	1.13	109/105	N	N
5	59	2.8	543	13	38.4	38.7	1.3	2000	40.2	7.78	106/102	PR3-ANCA	N
6	66	4.0	151	32.8	36.4	29.9	3.02	1850	94	1.88	99/98	ANA	N
7	91	5.1	338	15.6	36.5	26.3	1.41	1250	26.9	10.2	107/103	A-GBM	N
8	99	10.1	477	12.6	31.6	45.7	2.75	3000	35.5	10.2	127/122	Cryo	N
9	87	25.3	188	32.9	38.9	27.8	4.24	750	83.2	0.43	100/98	N	N
10	99	11.4	320	18.3	23.6	29.9	10.2	15	48.2	31.7	97/96	N	IgM, k
11	111	7.3	235	25.6	17.1	29.1	14.9	570	75.4	53.4	94/96	N	IgM, k
12	89	3.3	392	17.8	27.7	17.7	0.71	N	25.2	4.5	123/120	Cryo	IgM, k
13	135	8.8	158	46.3	44.2	29.7	0.39	N	20.2	10	167/146	N	N
14	98	5.6	166	37.2	40.6	27.4	0.84	N	32.4	3.44	114/110	N	N
15	113	4.2	168	34.2	38.3	15.5	1.24	47	21.1	0.13	103/101	N	N
16	107	10.6	77	103	36	18	0.68	50	25.7	0.1	106/101	N	N
17	109	4.5	74	103	34	40.3	0.41	N	26.2	0.93	129/120	N	IgM, k
18	78	9.4	50	95.8	27.2	18.8	0.7	230	82.3	0.84	111/110	Cryo	N
19	80	13.8	164	34.8	28.4	28.6	6.92	260	25	15.5	112/115	N	N
20	106	3.7	263	36.5	32.3	18.7	7.96	1100	119	11.9	112/106	N	IgM, k

Hb, hemoglobin; WBC, white blood count; BUN, blood urea nitrogen; SCr, serum creatinine; eGFR: estimated Glomerular Filtration Rate

NAG, N-acetyl-pD glucosaminidase enzyme, RBP: retinol-binding protein (RBP). ANA: antinuclear antibody, C-ANCA: antineutrophil cytoplasmic antibody, PR3-ANCA: anti-proteinase 3 ANCA, A-GBM: anti-glomerular basement membrane antibody, Cryo: cryoglobulinemia; SIFE: serum immunofixation electrophoresis, N negative

Table 3. Renal biopsy findings

	Glomerular Disease	Infiltrating cells		Immunofluorescence							Immunoperoxidase	
		Glomerular	PTC	IgG	IgA	IgM	C3	C1q	κ	λ	CD20(n/mm²)	CD68(n/mm²)
1	Crescent GN	>5	Y	-	-	-	-	-	-	-	NA	192
2	Crescent GN	2–3	Y	-	-	-	-	-	-	-	NA	NA
3	NSPA	2–3	No	+	-	+	-	-	-	-	96	NA
4	MCD	2–3	Y	-	-	-	-	-	-	-	Multifocal	152
5	NSPA	>3	Y	++	-	-	++	++	-	+	NA	624
6	MPGN	>10	Y	-	-	+	+	+	-	-	Diffuse	548
7	Crescent GN	>5	Y	++	-	-	-	-	-	+	Multifocal	Diffuse
8	Crescent GN	>5	Y	++	+	+	++	++	+	+	Multifocal	592
9	MPGN	>10	Y	++	+	++	++	+	++	+	Multifocal	152
10	MCD	3–5	Y	-	-	-	-	-	-	-	184	872
11	MCD	3–5	Y	-	-	-	-	-	-	-	72	356
12	ICMDD	3–5	Y	-	-	++	-	-	++	-	Diffuse	140
13	No glomerular	ND	Y	-	-	-	-	-	-	-	192	1192
14	Lymphoma	ND	Y	-	+	+	-	-	-	-	16	848
15	MPGN	>10	Y	++	+	++	+	++	+	++	NA	NA
16	MPGN	>10	No	++	++	-	++	-	+	+	144	NA
17	NSPA	3–5	Y	-	-	-	-	-	-	-	Multifocal	312
18	MPGN	>5	Y	-	++	-	++	-	+	-	Focal	268
19	MPGN	>10	No	++	-	-	+–	++	-	+	180	420
20	MPGN	>10	No	++	++	-	+–	-	++	+	NA	312

MPGN: Membranoproliferative glomerulonephritis. FSNGN: Focal segmental necrotizing glomerulonephritis. PTC: ICMDD: Intracapillary monoclonal IgM deposits. Lymphoma: Intraglomerular lymphoma. MCD: Minimal-change disease NSPA:No specific pathologic abnormalities; NA: not available. Immunofluorescence: -, negative; +, mild; ++, intense. λ: λ light chain; κ: κ light chain.

and/or immunoglobulins (paraprotein production) by secretory B-cell clones in patients with CLL/SLL.

In our series, the most common presentations of renal involvement in NHL patients were renal impairment and proteinuria. All patients presented with proteinuria, and 75% had impaired renal function; 30% had nephrotic syndrome and 25% had RPGN. It is difficult to distinguish lymphoma-associated glomerulonephritis from primary kidney disease in the clinic. Interestingly, at the time of the renal biopsy, only 10% patients in our series had an established diagnosis of current NHL. Therefore, renal biopsy may be suggested as the diagnostic method of choice.

The most common pattern of glomerular involvement in our series was glomerulonephritis with MPGN-like patterns. All seven cases of MPGN-like patterns were associated with B-cell neoplasm. Among these patients, three were positive for serum ANA, M-component or cryoglobulinemia. IgG deposition was not observed in two patients, which is different from typical MPGN. Moulin et al. [11] retrospectively analyzed 13 patients with glomerulonephritis and chronic lymphocytic leukemia (CLL) or B-cell lymphoma; MPGN was observed in eight patients, five patients had cryoglobulinemia and two patients had circulating M-component. Therefore, MPGN- like patterns associated with NHL may directly result from the lymphoma through a paraprotein deposition process that results in cryoglobulinemia or monoclonal immunoglobulin deposition disease, or it may be induced indirectly through immune-mediated mechanisms.

Four patients had crescent glomerulonephritis in our series; one patient with PR3-ANCA, one with anti-GBM antibody. Pauci-immune crescentic glomerulonephritis associated with NHL and ANCA has also been reported by Henriksen and Dussol [12–13]. However, we describe a previously unreported unique case of anti-GBM glomerulonephritis in a patient with CLL/SLL. Given that NHL patients have defective T-cell colony-forming capacity and T-cell regulatory function, the simultaneous presence of NHL, anti-GBM and crescentic glomerulonephritis may not be a coincidence.

Minimal-change nephrotic syndrome is described as a paraneoplastic manifestation of classical Hodgkin's lymphoma (HL) that occurs in 0.4% of Hodgkin's lymphoma patients but is a rare complication of NHL [14–15]. In our series, three patients presented with nephritic syndrome, and showed MCD by EM. Increased cytokine levels caused by T- or B-cell lymphoma cytokine-induced altered glomerular permeability and podocyte injury may be responsible for nephrotic syndrome [15]. In these patients, mononuclear cell infiltration into the PTC and lymphocytic infiltration of the tubule interstitium were also observed. It is not clear why patients with NHL associated renal injury have mononuclear cell infiltration into the PTC. One possibility would be that NHL induces the release of proinflammatory molecules, which induce infiltrating cells infiltration. These results suggest that the immune processes involved in the pathogenesis of NHL-associated MCD are different from those of idiopathic MCD.

ICMDD was defined as PAS-positive intracapillary thrombi in glomeruli that were sufficiently voluminous to occlude the capillary lumens and thrombi positive for IgM and either κ or λ LC by IF. This type of renal lesion was first reported in

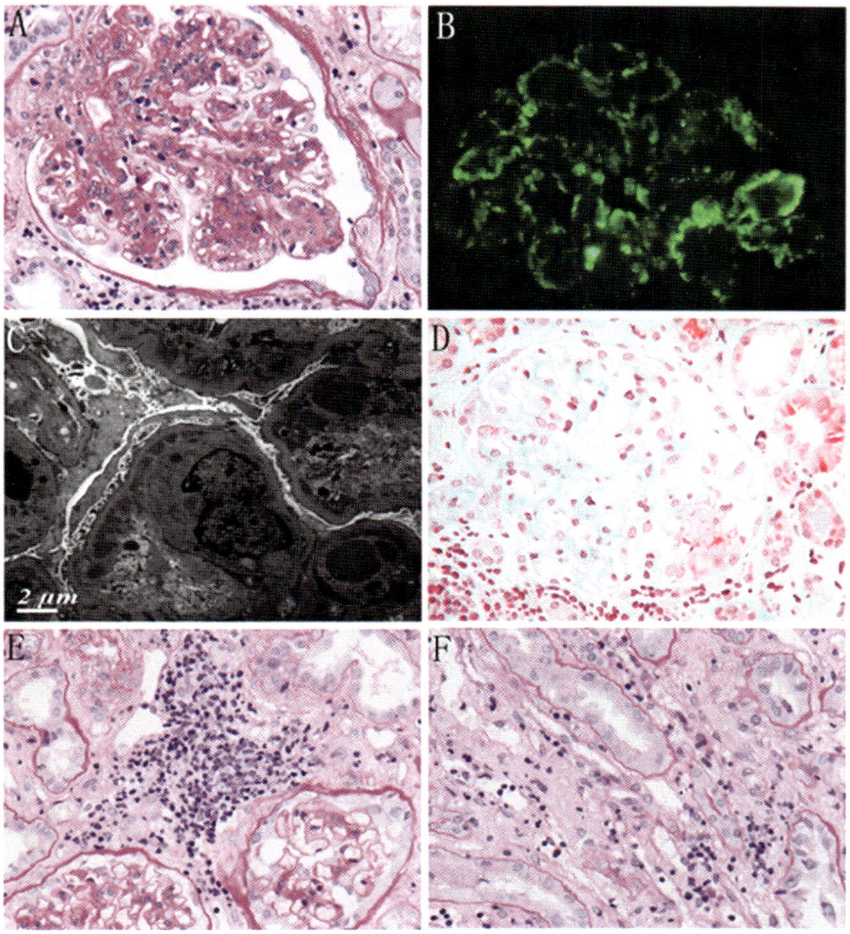

Figure 1. Representative renal histological change in patients with NHL. A Light microscopy showed increased cellularity in glomeruli and the accentuation of the lobular architecture (patient 9 PAS×400). B Immunofluorescence showed granular staining in a lobular pattern for IgG (patient 9 IF×400). C Electron microscopy showed fine subendothelial electron-dense deposits (patient 9 EM). D Glomeruli with focal segmental necrosis and lymphoid cell infiltration around glomeruli (patient 8 Masson×400). E Glomeruli without pathological abnormalities visualized by LM with lymphocyte-like cell infiltration in the interstitial tissue (patient 5 PAS×200). F Mononuclear cell infiltration in the peritubular capillaries (patient 5 PAS×400).

Waldenstrom macroglobulinemia (WM). However, Audard et al. [16] reported that only three of five patients with ICMDD had WM, whereas the two other patients had an IgM-related disorder and a B-cell lymphoma. In our study, patients with intraglomerular thrombi were found to have circulating monoclonal IgM and κ LC. Cellular proliferation in the glomeruli was absent or mild; no organized microtubular structures were visualized by EM, which suggests a diagnosis of ICMDD rather than cryoglobulinemic glomerulonephritis. Therefore, ICMDD may be applied to IgM-secreting B-cell lymphoma. In addition, κ and/or λ light chain staining was positive by immunofluorescence in 10 patients in our study. However, no linear deposits of κ or λ light chain staining within GBM and TBM was observed, which was the characteristic for light chain deposition disease (LCDD).

Renal involvement is rare in patients with diffuse large B-cell lymphoma (DLBCL). Villa et al. [17] identified renal involvement in only 2% (55/2656) of patients with DLBCL at the time of diagnosis. In the present study, computed tomography (CT) revealed markedly enlarged kidneys bilaterally in case 13, and the renal parenchyma was massively infiltrated by $CD20^{+}$ lymphoid cells; the lymphoma was classified as diffuse large B-cell lymphoma. Intravascular large B-cell lymphoma (IVLBCL) is a very rare subtype of NHL lymphoma. To the best of our knowledge, no more than 20 cases have been published in the literature [18–19]. The patients with intraglomerular large B-cell lymphoma may present with proteinuria, renal dysfunction, which may clinically mimic primary glomerulonephritis. The glomerular lesion may appear confusingly like endocapillary proliferative glomerulonephritis; only immunocytochemical characteristics can reveal the true lymphoid cells [20]. In such cases, kidney biopsy is the only way to establish the correct diagnosis.

In our study, 40% patients showed lymphomatous infiltration of the interstitium. All of these patients had B-cell lymphoma, and seven of eight presented with AKI. Lymphocytic infiltrations of the renal tubulointerstitium and AKI have been reported previously [2,6]. The mechanism of AKI due to lymphomatous infiltration of the kidneys is unknown; infiltrate may destruct of the normal renal architecture and cause intrarenal obstruction. The aggregates of inflammatory cells such as CD68+ cells can also be seen in these patients, which suggest to inflammatory response to lymphomatous infiltration. A monotonous appearance and aggregates of infiltrative pattern of the lymphomatous cell population in kidney

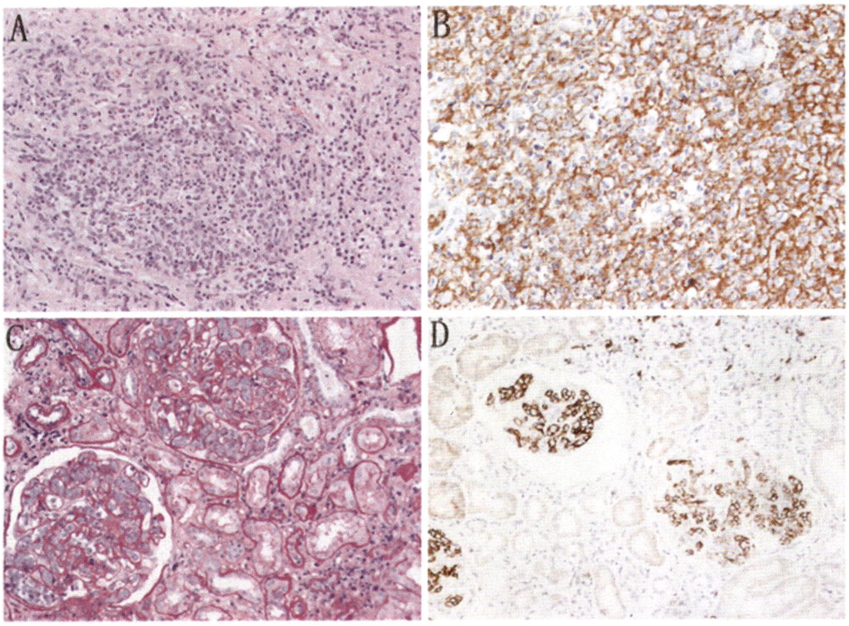

Figure 2. Diffuse infiltration into the renal parenchyma and intraglomerular lymphoma in DLBCL. A. Accumulation of large atypical lymphoid cells was observed in renal specimens (patient 13 PAS×400). B. Immunohistochemical staining showing strong staining for CD20 in the lymphoid cells (patient 13 IH×400). C. Glomerular capillary lumina containing atypical large cells in the enlarged glomeruli (patient 14 PAS ×400). D Immunohistochemistry showing strong staining for CD20 in lymphoid cells localized within the glomerular capillary lumina (patient 14 IH×400).

should prompt the examiner to perform an additional workup to rule out or confirm lymphoma.

The differentiation between a primary glomerular disease and lymphoma-associated glomerulonephritis is difficult. Therefore, we need to implement screening for the underlying hematological malignancy if a patient presents with (1) severe anemia, leukocytosis and/or thrombopenia; (2) enlarged lymph nodes and/or enlarged kidneys; (3) mononuclear cells in the PTC or

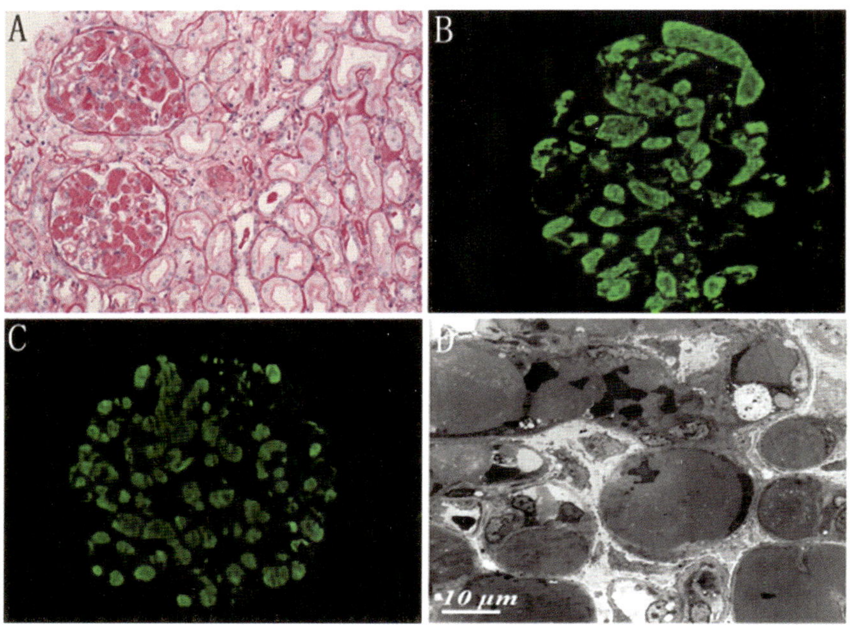

Figure 3. Intracapillary monoclonal deposition disease in an NHL patient (patient 12). A PAS-positive intracapillary thrombi in glomerulus (PAS, ×200). B Immunofluorescence showed bright staining of the intraglomerular thrombi for IgM. C Immunofluorescence showed bright staining of the intraglomerular thrombi for κ LC.D Electron microscopy showed that the glomerular capillary lumen was filled with granular electron-dense material. No organized structure was observed.

monomorphic lymphoid cells infiltration in renal parenchyma. If a patient has one or more of the above conditions, it is imperative that the patient undergo a full workup for lymphoma, which should include lymph node biopsy, bone marrow aspiration and biopsy, serum immunofixation studies and cryoglobulinemia detection. If these tests are positive, then a series of immunohistochemical staining studies is warranted to determine whether the kidney injury is caused by underlying lymphoma.

In conclusion, we confirmed that a wide spectrum of renal pathological findings can be observed in patients with NHL, and NHL may be first diagnosed by renal biopsies for evaluation of kidney injury or proteinuria. CLL/SLL were the most common types of NHL associated with renal injury, and the most common pattern of glomerular lesion was MPGN-like pattern. Renal biopsy is necessary to establish the underlying cause of renal involvement in NHL.

Author Contributions

Conceived and designed the experiments: S-JL Z-hL. Analyzed the data: Y-HC L-hZ Y-MT. Wrote the paper: S-JL H-PC.

References

1. Ronco PM. (1999) Paraneoplastic glomerulopathies: new insights into an old entity. Kidney Int 56:355–377.
2. Cohen LJ, Rennke HG, Laubach JP, Humphreys BD. (2010) The spectrum of kidney involvement in lymphoma: a case report and review of the literature. Am J Kidney Dis 56:1191–1196.
3. Rault R, Holley JL, Banner BF, el-Shahawy M.(1992) Glomerulonephritis and non-Hodgkin's lymphoma: a report of two cases and review of the literature. Am J Kidney Dis. 20:84–89.
4. Stokes MB, Wood B, Alpers CE. (2002) Membranoproliferative glomerulonephritis associated with low-grade B cell lymphoma presenting in the kidney. Clin Nephrol 57:303–309.
5. Da'as N, Polliack A, Cohen Y, Amir G, Darmon D, et al. (2001) Kidney involvement and renal manifestations in non-Hodgkin's lymphoma and lymphocytic leukemia: a retrospective study in 700 patients. Eur J Haematol 67:158–164.
6. Kowalewska J, Nicosia RF, Smith KD, Kats A, Alpers CE. (2011) Patterns of glomerular injury in kidneys infiltrated by lymphoplasmacytic neoplasms. Hum Pathol. 42:896–903.
7. Shi SF, Zhou FD, Zou WZ, Wang HY. (2012) Acute kidney injury and bilateral symmetrical enlargement of the kidneys as first presentation of B-cell lymphoblastic lymphoma. Am J Kidney Dis 60:1044–1048.
8. Yeo SC, Chuah KL, Lee HY, Liew A. (2013) An unusual case of glomerulonephritis in a patient with non-Hodgkin mucosal associated lymphoid tissue (MALT) B-cell lymphoma. BMC Nephrol 22;14:158
9. Swerdlow SH, Campo E, Harris NL, et al. (2008) WHO Classification of Tumours of Haematopoietic and Lymphoid Tissues. 4th ed. Lyon, France: IARC Press.
10. Sun J, Yang Q, Lu Z, He M, Gao L, et al. (2012) Distribution of lymphoid neoplasms in China: analysis of 4,638 cases according to the World Health Organization classification. Am J Clin Pathol 138:429–434.
11. Moulin B, Ronco PM, Mougenot B, Francois A, Fillastre JP, et al. (1992) Glomerulonephritis in chronic lymphocytic leukemia and related B-cell lymphomas. Kidney Int 42:127–135.
12. Dussol B, Brunet P, Vacher-Coponat H, Bouabdallah R, Chetaille P, et al. (1997) Crescentic glomerulonephritis with antineutrophil cytoplasmic antibodies associated with chronic lymphocytic leukaemia. Nephrol Dial Transplant 12:785–786.
13. Henriksen KJ, Hong RB, Sobrero MI, Chang A. (2011) Rare association of chronic lymphocytic leukemia/small lymphocytic lymphoma, ANCAs, and pauci-immune crescentic glomerulonephritis. Am J Kidney Dis 57:170–174.
14. Harper L, Adu D. (1997) Glomerulonephritis and non-Hodgkin lymphoma: Nephrol Dial Transplant 12:1520–1525.
15. Audard V, Larousserie F, Grimbert P,Abtahi M, Sotto JJ, et al. (2006) Minimal change nephrotic syndrome and classical Hodgkin's lymphoma: report of 21 cases and review of the literature. Kidney Int. 69:2251–2260.
16. Audard V, Georges B, Vanhille P, Toly C, Deroure B, et al. (2008) Renal Lesions Associated with IgM-Secreting Monoclonal Proliferations: Revisiting the Disease Spectrum. Clin J Am Soc Nephrol 3:1339–1349.
17. Villa D, Connors JM, Sehn LH, Gascoyne RD, Savage KJ. (2011) Diffuse large B-cell lymphoma with involvement of the kidney: outcome and risk of central nervous system relapse. Haematologica 96:1002–1007.
18. Bai X, Li X, Wan L, Wang G, Jia N, et al. (2011) Intravascular large B-cell lymphoma of the kidney: a case report. Diagn Pathol 6:86.
19. Kameoka Y, Takahashi N, Komatsuda A. (2009) Kidney-limited intravascular large B cell lymphoma: a distinct variant of IVLBCL? Int J Hematol 89:533–537.
20. Wood SM, Boyd SM, Taylor JE, Savill J. (1996) A case of non-Hodgkin lymphoma presenting primarily with renal failure. Nephrol Dial Transplant 11:535–536

SDF-1/CXCR4 Signaling Preserves Microvascular Integrity and Renal Function in Chronic Kidney Disease

Li-Hao Chen[1], Suzanne L. Advani[1], Kerri Thai[1], M. Golam Kabir[1], Manish M. Sood[2], Ian W. Gibson[3], Darren A. Yuen[1], Kim A. Connelly[1], Philip A. Marsden[1], Darren J. Kelly[4], Richard E. Gilbert[1], Andrew Advani[1]*

1 Keenan Research Centre for Biomedical Science and Li Ka Shing Knowledge Institute of St. Michael's Hospital, Toronto, Ontario, Canada, **2** Ottawa Hospital Research Institute, University of Ottawa, Ottawa, Ontario, Canada, **3** Health Sciences Centre, University of Manitoba, Winnipeg, Manitoba, Canada, **4** Department of Medicine, St. Vincent's Hospital, Melbourne, Victoria, Australia

Abstract

The progressive decline of renal function in chronic kidney disease (CKD) is characterized by both disruption of the microvascular architecture and the accumulation of fibrotic matrix. One angiogenic pathway recently identified as playing an essential role in renal vascular development is the stromal cell-derived factor-1α (SDF-1)/CXCR4 pathway. Because similar developmental processes may be recapitulated in the disease setting, we hypothesized that the SDF-1/CXCR4 system would regulate microvascular health in CKD. Expression of CXCR4 was observed to be increased in the kidneys of subtotally nephrectomized (SNx) rats and in biopsies from patients with secondary focal segmental glomerulosclerosis (FSGS), a rodent model and human correlate both characterized by aberration of the renal microvessels. A reno-protective role for local SDF-1/CXCR4 signaling was indicated by i) CXCR4-dependent glomerular eNOS activation following acute SDF-1 administration; and ii) acceleration of renal function decline, capillary loss and fibrosis in SNx rats treated with chronic CXCR4 blockade. In contrast to the upregulation of CXCR4, SDF-1 transcript levels were decreased in SNx rat kidneys as well as in renal fibroblasts exposed to the pro-fibrotic cytokine transforming growth factor β (TGF-β), the latter effect being attenuated by histone deacetylase inhibition. Increased renal SDF-1 expression was, however, observed following the treatment of SNx rats with the ACE inhibitor, perindopril. Collectively, these observations indicate that local SDF-1/CXCR4 signaling functions to preserve microvascular integrity and prevent renal fibrosis. Augmentation of this pathway, either purposefully or serendipitously with either novel or existing therapies, may attenuate renal decline in CKD.

Editor: Niels Olsen Saraiva Câmara, Universidade de Sao Paulo, Brazil

Funding: These studies were supported by grants from CIHR (grant MOP-97791) and the Canadian Diabetes Association (CDA, OG-3-10-2949-AA) to Dr. Advani. Mr. Chen was supported by a CIHR Frederick Banting and Charles Best Graduate Scholarship and a Banting and Best Diabetes Centre Graduate Studentship. Dr. Advani is a Canadian Diabetes Association Clinician Scientist and this work was supported, in part, by the Canadian Diabetes Association. Dr. Gilbert is a Canada Research Chair in Diabetes Complications. Dr. Yuen is a KRESCENT New Investigator and Canadian Diabetes Association Clinician Scientist. The funders had no role in study design, data collection and analysis, decision to publish, or preparation of the manuscript.

* E-mail: advania@smh.ca

Introduction

The progressive decline of renal function in chronic kidney disease (CKD) is characterized by both fibrotic scarring of the kidney and obliteration of the renal microvessels, these two pathogenetic hallmarks commonly occurring in tandem and enjoying a reciprocal relationship. On the one hand, microvascular loss may occur as a result of the occlusive actions of accumulating matrix proteins, whereas on the other hand the same process may itself contribute to organ fibrosis and progressive renal decline by predisposing the kidney to hypoxic injury [1]. Coupled with an increasing appreciation for the pivotal role that angiogenic factors may play in renal development [2], homeostasis [3] and disease [4,5], preservation of the glomerular and peritubular capillary architecture is thus a desirable characteristic of both existing and novel renoprotective therapies [6].

One pathway that has recently emerged as playing an essential role in renal vascular development is the stromal cell-derived factor-1α (SDF-1)/CXCR4 pathway [7]. SDF-1 is a CXC chemokine and the principal ligand for its cognate receptor, CXCR4, a seven transmembrane domain G-protein coupled receptor and the most prevalent chemokine receptor found in endothelial cells [8]. While originally defined for its role in maintenance of the hematopoietic stem cell niche and B-cell lymphopoiesis [9], the near ubiquitous tissue distribution of SDF-1 and its rapid degradation in blood indicate the capacity for much broader intra-organ specific functions [10]. The fundamental nature of the SDF-1/CXCR4 relationship is attested to by the development of identical defects in vasculogenesis and organogenesis that occur in the absence of either gene [11]. However, as with other angiogenic pathways [4,5,12], the role that SDF-1/CXCR4 signaling may play in the adult kidney appears to be context-dependent. For instance, studies in acute kidney injury support a reno-protective function for SDF-1/CXCR4 [13], whereas CXCR4-mediated hyperproliferation may actually contribute to the development of certain glomerular diseases [14].

Although reactivation of ontogenetic pathways is a common response of cells, tissues and organisms to a variety of injurious insults [15], the function of the developmentally essential SDF-1/CXCR4 pathway in CKD is unclear. Accordingly, in the present study we sought to combine studies conducted in experimental animals, cultured cells and human biopsy tissue to define the role of SDF-1/CXCR4 signaling in CKD, focusing on the bidirectional relationship between renal fibrosis and microvascular loss.

Materials and Methods

Ethics statement

Human biopsy studies were approved by the Institutional Research Board of the Health Sciences Centre, University of Manitoba. All patients gave written informed consent and the study was performed in accordance with the Declaration of Helsinki. All animal work was conducted according to the Canadian Council on Animal Care Guidelines. The specific experimental protocol, ACC 166, was approved by the Animal Care Committee of St. Michael's Hospital.

Human studies

Localization of CXCR4 and SDF-1 was determined in kidney sections from patients who had undergone nephrectomy for tumor, with tissue removed from the opposite pole [16]. For gene expression studies, kidney tissue was obtained from patients with either secondary focal segmental glomerulosclerosis (FSGS) or time zero live kidney donors.

Animals

Study 1. Expression of CXCR4 and SDF-1 was determined in the kidneys of sham (n = 6) and subtotally nephrectomized (SNx) (n = 8) rats after 8 weeks. Subtotal (5/6) nephrectomy or sham surgery was performed, in female Fischer 344 rats (F344, Charles River, Montreal, Quebec) aged 8 weeks, as previously described [17].

Study 2. For the study of chronic CXCR4 antagonism, female F344 rats aged 8 weeks underwent sham or subtotal nephrectomy surgery. Two days later, animals were randomized to receive either vehicle (PBS) or AMD3100 (1 mg/kg/day, Cayman Chemical, Ann Arbor, MI) s.c. and were followed for 8 weeks (sham, PBS n = 18, AMD3100 n = 12; SNx, PBS n = 14, AMD3100 n = 15). Glomerular filtration rate (GFR) was determined by FITC-inulin clearance [18]. Urine protein excretion was determined after 24 h metabolic caging. Systolic blood pressure (SBP) was measured with a 2F micro-manometer (Model SPR-838 Millar Instruments, Houston, TX) and analysed using Chart Software v5.6 (AD Instruments, NSW, Australia).

Study 3. In Study 3, we examined the effect of acute SDF-1 administration on glomerular signaling. Eight week old female F344 rats were first randomized to receive either PBS or AMD3100 (1 mg/kg) s.c. Four hours later, recombinant rat SDF-1 (10 μg/kg [19]; PeproTech, Rocky Hill, NJ) or vehicle (PBS) was delivered to the kidneys via the abdominal aorta (n = 6/group). To achieve this, the abdominal aorta was dissected, the right kidney was removed and the descending aorta was ligated distal and transiently ligated proximal to the renal artery. Either PBS or SDF-1 was delivered via an 18 G angiocath, circulation into the left kidney was then restored for 30 min before flushing the kidney with heparin (100 U), followed by 1 mL of PBS, with perfusion-exsanguination facilitated by severance of the external jugular vein. The kidney was then removed and glomeruli isolated by differential sieving [20].

Study 4. To determine whether either CXCR4 or SDF-1 mRNA were altered with ACE inhibition, real-time PCR was performed on mRNA isolated from the kidneys of sham (n = 8) and SNx (n = 7) Sprague Dawley rats after 12 weeks or SNx rats treated with the ACE inhibitor perindopril (8 mg/L in drinking water) (n = 8). The clinical characteristics of these rats have been previously described [21].

Immunohistochemistry

Immunohistochemistry was performed as previously described [4,16,22] with antibodies in the following concentrations: SDF-1 1:25 (R&D Systems, Minneapolis, MN), CXCR4 1:50 (Abcam, Cambridge, MA), collagen IV 1:100 (Southern Biotech, Birmingham, AL) and JG-12 1:1000 (Bender Medsystems GbdH, Vienna, Austria). For quantitation of JG-12 and collagen IV immunostaining, kidney sections were scanned with the Aperio ScanScope system (Aperio Technologies Inc., Vista, CA) and analyzed using ImageScope (Aperio Technologies Inc.). Glomerular endothelial (JG-12) immunostaining was determined in 30 glomerular profiles from each rat kidney section [4,23]. For estimation of peritubular JG-12 and tubulointerstitial collagen IV, the proportional area of positive immunostaining (excluding glomeruli) was determined in 10 randomly selected cortical fields (x100 magnification).

Glomerulosclerosis Index

A minimum of 50 glomeruli were examined in PAS-stained kidney sections from each rat. The degree of sclerosis was subjectively graded on a scale of 0 to 4 as previously described [4].

Fluorescent microangiography

Fluorescent microangiography (FMA) was performed in n≥3 rats/group as previously described [18]. Briefly, the abdominal aorta was ligated proximal to the renal artery and distally at the level of the aortic bifurcation and 1 ml of heparinized saline followed by 1 ml of 3% KCl were delivered, before perfusion with 100 ml 0.9% saline. A pre-warmed (40°C) agarose-fluorescent microbead mixture (1% low melting point agarose [Sigma] and 10% 0.02 μm fluospheres [Invitrogen, Carlsbad, CA]) was then delivered via an 18G angiocath. After infusion, the rat was cooled on ice and the kidney removed and fixed in 10% NBF. Subsequently, 200 μm thick kidney cross-sections were washed in PBS overnight and embedded in 95% 2,2′-thiodiethanol (Sigma). Serial images were collected with a confocal microscope (Leica TCS SL, Leica, Richmond Hill, ON) across the z-stack (0.8141 μm steps) in 6 glomeruli/rat. Glomerular capillary volume was calculated using ImageJ version 1.39 (National Institutes of Health, Bethesda, MD). Three dimensional reconstructions were generated using Neurolucida (MBF Bioscience, Williston, VT).

Cell culture

In vitro experiments were conducted in NRK-49F renal fibroblasts (ATCC, Manassas, VA) and human umbilical vein endothelial cells (HUVECs) [4,23]. NRK-49F cells were treated with 10 ng/ml recombinant rat transforming growth factor β (TGF-β) (R&D Systems) for 24 h, with or without pre-treatment with the histone deacetylase (HDAC) inhibitor vorinostat (5 μM) (Exclusive Chemistry, Obninsk, Russia) for 4 h. HUVECs were pre-incubated with 20 μM LY294002 (LC Laboratories, Woburn, MA), 1 μM AMD3100 or vehicle (0.1% DMSO) for 30 min before the addition of recombinant human SDF-1 (100 ng/ml) (R&D Systems) (or 1% BSA) for 30 min.

Immunoblotting

Immunoblotting was performed as previously described [23] with antibodies in the following concentrations: phospho-eNOS

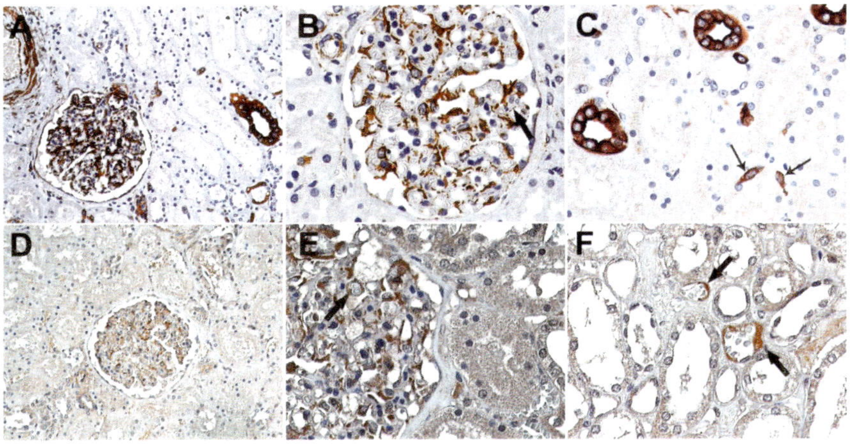

Figure 1. Immunostaining for SDF-1 (A–C) and CXCR4 (D–F) in adult human kidney. There is focal tubular (A and C) and glomerular podocyte staining for SDF-1. The thick arrows mark scattered positively staining glomerular and peritubular capillary endothelial cells; the thin arrows mark positively staining interstitial fibroblasts (C). (A and D) Original magnification x160. (B, C, E and F) Original magnification x400.

Ser1177 1:1000 (Cell Signaling, Danvers, MA), total eNOS 1:2500 (BD Transduction Laboratories, Lexington, KY). Densitometry was performed using Image J.

Real-time PCR

RNA was isolated from homogenized rat kidney tissue using TRIzol reagent (Life Technologies, Grand Island, NY). Total RNA (4 μg) was treated with RQ1 DNAse (1 U/μl) (Promega). For *in vitro* experiments, RNA isolation and DNase treatment of cultured cell extracts were performed using RNAspin Mini (GE Healthcare, Buckinghamshire, UK). DNase treated RNA (4 μg) was reverse-transcribed in a final volume of 25 μl using 0.5 μl AMV-RT (Roche Diagnostics, Laval, Quebec) in the manufacturer's buffer containing 1 mmol/L dNTPs, 0.5 μl RNase inhibitor (Roche) and 2 μg random hexamers (Amersham). Total RNA was extracted from human tissue using a Paradise Plus Reagent System (Arcturus, Mountain View, CA). SYBR green based real time PCR was performed on an ABI Prism 7900 HT Fast PCR System (Applied Biosystems, Foster City, CA) using the following primer sequences: rCXCR4, forward ATCATCTCCAAGCTGTCACACTCC, reverse GTGATGGAGATCCACTTGTGCAC; rSDF-1, forward GCTCTGCATCAGTGACGGTAAG, reverse TGGCGACATGGCTCTCAAA; rTGF-β, forward CACCCGCGTGCTAATGGT, reverse TGTGTGATGTCTTTGGTTTTGTCA; rRPL13a, forward GATGAACACCAACCCGTCTC, reverse CACCATCCGCTTTTTCTTGT; r18S, forward ATGTGGTGTTGAGGAAAGCAGAC, reverse GGATCTTGTATTGTCGTGGGTTCTG; hCXCR4, forward TGACGGACAAGTACAGGCTGC, reverse CCAGAAGGGAAGCGTGATGA; hSDF-1, forward AATTCTCAACACTCCAAACTGTGC, reverse TGCACACTTGTCTGTTGTTGTTC; hRPL32, forward CAACATTGGTTATGGAAGCAACA, reverse TGACGTTGTGGACCAGGAACT. Expression of the housekeeping genes did not differ between groups. Data analysis was performed using Applied Biosystems Comparative C_T method.

Statistics

Data are expressed as means ± SEM except numerical proteinuria data which are presented as geometric mean ×/÷ tolerance factor. Statistical significance was determined by one-way ANOVA with a Newman-Keuls post-hoc comparison or Student's t-test where appropriate. Statistical analyses were performed using GraphPad Prism 5 for Mac OS X (GraphPad Software Inc., San Diego, CA).

Results

CXCR4 and SDF-1 localization in the adult kidney

In our first experiments, we set out to define the sites of expression of SDF-1 and CXCR4 in the adult kidney. This initial immunostaining survey revealed constitutive expression of both SDF-1 and CXCR4 protein distributed prominently, although not exclusively, within the renal glomerulus (Figure 1). SDF-1 protein was notable within interstitial fibroblasts, podocytes, arteriolar smooth muscle and endothelial cells, epithelial cells of Bowman's capsule and scattered distal tubular cells, with weak, focal immunostaining within renal glomerular endothelial cells (Figure 1A-C). CXCR4 protein was present in glomerular podocytes and endothelial cells of the glomerular and peritubular capillaries (Figure 1D-F).

Altered expression of SDF-1/CXCR4 in subtotally nephrectomized rats

To elucidate the role of SDF-1/CXCR4 signaling in CKD we first determined gene expression of both receptor and ligand in the kidneys of rats that had undergone subtotal nephrectomy (SNx), a well-established model of progressive renal fibrosis. In these experiments, we observed an approximate two-fold increase in CXCR4 mRNA in the kidneys of SNx rats in comparison to sham-operated animals (Figure 2A). By way of contrast, SDF-1 mRNA was reduced in SNx kidneys (Figure 2B).

In exploring potential mechanisms that may mediate the downregulation of SDF-1 in SNx kidneys we considered the chemokine's prominent presence within interstitial fibroblasts and the sensitivity of these cells to the pro-fibrotic growth factor, TGF-β. TGF-β mRNA was increased >50% in the kidneys of SNx rats in comparison to sham animals (Figure 2C), whereas exposure of cultured NRK-49F renal fibroblasts to recombinant TGF-β resulted in an approximate 80% reduction in SDF-1 mRNA (Figure 2D). Consistent with an emerging recognition for the importance of post-translational protein acetylation in regulating the cellular response to TGF-β [24], SDF-1 downregulation was

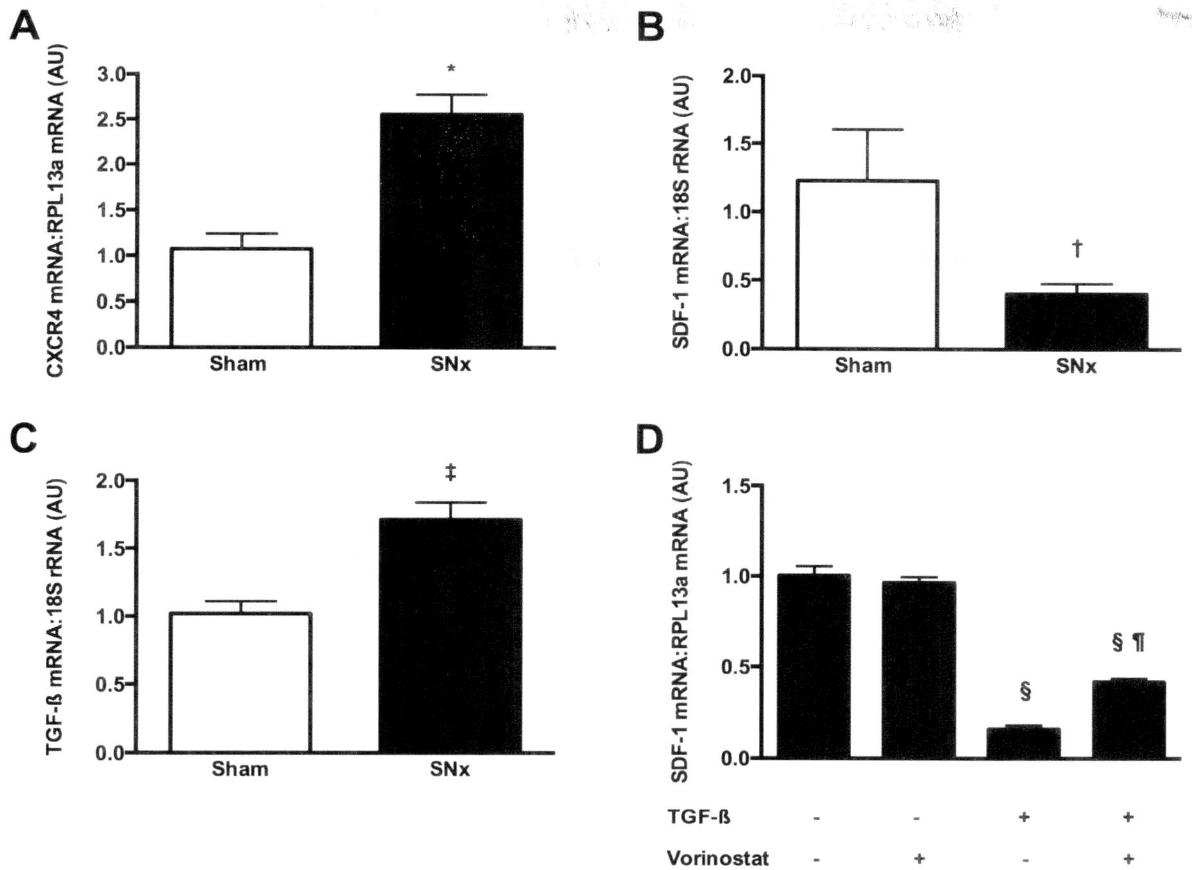

Figure 2. CXCR4 and SDF-1 mRNA in sham-operated and subtotally nephrectomized (SNx) rats. CXCR4 expression is increased in the kidneys of SNx rats (A), whereas SDF-1 is reduced (B). The kidneys of SNx rats also demonstrated an upregulation of the pro-fibrotic growth factor, transforming growth factor-β (TGF-β) (C). In cultured NRK-49F renal fibroblasts, recombinant TGF-β downregulated SDF-1 mRNA, with this effect being attenuated by HDAC inhibition with vorinostat (D). *$p<0.001$ vs. sham, †$p<0.05$ vs. sham, ‡$p<0.01$ vs. sham, §$p<0.001$ vs. control, ¶$p<0.001$ vs. TGF-β.

attenuated by pre-treatment of fibroblasts with the histone deacetylase (HDAC) inhibitor, vorinostat (Figure 2D).

Chronic CXCR4 antagonism accelerates renal decline in subtotally nephrectomized rats

Having identified a dysregulation in SDF-1/CXCR4 expression in the kidneys of SNx rats, we next sought to determine the role of this pathway in the chronically ischemic kidney. Sham and SNx rats were therefore randomized to receive either vehicle (PBS) or the CXCR4 antagonist AMD3100 (1 mg/kg/day s.c.) for eight weeks. AMD3100 is a non-peptide, highly specific antagonist of CXCR4 (IC_{50} for calcium flux 572±190 nM vs. >100 μM for CCR1, CCR2b, CXCR3, CCR4, CCR5 and CCR7 [25]) that binds to the receptor through three primary acid residues Asp^{171} (AspIV:20), Asp^{262} (AspVI:23) and Glu^{288} (GluVII:06) in an irreversible or slowly reversible manner [26]. At the end of the eight week study period, systolic blood pressure (SBP) and urine protein excretion were increased while GFR was decreased in SNx rats relative to sham animals (Table 1). Change in each of these parameters was augmented in SNx rats receiving AMD3100, with a rise in SBP and urine protein and decrease in GFR relative to vehicle-treated SNx rats (Table 1). AMD3100 had no effect on SBP, urine protein excretion or GFR in sham rats (Table 1). Examination of kidney sections by light microscopy revealed that SNx surgery was associated with an expected increase in glomerulosclerosis (Figure 3A–E) and tubulointerstitial collagen IV deposition (Figure 3F–J), with both of these indicators of renal fibrosis being augmented with CXCR4 antagonism in SNx rats (Figure 3).

CXCR4 blockade accelerates capillary loss in subtotally nephrectomized rats

As CXCR4 was detectable in the endothelial cells of both the glomerular and peritubular capillaries we next sought to determine the effect of CXCR4 antagonism on both capillary density and capillary volume in sham and SNx rats. To assess the density of the glomerular and peritubular capillaries, kidney sections were immunostained with the monoclonal antibody JG-12 that binds to endothelial cells of capillaries but not lymphatics in rat kidneys [27]. Endothelial immunostaining was reduced in both the glomerular and peritubular compartments eight weeks after SNx surgery, with a further reduction in capillary density noted in kidney sections of AMD3100-treated SNx rats (Figure 4A–J). To determine whether glomerular capillary volume was also affected, we used the novel technique of fluorescent microangiography (FMA) that allows the generation of virtual three dimensional

Table 1. Functional characteristics of sham and subtotal nephrectomy (SNx) rats treated with vehicle or AMD3100.

	Body weight (g)	Left kidney weight (g)	Left kidney weight / body weight (%)	SBP (mmHg)	GFR (ml/min/kg)	Urine protein excretion (mg/day)
Sham + vehicle	186±3	0.56±0.01	0.300±0.005	113±2	5.36±0.25	1.71×/÷1.12
Sham + AMD3100	185±5	0.54±0.02	0.296±0.005	112±3	5.29±0.28	2.37×/÷1.08
SNx + vehicle	172±3*†	0.67±0.04‡§	0.400±0.031§¶	145±7‡§	3.22±0.32‡§	20.42×/÷1.52‡§
SNx + AMD3100	180±3	0.67±0.03‡§	0.378±0.016†‡	165±5‡§‖	1.73±0.10‡§**	50.70×/÷1.26‡§‖

SBP = systolic blood pressure.
*$p<0.05$ vs. sham + vehicle, †$p<0.05$ vs. sham + AMD3100, ‡$p<0.01$ vs. sham + vehicle, §$p<0.01$ vs. sham + AMD3100, ¶$p<0.001$ vs. sham + vehicle, ‖$p<0.05$ vs. SNx + vehicle, **$p<0.01$ vs. SNx + vehicle.

glomerular microvascular casts following confocal optical sectioning [18]. Consistent with the hypertrophic response that accompanies renal mass ablation, glomerular volume was increased in vehicle-treated SNx rats in comparison to sham rats and this was also significantly reduced with CXCR4 blockade (Figure 4K-O).

Local SDF-1/CXCR4 signaling activates glomerular eNOS in the adult kidney

Since chronic CXCR4 antagonism accelerated renal decline and augmented capillary loss in SNx rats and since both the receptor and ligand were present in both the glomerular and tubulointerstitial compartments, we next sought to determine

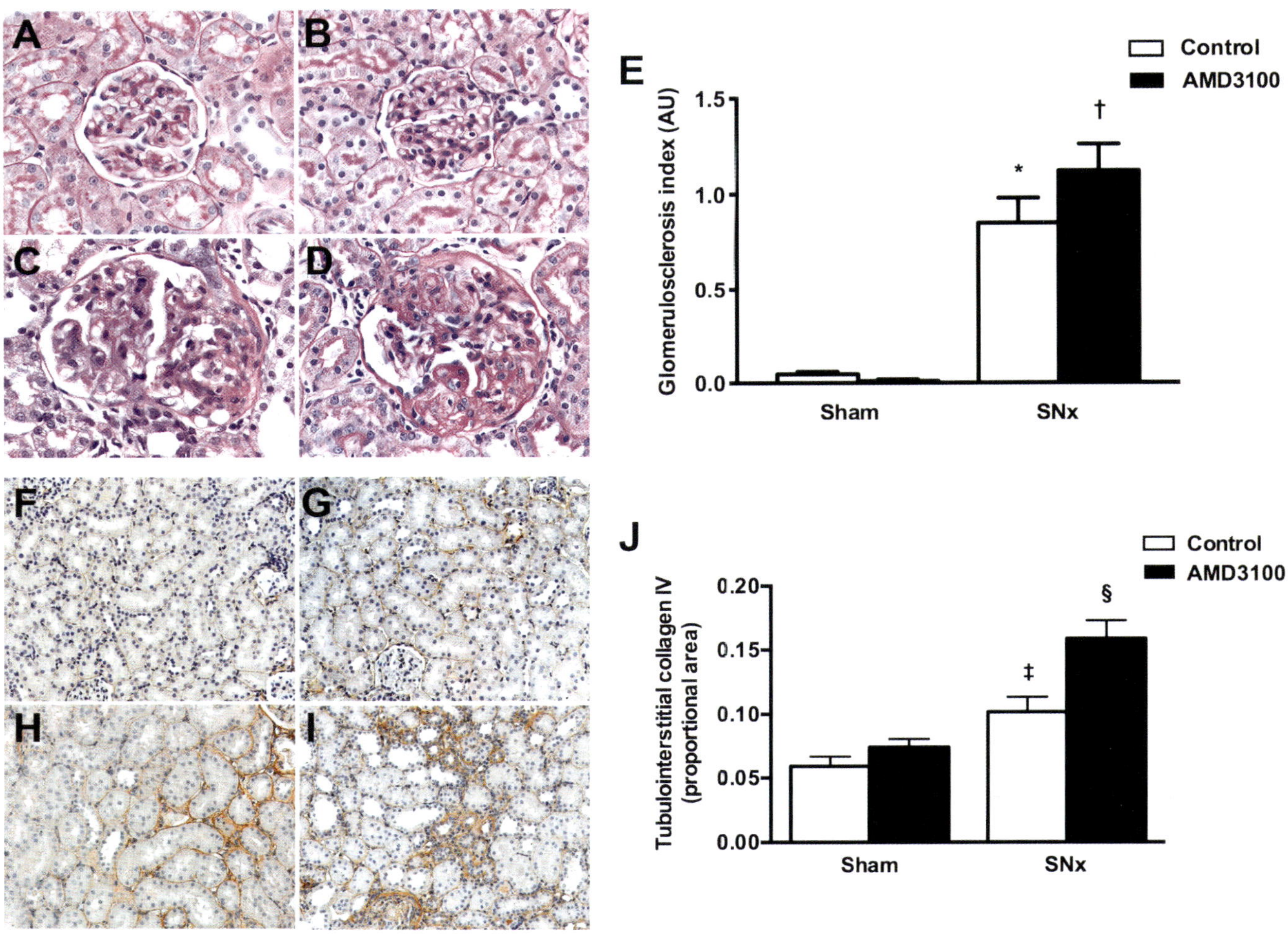

Figure 3. Effect of the CXCR4 antagonist, AMD3100 on glomerulosclerosis and renal fibrosis in subtotally nephrectomized (SNx) rats. PAS-stained kidney sections from sham (A and B) and SNx (C and D) rats treated with vehicle (A and C) or AMD3100 (B and D) for eight weeks. Original magnification x400. (E) Glomerulosclerosis index. Tubulointerstitial collagen IV immunostaining of kidney sections from sham (F and G) and SNx (H and I) rats treated with vehicle (F and H) or AMD3100 (G and I) for eight weeks. Original magnification x160. (J) Quantitation of tubulointerstitial collagen IV. AU = arbitrary units. *$p<0.001$ vs. sham, †$p<0.05$ vs. SNx + vehicle, ‡$p<0.05$ vs. sham, §$p<0.01$ vs. SNx + vehicle.

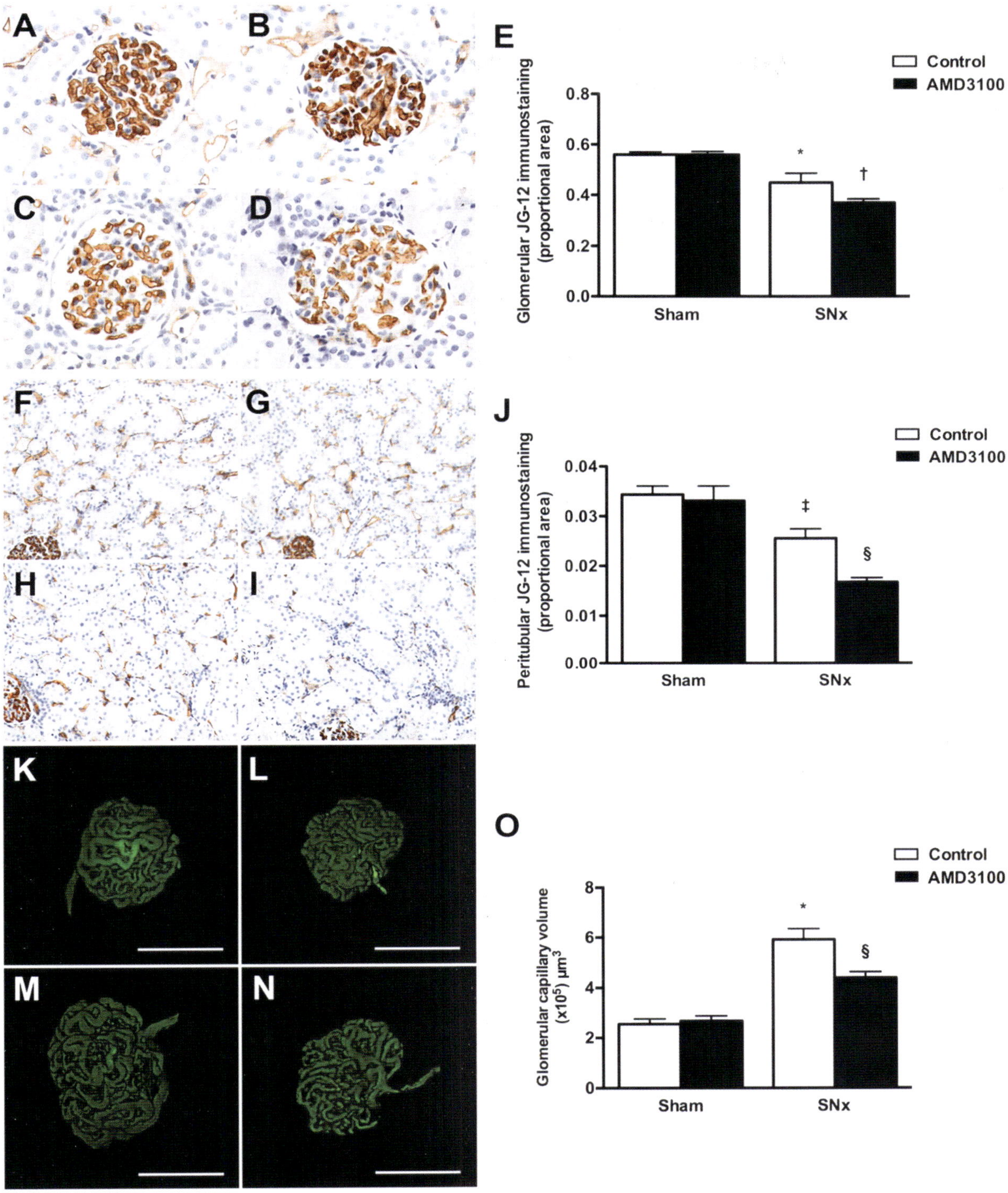

Figure 4. Effect of CXCR4 antagonism with AMD3100 on capillary loss in subtotally nephrectomized (SNx) rats. (A–D) Glomerular endothelial (JG-12) immunostaining of kidney sections from sham (A and B) and SNx (C and D) rats treated with vehicle (A and C) or AMD3100 (B and D) for eight weeks. Original magnification x400. (E) Quantitation of glomerular JG-12. (F–I) Peritubular JG-12 immunostaining of kidney sections from sham (F and G) and SNx (H and I) rats treated with vehicle (F and H) or AMD3100 (G and I). Original magnification x160. (J) Quantitation of peritubular JG-12. (K–N) Fluorescent microangiography (FMA) images of glomeruli from sham (K and L) and SNx (M and N) rats treated with vehicle (K and M) or AMD3100 (L and N) for eight weeks. (O) Glomerular capillary volume. *$p<0.001$ vs. sham, †$p<0.05$ vs. SNx + vehicle, ‡$p<0.01$ vs. sham, §$p<0.01$ vs. SNx + vehicle.

whether the SDF-1/CXCR4 axis may mediate local vascular signaling pathways in the adult kidney. One downstream regulator of the endothelial response to SDF-1, is endothelial nitric oxide synthase (eNOS) that may be activated by phosphorylation of its serine 1177 residue, through an Akt/phospho-inositide 3-kinase (PI3-kinase) dependent pathway [28]. To confirm the role of this pathway in endothelial eNOS activation, we first exposed cultured human umbilical vein endothelial cells (HUVECs) to recombinant SDF-1 with or without pre-treatment with either AMD3100 or the PI3-kinase antagonist, LY294002. Immunoblotting cell lysates confirmed that SDF-1 induced eNOS Ser1177 phosphorylation and that this was prevented by either CXCR4 or PI3-kinase inhibition (Figure 5A). To determine whether a similar signaling cascade is functional within the adult glomerulus, recombinant SDF-1 was next delivered to the kidneys of normal rats, via the abdominal aorta, with or without pre-treatment with AMD3100 (n = 6/group). Immunoblotting of glomeruli, isolated by differential sieving 30 min later, revealed that acute SDF-1 delivery induced an increase in eNOS Ser1177 phosphorylation and that this was antagonized by pre-treatment with AMD3100 (Figure 5B).

SDF-1/CXCR4 expression is altered in the biopsies of patients with secondary focal segmental glomerulosclerosis

Our experiments thus far had revealed that local SDF-1/CXCR4 signaling functions to preserve microvascular integrity and renal function in SNx rats, whereas the expression of both SDF-1 and CXCR4 is dysregulated following renal mass ablation, being characterized by downregulation of the former and upregulation of the latter. To determine whether the SDF-1/CXCR4 pathway is similarly dysregulated in human CKD, we examined gene expression of both receptor and ligand in biopsies from patients with secondary focal segmental glomerulosclerosis (FSGS) and time zero live kidney donor controls. FSGS is a common cause of progressive proteinuric kidney disease that bears pathophysiological similarity to the kidney injury that follows experimental renal mass ablation [29]. Sufficient archival formalin-fixed paraffin-embedded biopsy tissue was available to determine CXCR4 and SDF-1 expression in six samples from patients with biopsy-proven and clinically correlated obesity-related secondary FSGS compared with ten samples from time-zero live kidney donors. The clinical characteristics of patients with FSGS are shown in Table 2. All patients were hypertensive with an elevated urine protein excretion and two subjects had concomitant diabetes mellitus. For kidney donors, all patients were normotensive, with normal renal function and none of the donors had diabetes. In these studies, CXCR4 mRNA was observed to be increased approximately 5-fold in the kidneys of patients with FSGS relative to controls (Figure 6A), while there was a doubling in SDF-1 mRNA (Figure 6B).

ACE inhibition augments renal SDF-1 expression in CKD

Although CXCR4 expression was consistently increased in both experimental and human CKD, SDF-1 mRNA was more variable, with a decrease in expression in SNx kidneys and an increase in FSGS biopsies. In considering potential mechanisms that may contribute to this apparent discordance, we recognized that five of the six FSGS patients were treated with ACE inhibitors (Table 2). To determine whether either SDF-1 or CXCR4 expression may be altered by ACE inhibition, we finally examined mRNA levels in a separate cohort of rats that had been treated with the ACE inhibitor perindopril, as previously described [21].

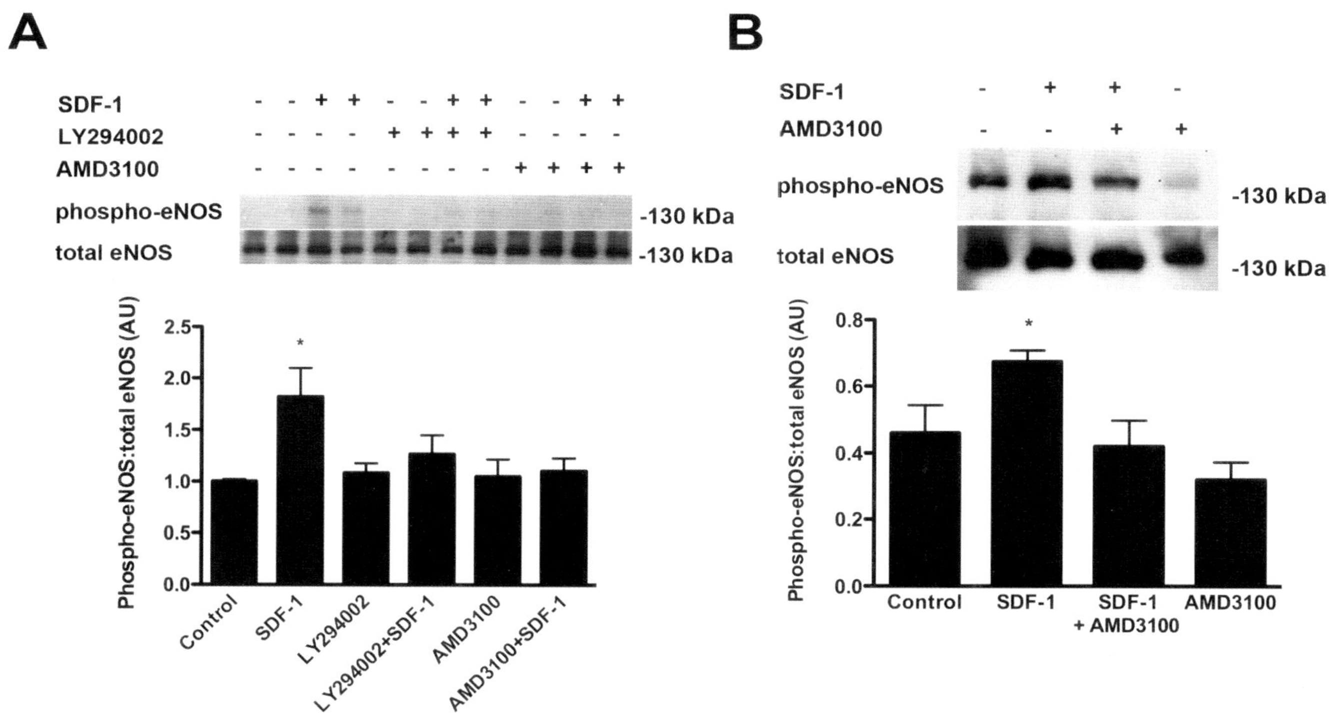

Figure 5. Phosphorylation of eNOS by SDF-1 at the activation site Ser1177. (A) Effect of SDF-1, the PI3-kinase inhibitor, LY294002 and the CXCR4 inhibitor, AMD3100 on eNOS Ser1177 phosphorylation in human umbilical vein endothelial cells (HUVECs). (B) Effect of acute SDF-1 administration on eNOS Ser1177 phosphorylation in sieved rat glomeruli following pre-treatment with PBS or the CXCR4 antagonist AMD3100. AU = arbitrary units. *$p<0.05$ vs. all other groups.

Table 2. Clinical characteristics of patients with secondary focal segmental glomerulosclerosis (FSGS).

Patient	Age (years)	Weight (kg)	Sex (M/F)	Hypertension (Y/N)	ACEi/ARB	Diabetes (Y/N)	Urine protein excretion	Serum creatinine (μmol/L)
1	13	102.6	M	Y	Enalapril 10 mg o.d.	N	Protein:creatinine ratio 400 mg/mmol	83
2	34	102.6	M	Y	Ramipril 10 mg o.d.	N	24 h urine protein excretion 1.87 g/24 h	300
3	55	106.6	M	Y	Ramipril 10 mg o.d.	Y	Protein:creatinine ratio 679 mg/mmol	108
4	34	104.5	F	Y	No	N	Protein:creatinine ratio 338mg/mmol	76
5	17	154.9	M	Y	Enalapril 10mg o.d.	Y	Protein:creatinine ratio 118mg/mmol	53
6	38	116	M	Y	Enalapril 20mg o.d.	N	Protein:creatinine ratio 120mg/mmol	98

These experiments revealed that CXCR4 mRNA was increased in SNx rats and, while reduced with perindopril-treatment, remained significantly elevated relative to sham rats (Figure 7A). Moreover, SDF-1 mRNA was markedly increased in the kidneys of perindopril-treated SNx rats when compared with either sham animals or SNx rats treated with vehicle, consistent with the change in gene expression observed in human FSGS biopsies (Figure 7B).

Discussion

Despite existing therapies and regardless of the underlying etiology, renal function continues to decline in the majority of people with CKD. Over recent years, the almost universal failure of novel anti-albuminuric therapies to meaningfully impact on clinical outcomes has encouraged investigators to direct their attention to pathogenetic processes that commonly occur during the later stages of CKD development. These pathogenetic processes include renal fibrosis and the associated disruption in the microvascular architecture, acting together and compounding the deleterious effects of one another in the relentless progression towards end-stage renal disease. In the present study, we identified a novel role for SDF-1/CXCR4 signaling in this reciprocal relationship, observing that local SDF-1/CXCR4 signaling preserves microvascular integrity and attenuates fibrogenesis, whereas the pro-fibrotic growth factor TGF-β, overelaborated in the CKD setting, downregulates SDF-1 expression. Augmentation of SDF-1/CXCR4 signaling by novel or existing agents, either purposefully or serendipitously, may thus slow the progression of renal decline in CKD.

SDF-1 signaling through CXCR4 promotes cell survival [30], migration [28], and proliferation [31], favoring neo-angiogenesis both through direct effects and through the creation of a permissive microenvironment that facilitates the actions of the angiogenic factor, vascular endothelial growth factor (VEGF) [32,33]. In the present study we observed that i) CXCR4 is expressed on the surface of endothelial cells in both the glomerular and peritubular compartments, ii) chronic CXCR4 blockade accelerates capillary loss in rats with CKD and iii) local SDF-1 delivery induces glomerular eNOS activation in a CXCR4-dependent manner. Moreover, accelerated disruption of the microvascular architecture with chronic CXCR4 blockade was associated with augmented renal decline and progressive renal fibrosis, analogous to the exacerbation of cardiac dysfunction with chronic CXCR4 blockade in the post-myocardial infarction setting [34]. Collectively, these observations highlight a hitherto unrecognized role for local SDF-1/CXCR4 signaling in preserving microvascular integrity and preventing coincident renal fibrosis in CKD.

In light of the detrimental effects observed with chronic CXCR4 blockade, the consistent upregulation of CXCR4 in the kidneys of SNx rats and in biopsies from patients with secondary FSGS is likely indicative of a compensatory response. CXCR4 upregulation has previously been described as a feature of a hypoxia-related glomerulopathy in patients with hypertensive nephrosclerosis [35]. Although both CXCR4 and SDF-1 are recognized as being hypoxia-responsive genes [36], their expression patterns were not indistinguishable in rat and human CKD. Whereas CXCR4 was consistently upregulated in both rats and humans with CKD, SDF-1 expression was more variable, the chemokine being notably downregulated in SNx kidneys of both female and male rats. In considering plausible mediators for SDF-1 downregulation in rats with CKD, we recognized the reciprocal relationship between fibrogenesis and capillary loss and hypoth-

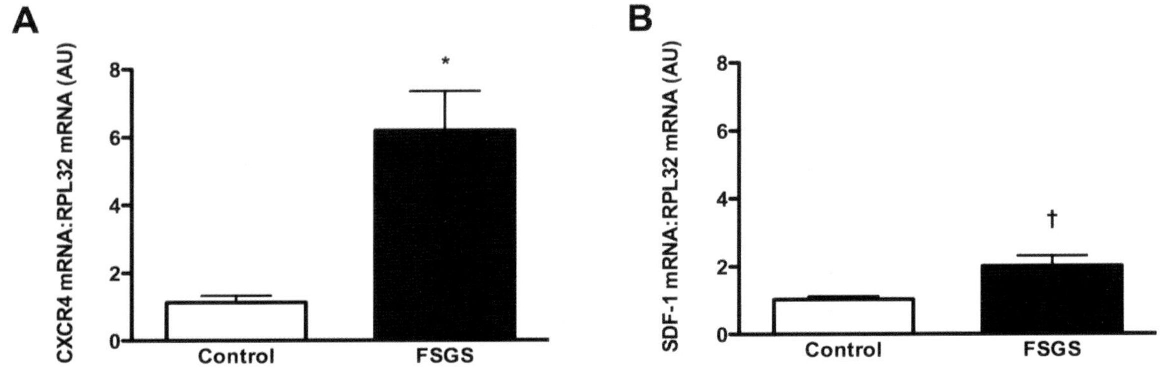

Figure 6. Real-time PCR for CXCR4 (A) and SDF-1 (B) mRNA in biopsies from time zero live kidney donors (Control, n = 10) and patients with secondary focal segmental glomerulosclerosis (FSGS, n = 6). AU = arbitrary units. *$p<0.001$, †$p<0.01$.

esized that decreased SDF-1 expression may occur as a consequence of the fibrotic process itself. TGF-β is a pro-sclerotic cytokine implicated in the fibrogenic response of many organs, including the kidney. Consistent with previous studies in oral myofibroblasts [37] and mimicking the changes in gene expression observed in the kidneys of SNx rats, exposure of cultured renal fibroblasts to recombinant TGF-β resulted in a marked downregulation in SDF-1 expression.

The post-translational modification of proteins, by the addition or removal of functional groups, is a common mechanism for controlling protein behaviour, perhaps most readily appreciated when considering the essential role that (de)phosphorylation plays in cellular homeostasis. More recently, post-translational protein modification through the addition or removal of acetyl groups has been recognized to rival phosphorylation in its diversity of substrates and the functional pathways affected [38]. (De)acetylation of proteins on lysine residues is regulated by the opposing actions of groups of enzymes called histone acetyltransferases and histone deacetylases (HDACs). In recent times, increasing evidence has begun to emerge for a pivotal role for HDACs in mediating both the progression of renal fibrosis and the response to TGF-β itself. For instance, work from our own group showed that HDAC inhibition attenuated glomerular matrix accumulation in diabetic mice [23], whereas acetylation may alter the cellular response to TGF-β through affecting Smad 2/3 activity [39], Smad7 stability [39] and/or the actions of downstream transcription factors [40] among other processes. Confirming that TGF-β mediated SDF-1 downregulation is under the regulatory control of protein acetylation, the decrement in SDF-1 transcript levels induced by TGF-β was attenuated by pre-treatment of cells with the HDAC inhibitor, vorinostat.

One of the challenges restricting the translation of promising experimental observations to the clinic is the limited ability of rodent models to recapitulate human disease. For instance, we observed that whereas SDF-1 expression was downregulated in SNx rats, the opposite effect occurred in biopsies from patients with secondary FSGS. This superficial discordance encouraged us to consider the differences between the human disease and experimental model. To account for the confounding effects of medication usage among patients, we therefore examined SDF-1 expression patterns in historical samples from SNx rats that had or had not been treated with the ACE inhibitor, perindopril [21]. In contrast to vehicle treatment, ACE inhibition, previously shown to decrease the overelaboration of TGF-β in SNx rats [41], resulted in a marked upregulation in SDF-1. Augmentation of SDF-1 activity may thus represent a novel mechanism by which renin angiotensin system blockade preserves the renal vasculature [42].

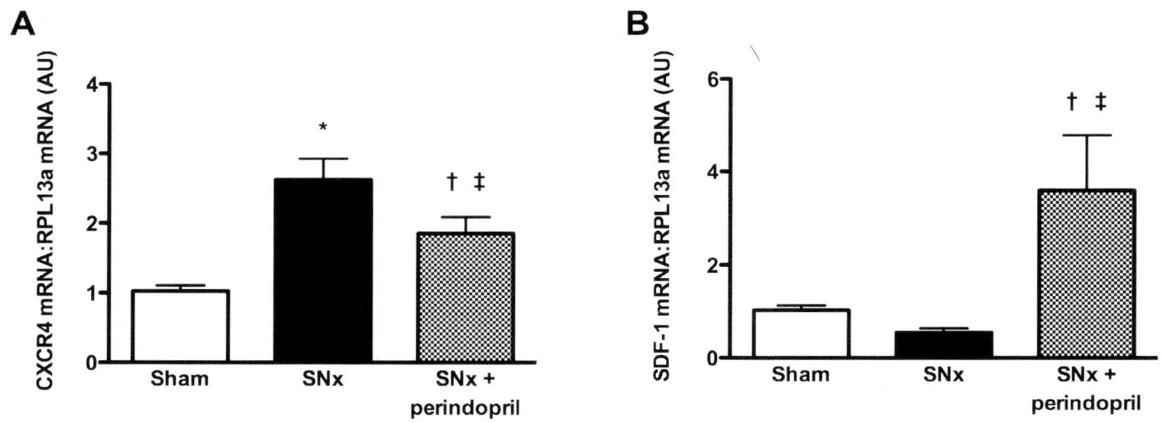

Figure 7. Real-time PCR for CXCR4 (A) and SDF-1 (B) mRNA in kidneys from sham rats, subtotally nephrectomized (SNx) rats and SNx rats treated with perindopril. *$p<0.001$ vs. sham, †$p<0.05$ vs. sham, ‡$p<0.05$ vs. SNx.

Although SDF-1/CXCR4 interaction was originally considered a monogamous relationship, more recent evidence suggests that this is not the case. CXCR4 also acts as a receptor for the HIV envelope receptor glycoprotein gp120 [43] and for the small protein ubiquitin [44], while SDF-1 may also bind to CXCR7. The renal actions of CXCR7 are complex with reports that the receptor signals in "renal multipotent progenitors" [45] while also functioning as a scavenger protein for SDF-1 [46]. Similarly, under some alternative conditions renal SDF-1/CXCR4 may play a potentially detrimental role through promoting podocyte proliferation [14], inflammatory cell recruitment [47] or, in the case of Shiga-toxin induced injury, endothelial phenotypic switch [48]. Thus, as with other angiogenic mediators [4,5], the role of renal SDF-1/CXCR4 is likely to be contextual, varying according to stage of development and the underlying injurious insult. The collective *in vitro*, acute and chronic *in vivo* and human correlative studies herein described indicate a reno-protective function for this pathway in CKD.

In summary, SDF-1/CXCR4 signaling is not only important for renal vascular development but the same system also plays a pivotal role in preserving microvascular integrity in CKD. Augmentation of this pathway by novel or existing therapies may attenuate renal fibrosis and slow the progression of renal decline in CKD.

Acknowledgments

The authors thank Ms. Bridgit Bowskill, Ms. Bailey Stead, Ms. Christine Kuliszewski, Ms. Krystina Vecchio and Ms. Katrina Zefkic for their excellent technical assistance.

Author Contributions

Conceived and designed the experiments: LHC DAY KAC PAM REG AA. Performed the experiments: LHC SLA KT MGK. Analyzed the data: LHC SLA KT MGK AA. Contributed reagents/materials/analysis tools: MMS IWG DJK. Wrote the paper: AA.

References

1. Fine LG, Orphanides C, Norman JT (1998) Progressive renal disease: the chronic hypoxia hypothesis. Kidney Int Suppl 65: S74–78.
2. Eremina V, Sood M, Haigh J, Nagy A, Lajoie G, et al. (2003) Glomerular-specific alterations of VEGF-A expression lead to distinct congenital and acquired renal diseases. J Clin Invest 111: 707–716.
3. Eremina V, Jefferson JA, Kowalewska J, Hochster H, Haas M, et al. (2008) VEGF inhibition and renal thrombotic microangiopathy. N Engl J Med 358: 1129–1136.
4. Advani A, Kelly DJ, Advani SL, Cox AJ, Thai K, et al. (2007) Role of VEGF in maintaining renal structure and function under normotensive and hypertensive conditions. Proc Natl Acad Sci U S A 104: 14448–14453.
5. Jeansson M, Gawlik A, Anderson G, Li C, Kerjaschki D, et al. (2011) Angiopoietin-1 is essential in mouse vasculature during development and in response to injury. J Clin Invest 121: 2278–2289.
6. Fogo AB (2005) New capillary growth: a contributor to regression of sclerosis? Curr Opin Nephrol Hypertens 14: 201–203.
7. Takabatake Y, Sugiyama T, Kohara H, Matsusaka T, Kurihara H, et al. (2009) The CXCL12 (SDF-1)/CXCR4 axis is essential for the development of renal vasculature. J Am Soc Nephrol 20: 1714–1723.
8. Gupta SK, Lysko PG, Pillarisetti K, Ohlstein E, Stadel JM (1998) Chemokine receptors in human endothelial cells. Functional expression of CXCR4 and its transcriptional regulation by inflammatory cytokines. J Biol Chem 273: 4282–4287.
9. Nagasawa T, Kikutani H, Kishimoto T (1994) Molecular cloning and structure of a pre-B-cell growth-stimulating factor. Proc Natl Acad Sci U S A 91: 2305–2309.
10. Janowski M (2009) Functional diversity of SDF-1 splicing variants. Cell Adh Migr 3: 243–249.
11. Tachibana K, Hirota S, Iizasa H, Yoshida H, Kawabata K, et al. (1998) The chemokine receptor CXCR4 is essential for vascularization of the gastrointestinal tract. Nature 393: 591–594.
12. Yuen DA, Stead BE, Zhang Y, White KE, Kabir MG, et al. (2012) eNOS deficiency predisposes podocytes to injury in diabetes. J Am Soc Nephrol 23: 1810–1823.
13. Stokman G, Stroo I, Claessen N, Teske GJ, Florquin S, et al. (2010) SDF-1 provides morphological and functional protection against renal ischaemia/reperfusion injury. Nephrol Dial Transplant 25: 3852–3859.
14. Ding M, Cui S, Li C, Jothy S, Haase V, et al. (2006) Loss of the tumor suppressor Vhlh leads to upregulation of Cxcr4 and rapidly progressive glomerulonephritis in mice. Nat Med 12: 1081–1087.
15. Floege J, Smeets B, Moeller MJ (2009) The SDF-1/CXCR4 axis is a novel driver of vascular development of the glomerulus. J Am Soc Nephrol 20: 1659–1661.
16. Advani A, Gilbert RE, Thai K, Gow RM, Langham RG, et al. (2009) Expression, localization, and function of the thioredoxin system in diabetic nephropathy. J Am Soc Nephrol 20: 730–741.
17. Yuen DA, Connelly KA, Advani A, Liao C, Kuliszewski MA, et al. (2010) Culture-modified bone marrow cells attenuate cardiac and renal injury in a chronic kidney disease rat model via a novel antifibrotic mechanism. PLoS One 5: e9543.
18. Advani A, Connelly KA, Yuen DA, Zhang Y, Advani SL, et al. (2011) Fluorescent microangiography is a novel and widely applicable technique for delineating the renal microvasculature. PLoS ONE 6: e24695.
19. Kanki S, Segers VF, Wu W, Kakkar R, Gannon J, et al. (2011) Stromal cell-derived factor-1 retention and cardioprotection for ischemic myocardium. Circ Heart Fail 4: 509–518.
20. Burlington H, Cronkite EP (1973) Characteristics of cell cultures derived from renal glomeruli. Proc Soc Exp Biol Med 142: 143–149.
21. Kelly DJ, Hepper C, Wu LL, Cox AJ, Gilbert RE (2003) Vascular endothelial growth factor expression and glomerular endothelial cell loss in the remnant kidney model. Nephrol Dial Transplant 18: 1286–1292.
22. Advani A, Kelly DJ, Cox AJ, White KE, Advani SL, et al. (2009) The (Pro)renin receptor: site-specific and functional linkage to the vacuolar H+-ATPase in the kidney. Hypertension 54: 261–269.
23. Advani A, Huang Q, Thai K, Advani SL, White KE, et al. (2011) Long-Term Administration of the Histone Deacetylase Inhibitor Vorinostat Attenuates Renal Injury in Experimental Diabetes through an Endothelial Nitric Oxide Synthase-Dependent Mechanism. Am J Pathol 178: 2205–2214.
24. Yuan H, Reddy MA, Sun G, Lanting L, Wang M, et al. (2013) Involvement of p300/CBP and epigenetic histone acetylation in TGF-beta1-mediated gene transcription in mesangial cells. Am J Physiol Renal Physiol 304: F601–613.
25. Fricker SP, Anastassov V, Cox J, Darkes MC, Grujic O, et al. (2006) Characterization of the molecular pharmacology of AMD3100: a specific antagonist of the G-protein coupled chemokine receptor, CXCR4. Biochem Pharmacol 72: 588–596.
26. Rosenkilde MM, Gerlach LO, Jakobsen JS, Skerlj RT, Bridger GJ, et al. (2004) Molecular mechanism of AMD3100 antagonism in the CXCR4 receptor: transfer of binding site to the CXCR3 receptor. J Biol Chem 279: 3033–3041.
27. Kim YG, Suga SI, Kang DH, Jefferson JA, Mazzali M, et al. (2000) Vascular endothelial growth factor accelerates renal recovery in experimental thrombotic microangiopathy. Kidney Int 58: 2390–2399.
28. Sameermahmood Z, Balasubramanyam M, Saravanan T, Rema M (2008) Curcumin modulates SDF-1alpha/CXCR4-induced migration of human retinal endothelial cells (HRECs). Invest Ophthalmol Vis Sci 49: 3305–3311.
29. Johnson RJ (1997) What mediates progressive glomerulosclerosis? The glomerular endothelium comes of age. Am J Pathol 151: 1179–1181.
30. Yano T, Liu Z, Donovan J, Thomas MK, Habener JF (2007) Stromal cell derived factor-1 (SDF-1)/CXCL12 attenuates diabetes in mice and promotes pancreatic beta-cell survival by activation of the prosurvival kinase Akt. Diabetes 56: 2946–2957.
31. De Falco V, Guarino V, Avilla E, Castellone MD, Salerno P, et al. (2007) Biological role and potential therapeutic targeting of the chemokine receptor CXCR4 in undifferentiated thyroid cancer. Cancer Res 67: 11821–11829.
32. Kanda S, Mochizuki Y, Kanetake H (2003) Stromal cell-derived factor-1alpha induces tube-like structure formation of endothelial cells through phosphoinositide 3-kinase. J Biol Chem 278: 257–262.
33. Grunewald M, Avraham I, Dor Y, Bachar-Lustig E, Itin A, et al. (2006) VEGF-induced adult neovascularization: recruitment, retention, and role of accessory cells. Cell 124: 175–189.
34. Dai S, Yuan F, Mu J, Li C, Chen N, et al. (2010) Chronic AMD3100 antagonism of SDF-1alpha-CXCR4 exacerbates cardiac dysfunction and remodeling after myocardial infarction. J Mol Cell Cardiol 49: 587–597.
35. Neusser MA, Lindenmeyer MT, Moll AG, Segerer S, Edenhofer I, et al. (2010) Human nephrosclerosis triggers a hypoxia-related glomerulopathy. Am J Pathol 176: 594–607.
36. Ceradini DJ, Kulkarni AR, Callaghan MJ, Tepper OM, Bastidas N, et al. (2004) Progenitor cell trafficking is regulated by hypoxic gradients through HIF-1 induction of SDF-1. Nat Med 10: 858–864.
37. Daly AJ, McIlreavey L, Irwin CR (2008) Regulation of HGF and SDF-1 expression by oral fibroblasts – implications for invasion of oral cancer. Oral Oncol 44: 646–651.
38. Kouzarides T (2000) Acetylation: a regulatory modification to rival phosphorylation? EMBO J 19: 1176–1179.

39. Simonsson M, Kanduri M, Gronroos E, Heldin CH, Ericsson J (2006) The DNA binding activities of Smad2 and Smad3 are regulated by coactivator-mediated acetylation. J Biol Chem 281: 39870–39880.
40. Chabane N, Li X, Fahmi H (2009) HDAC4 contributes to IL-1-induced mPGES-1 expression in human synovial fibroblasts through up-regulation of Egr-1 transcriptional activity. J Cell Biochem 106: 453–463.
41. Gilbert RE, Wu LL, Kelly DJ, Cox A, Wilkinson-Berka JL, et al. (1999) Pathological expression of renin and angiotensin II in the renal tubule after subtotal nephrectomy. Implications for the pathogenesis of tubulointerstitial fibrosis. Am J Pathol 155: 429–440.
42. Remuzzi A, Gagliardini E, Sangalli F, Bonomelli M, Piccinelli M, et al. (2006) ACE inhibition reduces glomerulosclerosis and regenerates glomerular tissue in a model of progressive renal disease. Kidney Int 69: 1124–1130.
43. Feng Y, Broder CC, Kennedy PE, Berger EA (1996) HIV-1 entry cofactor: functional cDNA cloning of a seven-transmembrane, G protein-coupled receptor. Science 272: 872–877.
44. Saini V, Marchese A, Majetschak M (2010) CXC chemokine receptor 4 is a cell surface receptor for extracellular ubiquitin. J Biol Chem 285: 15566–15576.
45. Mazzinghi B, Ronconi E, Lazzeri E, Sagrinati C, Ballerini L, et al. (2008) Essential but differential role for CXCR4 and CXCR7 in the therapeutic homing of human renal progenitor cells. J Exp Med 205: 479–490.
46. Naumann U, Cameroni E, Pruenster M, Mahabaleshwar H, Raz E, et al. (2010) CXCR7 functions as a scavenger for CXCL12 and CXCL11. PLoS One 5: e9175.
47. Chu PY, Zatta A, Kiriazis H, Chin-Dusting J, Du XJ, et al. (2011) CXCR4 antagonism attenuates the cardiorenal consequences of mineralocorticoid excess. Circ Heart Fail 4: 651–658.
48. Petruzziello-Pellegrini TN, Yuen DA, Page AV, Patel S, Soltyk AM, et al. (2012) The CXCR4/CXCR7/SDF-1 pathway contributes to the pathogenesis of Shiga toxin-associated hemolytic uremic syndrome in humans and mice. J Clin Invest 122: 759–776.

21

Temporal Profile of the Renal Transcriptome of HIV-1 Transgenic Mice during Disease Progression

Ying Fan[1], Chengguo Wei[2], Wenzhen Xiao[1], Weijia Zhang[2], Niansong Wang[1], Peter Y. Chuang[2], John Cijiang He[2]*

1 Department of Nephrology, Shanghai Jiao Tong University Affiliated Sixth People's Hospital, Shanghai, China, 2 Division of Nephrology, Department of Medicine, Icahn School of Medicine at Mount Sinai, New York, New York, United States of America

Abstract

Profiling of temporal changes of gene expression in the same kidney over the course of renal disease progression is challenging because repeat renal biopsies are rarely indicated in clinical practice. Here, we profiled the temporal change in renal transcriptome of HIV-1 transgenic mice (Tg26), an animal model for human HIV-associated nephropathy (HIVAN), and their littermates at three different time points (4, 8, and 12 weeks of age) representing early, middle, and late stages of renal disease by serial kidney biopsy. We analyzed both static levels of gene expression at three stages of disease and dynamic changes in gene expression between different stages. Analysis of static and dynamic changes in gene expression revealed that up-regulated genes at the early and middle stages are mostly involved in immune response and inflammation, whereas down-regulated genes mostly related to fatty acid and retinoid metabolisms. We validated the expression of a selected panel of genes that are up-regulated at the early stage (CCL2, CCL5, CXCL11, Ubd, Anxa1, and Spon1) by real-time PCR. Among these up-regulated genes, Spon1, which is a previously identified candidate gene for hypertension, was found to be up-regulated in kidney of human with diabetic nephropathy. Immunostaining of human biopsy samples demonstrated that protein expression of Spon1 was also markedly increased in kidneys of patients with both early and late HIVAN and diabetic nephropathy. Our studies suggest that analysis of both static and dynamic changes of gene expression profiles in disease progression avails another layer of information that could be utilized to gain a more comprehensive understanding of disease progression and identify potential biomarkers and drug targets.

Editor: Jian Fu, University of Kentucky, United States of America

Funding: This study is funded by NIH (R01-DK-88541, P01-DK-56492, and R01-DK-78897) http://report.nih.gov/ and Chinese 973 fund (2012CB517601). The funders had no role in study design, data collection and analysis, decision to publish, or preparation of the manuscript.

* E-mail: cijiang.he@mssm.edu

Introduction

Most patients with chronic kidney disease (CKD) progress to end stage renal failure (ESRD) despite medical intervention [1] [2]. One of the reasons is that biomarkers for early detection of the kidney disease are lacking. Therefore, we are unable to intervene early before irreversible damage. In order to identify early biomarkers and drug targets for progression of CKD, it is critical to understand the cellular and molecular mechanisms underlying the development and progression of disease.

Transcriptome-based approach has been widely applied for studying diabetic nephropathy (DN) [3] [4], focal segmental glomerulosclerosis [5], chronic kidney disease progression [6], and glomerular disease classification [7]. The transcriptiomic approach is one of the most promising and advanced methods for identifying biomarkers and studying disease pathogenesis. However, this approach is not without its limitations. First, access to renal biopsy samples are often limited due to the small volume of core needle sample and the relatively scarce number of routine biopsies performed in general nephrology practice. Second, most kidney biopsies are performed on patients with established disease. Hence, early changes in gene expression remain largely unknown. Third, in most cases repeat sampling of the kidney is not done if patients respond to therapy. Therefore, it is impossible to obtain a temporal change of gene profiles in patients over the entire course of the disease. Due to these factors, the clinical utility of current human transcriptomic data is limited. Some of these limitations, however, could be overcome by studying animal models of kidney disease. Here, we examined the temporal profile of gene expression over the course of disease progression by serial sampling of the kidney.

Many animal models have been used to study the pathogenesis and progression of kidney disease. However, most animal models develop only mild kidney disease without progression to renal failure, which is the case for almost all experimental models of diabetic nephropathy [8]. HIV-1 transgenic mouse model (Tg26) has been used extensively to study the pathogenesis of HIVAN because these mice develop renal disease mimicking human HIVAN [9]. Tg26 mice develop proteinuria as early as 4 weeks of age and proteinuria peaks at 8 weeks of age. Tg26 mice develop mild glomerulosclerosis (GS) at 4 weeks of age, moderate GS and mild tubulointerstitial injury at 8 weeks of age, and advanced GS and tubulointerstitial fibrosis, tubular atrophy and dilatation at 12 weeks of age [10]. Tg26 mice have rapid progression of kidney disease to renal failure and usually die from uremia between the ages of 2 to 6 months. Variability in disease progression is thought

Table 1. Proteinuria and histology of Tg26 mice at three time points.

	Albuminuria/Cr ratio	% Glomerulosclerosis	% Tubular atrophy/Interstitial Fibrosis
WT (n = 3)	0	0%	0%
Tg-4wks (n = 3)	0.6; 0.8; 1.2;	8%; 14%, 20%	0%; 0%; 0%
Tg-8wks (n = 3)	1.5; 1.8; 1.9	28%; 32%; 35%	5%; 8%; 10%
Tg-12wks (n = 3)	2.5; 2.8; 3.0	52%; 56%; 68%	20%; 25%; 28%

Summary of proteinuria and kidney histology: Proteinuria was measured by determination of urinary albumin to creatinine ratio. Periodic acid-Schiff (PAS)-stained kidney sections from *Tg26* mice and the littermates were graded by a renal pathologist blinded to genotypes as described in the method. Three numbers in each cell represent the data from three individual animals.

to be due to genetic penetrance [11]. Therefore, Tg26 mouse is a robust model to study the progression of kidney disease.

In the current study, we performed serial kidney biopsies in Tg26 mice and age and gender-matched control littermates at 4 weeks and 8 weeks of age and mice were sacrificed at 12 weeks of age. Gene expression profiles in the kidney cortices of Tg26 and their control littermates at these three time points were assessed by next-generation sequencing of mRNA extracted from the kidney cortex. Transcriptomic data were analyzed to identify temporal pattern of gene expression during disease progression. To determine cellular processes and genes that could be drivers of disease progression, we focused on the genes that are differentially regulated during the early stage of disease.

Results

Natural history of renal disease of HIV-1 transgenic, Tg26, mice

As shown in Table 1, Tg26 mice developed mild proteinuria at 4 weeks of age, moderate proteinuria at age of 8 weeks, and severe proteinuria at the age of 12 weeks, while control wild type (WT) littermates had no marked urinary albumin excretion. Kidney tissues from three Tg26 and three WT mice were obtained by open biopsies at ages of 4 and 8 weeks and when mice were sacrificed a 12 weeks of age. Tg26 mice developed mild GS without significant tubulointerstitial injury at 4 weeks of age, moderate GS with mild tubulointerstitial injury at 8 weeks of age, and severe GS and interstitial fibrosis and inflammation with tubular atrophy and dilatation at 12 weeks of age.

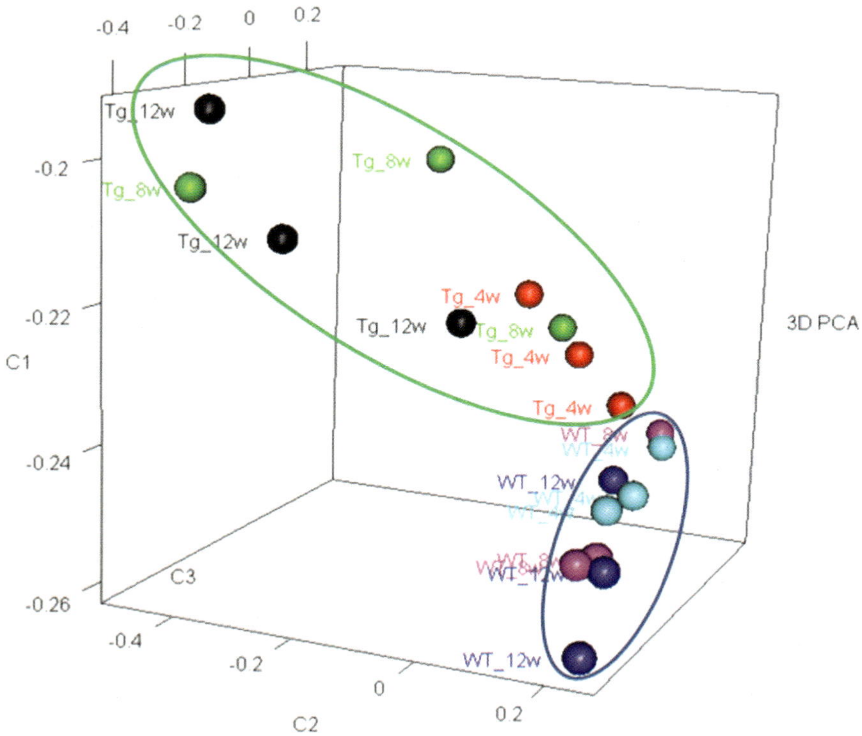

Figure 1. 3D snapshot of PCA analysis of samples distribution based on all the genes: The Tg26 samples were well separated from WT samples. Moreover, 8 wk and 12 wk Tg26 samples were farther away from WT samples than 4 w Tg26 samples, indicating dramatic transcriptomic changes in T26 mice after 8 weeks.

Figure 2. The Heat Map of gene expression profiles in the kidney of Tg26 mice at three time points: 4, 8, and 12 weeks of age when mice developed mild, moderate and severe kidney injury. The data were normalized by comparing to control littermate mice as described in the method.

Analysis of static levels of gene expression profiles in Tg26 kidneys at 4, 8, and 12 weeks

Messenger RNA was extracted from the renal cortices of three WT and three Tg26 mice at 4, 8, and 12 weeks of age for mRNA-sequencing. First, we analyzed the static levels of renal mRNA expression in Tg26 mice at three time points (4, 8, and 12 weeks). PCA was first performed to assess the sample correlations using the expression data of all the genes (Figure 1). Disease-specific changes in gene expression were determined by comparing against WT mice's gene expression to account for biopsy- and aging-related effects on gene expression. Comparisons of the gene expression profiles at three time points revealed several patterns of disease-specific changes in gene expression over the course of the disease (Figure 2). Gene ontology and pathway analyses were performed on datasets with more than 50 differentially expressed genes. We found that some genes were either consistently up-regulated or consistently down-regulated at all three time points (Figure 3 and 4). Genes that were consistently up-regulated at all three time points are involved in cytokine and Toll-like receptor pathways, immune response, inflammation, and defense mechanism (Tables S1 and S2 in File S1). Only 4 genes were consistently down-regulated at all three time points. Thirty-five genes and 1,583 genes were up-regulated only at the 4 week (Figure 5) and 12 week (Figure 6) time points, respectively. Much more genes were altered at the later stage (12 week) than early stage (4 week), possible due to secondary responses to the injury. Analyses of the dataset in Figures 6 found these genes were involved mostly in oxidative stress and RNA processing (Table S3 and S4 in File S1). In addition, we also identified a group of genes (313 genes) that were up-regulated transiently at 8 week (Figure 7). These genes are also involved in inflammation and immune defense, as well as regulation of cytoskeleton and cell adhesion (Table S5 and S6 in File S1). Twenty genes were down-regulated only at 4 week (Figure 8) and 484 genes were down-regulated only at 12 week (Figure 9). Both fatty acid and retinoid metabolisms have been shown to have renal protective effects [12] [13]. Interestingly, the 486 down-regulated genes at 12 week are involved mostly in fatty acid, retinoid, and vitamin A metabolism (Table S7 and S8 in File S1). There were a total of 54 genes which were down-regulated transiently at 8 week (Figure 10). These genes are mostly involved in cellular metabolism and immune response (Table S9 and S10 in File S1).

Dynamic changes in renal gene expression of Tg26 mice between 4 and 8 week and 8 and 12 week

Since we performed serial sampling of kidney tissue from each mouse, we were able to analyze the dynamic changes in gene expression over the course of the disease. We determined the average of changes in expression between 4 and 8 week and between 8 and 12 week for Tg26 and WT mice. This analysis identifies temporal changes in gene expression during disease progression in a dynamic manner. In addition, serial sampling of renal tissue from the same mouse permits pair-wise comparison of gene expression between different stages of the disease and avoids large inter-animal variations in gene expression. Using this analysis, we identified several patterns of changes of gene expression profiles (Figure 11). Eight four genes which were down-regulated from 4 to 8 week are involved mostly in lipid and fatty acid metabolism (Table S1 in File S2, Tables S11 and S12 in File S1). Two hundred and forty genes which were up-regulated from 4 to 8 week (Tables S2 in File S2, Tables S13 and S14 in File S1) and 66 genes which were up-regulated at both 4-to-8 week and 8-to-12 week intervals (Table S3 in File S2; Tables S15 and S16 in File S1) are all related to immune response and cytokine activation. Twenty five genes were up-regulated from 4 to 8 week but down-regulated from 8 to 12 week; and 14 genes were down-regulated from 4 to 8 week and up-regulated from 8 to 12 week (Tables S4-5 in File S2). The expression for forty two genes was not significantly different between 4 and 8 week, but was down-regulated from 8 to12 week (Table S6 in File S2). Sixty three genes were not different between 4 and 8 week, but was up-regulated from 8 to 12 weeks; and these genes are involved mostly in TGF-

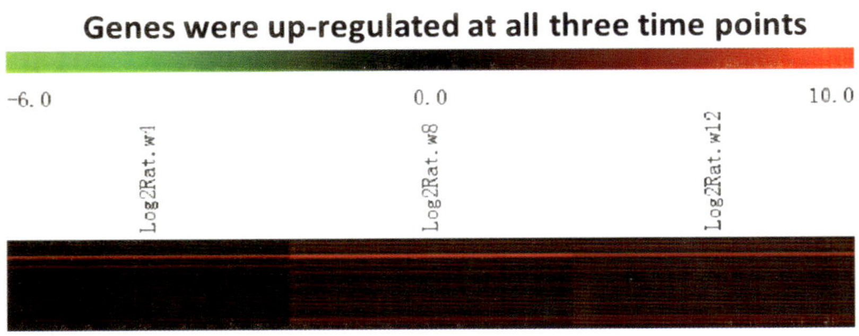

A total of 69 genes: 1110036O03Rik, 1700025G04Rik, Abcg1, Abp1, Ank, Anxa1, Apoe, Arhgap19, Arl4c, Atp8a2, Blnk, C530028O21Rik, Ccl2, Ccl22, Ccl5, Cd274, Clca1, Csrp1, Ctrl, Cxcl11, Cyp1b1, Dhrs7, Dkk3, Fam49a, Fcer1g, Figf, Gbp4, Gem, Gnb4, Golm1, Gpsm1, H2-gs10, H2-T24, Hfe, Ifi27l1, Iigp1, Irf9, Itpripl2, Klf4, Klf6, Lgals3bp, Lix1l, Maff, Mark1, Nbl1, Pamr1, Pik3ip1, Plbd1, Ptafr, Rasl11b, Rgs19, Rrad, Scube1, 8-Sep, Sepw1, Serpinb6b, Slc7a5, Snx10, Spon1, Spp1, Stk17b, Tacstd2, Tmem119, Tnfsf12, Tnfsf12-Tnfsf13, Tpm1, Tspan6, Ubd, Was

Figure 3. The Heat Map and the list of genes which were up-regulated at all three time points (4, 8, 12 weeks of age). There were a total of 69 genes in the list.

beta signaling and fibrosis (Tables S7 in File S2, Tables S17, and S18 in File S1).

Validation of gene expression by real-time PCR in mouse kidneys

We selected the top 6 genes (Ccl2, Ccl5, Cxcl11, Ubd, Anxa1, and Spon1) which were consistently higher in Tg26 than WT kidney at all 3 time points for validation because we believe these genes are likely to be involved in both disease initiation and progression. We confirmed that these genes were indeed higher in the disease Tg26 kidney than control WT kidney by real-time PCR (Figure 12). Ccl2 and Ccl5 are known to be involved in the regulation of inflammation [14] [15]. Ubd, which encodes a protein called Fat10, has been shown to be a pro-apoptotic and pro-inflammatory protein in HIVAN [16]. Interestingly, Anxa1 has been reported to display anti-inflammatory effects [17]. Spon1 is a novel candidate gene for hypertension [18]. However, its role in kidney disease has never been studied. When we queried the renal expression of Spon1 in human diabetic nephropathy deposited in a web-based database called Nephromine [19], we found that the mRNA level of Spon1 was significantly higher in kidneys from individuals with diabetic nephropathy compared to non-diabetic controls (Figure 13). By immunostaining, we confirmed that the protein levels of Spon1 were also markedly higher in kidneys of patients with both early and late DN, as well as HIVAN (Figure 14). Taken together, these data suggest that Spon1 may play a role in early disease development or/and late disease progression. However, the exact function of Spon1 needs to be further validated in the future studies.

Discussion

Mechanisms underlying CKD development and progression remain largely unknown. Treatment options that effectively prevent disease development or stop disease progression are lacking. Transcriptomics is a powerful tool for identifying potential new biomarkers and drug targets. However, the application of transcriptomics in kidney disease is limited because most renal transcriptome datasets were derived from kidney biopsies of patients with advanced kidney disease at a single point in time. Here, we evaluated the profile of gene expression changes over time in an animal model of kidney disease by serial sampling of the kidney. These data from animal models provided information that is not available for human kidney diseases, as protocol serial renal biopsies are not routinely performed. Our data suggest that findings from animal studies could help us to understand human kidney disease.

Time course experiments on gene expression are increasingly popular for exploring biological processes because temporal gene

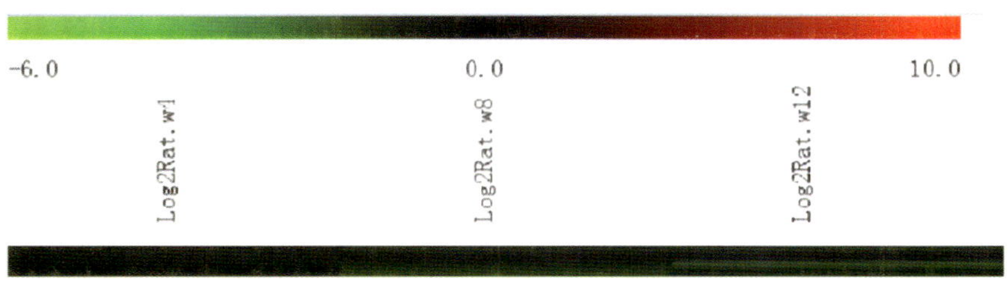

A total of 4 genes: BC021785, Nsdhl, Susd2, and Tpmt

Figure 4. The Heat Map and the list of genes which were down-regulated at all three time points (4, 8, 12 weeks of age). There were only 4 genes in the list.

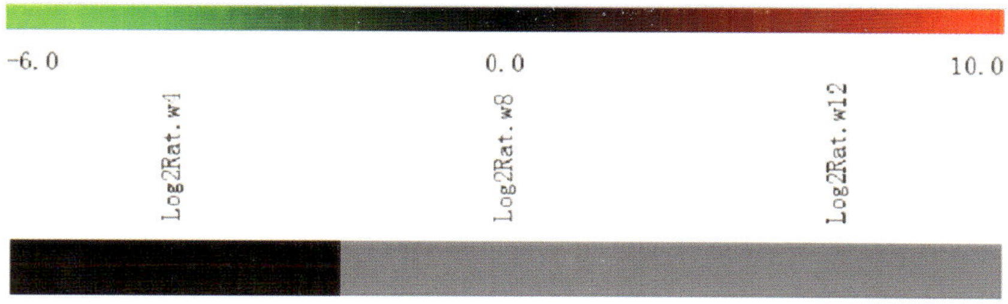

A total of 35 genes: 1810055G02Rik, 2610039C10Rik, 2610203C20Rik, Adm, Agpat9, Aqp2, Arid3b, Atp8b1, Bbox1, Cdkn1c, Cntfr, Eif5a2, Epha4, Igtp, Itga2, Mmp10, Mpa2l, Nsg1, Plagl1, Plek2, Ptbp2, Rab13, Rftn2, Samsn1, 6-Sep, Sspn, Synpo2, Tet2, Tm6sf2, Tmem79, Trim46, Trpm4, Usp13, Zfp354c, Zfp61

Figure 5. The Heat Map and the list of genes which were up-regulated at the early stage (4 weeks of age). There were a total of 35 genes in the list.

expression profiles provide an important characterization of gene function, as biological systems are both developmental and dynamic [20]. Temporal gene expression profiling could provide important information on disease progression. It is likely that the dynamic changes of gene expression could provide additional information that the static levels of gene expression could not give us. Potentially, dynamic changes of gene expression could serve as better biomarkers than static levels of gene expression. However, it is not routine clinically practice to obtain multiple kidney biopsies from the same individual during different phases of disease progression and clinical therapy. One potential alternative is to examine the dynamic changes of gene expression in peripheral blood cells or urinary cells.

Most studies examining temporal changes of gene expression are limited to in vitro cultured cells and yeasts [21] [22]. Data on the temporal pattern of gene expression in the kidney is scant. Here, we profiled the transcriptome of kidneys from Tg26 mice at three time points. These three time points reflect early, middle and late stages of kidney disease in Tg26 mice, allowing us to examine the temporal changes in gene expression. Kidney biopsy samples were also obtained from WT control mice and used to account for effects related to renal biopsy and aging-related changes in gene expression. We performed two types of analysis: static differences in gene expression between Tg26 and WT mice at different time points and dynamic changes of gene expression between different time points that are attributable to the disease. Dynamic changes in gene expression and differences in gene expression at a specific time point provide related, but non-redundant, layers of inform, which could be used to correlated with biochemical and histological parameters of the disease. We believe that this kind of comprehensive analysis could help us to better delineate disease

A total of 1583 genes: Abhd8, Abi3, Acd, Ache, Acin1, Acsbg1, Acsl5, Acta2, Actb, Actg1, Actg2, Actr3, Adam12, Adam15, Adamts1, Adamts10, Adamts5, Adar, Adcyap1r1, Ado, Adora2a, Adprh, Adprhl2, Adrbk1, Aen, Agap2, Agpat5, AI413582, AI429214, AI462493, AI506816, AI846148, Aif1, Aim2, Aimp2, Aip, Akap12, Akna, ...

Figure 6. The Heat Map and the list of genes which were up-regulated at the late stage (12 weeks of age). There were a total of 1583 genes in the list.

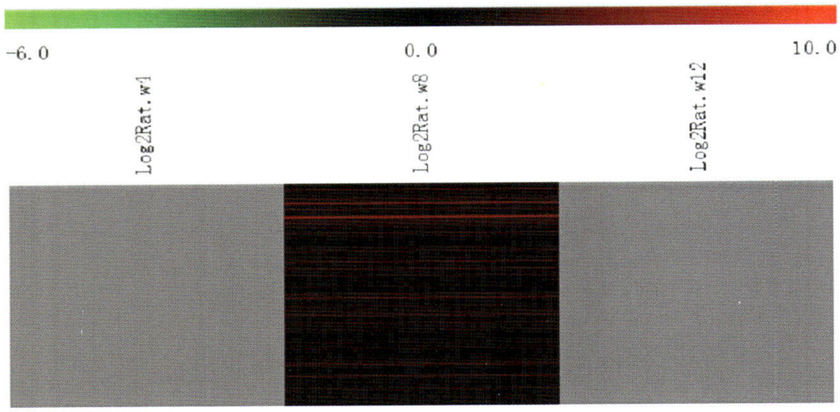

313 genes: 0610040J01Rik, 1200009I06Rik, 1700017B05Rik, 2310022B05Rik, 2610034B18Rik, 4930404N11Rik, 4930579G24Rik, 6330577E15Rik, 9830107B12Rik, A530064D06Rik, A630001G21Rik, Abcc3, Afap1l2, Ager, Agt, Ak5, Aldh3b1, Angpt2, Angptl4, Ankrd13d, Anxa6, Apob48r, Apobec1, Arc, Arg2, Arhgap23, Arntl, Art2a, Aurkb, BC005764, BC037703, BC061194, Bcl2l11, Bin1, Btk, Btnl2, C1qtnf1, C6, Capn5, Capzb, Card11, Card14, Cbfa2t3, Cbx6-Nptxr, Cchcr1, Ccl20, Ccnb1, Ccr4, Cd163, Cd33, Cd40, Cdc20, Cdc42ep1, Cdc6, Cdca2, Cdt1, Ch25h, Chaf1a, Chst1, Chtf18, Ckap2, Ckap2l, Cldn6, Clec14a, Clec5a, Clip3, Cnpy4, Coro2a, Cotl1.........

Figure 7. The Heat Map and the list of genes which were up-regulated transiently at the middle stage (8 weeks of age). There were a total of 313 genes in the list.

pathogenesis and identify potential new biomarkers and targets for therapy.

Analysis of static levels of gene expression profiles at early, middle, and late points identified several patterns of changes including genes up-regulated or down-regulated at all three time points, only at early stage, transiently at the middle stage, and only at the late stage. Genes that were differentially expressed at the early stage are likely to be involved in the development of the disease. Differentially expressed genes during the late stage are likely mediators or effectors of renal injury, including fibrosis. Genes increased transiently at the middle stage may serve as molecular intermediates during disease progression. However, these causal assignments of gene function in disease development and progression are purely speculative and will need further validation in future experiments. It was immediately obvious upon inspection of the data that more genes were perturbed at the late compared to the early stage of disease; and more genes were up-regulated than down-regulated in disease. We believe, on the first pass, it is more important to focus on genes that are perturbed early in disease. Therefore, we validated some of them by real-time PCR. In particularly, we were interested in Spon1, which has never been studied in kidney disease. Spon1 is a novel candidate gene for hypertension [18] and its polymorphism is associated with severity of dementia [23]. F-spondin, coded by Spon1 gene, is a multi-domain extracellular matrix (ECM) protein and a contact-repellent molecule that directs axon outgrowth and cell migration during development [24]. F-spondin is also involved in regulation of migration and differentiation of macrophages [25]. We found that Spon1 expression is significantly higher in the kidneys of subjects with diabetic nephropathy. We further validated that Spon1 protein expression was also increased in kidney biopsies from patients with DN as well as patients with both early and late stages of HIVAN. Our studies suggest that genes identified in animal models of kidney disease could provide relevant information about human kidney disease. The role of Spon1 in kidney disease requires further studies.

Genes were down-regulated only at 4 weeks.

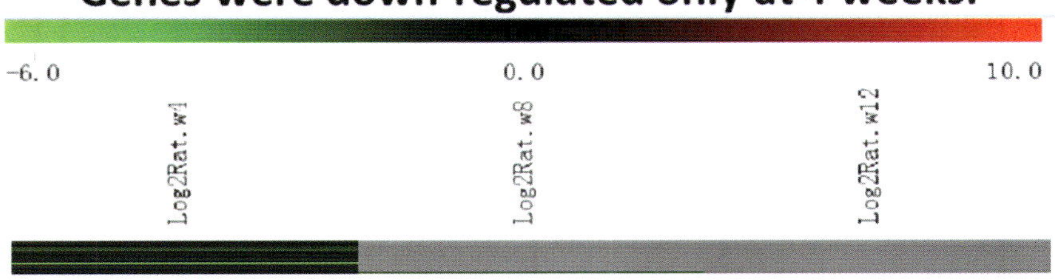

A total of 20 genes: 1810022C23Rik, Bdh1, Bhmt2, Cyp51, Ggct, Gm853, Hnf1b, Lpl, Lrrc67, Mep1b, Scrn3, Slc22a7, Slc7a13, Tmem63c, Ttbk1, Ubiad1, Usp20, Vps8, Mpv17l

Figure 8. The Heat Map and the list of genes which were down-regulated at the early stage (4 weeks of age). There were a total of 20 genes in the list.

A total of 486 genes: Abca6, Abcc2, Abl2, Acbd5, Acox3, Acss2, Acss3, Adam26b, Adcy9, Adk, Afmid, Agbl3, Agphd1, AI464131, AI747699, Aldh2, Aldh8a1, Aldh9a1, Alk, Alkbh8, Alox12b, Als2, Amot, Ankrd13c, Ankrd33b, Ano2, Aoah, Apeh, Ar, Arap2, Arhgef7, Arr3, Arsb, Arsg, Asah2, Asb13, Aspg, Atg2b, Atp10d, Atxn1, Atxn3, AU042651, Avl9, B3galnt2, BC031353, BC046331, Bco2, Bdh2, Bmpr2, Bnc2, Brd4, Brwd3, Btbd7, C1galt1, C1ql3, C78339, Cabc1, Capn8, Caprin1, Casc4, Cat, Catsperg2, Ccdc132, Ccdc38, Ccdc6, Ccdc90a, Cdcp1, Cdk12, Cdk15, Cdk5rap1, Cenpk, Chadl, Cideb, Cit, Cldn12, Clec2h, Clec4a4, Cmbl, Cml1, Cml3, Cmtm4, Cnga2, Coasy, Col4a3bp, Col6a6, Copg, Cpox, Cpt1a, Creb3l2, Csnk1g3, Ctage5, Ctbs, Ctnna2, Ctnna3, Cul3, Cux1, Cyb5d1, Cyp26b1, Cyp2b23, D18Ertd653e, D4Bwg0951e, D9Ertd402e, Dab2, Dars, Dcaf8, Ddah1, Ddi2, Ddx59, Dennd1a, Dennd5b, Depdc7, Dgkg, Dgkq, Dhdpsl, Dhtkd1, Dnajb12, Dnajc12, Dnajc13, Dock3, Dusp16, Dusp7, Dyrk2, Egfr, Ehhadh........

Figure 9. The Heat Map and the list of genes which were down-regulated at the late stage (12 weeks of age). There were a total of 486 genes in the list.

In addition, analysis of dynamic in gene expression from individual mouse could help to identify genes that are associated with the progression of disease in Tg26 mice. Consistent with analysis on the static levels of gene expression, dynamic analysis revealed that the up-regulated genes are involved in immune response and down-regulated genes are involved in metabolism. Genes up-regulated at the late stage are involved in renal fibrosis. Future studies are required to determine the role of these genes in disease progression.

Several important candidate pathways and genes were identified in our studies. The function of these genes and pathways need to be further studied because they may play important role in either or both disease development and progression. In addition, genes that are differentially expression at the early stage of disease could be used as biomarkers for predicting disease progression or drug targets for early intervention. It is critical for us to understand the function of different clusters of genes during disease progression because this could help us to develop specific

A total of 54 genes: 4833424O15Rik, A830010M20Rik, Aacs, Anxa13, Aqp4, Aspa, Astn1, BC024386, Cct6b, Cdr2, Chac2, Dhdds, Esm1, Etfa, Fam57b, Fbxo8, Fhl1, Galnt14, Gm129, Grik2, Hsd3b3, Hspd1, Ivd, Kcnj12, Klk7, Letm1, Lypla1, Mapt, Mlx, Nags, Nqo1, Nr1h4, Ovol1, Paqr9, Pdzrn4, Proz, Ptpru, Satb2, Sh3gl2, Slc18a1, Slco1a4, Sptlc1, Sypl, Tcp10a, Tfrc, Tmem161b, Tmem25, Tmem38b, Tmie, Tmlhe, Unc119b, Wfikkn1, Zfp655, Zfp706

Figure 10. The Heat Map and the list of genes which were down-regulated transiently at the middle stage (8 weeks of age). There were a total of 54 genes in the list.

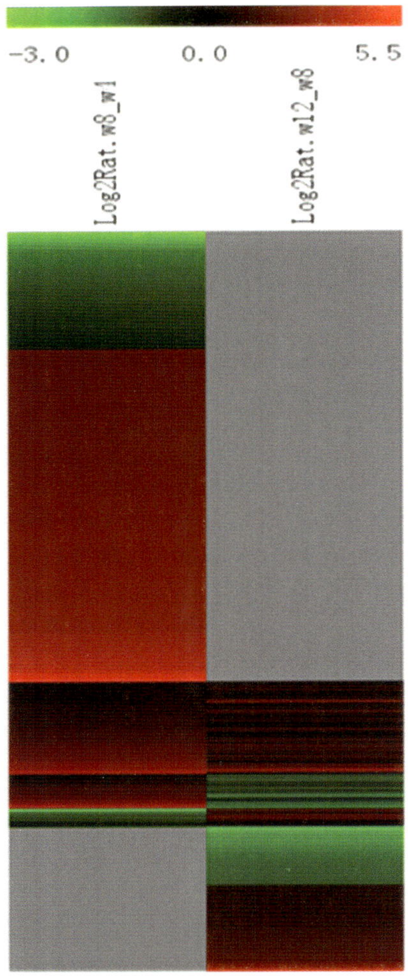

Figure 11. The Heat Map of the genes with dynamic changes between 4–8 weeks and 8–12 weeks of age.

treatment for different stages of disease by targeting a specific subnetwork of genes or pathways.

In summary, we present here data on static levels and dynamic changes of gene expression over the disease progression in Tg26 mice. Several candidate genes and pathways were identified through our analysis. They need to be further characterized to see if they can be used as biomarkers and drug targets for prevention and treatment of kidney disease. The function and pathways associated with these differentially expressed genes and their relevance in human disease will need to be further validated in the future studies.

Methods

Animal studies

Derivation of a transgenic mouse line (Tg26 mice) that bears a defective HIV-1 provirus lacking gag-pol (Tg26) has been described [9]. Genotyping by tail prep and PCR were performed at 2 weeks of age as described [26]. Three Tg26 mice and three control mice generated from the same litter were used in the studies. Each mouse underwent serial renal biopsies at the age of 4 weeks, 8 weeks, and then was sacrificed at age of 12 weeks by cervical dislocation after been anesthetized with ketamine. Unrestricted food and water were provided throughout the duration of the experiment. Urine samples were collected at each time point (4, 8, and 12 wk). All animal studies were performed according to the protocols approved by Institutional Animal Care and Use Committee at the Mount Sinai School of Medicine.

Serial Renal Biopsies

Renal biopsies were performed at 4 and 8 weeks of age. Ketamine (70 mg/kg) and xylazine (12 mg/kg) mixture was used for anesthesia. Before the surgery, the back hair was shaved and the skin was disinfected with a povidone-iodine solution. An incision of approximately 10 mm was made in the lower back and the kidney was pulled out using small forceps. A slice of the kidney was removed using a sharp surgical scissor. Strict hemostasis was performed before closing the abdominal cavity. A small piece from the lower pole of the right kidney was removed at 4 weeks of age and another small piece was removed from the upper pole of the right kidney at 8 week of age. Because the similar amount of tissues was removed from the lower or upper pole of kidney the proportions of glomeruli and tubuli in these samples were similar among individual animals. This was also confirmed by the kidney histology. On the day of sacrifice at 12 week of age, the left side of the kidney (un-biopsied sided) was collected after the perfusion with PBS. All the tissue samples were submerged in RNAlater Stabilization Reagent (Qiagen 76104) immediately after biopsies and then stored at −80°C before use.

RNA Preparation for Sequencing

Total RNA was isolated from kidney tissues by using RNeasy mini kit (Qiagen 74104) according to the manufacturer's protocol. RNA concentrations were quantified using a Nano-drop Spectrophotometer at a wavelength of 260 nm. RNA samples were then analyzed by Bioanalyzer at a concentration of 100–200 ng/ul to verify the concentration and the purity of samples. Only the samples with RNA integrity (RIN) values of >7.0 were used for mRNA sequencing at the core facility of Mount Sinai School of Medicine.

Bioinformatics Analysis of mRNA sequence data

The RNAseq data was analyzed by following the procedure described below. Briefly, after sequence quality filtering at a cutoff of a minimum quality score Q20 in at least 90% bases, the good quality reads were aligned to several mouse reference databases including mm9 genome, RefSeq exons, splicing junction sequences as well as contamination sequences of mouse ribosomes, mitochondria and phix genome using BWA alignment algorithm [27]. The alignments with more than 2 mismatched were discarded. After filtering out the reads that aligned to contamination sequences, the reads that are uniquely aligned to the exon and splicing-junction sites for each transcript were combined to calculate as expression level for a corresponding transcript and further normalized based on reads per kilobase per million reads(RPKM) [28] in order to compare transcription levels among samples. Gene expression value was transformed to the log 2 base scale. PCA was first performed to assess the sample correlations using the expression data of all the genes. The differentially expressed genes in biopsy in Tg26 mice compared to wild type mice were identified by the R package DEGseq [29] and ANOVA for multiple group comparisons and subjected to Gene Ontology enrichment by fisher-exact test and pathway analysis using Enrichr program [30]. The gene regulation model for disease progression was built using the statistically significant expression genes at early (4 weeks), middle (8 weeks), and late (12 weeks) stages and gene clusters with same change tendency in 3 different time points were

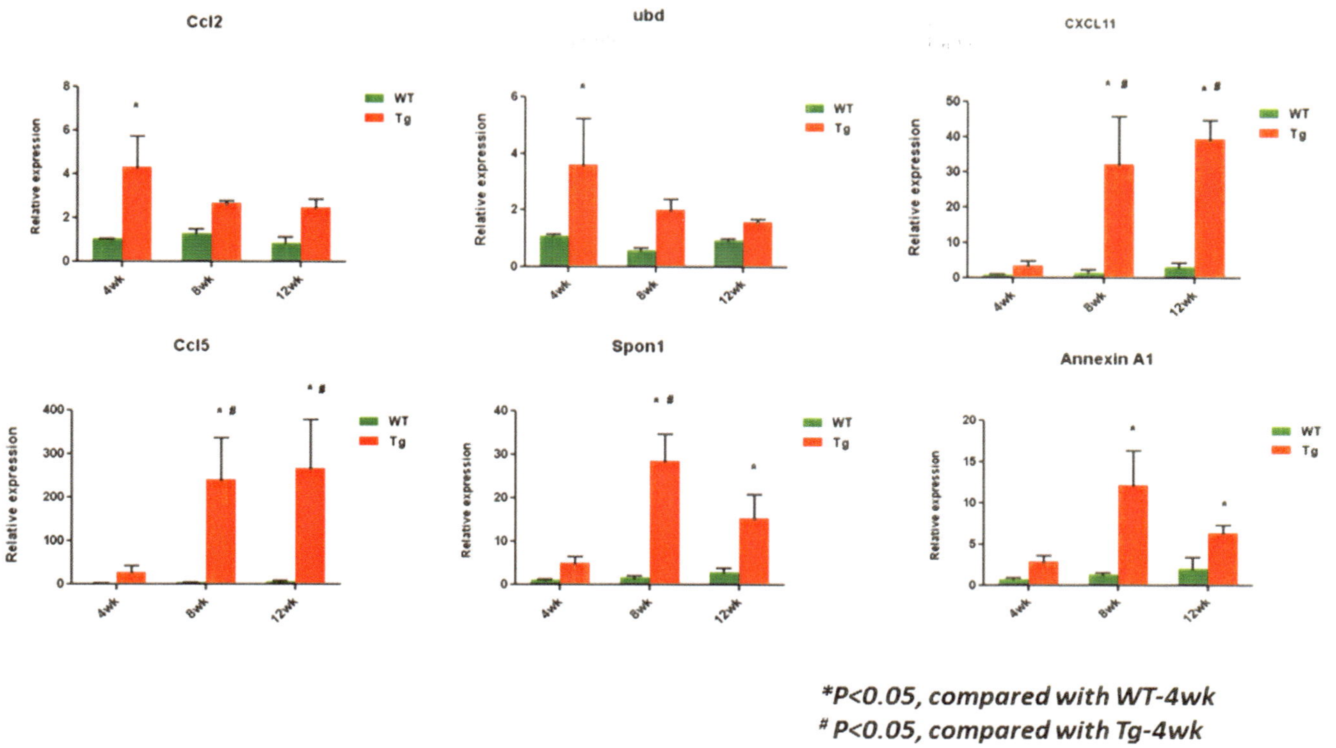

Figure 12. Validation of the selected genes from those up-regulated at all three time points by real-time PCR in kidney cortices of these mice. *P<0.05, compared with WT-4wk; #P<0.05, compared with Tg-4wk; n = 3.

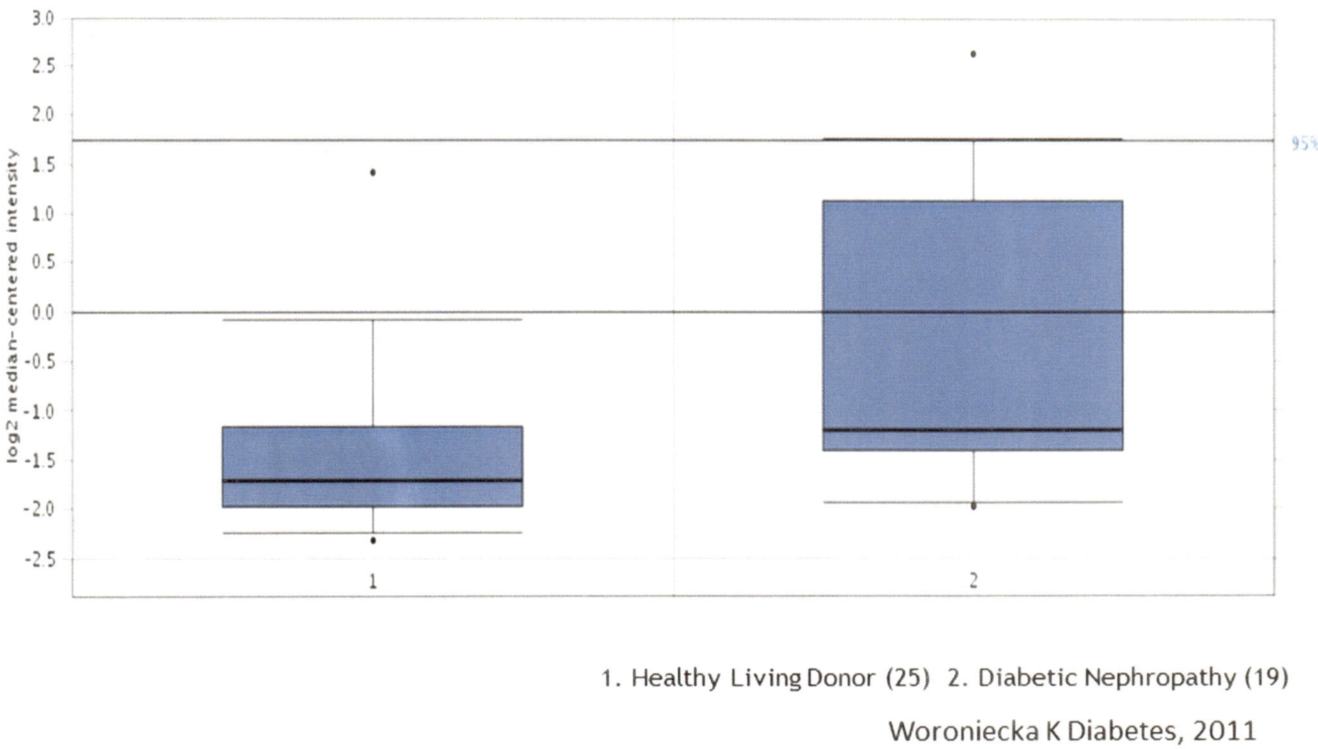

Figure 13. mRNA levels of Spon1 between diabetic kidneys and control kidneys. The data were obtained from Nephromine.org based on the datasets from the published studies [19].

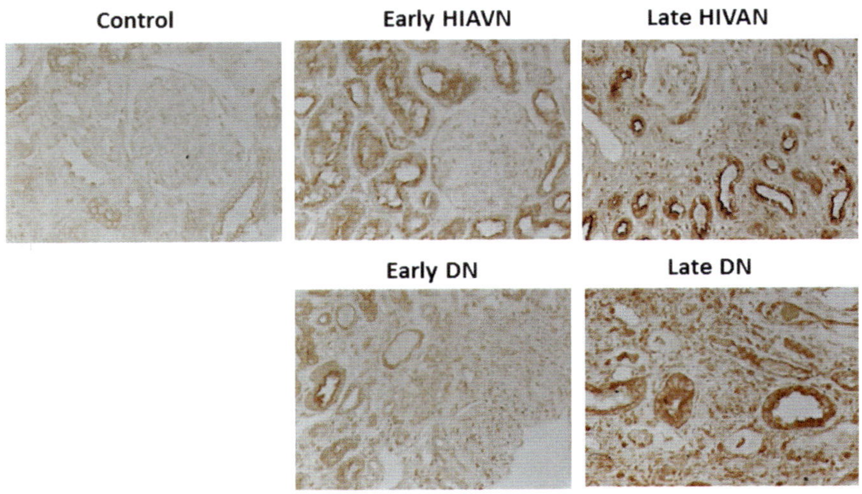

Figure 14. Immunostaining of Spon1 in kidney biopsies from patients with nephrectomy (control), early and late HIVAN and DN. The representative pictures from five individual patients are shown.

identified and subjected to Gene Ontology enrichment and pathway analysis. The read coverage of gene functional elements was also visualized by IGV tool (Integrative Genome Viewer, http://www.broadinstitute.org/igv/) from the genome alignment file.

Also, we analyzed the dynamic changes of genes between different time points in individual mice. In brief, the changes of gene expression of individual mice between week 8 and week 4 and between week 12 and week 8 were obtained for each gene, defined as Δ_week8_week4 and Δ_week12_week8. Then, unpaired limma test [31] was used to compare the delta values between Tg26 and WT mice with a $p < 0.05$ as significant difference. The gene lists with different patterns of changes were subjected to Gene Ontology enrichment and pathway analysis.

Urinary albuminuria excretion

Urine albumin was quantified by ELISA using a kit from Bethyl Laboratory Inc. (Houston, TX, USA). Urine creatinine levels were measured in the same samples using QuantiChrom^{TM} Creatinine Assay Kit (DICT-500) (BioAssay Systems) according to the manufacturer instruction. The urine albumin excretion rate was expressed as the ratio of albumin to creatinine.

Histology

After fixation with 4% paraformaldehyde overnight, kidney tissues were embedded in paraffin by American Histolabs (Gaithersberg, MD) and 3 μm thick sections were used for staining with H&E and periodic acid-Schiff (PAS) (Sigma). Histologic changed were scored by a pathologist blind to mouse genotype. The percentage of glomerulosclerosis was obtained by identifying the total number of glomeruli with any sclerosis and dividing this number by the total number of glomeruli seen. The percentage of tubular atrophy/fibrosis score was obtained by the number of tubules with either tubular atrophy or microcystic dilatation divided by the total number of tubular cross sections in a representative area or the percentage of area with fibrosis divided by the total area examined in a cross section.

Table 2. Real Time PCR Primers.

Gene	Forward	Reverse
Ccl2	TTAAAAACCTGGATCGGAACCAA	GCATTAGCTTCAGATTTACGGGT
Ccl5	GCTGCTTTGCCTACCTCTCC	TCGAGTGACAAACACGACTGC
Ccl11	AGATGCACCCTGAAAGCC	AGCCAAGTCCTTGGGCGAC
Ubd	ACAGACATGGCTTCTGTCCG	TTTCGATGGGGCTTGAGGA
Anxa 1	TGTTGCTGCCTTGCACAAAGC	AGTACGCGGCCTTGATCTG
Spon 1	AGGGCTCCCTGACCAAGAAG	TACTTGGCAGTTCCACAGGC

Real-time PCR

First strand cDNA was prepared from total RNA (1.5 ug) using the SuperScript^{TM} III First-Strand Synthesis Kit (Invitrogen) and cDNA (1 μl) was amplified in triplicate using SYBR GreenER qPCR Supermix on an ABI PRISM 7900 HT (Applied Biosystems, Foster City, CA, USA). Primers were designed using PrimerBlast (http://www.ncbi.nlm.nih.gov/tools/primer-blast/) and purchased through Sigma (Table 1). The sequences of the primers are listed in the Table 2. Light cycler analysis software was used to determine crossing points using the second derivative method. Efficiency was calculated for all the designed primers using relative standard curve method. Data was normalized to housekeeping gene (GAPDH) and presented as fold increase compared to RNA isolated from WT animals using the Pfaffl method [32].

Immunohistochemistry

Archival Human biopsy specimens of healthy donor nephrectomies, HIVAN, and DN for IHC were collected at Mount Sinai School of Medicine under a protocol approved by its Institutional Review Board. Specimens were initially baked for 20 minutes in 55–60°C oven and then processed as previously described below. Briefly formalin-fixed and paraffin embedded sections were deparaffinized, and endogenous peroxidase was inactivated with H_2O_2. Sections were then blocked in 2% goat serum in phosphate buffered saline (PBS) for 1 hour at room temperature and then incubated with a rabbit anti-Spon1 antibody (Abcam) at 4°C overnight. The next day, sections were washed three times with PBS and then incubated with secondary antibody for 30 minutes.

Positive staining was revealed by peroxidase-labeled streptavidin and diaminobenzidine substrate.

Statistical analysis

Data were expressed as mean±standard deviation (X±SEM). The unpaired t-test was used to analyze data between two groups. The ANOVA followed by Bonferroni correction was used when more than two groups were present. All experiments were repeated at least three times, and representative experiments are shown. Statistical significance will be considered when $P<0.05$.

Supporting Information

File S1 Pathway analysis of differentially regulated genes. Table S1: The 69 genes, which were up-regulated at all three time points, were analyzed by using Enrichr KEGG program. **Table S2**: The 69 genes, which were up-regulated at all three time points, were further analyzed by using Enrichr GO Biological Process program. **Table S3**: The 1583 genes, which were up-regulated at late stage (12 weeks), were analyzed further by using Enrichr KEGG program. **Table S4**: The 1583 genes, which were up-regulated at late stage (12 weeks), were analyzed further by using Enrichr GO Biological Process. **Table S5**: The 313 genes, which were up-regulated transiently at the middle stage (8 weeks), were analyzed further by using Enrichr KEGG program. **Table S6**: The 313 genes, which were up-regulated transiently at the middle stage (8 weeks), were analyzed further by using Enrichr GO Biological Process program. **Table S7**: The 486 genes, which were down-regulated at the late stage (12 weeks), were analyzed further by using Enrichr KEGG program. **Table S8**: The 486 genes, which were down-regulated at the late stage (12 weeks), were analyzed further by using Enrichr GO Biological Process. **Table S9**: The 54 genes, which were down-regulated transiently at 8 weeks of age, were analyzed further by using Enrichr KEGG program. **Table S10**: The 54 genes, which were down-regulated transiently at 8 weeks of age, were analyzed further by using Enrichr GO Biological Process. **Table S11**: 84 genes which were down-regulated between 4–8 weeks but no changes between 8–12 weeks further analyzed for Enrichr KEGG. **Table S12**: 84 genes which were down-regulated between 4–8 weeks but no changes between 8–12 weeks further analyzed for Enrichr Go Biological Process. **Table S13**: 240 genes which were up-regulated between 4–8 weeks but no changes between 8–12 weeks further analyzed for Enrichr KEGG. **Table S14**: 240 genes which were up-regulated between 4–8 weeks but no changes between 8–12 weeks further analyzed by GO Biological Process. **Table S15**: 66 genes which were up-regulated between 4–8 weeks and between 8–12 weeks further analyzed for Enrichr KEGG. **Table S16**: 66 genes which were up-regulated between 4–8 weeks and between 8–12 weeks further analyzed by GO Biological Process. **Table S17**: 63 genes which were no changes between 4–8 weeks but up-regulated between 8–12 weeks further analyzed for Enrichr KEGG. **Table S18**: 63 genes which were no changes between 4–8 weeks but up-regulated between 8–12 weeks further analyzed for Enrichr GO Biological Process.

File S2 Lists of genes differentially regulated between different time points (dynamic changes). Table S1: Genes down-regulated from 4 to 8 weeks but no changes from 8 weeks to 12 weeks. **Table S2**: Genes up-regulated from 4 to 8 weeks but no changes from 8 weeks to 12 weeks. **Table S3**: Genes up-regulated from 4 to 8 weeks and from 8 weeks to 12 weeks. **Table S4**: Genes up-regulated from 4 to 8 weeks but down-regulated from 8 weeks to 12 weeks. **Table S5**: Genes down-regulated from 4 to 8 weeks but up-regulated from 8 weeks to 12 weeks. **Table S6**: Genes no changes from 4 to 8 weeks but down-regulated from 8 weeks to 12 weeks. **Table S7**: Genes no changes from 4 to 8 weeks but up-regulated from 8 weeks to 12 weeks.

Author Contributions

Conceived and designed the experiments: JCH PYC YF NW. Performed the experiments: YF WX CW. Analyzed the data: YF CW WZ. Contributed reagents/materials/analysis tools: JCH WZ NW. Wrote the paper: JCH PYC YF.

References

1. Appel LJ, Wright JT, Jr., Greene T, Kusek JW, Lewis JB, et al. (2008) Long-term effects of renin-angiotensin system-blocking therapy and a low blood pressure goal on progression of hypertensive chronic kidney disease in African Americans. Arch Intern Med 168: 832–839.
2. Sharma P, Blackburn RC, Parke CL, McCullough K, Marks A, et al. (2011) Angiotensin-converting enzyme inhibitors and angiotensin receptor blockers for adults with early (stage 1 to 3) non-diabetic chronic kidney disease. Cochrane Database Syst Rev: CD007751.
3. Martini S, Eichinger F, Nair V, Kretzler M (2008) Defining human diabetic nephropathy on the molecular level: integration of transcriptomic profiles with biological knowledge. Rev Endocr Metab Disord 9: 267–274.
4. Berthier CC, Zhang H, Schin M, Henger A, Nelson RG, et al. (2009) Enhanced expression of Janus kinase-signal transducer and activator of transcription pathway members in human diabetic nephropathy. Diabetes 58: 469–477.
5. Hodgin JB, Borczuk AC, Nasr SH, Markowitz GS, Nair V, et al. (2010) A molecular profile of focal segmental glomerulosclerosis from formalin-fixed, paraffin-embedded tissue. Am J Pathol 177: 1674–1686.
6. Ju W, Eichinger F, Bitzer M, Oh J, McWeeney S, et al. (2009) Renal gene and protein expression signatures for prediction of kidney disease progression. Am J Pathol 174: 2073–2085.
7. Bhavnani SK, Eichinger F, Martini S, Saxman P, Jagadish HV, et al. (2009) Network analysis of genes regulated in renal diseases: implications for a molecular-based classification. BMC Bioinformatics 10 Suppl 9: S3.
8. Brosius FC, 3rd, Alpers CE, Bottinger EP, Breyer MD, Coffman TM, et al. (2009) Mouse models of diabetic nephropathy. J Am Soc Nephrol 20: 2503–2512.
9. Dickie P, Felser J, Eckhaus M, Bryant J, Silver J, et al. (1991) HIV-associated nephropathy in transgenic mice expressing HIV-1 genes. Virology 185: 109–119.
10. Lu TC, He JC, Klotman P (2006) Animal models of HIV-associated nephropathy. Curr Opin Nephrol Hypertens 15: 233–237.
11. Kopp JB, Klotman ME, Adler SH, Bruggeman LA, Dickie P, et al. (1992) Progressive glomerulosclerosis and enhanced renal accumulation of basement membrane components in mice transgenic for human immunodeficiency virus type 1 genes. Proc Natl Acad Sci U S A 89: 1577–1581.
12. Ratnam KK, Feng X, Chuang PY, Verma V, Lu TC, et al. Role of the retinoic acid receptor-alpha in HIV-associated nephropathy. Kidney Int 79: 624–634.
13. Wang H, Liu H, Jia Z, Olsen C, Litwin S, et al. (2010) Nitro-oleic acid protects against endotoxin-induced endotoxemia and multiorgan injury in mice. Am J Physiol Renal Physiol 298: F754–762.
14. Tesch GH (2008) MCP-1/CCL2: a new diagnostic marker and therapeutic target for progressive renal injury in diabetic nephropathy. Am J Physiol Renal Physiol 294: F697–701.
15. Krensky AM, Ahn YT (2007) Mechanisms of disease: regulation of RANTES (CCL5) in renal disease. Nat Clin Pract Nephrol 3: 164–170.
16. Gong P, Canaan A, Wang B, Leventhal J, Snyder A, et al. (2009) The ubiquitin-like protein FAT10 mediates NF-kappaB activation. J Am Soc Nephrol 21: 316–326.
17. Araujo LP, Truzzi RR, Mendes GE, Luz MA, Burdmann EA, et al. (2010) Interaction of the anti-inflammatory annexin A1 protein and tacrolimus immunosuppressant in the renal function of rats. Am J Nephrol 31: 527–533.
18. Clemitson JR, Dixon RJ, Haines S, Bingham AJ, Patel BR, et al. (2007) Genetic dissection of a blood pressure quantitative trait locus on rat chromosome 1 and gene expression analysis identifies SPON1 as a novel candidate hypertension gene. Circ Res 100: 992–999.
19. Woroniecka KI, Park AS, Mohtat D, Thomas DB, Pullman JM, et al. (2011) Transcriptome analysis of human diabetic kidney disease. Diabetes 60: 2354–2369.
20. Bar-Joseph Z (2004) Analyzing time series gene expression data. Bioinformatics 20: 2493–2503.

21. Sharif O, Bolshakov VN, Raines S, Newham P, Perkins ND (2007) Transcriptional profiling of the LPS induced NF-kappaB response in macrophages. BMC Immunol 8: 1.
22. Spellman PT, Sherlock G, Zhang MQ, Iyer VR, Anders K, et al. (1998) Comprehensive identification of cell cycle-regulated genes of the yeast Saccharomyces cerevisiae by microarray hybridization. Mol Biol Cell 9: 3273-3297.
23. Jahanshad N, Rajagopalan P, Hua X, Hibar DP, Nir TM, et al. (2013) Genome-wide scan of healthy human connectome discovers SPON1 gene variant influencing dementia severity. Proc Natl Acad Sci U S A 110: 4768-4773.
24. Tan K, Lawler J (2011) The structure of the Ca(2)+-binding, glycosylated F-spondin domain of F-spondin - A C2-domain variant in an extracellular matrix protein. BMC Struct Biol 11: 22.
25. Oka H, Mori M, Kihara H (2011) F-spondin inhibits migration and differentiation of osteoclastic precursors. J Periodontol 82: 1776-1783.
26. Feng X, Lu TC, Chuang PY, Fang W, Ratnam K, et al. (2009) Reduction of Stat3 Activity Attenuates HIV-Induced Kidney Injury. J Am Soc Nephrol.
27. Li H, Durbin R (2009) Fast and accurate short read alignment with Burrows-Wheeler transform. Bioinformatics 25: 1754-1760.
28. Mortazavi A, Williams BA, McCue K, Schaeffer L, Wold B (2008) Mapping and quantifying mammalian transcriptomes by RNA-Seq. Nat Methods 5: 621-628.
29. Wang L, Feng Z, Wang X, Zhang X (2010) DEGseq: an R package for identifying differentially expressed genes from RNA-seq data. Bioinformatics 26: 136-138.
30. Chen EY, Tan CM, Kou Y, Duan Q, Wang Z, et al. (2013) Enrichr: interactive and collaborative HTML5 gene list enrichment analysis tool. BMC Bioinformatics 14: 128.
31. Berger DK, Crampton BG, Hein I, Vos W (2007) Screening of cDNA libraries on glass slide microarrays. Methods Mol Biol 382: 177-203.
32. Pfaffl MW (2001) A new mathematical model for relative quantification in real-time RT-PCR. Nucleic Acids Res 29: e45.

22

Clonal, Self-Renewing and Differentiating Human and Porcine Urothelial Cells, a Novel Stem Cell Population

Hans M. Larsson[1], Francois Gorostidi[2,3], Jeffrey A. Hubbell[1], Yann Barrandon[2,3], Peter Frey[1,4]*

1 Laboratory for Regenerative Medicine and Pharmacobiology, Institute for Bioengineering, School of Life Sciences and School of Engineering, Ecole Polytechnique Fédérale de Lausanne, Lausanne, Switzerland, **2** Laboratory of Experimental Surgery, Department of Experimental Surgery, Centre Hospitalier Universitaire Vaudois, Lausanne, Switzerland, **3** Laboratory of Stem Cell Dynamics, Institute for Bioengineering, School of Life Sciences, Ecole Polytechnique Fédérale de Lausanne, Lausanne, Switzerland, **4** Laboratory of Experimental Pediatric Urology, Department of Pediatric Urology, Centre Hospitalier Universitaire Vaudois, Lausanne, Switzerland

Abstract

Although urothelial progenitor-like cells have been described in the human urinary tract, the existence of stem cells remains to be proven. Using a culture system that favors clonogenic epithelial cell growth, we evaluated and characterized clonal human urothelial cells. We isolated human urothelial cells that were clonogenic, capable of self-renewal and could develop into fully differentiated urothelium once re-implanted into the subcapsular space of nude mice. In addition to final urothelial cell differentiation, spontaneous formation of bladder-like microstructures was observed. By examining an epithelial stem cell signature marker, we found p63 to correlate with the self-renewal capacity of the isolated human urothelial clonal populations. Since a clinically relevant, long-term model for functional reconstitution of human cells does not exist, we sought to establish a culture method for porcine urothelial cells in a clinically relevant porcine model. We isolated cells from porcine ureter, urethra and bladder that were clonogenic and capable of self-renewal and differentiation into fully mature urothelium. In conclusion, we could isolate human and porcine cell populations, behaving as urothelial stem cells and showing clonogenicity, self-renewal and, once re-implanted, morphological differentiation.

Editor: Zoran Ivanovic, French Blood Institute, France

Funding: This work was funded by the European Framework Program 6 EuroSTEC (Soft tissue engineering for congenital birth defects in children; reference: LSHB- CT-2006–037409, URL: http://ec.europa.eu/research/fp6/index_en.cfm). The funders had no role in study design, data collection and analysis, decision to publish, or preparation of the manuscript.

* E-mail: peter.frey@epfl.ch

Introduction

Adult stem cells are currently used to treat patients with severe burns and hematological diseases [1,2,3]. To date, such adult stem cells displaying clonogenicity, self-renewal and differentiation capacity have not been characterized in human urothelium. Urothelial stem cells have been described in mice and were found to express sonic-hedgehog proteins in the basal cell layers of the bladder urothelium [4]. A more recent report has demonstrated that mouse urothelial stem cells are p63-positive as well [5]. This has not been shown in larger-animal models or humans, although the existence of human urothelial progenitor-like cells have been described in the human urinary tract by multiple groups [6,7]. Clonogenic cell growth, however, ultimately proving the existence of human urothelial stem cells, has not been demonstrated *in vitro*. In larger-animal models, both porcine and bovine urothelial cells have been shown to be capable of forming colonies and to differentiate *in vitro* [8,9].

To establish whether the human urinary tract possesses a stem cell capable of clonogenicity, self-renewal and differentiation *in vivo*, we used an established culture system for human epithelial stem cells: the 3T3-J2 culture system [10]. In parallel, we also explored porcine urothelial cells from different anatomical locations of the urinary tract, to have a clinically relevant animal model for investigations in urinary tract repair intended for human patients. Our criteria for human and porcine urothelial stem cells were clonogenicity, self-renewal *in vitro* and full urothelium differentiation capacities *in vivo*.

Materials and Methods

Ethical Human and Animal Research Approval

Ethical approval for working with human biopsies was given by the ethical board of the "Centre Hospitalier Universitaire Vaudois" (CHUV, Lausanne, CH). Furthermore, urinary tract biopsies were harvested following signed consent by the patients or their guardians. The "Office Vétérinaire Cantonal", Vaud, Switzerland, approved all animal procedures.

3T3-J2 Cell Culture

Human and porcine urothelial cells were cultured on feeder layers of lethally irradiated 3T3-J2 cells as previously described by Rheinwald *et al.* [10]. 3T3-J2 fibroblasts in passage 4–12 were cultivated in Dulbecco-Vogt's modification of Eagle's medium (DMEM) (Life Technologies, CH) supplemented with 10% of fetal bovine serum (Life Technologies, CH). 3T3-J2 fibroblasts were grown in T162 flasks (Costar, USA) in a 10% CO_2 atmosphere at 37°C 7 days after seeding, or when confluent. 3T3-J2 cells were dissociated with 0.05% trypsin and 0.01% EDTA and re-seeded. One day prior to seeding of the epithelial cells, 3T3-J2 cells were lethally irradiated by gamma radiation (60 Gy dose, MDS

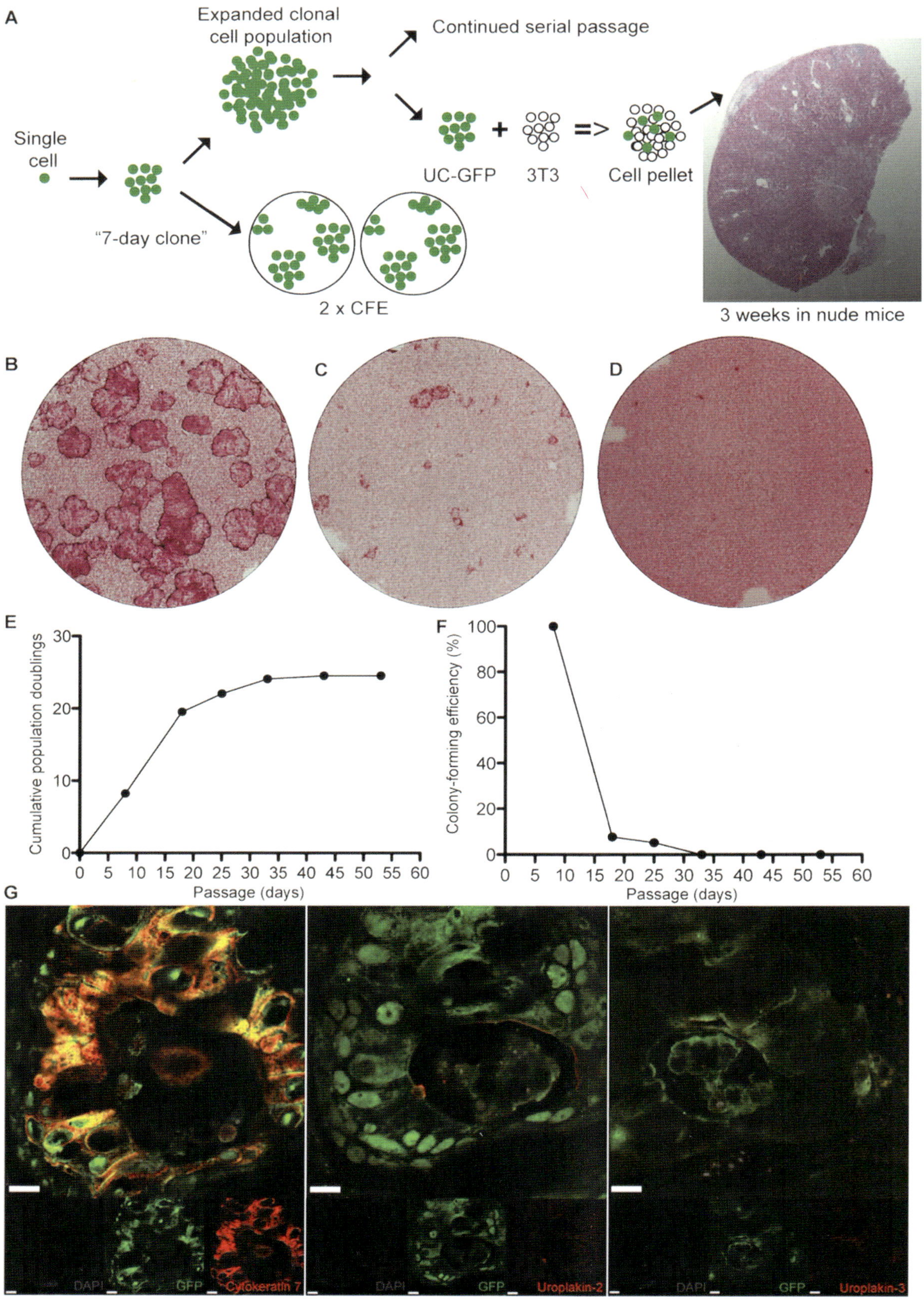

Figure 1. Human clonal urothelial cells arising from single ureteral cell. (A) Schematics showing the passage from the single selected cell to the in vivo implantated clonal cell pellet. (B,C and D) Human urothelial holoclone, meroclone and paraclone cultures arising from one single ureteral

cell. (E and F) Growth curve of a human urothelial holoclone (G) *In vivo* urothelial differentiation of human ureteral urothelial holoclone pellets implanted into the subcapsular space of the Swiss nu/nu mice, expressing cytokeratin 7, uroplakin-2 and uroplakin 3 (scale bars, 10 μm). Note the "micro-bladder" like structure.

Nordion Gammacell 3000 irradiator, Best Theratronics, UK) and seeded at a density of 2×10^4 cells/cm^2.

Human Urothelial Cell Isolation and Culture

Human urothelial cells were isolated from ureteral biopsies from pediatric donors undergoing open surgeries for non-malignant congenital anomalies (Table S1A). Primary human urothelial cell isolation was carried out as previously described by Southgate *et al.* [6]. The urinary tract biopsies were incubated for 16 h at 4°C in HBSS buffer supplemented with 0.1% EDTA (Sigma, CH), 10 mM HEPES (Life Technologies, CH) and aprotinin (1X, Roche, CH). Using forceps, the tissue was mechanically scraped. Scraped tissue was incubated with 2 mL collagenase IV (100 U/mL, Sigma, CH) at 37°C for 20 min. Finally, cells were strained through a 100 μm cell-strainer (Falcon, BD, CH) before being seeded onto the lethally irradiated 3T3-J2 cells. Human urothelial cells were cultured in a 10% CO_2 atmosphere at 37°C in cFAD medium, which consists of DMEM and Ham's F12 (Life Technologies, CH) medium (v/v 3:1), supplemented with 20% of fetal bovine serum (FBS) (Life Technologies, Australia), adenine (24.3 μg/mL, Merck, CH), insulin (5 μg/mL, Sigma, CH), 3,3,5-triiodo-L-thyronine (T3) (2×10^{-9} M, Sigma, CH), hydrocortisone (0.4 μg/mL, Sigma, CH), cholera toxin (1×10^{-10} M, Sigma, CH), and 1% penicillin/streptomycin (Life Technologies, CH). All urothelial cultures were fed cFAD-containing FBS originating from the same batch. The urothelial cells were fed with cFAD supplemented with Epidermal growth factor (EGF) (10 ng/mL, Roche, CH) every 4 days or when the medium became acidic.

Porcine Urothelial Cell Isolation and Culture

Porcine urinary tract biopsies for cell isolation were kindly donated from the University of Bern Veterinarian School and the CHUV. GFP-porcine urothelial cells were isolated from urinary tract biopsies of a 12-month-old transgenic pig constitutively expressing eGFP bought from the Institute of Molecular Animal Breeding/Gene Center (LMU, Munich, Germany) [11]. Details of the porcine donors can be found elsewhere (Table S1). Bladder biopsies were taken from the bladder trigone and the bladder dome, while urethral biopsies were taken from the proximal urethra and ureteral biopsies were taken from mid distance between the ureteral meatus and the kidney. Porcine epithelial cells were isolated and cultured as previously described by Grasset *et al.* [12]. Biopsies were minced into small pieces (1–3 mm^2) and incubated in a cell isolation solution (trypsin (0.02%), EDTA (0.1%) and collagenase A (1 mg/mL, Roche, CH)) at 37°C under gentle stirring. Every hour, the cell isolation solution was replaced. Each batch of recovered cell isolation media was centrifuged (1300 rpm, 5 min) and filtered through a 100 μm cell-strainer before being seeded into dishes or flasks containing lethally irradiated 3T3-J2 cells. Porcine epithelial cells were grown in the same culture condition as the human urothelial cells, except using 10% of the same batch of FBS.

During harvesting of porcine tissues for cell isolation, biopsies of native porcine tissues were taken and fixed in 10% natural buffered formalin (NBF 10%). Paraffin embedded native porcine tissues were later used as controls for immunohistochemistry. Porcine skin epithelial tissue was used as negative control in immunohistochemistry. Cultured porcine keratinocytes and thymus cells were used as negative controls in immunofluorescence.

Mass-cultivation of Urothelial Cells

Mass-cultivated urothelial cells were seeded at a density of 5×10^4–2×10^5 cells into 30 mm, 60 mm or T25 flasks containing lethally irradiated 3T3-J2 cells. Cells were passaged every week by dissociating growing epithelial cells in 0.05% trypsin/0.1% EDTA and then by re-plating them at the appropriate density to achieve cell confluence within 7 days. Population doubling (PD) was calculated using the following formula: $PD = Log(N/N0)/Log(2)$, where N0 is the number of seeded viable cells and N is the number of viable cells at the time of passage counted, using a hemocytometer.

Colony-forming Assay

Each time a new urothelial cell population was passaged, a colony-forming assay was performed. The colony-forming assay consisted of seeding urothelial cells at a density of 50 to 5000 cells into duplicated 60 mm or 100 mm indicator culture dishes, containing lethally irradiated 3T3-J2 cells. The cells were cultivated for 12 days as described above, before being fixed in NBF 10% and stained with rhodamine-B (1%, Sigma, Germany). Colony-forming efficiencies (CFE) were calculated by dividing the number of colonies by the initial number of seeded cells in each plate.

Clonal Analysis

Single cells from passages 1–3 were aspirated into a Pasteur pipette under a Zeiss Axiovert inverted microscope (Germany) using a 10x objective and were subsequently inoculated into a tissue culture dish containing lethally irradiated 3T3-J2 cells. Small and round cells were selected following the rationale of Barrandon et al [13]. Cultures were fed every 3–4 days with cFAD medium supplemented with 10 ng/mL human recombinant EGF, as described above. After 7 days, adherent single cells that formed colonies were identified and imaged with an inverted microscope (Zeiss, Germany). Areas of 7-day clones were measured with the ImageJ software (Clonal Area = CA), while cell numbers in the 7-day colonies were counted manually (Estimated cell number = -Estim CN). Population doubling for each 7-day clones (Generation number = GN) was calculated from using the same formula as previously described in the method section, but with N0 = 1 and N = Estim CN. Generation time was calculated dividing the time of culture (7 days = 168 h) with the generation number. Clones were detached from the dishes with 0.05% trypsin and 0.01% EDTA and re-seeded, 2 dishes were inoculated each with 1/7 of cell suspensions obtained (for CFE). The rest (= 5/7 of cell suspensions) was inoculated for clonal population expansion (Figure 1A).

Human and porcine clones arising from epidermal single cells can be classified as holoclones, meroclones or paraclones depending on the clone's capacity to form aborted colonies [12,14]. We used the following similar criteria to classify aborted and growing urothelial colonies under a binocular microscope defining "Growing" as having a colony diameter of ≥2 mm, "Aborted" of <2 mm, and "Aborted" as having a highly irregular colony shape.

Clones that formed 0–5% aborted colonies were classified as urothelial holoclones. Conversely, if a clone formed 100% aborted colonies or no colonies, it was classified as an urothelial paraclone.

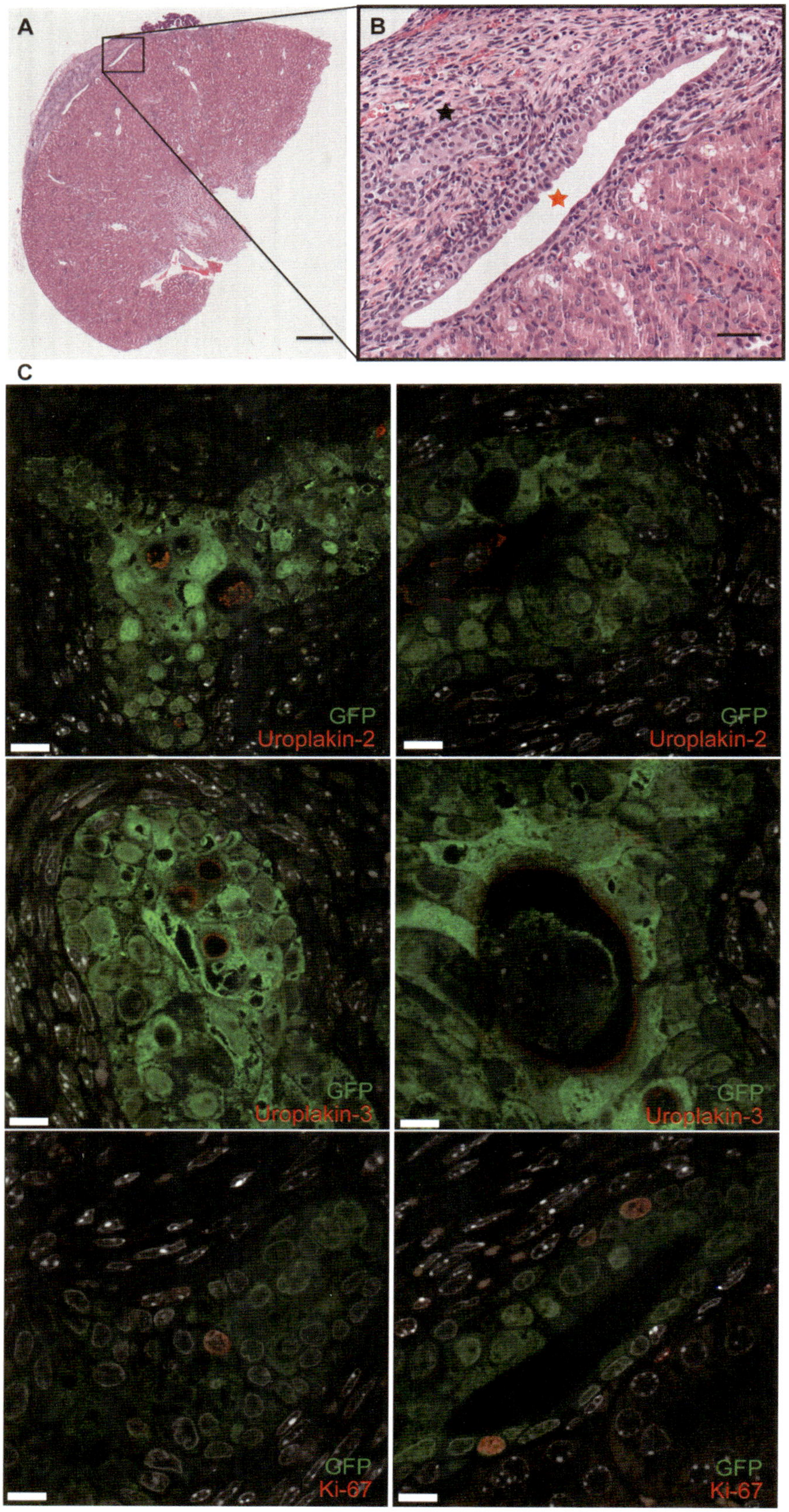

Figure 2. Urothelial cell differentiation and "micro-bladder" formation in mice. (A and B) Hematoxylin & eosin (H&E) staining of an implanted mass-cultured, native porcine bladder urothelial cell pellet into the subcapsular space of a Swiss nu/nu mice kidney (A: scale bar 500 μm, B:

scale bar 50 μm, urothelial bundle-like structure indicated with black star and epithelial "micro-bladder" like structure indicated with red star). (C–H) Immunohistochemistry of the implanted urothelial pellet forming urothelial bundle-like structures (C, E and G) and "micro-bladder" like structures (D, F and H) using antibodies against uroplakin-2 (C and D), uroplakin-3 (E and F) and Ki-67 (G and H) (scale bars, 10 μm).

Clones that formed more than 5% but fewer than 100% aborted colonies were classified as urothelial meroclones.

Lentiviral Infection for Human Urothelial Cell GFP Transduction

Titers of lentivirus containing the hPGK-GFP lentivector were kindly donated from Professor D. Trono (EPFL, Switzerland). 1 μL of lentivirus (titer $5*10^9$ TU/mL) was applied to 75% confluent human urothelial cells cultured in 6 well plate at passage 1.

Immunohistochemistry/Fluorescence

Biopsies were fixed in 10% NBF and embedded in paraffin. Sections were prepared at a thickness of 8 μm. Hematoxylin and eosin staining was performed on all biopsies. Primary antibodies used for immunohistochemistry/fluorescence were donkey anti-goat uroplakin-2 (1:500 dilution, Labforce, CH), mouse anti-uroplakin-3 (1:50 dilution, Progen, Germany), mouse anti-cytokeratin 7 (1:1000 dilution, Abcam, CH), rabbit anti-GFP (1:500 dilution, Life Technologies, CH), mouse anti-Ki67 (1:100 dilution, BD Pharmingen, CH) and mouse anti-p63 (1:100 dilution, Neomarker, US). Secondary antibodies used were Alexa-Fluor 488, Alexa-Fluor 568, or Alexa-Fluor 647 (Molecular Probes, Life Technologies, CH).

For immunofluorescence, cells were cultured on glass cover slips in 12-well plates and fixed in 10% NBF (20 min, at 4°C) after 8–12 days. Cells were permeabilized with 0.4% saponin (Applichem, CH) in D-PBS (Life Technologies, CH) for 30 min. After blocking for 1 h (3% BSA and 0.4% saponin in D-PBS), the cells were incubated with primary antibodies at room temperature for 2 h. After washing, the cells were incubated with secondary antibodies for 2 h. After multiple washing steps, Hoechst 33342 (Life Technologies, CH) was added to the cells and incubated for 10 min before imaging. Images were taken with a LSM 700 confocal laser-scanning microscope (Zeiss, Germany). For negative controls, the primary antibody was omitted.

In vivo Nude Mice Experiments

The renal subcapsular space of Swiss nu/nu mice (Charles-River Breeding laboratories, France) was used as an ectopic location for implanted urothelial pelleted cells. The implanted urothelial pelleted cells were a mix of $2.5*10^5$ GFP positive urothelial cells plus $2.5*10^5$ non-lethally irradiated 3T3-J2 cells. After 3 wk, kidneys were harvested and imaged with a fluorescence stereomicroscope (Leica, Germany) to locate GFP positive cells. Kidneys were fixed in 10% NBF and embedded in paraffin for histological analysis.

The dorsal subdermal space of Swiss nu/nu mice was also used as an ectopic location for implanted urothelial sheets following the technique described in Barrandon *et al.* [15]. The implanted sheets consisted of 12 day cultured urothelial cells treated with Dispase-II (Roche, CH), initially seeded at a density of $1*10^5$ GFP positive urothelial cells. After 3 wk, the subdermal implant was harvested and imaged with a fluorescence stereomicroscope (Leica, Germany) to locate GFP positive cells. The tissue segments were fixed in 10% NBF and embedded in paraffin for histological analysis.

Results

Characterization of Mass-cultured Human and Porcine Urothelial Cells

We observed that both human and porcine urothelial cells arising from respective biopsies were capable of forming colonies in culture (Figure S1). Urothelial cells of human native ureters as well as native porcine bladder and ureter expressed uroplakin-2 and uroplakin-3 (Figure S2C, S3C, S4C and S5C). In contrast, the urothelial cells of native porcine urethral tissue only expressed uroplakin-2 but not uroplakin-3 (Figure S6C). We also found that human and porcine urothelial cells cultured *in vitro* for 8 days widely expressed a general marker of urothelial cells, cytokeratin-7, but only expressed uroplakin-2 spot-wise in a sparse manner (Figure S2D, S3D, S4D, S5D and S6D). However, none of the human or porcine urothelial cells cultured *in vitro* for this period expressed uroplakin-3 (Figure S2D, S3D, S4D, S5D and S6D).

We sought to develop an *in vivo* model to study full differentiation of the urothelium. We tested two ectopic locations to implant GFP positive porcine mass-cultured urothelial cells in Swiss nu/nu mice. Dispase-treated sheets of urothelial cells cultured for 12 days were implanted into the dorsal sub-dermal space of the nude mice and were compared to urothelial cells implanted as a pellet under the kidney capsule. We sacrificed the animals after 3 wk and studied the expression of uroplakin-2 and uroplakin-3 in GFP positive cells. The urothelial sheets on the back of the mice formed a uniform sheet expressing uroplakin-2, but not uroplakin-3 (Figure S7). On the other hand the pellets implanted beneath the renal capsule formed urothelial bundle-like and urothelial "micro-bladder"-like structures with a lumen (Figure 2A and 2B). Both of these structures expressed uroplakin-2 and uroplakin-3 (Figure 2C). Furthermore we observed that they expressed a proliferation

Table 1. Clonal analysis of human ureteral cells.

Clone	CA day 7 (mm^2)	Estim CN	GT (h)	GN	CFE (%)	GC (nb)	AB (nb)	AB (%)	Clonal type
1	1.295	1634	15.7	10.6	31.2	97	5	4.90	Holoclone
2	0.733	1209	16.4	10.2	19.9	46	2	4.17	Holoclone
3	0.243	330	20.1	8.36	3.04	0	2	100	Paraclone
4	1.378	1243	16.3	10.3	6.84	3	14	82.3	Meroclone
5	1.294	2661	14.8	11.4	4.51	12	12	50.0	Meroclone

(CA = clone area, Estim CN = estimated cell number, GT = generation time, GN = generation number, GC = growing colony, nb = number, AB = aborted).

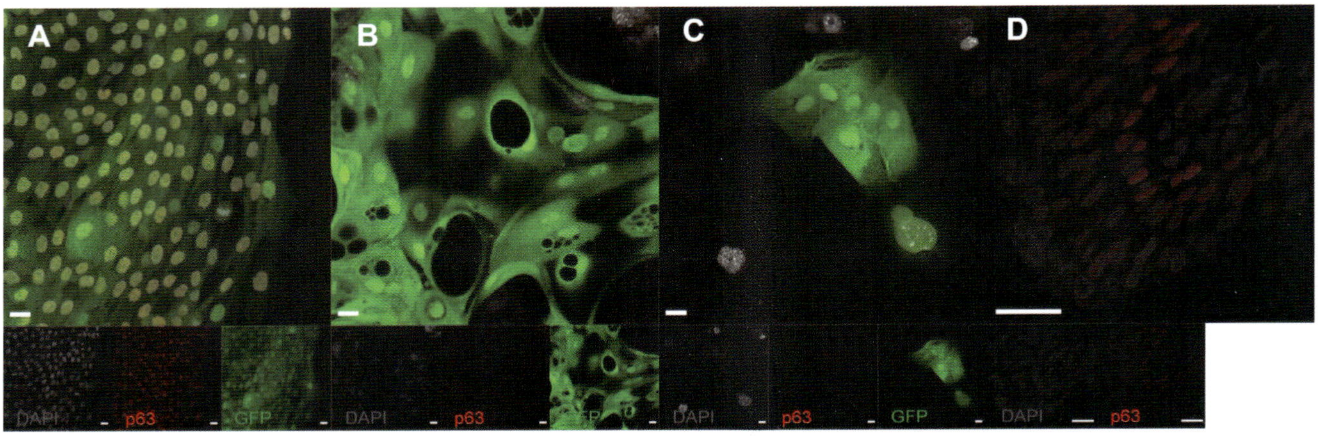

Figure 3. p63 expression in clonal human urothelial cells and urothelium. (A) p63-expression in a human urothelial holoclone culture at passage 2. (B) p63-expression in a human urothelial holoclone culture at passage 5. (C) p63-expression in a human urothelial meroclone culture at passage 2. (D) p63-expression in a human ureter biopsy (scale bars, 10 µm). Note the DAPI positive together with GFP negative cells are 3T3-J2 cells and DAPI positive together with GFP positive cells are urothelial cells.

marker, Ki-67, suggesting that the GFP-urothelial cells were proliferating beneath the kidney capsule (Figure 2C).

We found that porcine ureteral, urethral, bladder dome and trigone cells grew well in the 3T3-J2 culture system, showing high colony-forming efficiencies for all the isolated biopsies (independent on age of donors) (Figure S3A–B, S4A–B, S5A–B and S6A–B). We did not observe any major growth differences between the different anatomical harvesting locations. Next, we investigated whether the porcine ureteral, urethral, bladder dome and trigone urothelial cells had similar differentiation capacities in the mouse kidney capsule model. We observed that the porcine ureteral, bladder dome and trigone cells formed fully differentiated urothelium, expressing uroplakin-2 and uroplakin-3 (Figure S3E, S4E and S5E). Interestingly, implanted urethral urothelial cells expressed uroplakin-2, following the protein expression pattern of native urethral tissue (Figure S6C and S6E), but as would be expected did not express uroplakin-3. Confirming the specificity of these antibodies for urothelium, we also found porcine skin biopsies as well as 8-day *in vitro* cultured porcine keratinocytes and thymus, to be negative for cytokeratin-7, uroplakin-2 and uroplakin-3 (Figure S8).

Clonogenicity, Self-renewal in vitro and Urothelial Differentiation *in vivo* of Human Urothelial Cells Isolated from the Ureter

We explored whether handpicked cells with an elongated Pasteur pipette under an inverted microscope could initiate clonal growth. Following the rationale of Barrandon *et al.* [13], we selected small and round urothelial cells, and observed the development of clonal populations with different growth capacities. Applying the similar definitions for classifying the clonal type, based on aborted colony percentages as previously used for human epidermal, hair-follicle and corneal epithelial clonal cells [14,16,17], we observed that the selected clonal populations formed urothelial holoclones, meroclones and paraclones (Figure 1B, 1C and 1D) (Table 1).

The human urothelial holoclone could not be serially passaged longer than 25 population doublings with a decreased colony-forming efficiency over 45 days of culture, after which senescence occurred (Figure 1E and 1F). We observed that cells of human urothelial holoclones stained strongly and homogenously for p63 at an early passage (passage 2), while at later passage (passage 5) the urothelial holoclones expression of p63-expression was weak or not even present in colonies (Figure 3A and 3B). Evident from these images are the cell morphology differences going from a non-stretched cell morphology at passage 2 (characteristic of a proliferative urothelial phenotype) to a stretched cell morphology at passage 5 (characteristic of a differentiated/senescent urothelial cell phenotype) (Figure 3A and 3B). When we examined urothelial meroclones at an early passage (passage 2), we observed mixed p63-expression, ranging from strong, weak to no expression (Figure 3C). Interestingly, in human ureter biopsies we saw a strong p63-expression in the basal cells in the urothelium, a weak

Table 2. Clonal analysis of porcine ureteral cells.

Clone	CA day 7 (mm^2)	Estim CN	GT (h)	GN	CFE (%)	GC (nb)	AB (nb)	AB (%)	Clonal type
1	0.875	721	17.7	9.49	99.9	142	2	1.38	Holoclone
2	1.405	895	17.1	9.81	67.0	118	3	2.48	Holoclone
3	0.891	304	20.4	8.24	4.95	0	3	100	Paraclone
4	1.765	1310	16.2	10.4	39.3	54	49	47.6	Meroclone
5	0.284	639	18.0	9.32	33.7	21	22	51.2	Meroclone

(CA = clone area, Estim CN = estimated cell number, GT = generation time, GN = generation number, GC = growing colony, nb = number, AB = aborted).

Table 3. Clonal analysis of porcine bladder cells.

Clone	CA day 7 (mm^2)	Estim CN	GT (h)	GN	CFE (%)	GC (nb)	AB (nb)	AB (%)	Clonal type
1	8.372	2500	14.9	11.3	56.0	272	8	2.86	Holoclone
2	0.098	185	22.3	7.53	81.1	29	1	3.33	Holoclone
3	0.009	12	46.9	3.58	83.3	0	2	100	Paraclone
4	0.035	90	25.9	6.49	55.5	8	2	20.0	Meroclone
5	0.155	140	23.6	7.13	39.3	8	3	27.3	Meroclone

(CA = clone area, Estim CN = estimated cell number, GT = generation time, GN = generation number, GC = growing colony, nb = number, AB = aborted).

p63-expression in the intermediate cells and no p63 expression in the superficial cells (Figure 3D).

When we implanted the GFP-positive human urothelial holoclones in the kidney capsule model, we also found that these had the capacity to form "micro-bladder"-like structures, expressing uroplakin-2 and uroplakin-3, protein markers for fully differentiated urothelium (Figure 1G).

Clonogenicity, Self-renewal in vitro and Urothelial Differentiation *in vivo* of Porcine Urothelial Cells Isolated from the Ureter, Bladder and Urethra

Studying the *in vitro* behavior of cells harvested from the porcine bladder, ureter and urethra, we observed the same clonogenic capacity as the cells harvested from the human ureter. Porcine clonogenic urothelial cells were, as for the human cells, classified as urothelial holoclones, meroclones or paraclones, depending on the growth capacities. (Figure 4A–C, 5A–C and 6A–C) (Table 2, 3 and 4). Compared to human holoclones, porcine holoclones had a much greater growth capacity. It could be demonstrated that after 38 days of passaging, porcine urothelial holoclone showed 30 population doublings and thereafter were still in a growing phase (Figure 4D–E, 5D–E and 6D–E).

Next we analyzed the differentiation capacity of the porcine bladder-, porcine ureter-, and porcine urethra-holoclones in the kidney capsule model. We observed that all the implanted holoclones had the capacity to form "micro-bladder"-like structures. The porcine ureteral- and bladder-holoclones expressed both uroplakin-2 and uroplakin-3 (4F and 5F). Interestingly, in one of the three kidneys harvested from animals with implanted urethral holoclones, one micro-bladder was observed to express uroplakin-3 (Figure 6G), however, all other micro-bladders formed by the urethral holoclones only expressed uroplakin-2 and not uroplakin-3 (Figure 6F).

Discussion

Human and porcine cell populations derived from a single urothelial cell, can self-renew *in vitro* and differentiate into mature urothelium *in vivo*, and therefore represent clonogenic urothelial stem cell populations. First, we aimed at reproducing the findings that urothelial cells had the capacity to form colonies at low cell seeding density when seeded using the 3T3-J2 culture system, as reported by Wu in the 1980's [18]. These results encouraged us to perform clonal analysis of urothelial cells. The commonly applied urothelial cell culture technique uses a feeder cell-free culturing system [6], which does not allow clonal cell analysis. Using the 3T3-J2 culture system, we demonstrated that both human and porcine urothelial cells could initiate colony growth when seeded at low densities and clonal cell populations based on single cell seeding. However, the decrease of CFE, the premature change of morphology together with the loss of p63 expression indicates that the 3T3-J2 culture system can be improved for human urothelial stem cells expansion.

Further we evaluated if cultured urothelial cells can differentiate into a superficial urothelial cell type, representing the mature urothelial umbrella cells, being in contact with urine. In these cells, uroplakins are the main responsible molecules for the barrier function, forming protein plaques and preventing the urine from entering surrounding tissues. The uroplakin family consists of four proteins that make up these plaques, consisting of pairs of uroplakin-1a with uroplakin-2 and uroplakin-1b with uroplakin-3 [19]. We observed that after implantation of human and porcine urothelial cell pellets, generated from a single urothelial cells, into the renal subcapsular space of Swiss nu/nu mice, uroplakin-2 and uroplakin-3 expression were initiated. However, implanting urothelial sheets into the dorsal subdermal space of nude mice, only the expression of uroplakin-2 but not of uroplakin-3 was observed during the observation period of 3 weeks. It seems that urothelial cell pellets implanted into the renal subcapsular space favor differentiation into mature urothelial cells, making it a more suitable assay to study urothelial differentiation. We noticed that

Table 4. Clonal analysis of porcine urethral cells.

Clone	CA day 7 (mm^2)	Estim CN	GT (h)	GN	CFE (%)	GC (nb)	AB (nb)	AB (%)	Clonal type
1	1.156	990	16.9	9.95	79.9	151	7	4.43	Holoclone
2	0.072	220	21.6	7.78	2.28	0	1	100	Paraclone
3	0.069	371	19.7	8.53	13.5	5	5	50.0	Meroclone
4	0.140	289	20.6	8.17	27.7	12	4	25.0	Meroclone

(CA = clone area, Estim CN = estimated cell number, GT = generation time, GN = generation number, GC = growing colony, nb = number, AB = aborted).

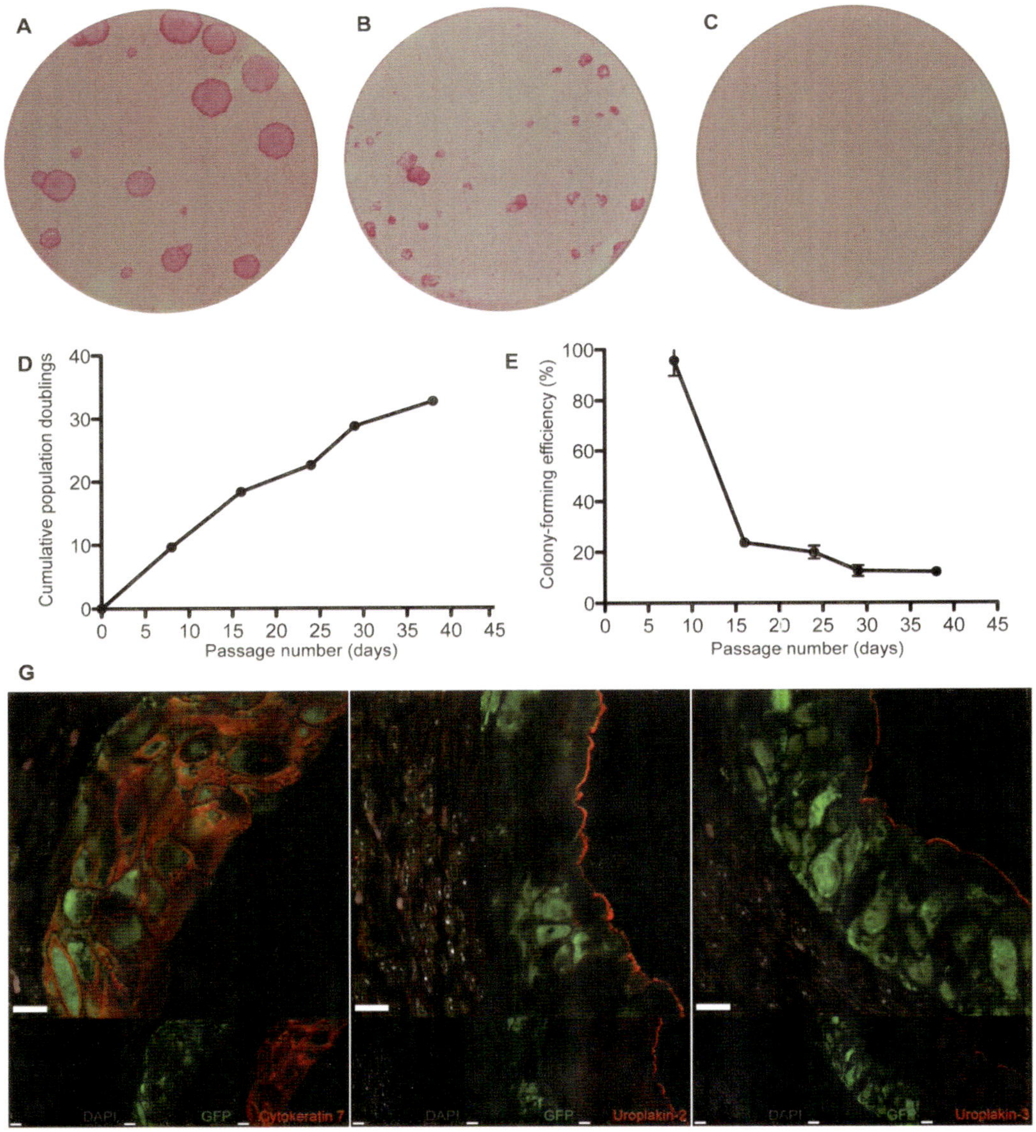

Figure 4. Porcine clonal urothelial cells arising from a single ureteral cell. (A, B and C) Porcine urothelial holoclone, meroclone and paraclone cultures arising from a single ureteral cell. (D and E) Growth curves of a porcine urothelial holoclone. (F) *In vivo* urothelial differentiation of porcine ureteral urothelial holoclone pellets implanted into the subcapsular space of the Swiss nu/nu mice, expressing cytokeratin 7, uroplakin-2 and uroplakin 3 (scale bars, 10 μm). Note the "micro-bladder" like structure.

uroplakin-3 expression was only found after vacuole formation within urothelial bundle structures and at a later state within the "micro-bladder" like structures but not in the tight urothelial bundles. It can be speculated that an up-regulation of the PPARγ signal pathway and a down-regulation of EGF-pathway seen in *in vitro* cultured urothelial cells is due to the 3T3-J2 cells in the cell pellet [20]. We have not observed that rat or human thymic epithelial cells form these "micro-bladder" structures when implanted into the renal subcapsular space [21]. Indicating the "micro-bladder" like structures are specific for implanting urothelial cells. However, in literature it has been described that mouse embryonic stem cells are able to form similar "micro-bladder" like structures, when implanted together with micro dissected embryonic rat urogenital sinus into the renal subcapsular space [22]. Mouse bladder urothelial cells together with embryonic rat urogenital sinus also forms the "micro-bladder" like structures [23]. From these data it seems that "micro-bladder" like structures, can be formed either with 3T3-J2 cells or micro dissected embryonic rat urogenital sinus as carriers.

We aimed to establish whether there is a difference in porcine urothelial cell growth and differentiation capacities between different cell harvesting locations, as previously reported for bovine urothelial cells by Liang *et al.* [9]. This might become important if isolation of urothelial cells from a disease-free location of the urinary tract is performed to replace neoplastic or diseased tissues. From our porcine *in vitro* and *in vivo* data, we could not observe any difference in cell growth and differentiation between cells harvested from the ureter and the bladder. The *in vitro* cell growth and differentiation capacity of urothelial cells harvested from the urethra was comparable to the one of cells harvested

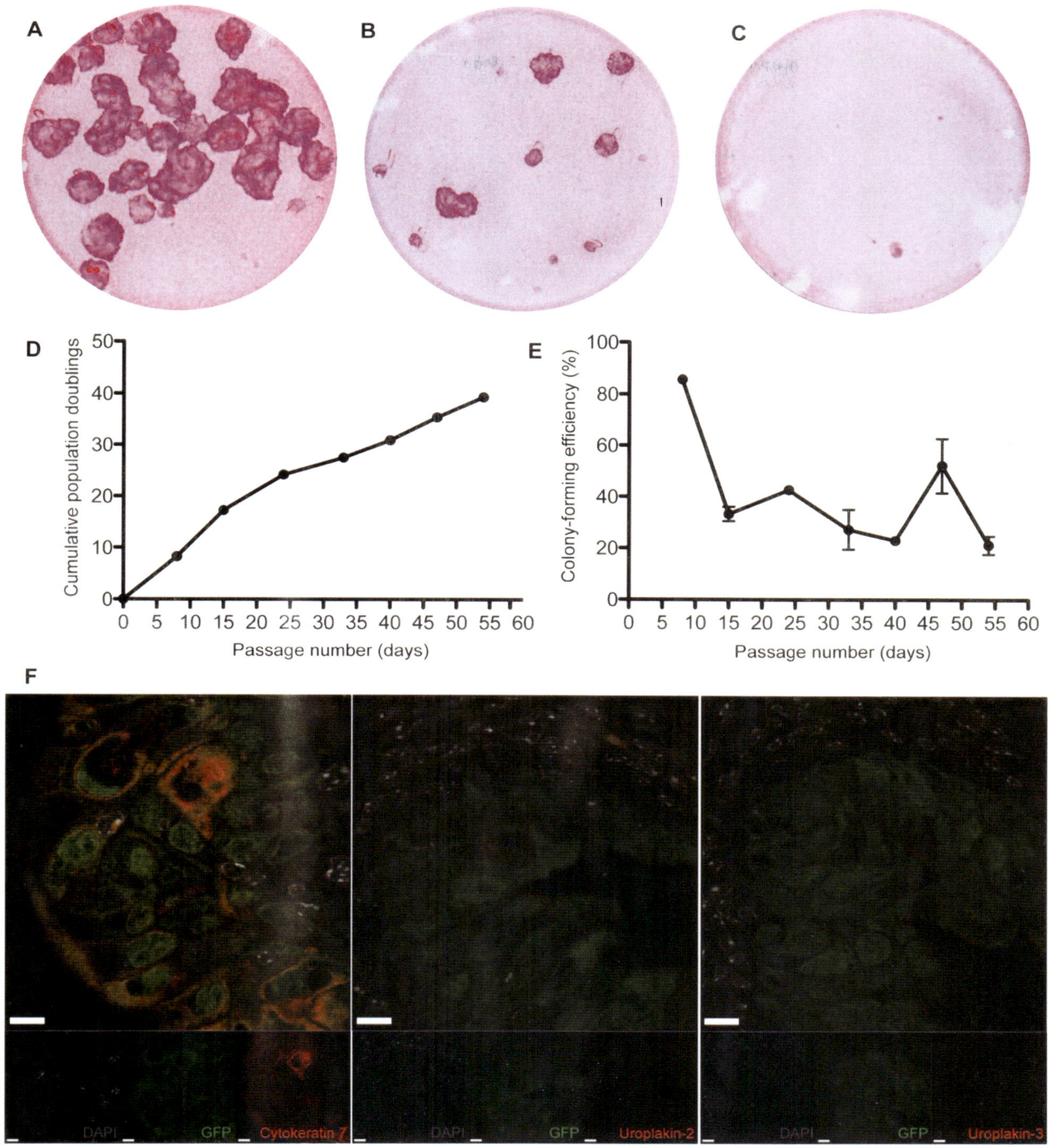

Figure 5. Porcine clonal urothelial cells arising from a single bladder cell. (A, B and C) Porcine urethelial holoclone, meroclone and paraclone cultures arising from a single bladder cell. (D and E) Growth curves of a porcine urothelial holoclone. (F) *In vivo* urothelial differentiation of porcine bladder urothelial holoclone pellets implanted into the subcapsular space of the Swiss nu/nu mice, expressing cytokeratin 7, uroplakin-2 and uroplakin 3 (scale bars, 10 μm). Note the "micro-bladder" like structure.

from the bladder. However, we observed that native urethral biopsies and the implanted mass-cultured urethral cells did not express uroplakin-3 in Swiss nu/nu mice, apart from the expression in one single "micro-bladder"-like structure, arising from a urethral holoclone. This lets us assume that urothelial umbrella cells arising from urethral holoclones can express uroplakin-3 if implanted underneath the kidney capsule, although it is not expressed in the native urethra. Indicating that urethral holoclones can under certain condition have a broaden differentiation capacity.

We also investigated if there is a difference in the behavior of urothelial cells harvested from the bladder dome or the trigone. As

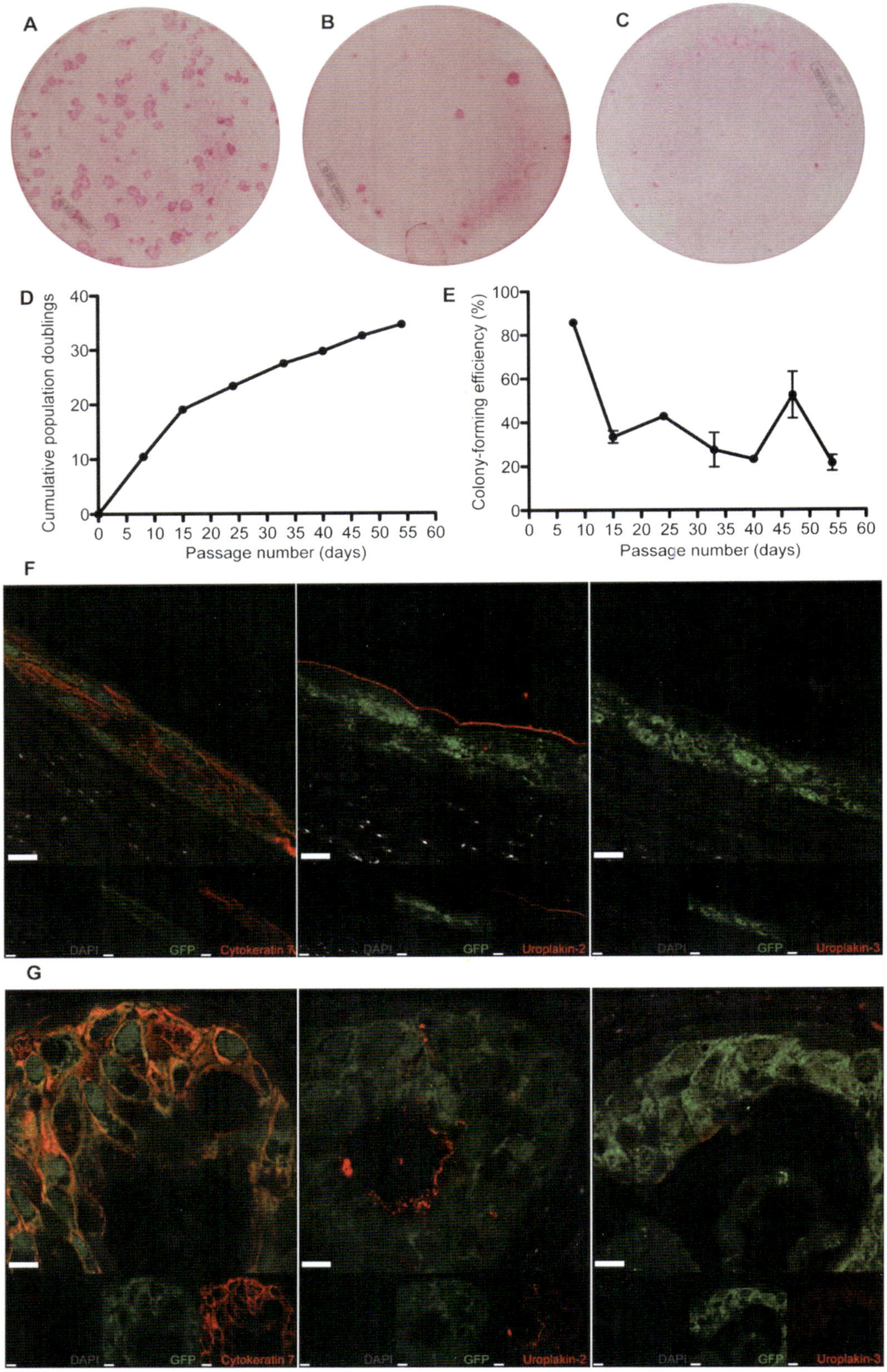

Figure 6. Porcine clonal urothelial cells arising from a single urethral cell. (A, B and C) Porcine urethelial holoclone, meroclone and paraclone cultures arising from a single urethral cell. (D and E) Growth curves of a porcine urothelial holoclone. (F, G) *In vivo* urothelial differentiation of porcine urethral urothelial holoclonal cell pellets implanted into the subcapsular space of the Swiss nu/nu mice, expressing cytokeratin 7, uroplakin-2 and uroplakin 3 (scale bars, 10 μm). Note the "micro-bladder" like structure.

it has been reported that urothelial cancers often develops in the trigone, it could be speculated that the trigonal region has an increased stem cell pool and would therefore be optimal for cell harvesting [24]. However, we observed no difference in the cell growth and differentiation capacity of cells from the two harvest locations. These data correlate well with histological assessments of the human bladder, where clonal patches were found to replenish urothelium in all regions of the bladder, and not particularly from the trigone [25].

Porcine clonogenic urothelial cells seem to favor the 3T3-J2 culture system for continuous self-renewal, in contrary to human clonogenic urothelial cells. We can exclude a potential lentiviral bias for the human urothelial senescence since also non-transduced clonogenic human urothelial cells senesced. Thus, we observe an epithelial tissue difference between human keratinocytes and human urothelial cells, where *in vitro* cultured human clonal keratinocytes can reach 180 population doublings while clonal human urothelial cells can only reach 25 population doublings [26]. We argue that this is not only because of the 3T3-J2 culture system is optimized for keratinocyte growth, but that normal *in vivo* human urothelium cell turnover is also estimated to be slower (6–11 months), and inherently human urothelial cells should have a lower growth potential than the human keratinocytes (20 days epidermal cell turnover) [27,28]. However, the 3T3-J2 culture system allows us, during a period of two weeks, to evaluate human urothelial cell self-renewal and to study which molecular signatures, such as p63, are important for self-renewal [29]. Since p63 has been reported in keratinocyte and cornea holoclones and more recently has been implicated as an *in vivo* signature of mouse bladder stem cells, we saw this as a likely molecular signature of human urothelial holoclones [5,30,31]. Proliferation data from holoclones showed that they senesced at a late passage and this correlated with a mixed and weak expression of p63 in the few occurring urothelial colonies. However, the urothelial holoclones at an early passage (in a self-renewing phase) expressed p63 homogenously and strongly in the urothelial colonies. We also observed that the clonal hierarchy reflected the level of p63 expression, where the holoclone had a more homogenous expression of p63 compared to the meroclone. It is tempting to infer from the biopsy data of p63 expression in native human ureter, where the p63 expression from basal to superficial cell goes from high to none, that the urothelial holoclones are derived from the basal layer of the urothelium and that the *in vitro* 3T3-J2 culture system reflects what we partially observe *in vivo*, similar to what has been described for skin model system [30]. We believe that further investigation in understanding the molecular mechanism for continuous human urothelial self-renewal is of importance to learn to retain stemness in long-term cell culture, which could be useful for potential clinical regenerative medicine applications.

We further plan to implant clonal cell populations into an orthotopic bladder model to determine if they can induce long-term functional reconstitution. Due to ethical concerns, clinical trials must be preceded by porcine functional reconstitution studies. Our finding that clonogenic porcine urothelial cells can be captured *in vitro* will allow us to perform long-term functional reconstitution experiments to determine how these single cell populations behave.

To date, only epidermal, corneal and blood-derived adult stem cell populations have been successfully used in long-term functional reconstitution for the treatment of severe diseases in human patients [1,2,3]. Our results suggest that clonogenic urothelial stem cell populations could potentially represent an additional adult stem cell population, to be used for functional regeneration of the diseased human urinary tract.

Conclusions

Human clonogenic urothelial stem cells have not previously been studied *in vitro* or *in vivo*. We showed that isolated clonogenic, human ureteral urothelial cells are able to self-renew *in vitro* and to fully differentiate *in vivo*. Future larger-animal functional reconstitution studies of *in vitro* cultured clonogenic urothelial stem cells will be useful before initiating clinical trials in human patients. Toward this end, we showed that porcine clonogenic urothelial stem cells exist and therefore can be used for such studies.

Supporting Information

Figure S1 Colony forming capacity of mass-cultured human and porcine urothelial cells. (A) Isolated human ureteral cells, (B) porcine ureteral cells, (C) porcine urethral cells, (D and E) porcine bladder dome and trigonal cells.

Figure S2 *In vitro* and *in vivo* behavior of mass-cultured human ureteral cells. (A and B) Growth curves and colony forming capacity of isolated human ureteral urothelial cells. (C) Cytokeratin 7, uroplakin-2 and uroplakin-3 expression in native human ureteral tissue. (D) Cytokeratin 7, uroplakin-2 and uroplakin-3 expression of *in vitro* cultured human ureteral urothelial cells after 8 days. (E) Cytokeratin 7, uroplakin-2 and uroplakin-3 expression of *in vivo* implanted human ureteral urothelial cells after 3 wk (scale bars, 20 μm).

Figure S3 *In vitro* and *in vivo* behavior of mass-cultured porcine ureteral cells. (A and B) Growth curves and colony forming capacity of isolated porcine ureteral urothelial cells. (C) Cytokeratin 7, uroplakin-2 and uroplakin-3 expression in native porcine ureteral tissue. (D) Cytokeratin 7, uroplakin-2 and uroplakin-3 expression of *in vitro* cultured porcine ureteral urothelial cells after 8 days. (E) Cytokeratin 7, uroplakin-2 and uroplakin-3 expression of *in vivo* implanted porcine ureteral urothelial cells after 3 wk (scale bars, 20 μm).

Figure S4 *In vitro* and *in vivo* behavior of mass-cultured porcine bladder dome cells. (A and B) Growth curves and colony forming capacity of isolated porcine bladder dome urothelial cells. (C) Cytokeratin 7, uroplakin-2 and uroplakin-3 expression in native porcine bladder dome tissue. (D) Cytokeratin 7, uroplakin-2 and uroplakin-3 expression of *in vitro* cultured porcine bladder dome urothelial cells after 8 days. (E) Cytokeratin 7, uroplakin-2 and uroplakin-3 expression of *in vivo* implanted porcine bladder dome urothelial cells after 3 wk (scale bars, 20 μm).

Figure S5 *In vitro* and *in vivo* behavior of mass-cultured porcine bladder trigone cells. (A and B) Growth curves and colony forming capacity of isolated porcine bladder trigone urothelial cells. (C) Cytokeratin 7, uroplakin-2 and uroplakin-3 expression in native porcine bladder trigone tissue. (D) Cytokeratin 7, uroplakin-2 and uroplakin-3 expression of *in vitro* cultured porcine bladder trigone urothelial cells after 8 days. (E) Cytokeratin 7, uroplakin-2 and uroplakin-3 expression of *in vivo* implanted porcine bladder trigone urothelial cells after 3 wk (scale bars, 20 μm).

Figure S6 *In vitro* and *in vivo* behavior of mass-cultured porcine urethral cells. (A and B) Growth curves and colony forming capacity of isolated porcine urethral urothelial cells. (C) Cytokeratin 7, uroplakin-2 and uroplakin-3 expression in native porcine urethral tissue. (D) Cytokeratin 7, uroplakin-2 and uroplakin-3 expression of *in vitro* cultured porcine urethral urothelial cells after 8 days. (E) Cytokeratin 7, uroplakin-2 and uroplakin-3 expression of *in vivo* implanted porcine urethral urothelial cells after 3 wk (scale bars, 20 μm).

Figure S7 Back skin model for *in vivo* urothelial differentiation. (A and B) Hematoxylin & eosin (H&E) staining of an implanted urothelial sheet into the dorsal subdermal space of Swiss nu/nu mice (A: scale bar 500 μm, B: scale bar 50 μm). (C and D) Immunohistochemistry of an implanted urothelial sheet using antibodies against uroplakin-2 and uroplakin-3. Note no uroplakin-3 expression (D).

Figure S8 Immunohistochemistry of skin and thymus acting as negative control. (A) Cytokeratin 7, uroplakin-2 and uroplakin-3 expression in native porcine skin tissue. (B) Cytokeratin 7, uroplakin-2 and uroplakin-3 expression of *in vitro* cultured porcine keratinocytes after 8 days. (C) Cytokeratin 7, uroplakin-2 and uroplakin-3 expression of *in vitro* cultured porcine epithelial thymus epithelial cells after 8 days.

Table S1 Tissue donor information. (A) Human donor information. (B) Porcine donor information.

Acknowledgments

The authors thank the Histology Core Facility, the Transgenic Core Facility, the Flow Cytometry Core Facility and the Bioimaging and Optics Platform of EPFL for their assistance. The authors also wish to thank Professor W. Zimmermann (Bern University, Bern, Switzerland) for donating porcine tissue, Professor D. Trono (EPFL) for providing the GFP-lentivector used in this study, Professor C. Brisken (EPFL) for providing the p63-antibody, Dr. Rochat (CHUV) and Dr. Amici (CHUV) for discussions and teaching of techniques.

Author Contributions

Conceived and designed the experiments: HML FG JAH YB PF. Performed the experiments: HML FG. Analyzed the data: HML FG JAH YB PF. Contributed reagents/materials/analysis tools: JAH YB PF. Wrote the paper: HML FG JAH YB PF.

References

1. Ronfard V, Rives JM, Neveux Y, Carsin H, Barrandon Y (2000) Long-term regeneration of human epidermis on third degree burns transplanted with autologous cultured epithelium grown on a fibrin matrix. Transplantation 70: 1588–1598.
2. Rama P, Matuska S, Paganoni G, Spinelli A, De Luca M, et al. (2010) Limbal stem-cell therapy and long-term corneal regeneration. The New England journal of medicine 363: 147–155.
3. Daley GQ (2012) The promise and perils of stem cell therapeutics. Cell stem cell 10: 740–749.
4. Shin K, Lee J, Guo N, Kim J, Lim A, et al. (2011) Hedgehog/Wnt feedback supports regenerative proliferation of epithelial stem cells in bladder. Nature 472: 110–114.
5. Pignon JC, Grisanzio C, Geng Y, Song J, Shivdasani RA, et al. (2013) p63-expressing cells are the stem cells of developing prostate, bladder, and colorectal epithelia. Proceedings of the National Academy of Sciences of the United States of America 110: 8105–8110.
6. Southgate J, Hutton KA, Thomas DF, Trejdosiewicz LK (1994) Normal human urothelial cells in vitro: proliferation and induction of stratification. Laboratory investigation; a journal of technical methods and pathology 71: 583–594.
7. Cilento BG, Freeman MR, Schneck FX, Retik AB, Atala A (1994) Phenotypic and cytogenetic characterization of human bladder urothelia expanded in vitro. The Journal of urology 152: 665–670.
8. Thangappan R, Kurzrock EA (2009) Three clonal types of urothelium with different capacities for replication. Cell proliferation 42: 770–779.
9. Liang FX, Bosland MC, Huang H, Romih R, Baptiste S, et al. (2005) Cellular basis of urothelial squamous metaplasia: roles of lineage heterogeneity and cell replacement. The Journal of cell biology 171: 835–844.
10. Rheinwald JG, Green H (1975) Serial cultivation of strains of human epidermal keratinocytes: the formation of keratinizing colonies from single cells. Cell 6: 331–343.
11. Hofmann A, Kessler B, Ewerling S, Weppert M, Vogg B, et al. (2003) Efficient transgenesis in farm animals by lentiviral vectors. EMBO reports 4: 1054–1060.
12. Grasset N (2008) Understanding engraftment of cultured epidermal stem cells: EPFL.
13. Barrandon Y, Green H (1985) Cell size as a determinant of the clone-forming ability of human keratinocytes. Proceedings of the National Academy of Sciences of the United States of America 82: 5390–5394.
14. Barrandon Y, Green H (1987) Three clonal types of keratinocyte with different capacities for multiplication. Proceedings of the National Academy of Sciences of the United States of America 84: 2302–2306.
15. Barrandon Y, Li V, Green H (1988) New techniques for the grafting of cultured human epidermal cells onto athymic animals. The Journal of investigative dermatology 91: 315–318.
16. Rochat A, Kobayashi K, Barrandon Y (1994) Location of stem cells of human hair follicles by clonal analysis. Cell 76: 1063–1073.
17. Pellegrini G, Golisano O, Paterna P, Lambiase A, Bonini S, et al. (1999) Location and clonal analysis of stem cells and their differentiated progeny in the human ocular surface. The Journal of cell biology 145: 769–782.
18. Wu YJ, Parker LM, Binder NE, Beckett MA, Sinard JH, et al. (1982) The mesothelial keratins: a new family of cytoskeletal proteins identified in cultured mesothelial cells and nonkeratinizing epithelia. Cell 31: 693–703.
19. Wu XR, Kong XP, Pellicer A, Kreibich G, Sun TT (2009) Uroplakins in urothelial biology, function, and disease. Kidney international 75: 1153–1165.
20. Varley CL, Stahlschmidt J, Lee WC, Holder J, Diggle C, et al. (2004) Role of PPARgamma and EGFR signalling in the urothelial terminal differentiation programme. Journal of cell science 117: 2029–2036.
21. Bonfanti P, Claudinot S, Amici AW, Farley A, Blackburn CC, et al. (2010) Microenvironmental reprogramming of thymic epithelial cells to skin multipotent stem cells. Nature 466: 978–982.
22. Oottamasathien S, Wang Y, Williams K, Franco OE, Wills ML, et al. (2007) Directed differentiation of embryonic stem cells into bladder tissue. Developmental biology 304: 556–566.
23. Tanaka ST, Ishii K, Demarco RT, Pope JCt, Brock JW, 3rd, et al. (2010) Endodermal origin of bladder trigone inferred from mesenchymal-epithelial interaction. The Journal of urology 183: 386–391.
24. Nguyen MM, Lieu DK, deGraffenried LA, Isseroff RR, Kurzrock EA (2007) Urothelial progenitor cells: regional differences in the rat bladder. Cell proliferation 40: 157–165.
25. Gaisa NT, Graham TA, McDonald SA, Canadillas-Lopez S, Poulsom R, et al. (2011) The human urothelium consists of multiple clonal units, each maintained by a stem cell. The Journal of pathology 225: 163–171.
26. Barrandon Y, Grasset N, Zaffalon A, Gorostidi F, Claudinot S, et al. (2012) Capturing epidermal stemness for regenerative medicine. Seminars in cell & developmental biology 23: 937–944.
27. Hicks RM (1975) The mammalian urinary bladder: an accommodating organ. Biological reviews of the Cambridge Philosophical Society 50: 215–246.
28. Bickenbach JR, Chism E (1998) Selection and extended growth of murine epidermal stem cells in culture. Experimental cell research 244: 184–195.
29. Dabelsteen S, Hercule P, Barron P, Rice M, Dorsainville G, et al. (2009) Epithelial cells derived from human embryonic stem cells display p16INK4A senescence, hypermotility, and differentiation properties shared by many P63+ somatic cell types. Stem cells 27: 1388–1399.
30. Pellegrini G, Dellambra E, Golisano O, Martinelli E, Fantozzi I, et al. (2001) p63 identifies keratinocyte stem cells. Proceedings of the National Academy of Sciences of the United States of America 98: 3156–3161.
31. Di Iorio E, Barbaro V, Ruzza A, Ponzin D, Pellegrini G, et al. (2005) Isoforms of DeltaNp63 and the migration of ocular limbal cells in human corneal regeneration. Proceedings of the National Academy of Sciences of the United States of America 102: 9523–9528.

23

Detection of Puumala Hantavirus Antigen in Human Intestine during Acute Hantavirus Infection

Joerg Latus[1], Klara Tenner-Racz[2], Paul Racz[2], Daniel Kitterer[1]*, Daniel Cadar[2], German Ott[3], M. Dominik Alscher[1], Jonas Schmidt-Chanasit[2,4], Niko Braun[1]

1 Department of Internal Medicine, Division of Nephrology, Robert-Bosch Hospital, Auerbachstrasse 110, Stuttgart, Germany, **2** Bernhard Nocht Institute for Tropical Medicine, WHO Collaborating Centre for Arbovirus and Haemmorrhagic Fever Reference and Research, Bernhard-Nocht-Strasse 74, Hamburg, Germany, **3** Department of Diagnostic Medicine, Division of Pathology, Robert-Bosch Hospital, Auerbachstrasse 110, Stuttgart, Germany, **4** German Centre for Infection Research (DZIF), partner site Hamburg-Luebeck-Borstel, Hamburg, Germany

Abstract

Background: Puumala virus (PUUV) is the most important hantavirus species in Central Europe. Nephropathia epidemica (NE), caused by PUUV, is characterized by acute renal injury (AKI) with thrombocytopenia and frequently gastrointestinal symptoms.

Methods: 456 patients with serologically and clinically confirmed NE were investigated at time of follow-up in a single clinic. The course of the NE was investigated using medical reports. We identified patients who had endoscopy with intestinal biopsy during acute phase of NE. Histopathological, immunohistochemical and molecular analyses of the biopsies were performed.

Results: Thirteen patients underwent colonoscopy or gastroscopy for abdominal pain, diarrhea, nausea and vomiting during acute phase of NE. Immunohistochemistry (IHC) revealed PUUV nucleocapsid antigen in 11 biopsies from 8 patients; 14 biopsies from 5 patients were negative for PUUV nucleocapsid antigen. IHC localized PUUV nucleocapsid antigen in endothelial cells of capillaries or larger vessels in the lamina propria. Rate of AKI was not higher and severity of AKI was not different in the PUUV-positive compared to the PUUV-negative group. All IHC positive biopsies were positive for PUUV RNA using RT-PCR. Phylogenetic reconstruction revealed clustering of all PUUV strains from this study with viruses previously detected from the South-West of Germany. Long-term outcome was favorable in both groups.

Conclusions: In patients with NE, PUUV nucleocapsid antigen and PUUV RNA was detected frequently in the intestine. This finding could explain frequent GI-symptoms in NE patients, thus demonstration of a more generalized PUUV infection. The RT-PCR was an effective and sensitive method to detect PUUV RNA in FFPE tissues. Therefore, it can be used as a diagnostic and phylogenetic approach also for archival materials. AKI was not more often present in patients with PUUV-positive IHC. This last finding should be investigated in larger numbers of patients with PUUV infection.

Editor: Niklas K. Björkström, Karolinska Institutet, Sweden

Funding: The authors have no support or funding to report.

* E-mail: Daniel.Kitterer@rbk.de

Introduction

Hantaviruses are rodent-borne zoonotic viruses of the *Bunyaviridae* family [1] that can cause Hemorrhagic Fever with Renal Syndrome (HFRS) in Asia and Europe and Hantavirus Cardiopulmonary Syndrome in the Americas with reported case fatality rates up to 35% [2–5]. Puumala virus (PUUV) is the main hantavirus species in Central Europe and is known to cause a milder form of HFRS, which also is called nephropathia epidemica (NE) [6–11]. The clinical picture in NE includes acute kidney injury (AKI), thrombocytopenia, proteinuria and hematuria caused by tubular and glomerular involvement [12]. Both renal tubular and glomerular cells are affected by infection that leads to breakdown of cell-to cell contacts [13]. Therefore, the urinary sediment of patients with hantavirus infection contains tubular cells, with enlarged nucleoli, that are positive for hantavirus antigen [14–16]. At the level of histopathology, hantavirus infection leads to mild tubular interstitial changes and moderate interstitial infiltration with mononuclear cells [13,17]. Up to now, hantavirus antigen has been found only in the cytoplasm of tubular epithelial cells from kidney biopsies of infected patients [16,18–21]. In 1992, Nuutinen et al. [22] were the first who performed endoscopy (gastroscopy or colonoscopy) in 10 patients with acute NE (within 1–4 weeks after beginning of symptoms). In every case, hemorrhagic gastropathy was observed. Histopathological analysis of the intestinal biopsies showed that the hemorrhagic lesions were associated with edema in the lamina propria. No inflammatory changes could be detected within the biopsies [22].

A high percentage of patients with PUUV infection have severe gastrointestinal (GI) symptoms, e.g. abdominal pain, nausea and vomiting [12,23,24]. Recently we demonstrated PUUV antigen in the appendix of a NE patient with severe AKI, who underwent surgery due to severe abdominal pain. Immunohistochemistry (IHC) of the appendix from this patient showed PUUV antigen in capillary and large vessel endothelium. The capillaries with PUUV-positive, endothelial cells were located mainly in the lamina propria, including the gut associated lymphoid tissue (GALT). PUUV antigen in larger vessels was present mainly in the serosa and mesoappendix [25]. Rarely, viral antigen was found in lymphoreticular cells. In the present study, our aim was to investigate whether GI symptoms in some patients with NE is associated with PUUV infection of intestine. We have performed histopathological, immunohistochemical and molecular analyses of biopsies of the human intestine of 13 patients with NE and severe GI symptoms. The course of the disease and long- term outcome was investigated in these patients.

Materials and Methods

Patients

Since 2001, German laboratories report diagnosed PUUV infections to the local health authorities. All serologically and clinically confirmed NE patients from four selected local health authorities in southern Germany were contacted by mail. We identified 1.570 patients with NE between who became ill between 2001 and 2012. These patients were asked to attend the outpatient clinic between September 2012 and April 2013. Overall 456 NE patients could be followed at the outpatient department at the Robert-Bosch-Hospital Stuttgart, Germany. Three patients were excluded by age <18 years at the time of NE. All patients gave written informed consent before participating in the study, which was approved by the Ethics Committee of the Ethics Commission of the State Chamber of Medicine in Baden- Wuerttemberg (Stuttgart) (F-2012-046). Studies were conducted in concordance with the Declaration of Helsinki.

Data acquisition

Clinical and laboratory data during the acute phase of NE were obtained from medical reports and files from each patient or reported by the patient at time of follow-up. We identified patients who underwent colonoscopy or gastroscopy including biopsies during acute PUUV- infection. At time of follow-up at the outpatient department at the Robert-Bosch-Hospital Stuttgart, Germany detailed past and current medical histories were obtained, and a careful physical examination was done. AKI was classified on the basis of the RIFLE criteria [26]. Mild/ moderate AKI was defined in patients with no AKI and AKI Risk (R) and severe AKI was classified as RIFLE Injury (I) and RIFLE Failure (F). Information on pre-hospital baseline serum creatinine levels was available for all patients. Blood pressure was measured in all patients twice as recommended by the American Heart Association [27]. Hypertension stage 1 was defined by SBP of 140–159 mm Hg or DBP 90–99 mmHg and hypertension stage 2 by SBP >160 mm Hg or DBP >100 mmHg according to the classification of blood pressure for adults of the Seventh Report of the Joint National Committee on Prevention, Detection, Evaluation, and Treatment of High Blood Pressure [28].

All serum samples at time of follow-up were analyzed for PUUV-specific IgM and IgG in all patients using a strip-immunoblotassay (recomLine Bunyavirus IgG/IgM, Mikrogen, Germany) [29]. Hematuria was defined as a positive dipstick test for erythrocytes and over two erythrocytes per high-power field. Proteinuria was defined by an albumin/creatinine ratio (ACR)> 0.25 g/g creatinine in spot urine sample [30].

Biopsies and IHC

All patients had given their informed consent regarding a scientific work-up of tissues taken during routine procedures and eight different departments of pathology were involved in the routine pathological work-up of the biopsies. Twenty-five intestinal biopsies were fixed in 10% neutral-buffered formalin solution and embedded in paraffin. Five µm-thick sections were prepared and placed on slides coated with 3-amino-propyl-trethosilane. After deparaffinizing through xylene the sections were boiled in a domestic pressure cooker in citrate buffer pH 6 for 3 minutes and chilled down to room temperature. The sections were incubated with a PUUV monoclonal antibody raised against nucleocapsid protein (clone A1C5; dilution: 1:30; Progen Biotechnik, Heidelberg, Germany) for 30 min. Binding of antibody was visualized using the kit DCS Detection Line (DCS Innovative Diagnostik System, Hamburg, Germany) containing a secondary antibody coupled with biotin and a conjugate Streptavidin and horseradish peroxidase. The slides were developed using DAB (3,3′diaminobenzidine), counterstained with haematoxylin and mounted. To delineate the cells containing PUUV nucleocapsidantigen, immunohistochemical double labelling was applied. After developing the DAB step, the sections were then heat treated again for 2 min and incubated with the monoclonal antibody CD34 (dilution: 1:100; Dako) for overnight. The second antibody was visualized with alkaline phosphatase (Dako) Fast Blue salt. The sections were examined using an AxioImager M1 microscope (Carl Zeiss, Jena, Germany). Vero E6 cells infected with PUUV strain Sotkamo served as positive control.

Molecular detection and phylogenetic characterization of PUUV from biopsies

A total of 8 biopsies from different patients (7 gastric and 1 colon), which were detected as positive by IHC, have been subjected to molecular investigation. In parallel, we used formalin fixed and paraffin embedded (FFPE) PUUV uninfected and infected Vero E6 cells as controls. Four 10-micron thickness sections from each FFPE biopsies were used for RNA extraction. Whole viral RNA was extracted from tissues by use of RNeasy FFPE Kit (Qiagen, Hilden, Germany) according to the manufacturer's instructions. RNA was then subjected to RT-PCR to recover partial S segment (144 bp) using a degenerate forward primer PUMAGJ1-F 5′-CAACMCGTGGGAGACARACTGT-3′ at position 429 and reverse primer PUMAGJ1-R 5′-CYTTCATRGTTGAYTGAGCAGT-3′ at position 572 both positions according to the complete nucleocapsid gene protein sequence of the Bavaria CG 33/04 strain (GenBank acc. no. DQ016430) designed based on all available European PUUV strains retrieved from the GenBank. Reverse transcription and PCR amplification (RT-PCR) of the 144 bp segment of the nucleocapsid gene was performed using the SuperScript III One-Step RT-PCR System with Platinum Taq High Fidelity (Invitrogen). The PCR was performed in a 50-ml volume containing 5 µl of sample RNA, 25 µl of 2x Reaction Mix, 2.5 µl of each primer (PUMAGJ1 and PUMAGJ2), 2 µl High Fidelity Enzym-Mix and ddH2O up to 50 µl. The reaction was then incubated in a thermocycler under the following conditions: 50°C for 50 minutes and 94°C as cDNA synthesis and pre-denaturation step; 45 cycles of 94°C for 20 seconds (denaturation), 55°C for 45 seconds (annealing), 72°C for 1 minute (extension) with a final elongation step at 72 °C for 10 min. The PCR product was visualized on a UV transilluminator following separation on 2.5% agarose gels containing ethidium bromide. Amplicons were sent to the company LGC Genomics for Sanger sequencing. Sequence data were analyzed using Geneious 7.4.1 program for multiple alignments. Phylogenetic analyses of the obtained sequences were performed in comparison to the strains belonging to different geographical regions as retrieved from GenBank. Evolutionary tree and distances (number of base substitutions per site) were generated by PhyML v3.1 [31]with the General-Time-Reversible model of sequence evolution with gamma-distributed rate variation among sites and proportion of invariable sites (GTR + Γ+I) found to be most appropriate model according to Akaike information criteria included in the jModelTest [32]. The PUUV sequences were shown in File S1.

Statistical analysis

Data are reported as median and range unless otherwise specified. All continuous variables were tested for normality using the Kolmogorov-Smirnov test. Comparisons between different groups were performed with the Mann-Whitney test or the Fisher's exact test, as appropriate. Analysis was performed using GraphPad statistical software package (San Diego, California, USA). A p value <0.05 was considered statistically significant.

Results

Overall, 456 patients were followed-up at our outpatient clinic with a median follow up time of 10 (7–29) months after acute NE. All patients lived in southern Germany and had laboratory and clinically confirmed NE between 2001 and 2012.Thirteen patients had colonoscopy or gastroscopy with biopsies during their acute PUUV- infection. Endoscopy was done 12 (9–15) days in the PUUV-positive group and 7 (4–9) days in the PUUV-negative group after beginning of symptoms associated with NE. The indications for endoscopy were severe abdominal pain, diarrhea, nausea and vomiting. Gastroscopy revealed gastritis with subepithelial hemorrhages and telangiectasia in all patients. The most prominent hemorrhagic findings were found in the antrum. In the PUUV-positive group, in two patients gastritis was associated with *Helicobater pylori* infection, whereas in the PUUV-negative group no *Helicobater pylori* infection could be found. In the PUUV-negative group, two patients had mild gastro-esophageal reflux disease and in one patient thrush esophagitis was present. Colonoscopy was done in 3 patients revealing spotty hemorrhage in all biopsies without any signs of inflammation.

IHC was done on 25 intestinal biopsies. Twenty-one of these were gastric; 1 was esophageal; and 3 were from colon. PUUV nucleocapsid antigen was detected in eleven biopsies from eight patients (9 gastric and 2 colon). Fourteen biopsies (12 gastric, 1 esophageal and 1 colon) from 5 patients were negative for PUUV nucleocapsid antigen. PUUV nucleocapsid antigen was mainly found in endothelial cell of capillaries or larger vessels in the lamina propria of biopsies from stomach or colon (see Figure 1 and 2). The intense immunohistochemical staining of cells expressing PUUV nucleocapsid antigen deposited in a granular pattern documents the involvement of the human intestine in PUUV infection. Biopsies from all patients, which were detected as positive by IHC, have been subjected to molecular investigation. All IHC positive biopsies were positive for PUUV RNA using RT-PCR.

Four out of eight patients in the PUUV-positive and three out of five patients in the PUUV-negative group presented with abdominal pain at time of diagnosis. Nausea and vomiting were present in five out of eight patients in the PUUV-positive and in three out of five patients in the PUUV negative group. In total, ten out of thirteen patients had AKI during PUUV infection. Neither higher rates of AKI, nor differences regarding severity of AKI could be detected in the PUUV-positive compared to the PUUV-negative group. At time of follow-up, kidney function was within the normal range in all patients. The prevalence of hypertension, proteinuria, hematuria and co-morbidities as long-term consequences after PUUV infection was not different between both groups. A detailed summary of study population including laboratory values during acute course of the disease and at time of follow-up is given in table 1 and table 2. Due to a possible selection bias, we compared baseline characteristics during acute course of the disease (e.g. laboratory values, severity of AKI, symptoms during acute course of the disease) and outcome data between the patients who underwent endoscopy with biopsies ($n = 13$) and the study population without endoscopy ($n = 443$ patients). No statistical significant differences could be observed between the groups (data not shown).

Phylogenetic reconstruction revealed clustering of all PUUV strains from this study with viruses previously detected from the South-West of Germany (Figure 3) [33].

Discussion

We investigated biopsies of the human intestine in patients with acute PUUV infection in order to understand why a majority of patients with NE have severe abdominal pain [23], for which there is no pathophysiologic explanation. We found 13 patients who had an endoscopy at time of acute Hantavirus infection due to severe gastrointestinal symptoms. Endoscopy was carried out during acute phase of NE and gastritis with hemorrhage could be observed in all patients. In line with the results from to the study of Nuutinen et al. [22], the hemorrhagic changes were more prominent in the proximal compared to the distal part of the stomach. In contrast, signs of inflammation could be detected in all intestinal biopsies in our study.

IHC demonstrated PUUV nucleocapsid antigen in 62% of the analyzed biopsies. PUUV nucleocapsid antigen was located mainly in endothelial cells of capillaries or larger vessels in the lamina propria. This finding accords with previous reports from patients with HCPS, with experimental PUUV infection in cynomolgus macaques and from our recent report [25,34,35]. Almost all hantavirus infections (especially southern Germany) are caused by PUUV [7,33], although Tula virus and Dobrava-Belgrade virus circulates in Germany and might cause symptomatic infections in humans [36–39].

Regarding clinical course of the disease, twelve out of thirteen patients had to be admitted to hospital. Duration of hospital stay was more than one week and ten out of thirteen patients had AKI, indicating that PUUV causes severe disease in most patients with NE. Although the number of patients is relatively small, a possible explanation could be an enhanced inflammatory response caused by a generalized PUUV infection. This systemic infection could be reflected by the presence of PUUV nucleocapsid antigen in human intestine and might explain the clinical phenotype of severe GI-symptoms. Further studies in larger numbers of NE patients are needed to investigate whether detection of PUUV nucleocapsid antigen in the human intestine might be a risk factor for severe course of the disease.

Remarkably, all IHC positive biopsies were positive for PUUV RNA using RT-PCR. Thus, the RT-PCR technique could be used to detect infection from archival or fixed materials. As an auxiliary advantage of RT-PCR, it is possible to sequence the amplicon, enabling more extensive molecular analyses. In this study, the nucleocapsid gene was chosen for amplification because it provides valuable information regarding the possible origin of the PUUV. The success of the development of this RT-PCR from FFPE biopsies enables work on PUUV in more flexible conditions

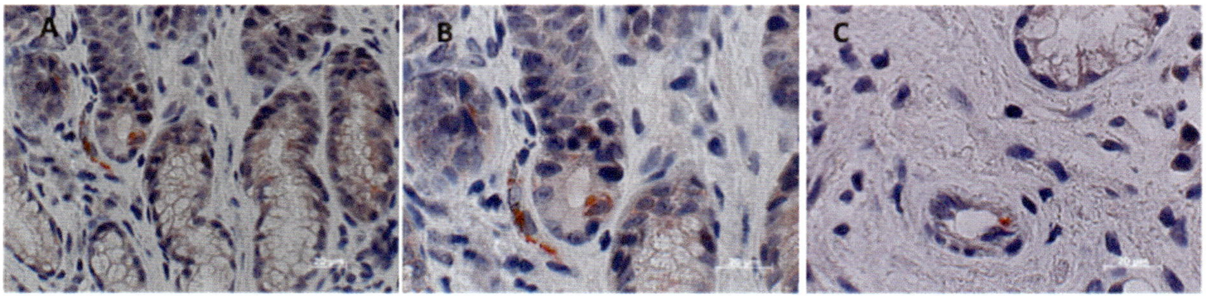

Figure 1. Detection of PUUV nucleocapsid antigen in the capillaries in the lamina propria of a gastric biopsy 8 days after beginning of symptoms associated with NE (fever, abdominal pain, nausea and vomiting) A Higher magnification demonstrates capillaries with positive endothelial cells in the lamina propria (same patient) B Endothelial cell with PUUV nucleocapsid antigen (same patient) C.

because FFPE could be handled without biosecurity concerns. In this study, phylogenetic reconstruction revealed clustering of all PUUV strains with viruses previously detected from South-West of Germany [33]. Based on Ettinger et al. [33] the German PUUV strains formed 6 distinct clades comprising strains of human and vole origin corresponding to a different outbreak region. High similarities between human and rodent-derived PUUV strains from the same region and distinct from the others highlight the

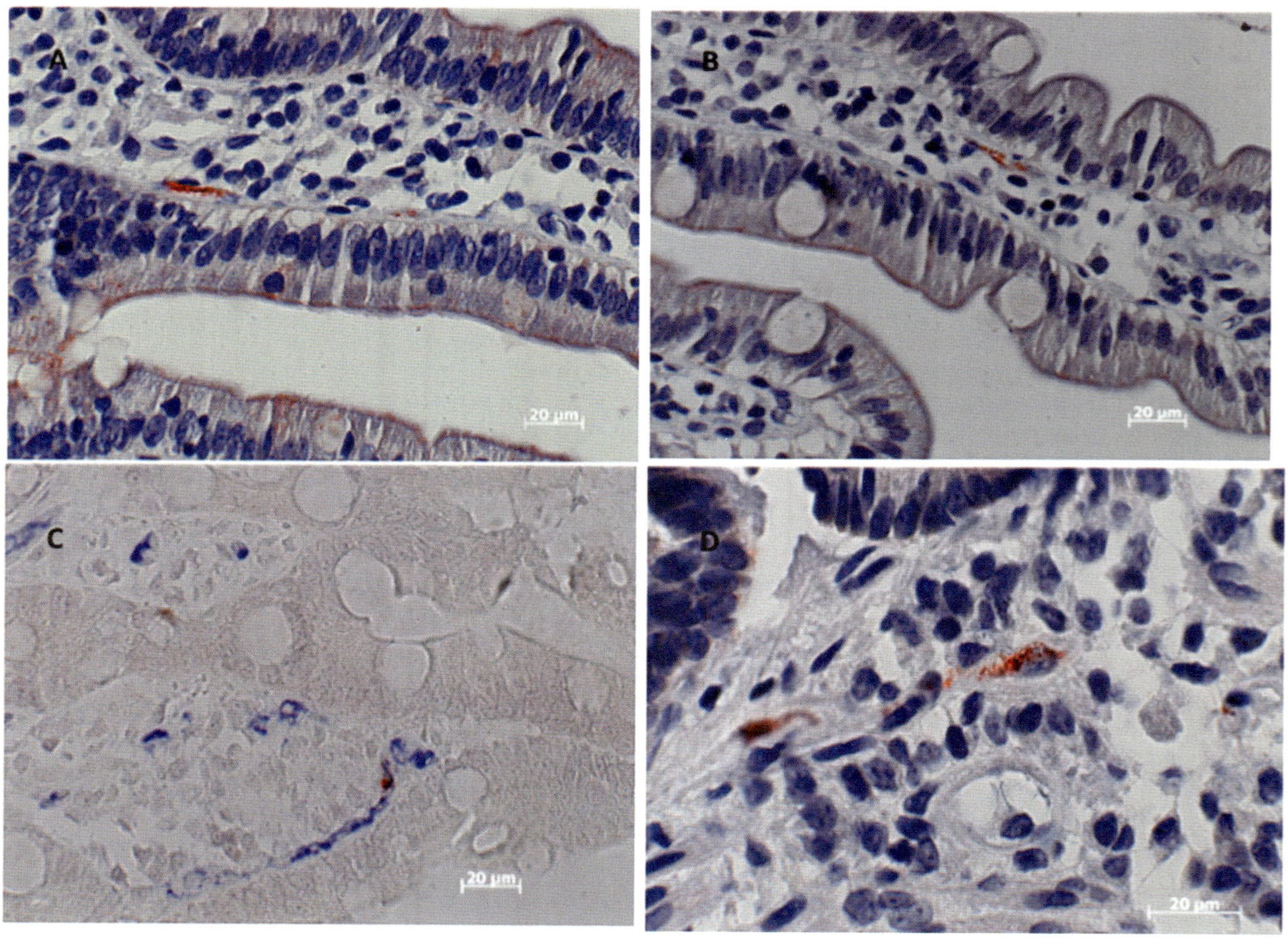

Figure 2. Detection of PUUV nucleocapsid antigen in the capillaries in the lamina propria (gastric biopsy) 10 days after beginning of symptoms A and B Immunohistochemical double labeling with the monoclonal antibody A1C5 (brown) and the monoclonal antibody to CD34 reacting the endothelial cells (blue). The PUUV nucleocapsid antigen is granular C Detection of PUUV nucleocapsid antigen in interstitial cells (gastric biopsy) D.

Table 1. Baseline characteristics of study population during acute phase of NE.

Variable	PUUV nucleocapsid antigen positive (n = 8)	PUUV nucleocapsid antigen negative (n = 5)
n	8	5
Female/male	4/4	1/4
Age at diagnosis (years)	55 (48–65)	51 (38–63)
In-patients/outpatients	8/0	4/1
Duration of hospital stay	9 (7–13)	11 (9–12)
Assumed path of infection		
- Occupational	0	1
- During leisure time	8	4
Symptoms		
Abdominal pain	4/8	3/5
Back pain	3/8	4/5
Pain of the limbs	6/8	3/5
Headache	6/8	4/5
Visual disorders	1/8	0/5
Diarrhea	2/8	2/5
Nausea/Vomiting	5/8	3/5
Clinical signs		
Fever	7/8	5/5
Hemorrhage	0/8	0/5
Urinary analysis at admission	6/8	4/4
- Proteinuria	5/6	3/5
- Hematuria	4/6	1/5
- Leucocyturia	1/6	0/5
Acute Kidney Injury		
Acute Kidney Injury according to RIFLE classification	7/8	3/5
- Risk	5	1
- Injury	0	1
- Failure	2	1

Table 2. Baseline characteristics of study population at follow-up.

Variable	PUUV nucleocapsid antigen positive (n = 8)	PUUV nucleocapsid antigen negative (n = 5)
Number of patients	8	5
Follow-up (months)	10 (7–33)	19 (10–28)
Laboratory findings		
Creatinine (mg/dl [0.5–1.4])	0.9 (0.8–1.0)	0.9 (0.8–0.9)
Platelets (10^9/L [>150])	238 (220–256)	241 (216–258)
Urinary analysis		
- Proteinuria	0/8	0/5
- Hematuria	2/8	0/5
- Leucocyturia	2/8	0/5
- Presence of bacteria	0/8	0/5
Hypertension		
Hypertension at time of presentation	1/8	1/5

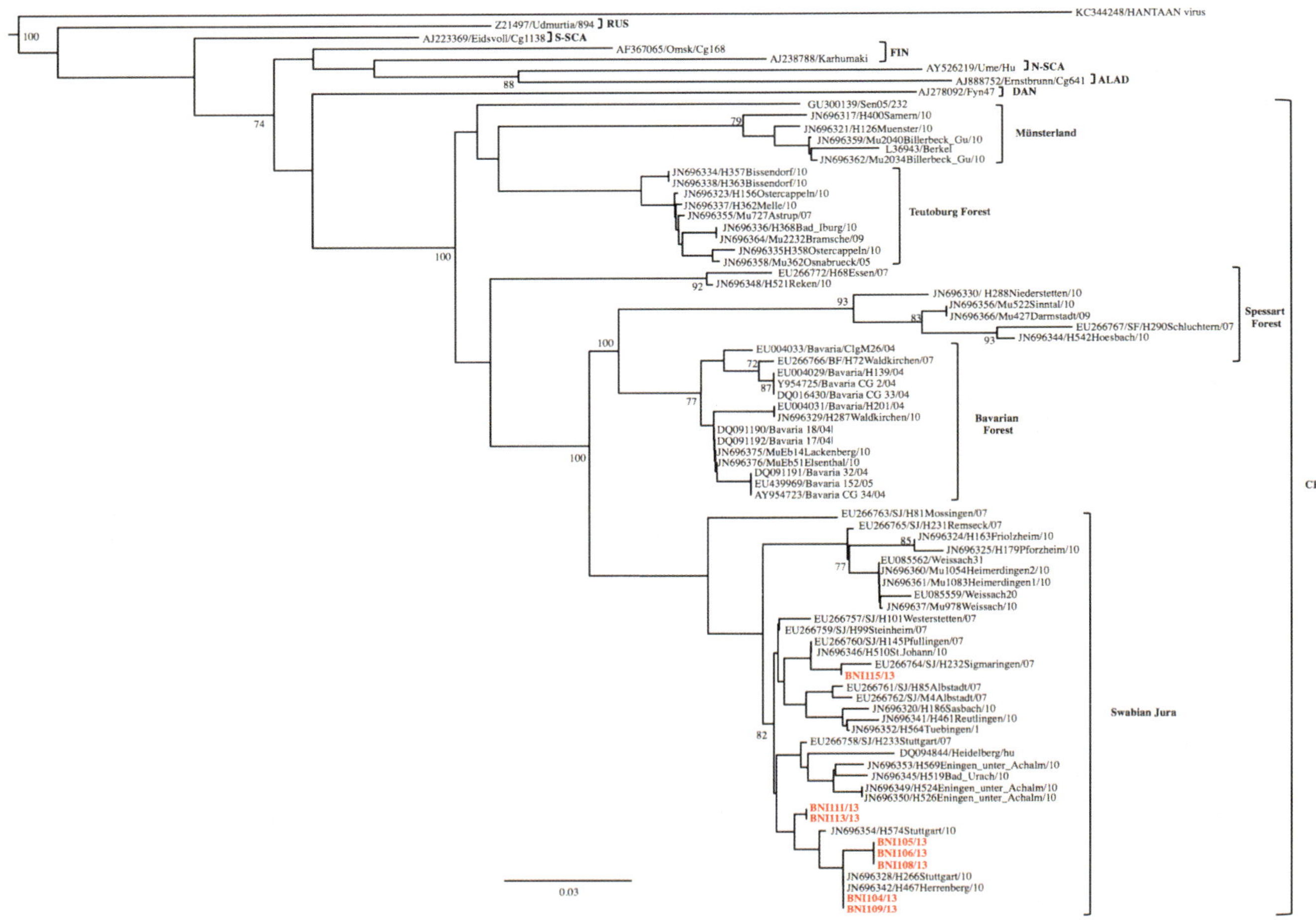

Figure 3. Maximum-likelihood phylogenetic tree of PUUV based on partial (144 bp) sequences of the small segment showing the placement of the PUUV strains from this study into the German subtypes. Bootstrap values >70%, calculated from 10,000 replicates are shown at the tree branches. For clarity, the Central European PUUMV clade include only German strains. Previously characterized PUUMV clades: **ALAD**, Alpe-Adrian; **CE**, Central European; **S-SCA**, South Scandinavian; **FIN**, Finnish; **RUS**, Russian; **N-SCA**, North Scandinavian; **DAN**, Dannish. The tree was rooted using murine-associated hantavirus: Hantaan virus (HNTV). Scale bar indicates mean number of nucleotide substitutions per site. GenBank accession numbers and the name of the strains are shown.

fact that the 2010 epidemic was associated with increased densities and infection rates of the bank voles in several regions of Germany and not determined by countrywide spread of the same PUUV strain [33]. In conclusion, we successfully developed a method to detect PUUV in FFPE tissues by RT-PCR and demonstrated its use as potential diagnostic tool as well as for PUUV molecular epidemiology investigations. Furthermore, it is possible to perform retrospective studies of archived materials from patients where PUUV was not the initial diagnosis.

This is the first study, which investigated biopsies of the human intestine in patients with NE using IHC and molecular approaches. PUUV nucleocapsid antigen and PUUV RNA were frequently detected. This finding might be an expression of a more generalized infection, which is emphasized by high rates of AKI in this study population. The presence of PUUV antigen was not correlated with the extension of abdominal complains. We suggest that a larger patient cohort should be analyzed in future studies to demonstrate possible significant differences and correlations.

Author Contributions

Conceived and designed the experiments: NB JL JSC DC. Performed the experiments: NB JL JSC DK MDA GO KTR PR DC. Analyzed the data: JL NB DK MDA JSC DC. Contributed reagents/materials/analysis tools: KTR PR GO DC. Wrote the paper: JL NB MDA DK JSC DC.

References

1. Schmaljohn CS, Dalrymple JM (1983) Analysis of Hantaan virus RNA: evidence for a new genus of bunyaviridae. Virology 131: 482–491.
2. Kruger DH, Schonrich G, Klempa B (2011) Human pathogenic hantaviruses and prevention of infection. Hum Vaccin 7: 685–693.
3. Lee HW, van der Groen G (1989) Hemorrhagic fever with renal syndrome. Prog Med Virol 36: 62–102.
4. Mertz GJ, Hjelle B, Crowley M, Iwamoto G, Tomicic V, et al. (2006) Diagnosis and treatment of new world hantavirus infections. Curr Opin Infect Dis 19: 437–442.

5. Peters CJ, Simpson GL, Levy H (1999) Spectrum of hantavirus infection: hemorrhagic fever with renal syndrome and hantavirus pulmonary syndrome. Annu Rev Med 50: 531–545.
6. Vapalahti O, Mustonen J, Lundkvist A, Henttonen H, Plyusnin A, et al. (2003) Hantavirus infections in Europe. Lancet Infect Dis 3: 653–661.
7. Kruger DH, Ulrich RG, Hofmann J (2013) Hantaviruses as zoonotic pathogens in Germany. Dtsch Arztebl Int 110: 461–467.
8. Hofmann J, Meisel H, Klempa B, Vesenbeckh SM, Beck R, et al. (2008) Hantavirus outbreak, Germany, 2007. Emerg Infect Dis 14: 850–852.
9. Heyman P, Thoma BR, Marie JL, Cochez C, Essbauer SS (2012) In Search for Factors that Drive Hantavirus Epidemics. Front Physiol 3: 237.
10. Mertens M, Wolfel R, Ullrich K, Yoshimatsu K, Blumhardt J, et al. (2009) Seroepidemiological study in a Puumala virus outbreak area in South-East Germany. Med Microbiol Immunol 198: 83–91.
11. Essbauer SS, Schmidt-Chanasit J, Madeja EL, Wegener W, Friedrich R, et al. (2007) Nephropathia epidemica in metropolitan area, Germany. Emerg Infect Dis 13: 1271–1273.
12. Krautkramer E, Zeier M, Plyusnin A (2013) Hantavirus infection: an emerging infectious disease causing acute renal failure. Kidney Int 83: 23–27.
13. Krautkramer E, Grouls S, Stein N, Reiser J, Zeier M (2011) Pathogenic old world hantaviruses infect renal glomerular and tubular cells and induce disassembling of cell-to-cell contacts. J Virol 85: 9811–9823.
14. Zeier M, Ritz E (1996) [Hantavirus-induced acute renal failure]. Internist (Berl) 37: 1092–1095.
15. Mustonen J, Helin H, Pietila K, Brummer-Korvenkontio M, Hedman K, et al. (1994) Renal biopsy findings and clinicopathologic correlations in nephropathia epidemica. Clin Nephrol 41: 121–126.
16. Groen J, Bruijn JA, Gerding MN, Jordans JG, Moll van Charante AW, et al. (1996) Hantavirus antigen detection in kidney biopsies from patients with nephropathia epidemica. Clin Nephrol 46: 379–383.
17. Muranyi W, Bahr U, Zeier M, van der Woude FJ (2005) Hantavirus infection. J Am Soc Nephrol 16: 3669–3679.
18. Hautala T, Sironen T, Vapalahti O, Paakko E, Sarkioja T, et al. (2002) Hypophyseal hemorrhage and panhypopituitarism during Puumala Virus Infection: Magnetic Resonance Imaging and detection of viral antigen in the hypophysis. Clin Infect Dis 35: 96–101.
19. Hung T, Zhou JY, Tang YM, Zhao TX, Baek LJ, et al. (1992) Identification of Hantaan virus-related structures in kidneys of cadavers with haemorrhagic fever with renal syndrome. Arch Virol 122: 187–199.
20. Kim S, Kang ET, Kim YG, Han JS, Lee JS, et al. (1993) Localization of Hantaan viral envelope glycoproteins by monoclonal antibodies in renal tissues from patients with Korean hemorrhagic fever H. Am J Clin Pathol 100: 398–403.
21. Temonen M, Mustonen J, Helin H, Pasternack A, Vaheri A, et al. (1996) Cytokines, adhesion molecules, and cellular infiltration in nephropathia epidemica kidneys: an immunohistochemical study. Clin Immunol Immunopathol 78: 47–55.
22. Nuutinen H, Vuoristo M, Farkkila M, Kahri A, Seppala K, et al. (1992) Hemorrhagic gastropathy in epidemic nephropathy. Gastrointest Endosc 38: 476–480.
23. Braun N, Haap M, Overkamp D, Kimmel M, Alscher MD, et al. (2010) Characterization and outcome following Puumala virus infection: a retrospective analysis of 75 cases. Nephrol Dial Transplant 25: 2997–3003.
24. Vaheri A, Strandin T, Hepojoki J, Sironen T, Henttonen H, et al. (2013) Uncovering the mysteries of hantavirus infections. Nat Rev Microbiol 11: 539–550.
25. Latus J, Fritzenkotter M, Schmidt-Chanasit J, Tenner-Racz K, Leibold T, et al. (2012) Hantavirus and acute appendicitis – the diagnosis behind the diagnosis? J Clin Virol 53: 156–158.
26. Bellomo R, Ronco C, Kellum JA, Mehta RL, Palevsky P (2004) Acute renal failure - definition, outcome measures, animal models, fluid therapy and information technology needs: the Second International Consensus Conference of the Acute Dialysis Quality Initiative (ADQI) Group. Crit Care 8: R204–212.
27. Pickering TG, Hall JE, Appel LJ, Falkner BE, Graves J, et al. (2005) Recommendations for blood pressure measurement in humans and experimental animals: Part 1: blood pressure measurement in humans: a statement for professionals from the Subcommittee of Professional and Public Education of the American Heart Association Council on High Blood Pressure Research. Hypertension 45: 142–161.
28. Chobanian AV, Bakris GL, Black HR, Cushman WC, Green LA, et al. (2003) The Seventh Report of the Joint National Committee on Prevention, Detection, Evaluation, and Treatment of High Blood Pressure: the JNC 7 report. JAMA 289: 2560–2572.
29. Zoller LG, Yang S, Gott P, Bautz EK, Darai G (1993) A novel mu-capture enzyme-linked immunosorbent assay based on recombinant proteins for sensitive and specific diagnosis of hemorrhagic fever with renal syndrome. J Clin Microbiol 31: 1194–1199.
30. Schwab SJ, Christensen RL, Dougherty K, Klahr S (1987) Quantitation of proteinuria by the use of protein-to-creatinine ratios in single urine samples. Arch Intern Med 147: 943–944.
31. Guindon S, Dufayard JF, Lefort V, Anisimova M, Hordijk W, et al. (2010) New algorithms and methods to estimate maximum-likelihood phylogenies: assessing the performance of PhyML 3.0. Syst Biol 59: 307–321.
32. Darriba D, Taboada GL, Doallo R, Posada D (2012) jModelTest 2: more models, new heuristics and parallel computing. Nat Methods 9: 772.
33. Ettinger J, Hofmann J, Enders M, Tewald F, Oehme RM, et al. (2012) Multiple synchronous outbreaks of Puumala virus, Germany, 2010. Emerg Infect Dis 18: 1461–1464.
34. Clement J, Maes P, van Ypersele de Strihou C, van der Groen G, Barrios JM, et al. (2010) Beechnuts and outbreaks of nephropathia epidemica (NE): of mast, mice and men. Nephrol Dial Transplant 25: 1740–1746.
35. Sironen T, Klingstrom J, Vaheri A, Andersson LC, Lundkvist A, et al. (2008) Pathology of Puumala hantavirus infection in macaques. PLoS One 3: e3035.
36. Maes P, Clement J, Gavrilovskaya I, Van Ranst M (2004) Hantaviruses: immunology, treatment, and prevention. Viral Immunol 17: 481–497.
37. Klempa B, Meisel H, Rath S, Bartel J, Ulrich R, et al. (2003) Occurrence of renal and pulmonary syndrome in a region of northeast Germany where Tula hantavirus circulates. J Clin Microbiol 41: 4894–4897.
38. Klempa B, Schutt M, Auste B, Labuda M, Ulrich R, et al. (2004) First molecular identification of human Dobrava virus infection in central Europe. J Clin Microbiol 42: 1322–1325.
39. Ulrich RG, Imholt C, Kruger DH, Krautkramer E, Scheibe T, et al. (2013) [Hantaviruses in Germany: threat for zoo, pet, companion and farm animals?]. Berl Munch Tierarztl Wochenschr 126: 514–526.

24

Smoking Is a Risk Factor for the Progression of Idiopathic Membranous Nephropathy

Makoto Yamaguchi[1], Masahiko Ando[2], Ryohei Yamamoto[3], Shinichi Akiyama[1], Sawako Kato[1], Takayuki Katsuno[1], Tomoki Kosugi[1], Waichi Sato[1], Naotake Tsuboi[1], Yoshinari Yasuda[1], Masashi Mizuno[1], Yasuhiko Ito[1], Seiichi Matsuo[1], Shoichi Maruyama[1]*

1 Department of Nephrology, Nagoya University Graduate School of Medicine, Nagoya, Japan, **2** Center for Advanced Medicine and Clinical Research, Nagoya University Hospital, Nagoya, Japan, **3** Department of Geriatric Medicine and Nephrology, Osaka University Graduate School of Medicine, Suita, Japan

Abstract

Background: Multiple studies have shown cigarette smoking to be a risk factor for chronic kidney disease. However, it is unknown whether smoking similarly increases the risk for progression of membranous nephropathy.

Methods: This study used the Nagoya Nephrotic Syndrome Cohort Study (N-NSCS), including 171 patients with idiopathic membranous nephropathy (IMN) from 10 nephrology centers in Japan. The dose-response relationships between cigarette smoking and the outcomes were assessed by using multivariate Cox proportional hazards models adjusted for clinically relevant factors. The primary outcome was a 30% decline in the estimated glomerular filtration rate (eGFR). The secondary outcome was first complete remission (CR) of proteinuria.

Results: During the observation period (median, 37 months; interquartile range, 16–71 months), 37 (21.6%) patients developed a 30% decline in eGFR and 2 (1.2%) progressed to ESRD. CR occurred in 103 (60.2%) patients. Multivariate Cox proportional hazards models revealed current smoking (adjusted hazard ratio [HR], 7.81 [95% confidence interval (CI), 3.17–19.7]), female sex (adjusted HR, 3.58 [95% CI, 1.87–8.00]), older age (adjusted HR, 1.71 [95% CI, 1.13–2.62] per 10 years), the number of cigarettes smoked daily (adjusted HR, 1.61 [95% CI, 1.23–2.09] per 10 cigarettes daily), and cumulative smoking of ≥40 pack-years (adjusted HR, 5.56 [95% CI, 2.17–14.6]) to be associated with a 30% decline in eGFR. However, smoking was not associated with CR.

Conclusion: Smoking is a significant and dose-dependent risk factor for IMN progression. All patients with IMN who smoke should be encouraged to quit.

Editor: Chris Bullen, The University of Auckland, New Zealand

Funding: This study was supported by a Grant-in-Aid for Progressive Renal Diseases Research, Research on Rare and Intractable Disease, from the Ministry of Health, Labour, and Welfare of Japan. The funders had no role in study design, data collection and analysis, decision to publish, or preparation of the manuscript.

* Email: marus@med.nagoya-u.ac.jp

Introduction

Membranous nephropathy (MN) is a very common cause of nephrotic syndrome in adults [1,2]. Spontaneous remission occurs in 30–50% of patients, whereas another 30–50% experience progressive renal failure [3,4]. Previously identified clinical predictors of poor renal survival include older age, male sex, elevated serum creatinine level at the time of diagnosis, and the severity of proteinuria at the time of disease onset and during follow-up [5–9]. However, most of these cannot be modified, and the long-term outcome is not unfavorable regardless: the 10-year renal survival ranges from 60 to 80% [10,11]. The optimal management strategy for MN remains unclear.

It has recently become apparent that cigarette smoking, in addition to promoting cardiovascular disease (CVD), is an important independent renal risk factor [12–21]. However, these studies included patients with heterogeneous causes of CKD, such as diabetes, nephrosclerosis, and other diseases. Therefore, it was uncertain whether all kidney diseases were equally exacerbated by cigarette smoking. Elisabeth et al. reported in a nationwide population-based case-control study that the relationship between cigarette smoking and kidney impairment varied with the underlying kidney disease [22].

Yamamoto et al. reported in a large-scale retrospective cohort study that cigarette smoking was a key, dose-dependent prognostic factor in patients with IgA nephropathy [23]. The link between smoking and nephrotic syndrome has been investigated in only one case-control study of 80 patients with MN [24]. Although that study showed no relationship between smoking and MN, it was limited by the omission of two potentially significant independent variables, baseline proteinuria and kidney function at the time of study entry.

This study aimed to determine whether a history of smoking is an independent risk factor for the progression of MN and whether such risk is dose-dependent. This multicenter observational cohort study was organized as part of the Nagoya Nephrotic Syndrome Cohort Study (N-NSCS) based at 10 major nephrology centers in Nagoya, Japan.

Subjects and Methods

Study Population and Data Source

This cohort study included patients aged >18 years who had been diagnosed with membranous nephropathy (MN) on the basis of kidney biopsy between January 2003 and December 2012 at Nagoya University, Chubu Rosai Hospital, Japanese Red Cross Nagoya Daiichi Hospital, Tsushima City Hospital, Kasugai Municipal Hospital, Nagoya Kyoritsu Hospital, Anjo Kosei Hospital, Ichinomiya Municipal Hospital, Handa City Hospital, or Tosei General Hospital. Of the 272 such patients, we excluded patients with conditions generally considered to cause secondary MN, such as exposure to drugs associated with MN, diabetes mellitus, systemic lupus erythematosus, malignancy, or any other systemic disease known to be associated with secondary MN [25].

After exclusion of an additional 7 (3.9%) patients with missing data related to smoking status, 171 (62.9%) patients with idiopathic membranous nephropathy (IMN) were enrolled and followed up until September 2013. Clinically relevant factors at the baseline of those excluded (n = 7) and enrolled (n = 171) were not significantly different.

Our study was conducted by using linkable anonymous data set. No informed consent was obtained. The study protocol and consent procedure were approved by the ethics committees of Nagoya University, Chubu Rosai Hospital, Japanese Red Cross Nagoya Daiichi Hospital, Tsushima City Hospital, Kasugai Municipal Hospital, Nagoya Kyoritsu Hospital, Anjo Kosei Hospital, Ichinomiya Municipal Hospital, Handa City Hospital, and Tosei General Hospital Approval number:2012–0268.

Data Collection

Data pertaining to the patients' clinical characteristics at baseline were collected retrospectively from their medical records. The time of kidney biopsy was used as the baseline if the patient had not received immunosuppressive therapy or had received immunosuppressive therapy only after kidney biopsy. In patients who had received immunosuppressive therapy before kidney biopsy, the time of the initiation of immunosuppressive treatment was used as the baseline. The clinical characteristics included age, sex, body mass index, systolic and diastolic blood pressure, serum total cholesterol level, serum creatinine level, glomerular filtration rate (GFR; estimated using the equation recently generated by the Japanese Society of Nephrology: eGFR [mL/min/1.73 m^2] $= 194 \times Scr^{-1.094} \times Age^{-0.287} \times 0.739$ [if female] [26]), serum albumin level, 24-hour urinary protein excretion or urinary protein-to-creatinine ratio, smoking status, use of any antihypertensive drugs, and initial use of corticosteroids and/or other immunosuppressive agents. Urinary protein excretion and eGFR data were collected from the medical record at each checkup in 1 to 3 month intervals.

We obtained detailed information about each patient's smoking status at the time of kidney biopsy, including the amount smoked (cigarettes/day), starting and stopping dates, and changes in use over time, from the medical records. The relationships between smoking and outcome measures were then studied for the following variables: (1) smoking status (all patients): never smoked, ex-smoker, or current smoker; (2) number of cigarettes smoked daily (current and ex-smokers); and (3) cumulative quantity smoked (current and ex-smokers): 0, 1–20, 21–39, or ≥40 pack-years (PY; 1 PY = 1 pack of 20 cigarettes/day ×1 year). Because we were most interested in whether a history of smoking was a risk factor for the progression of IMN, current smokers and ex-smokers were combined into a single group (current/ex-smokers).

The antihypertensive drugs used in this cohort were angiotensin-converting enzyme (ACE) inhibitors or angiotensin II receptor blockers (ARB), calcium channel blockers, β-blockers, and thiazides. The drugs used for therapeutic intervention, including the prescription of ACE inhibitors/ARB and corticosteroids or other immunosuppressive agents within 6 months of kidney biopsy, were also examined.

Nephrotic syndrome was defined as urinary protein excretion of ≥3.5 g/day (or a urinary protein/creatinine ratio of ≥3.5) and a serum albumin level of <3.0 mg/dL.

Complete remission (CR) of proteinuria was defined as urinary protein excretion of <0.3 g/day, a urinary protein/creatinine ratio of <0.3, and/or a negative/trace result for urinary protein on a dipstick test.

Partial remission (PR) of proteinuria was defined as urinary protein excretion of <3.5 g/day and a urinary protein/creatinine ratio of <3.5.

Relapse was defined as urinary protein excretion of ≥1.0 g/day, a urinary protein/creatinine ratio of ≥1.0, or a urinary protein dipstick result of ≥2+ on at least 2 occasions after achievement of CR.

The rate of decline in eGFR per year (mL/min per 1.73 m^2/year) was determined by plotting the eGFR against the observation time.

The anonymous data set is available in the Table S4.

Outcomes

The primary outcome was a 30% decline in eGFR before end-stage renal disease (ESRD). The secondary outcome was first CR.

The serum creatinine level was measured as required for each patient. Patients were followed up until September 2013 and censored at the time of death (if before ESRD or CR) or as of the last serum creatinine measurement before September 2013.

Statistical Analysis

Differences in clinical characteristics between those who had never smoked and current-/ex-smokers were compared by using the Wilcoxon rank-sum test or Fisher's exact test. To identify predictors independently associated with each outcome, potential covariates were examined by using the log-rank test and/or univariate and multivariate Cox proportional hazards models. The proportional hazards assumption for covariates was tested by using scaled Schoenfeld residuals. For continuous variables, the Wilcoxon rank-sum test was performed to assess the significance of inter-group differences. Categorical variables were expressed as percentages and compared by using Fisher's exact test. The rate of survival without a 30% decline in eGFR and the cumulative probability of achieving a first CR were calculated by using the Kaplan-Meier method and the log-rank test. The trend in each outcome with respect to the cumulative quantity smoked was examined statistically by scoring never smoking as 0 and current-/ex-smokers with 1–20, 21–39, and ≥40 pack-years' exposure as 1, 2, and 3, respectively; the resulting scores were then included in the regression model. The level of statistical significance was set at $P<0.05$. All statistical analyses were performed by using JMP version 10.0.0 (SAS Institute, Cary, NC, USA; www.jmp.com) and STATA version 13.0 (STATA Corp, www.stata.com).

Results

Study participants and clinical characteristics

The present study included 171 patients with IMN, of whom 108 (63.2%) had never smoked, 28 (16.4%) were ex-smokers, and 35 (20.5%) were current smokers. The clinical characteristics of the two groups (those who had never smoked and current/ex-smokers) are summarized in Table 1.

The two groups differed significantly in age, proportion of males, body mass index, urinary protein excretion, and rate of therapeutic intervention with an ACE inhibitor or ARB within 6 months of kidney biopsy. At baseline, 114 patients (66.7%) had nephrotic syndrome as previously defined. The median follow-up period of those who had never-smoked, ex-smokers, and current-smokers was 36 (15–71), 33 (16–63), and 46 (18–87) months, respectively ($P = 0.288$).

We obtained the number of cigarettes smoked daily for 62 (98.4%) of the current/ex-smokers (1–10 cigarettes for 10 [16.1%], 11–20 cigarettes for 32 [51.6%], 21–30 cigarettes for 9 [14.5%], and 31–50 cigarettes for 11 [17.7%] patients) and the cumulative smoking dose for 60 (95.2%) of the current-/ex-smokers (≤20 pack-years for 11 [18.3%], 21–39 pack-years for 15 [25.0%], and ≥40 pack-years for 34 [56.7%] patients).

Table 1. Clinical Characteristics of the 171 Patients with IMN.

	Never smoked	Smokers (Current/Ex-)	*P* value
Number	108	63 (35/28)	
Baseline characteristics			
Age (years)	66 (59–73)	63 (53–68)	0.012
Male [n (%)]	63 (58.3)	55 (87.3)	<0.001
Body mass index (kg/m^2)	22.9 (21.1–24.7)	23.5 (22.3–26.2)	0.046
Systolic blood pressure (mmHg)	130 (120–145)	132 (121–143)	0.873
Diastolic blood pressure (mmHg)	76 (70–84)	79 (72–86)	0.156
Serum creatinine (mg/dL)	0.78 (0.66–1.00)	0.80 (0.71–1.00)	0.171
eGFR (mL/min/1.73 m^2)	76 (58–92)	76 (63–86)	0.639
Serum albumin (g/dL)	2.6 (2.1–3.2)	2.4 (2.0–3.2)	0.518
Urinary protein (g/day)	3.9 (2.4–6.1)	4.8 (3.2–8.4)	0.025
Urinary protein >3.5 (g/day) [n (%)]	68 (63.0)	46 (73.0)	0.239
Total cholesterol (mg/dL)	283 (238–375)	295 (247–368)	0.617
Use of antihypertensive drugs [n (%)]	33 (30.6)	25 (39.7)	0.244
Smoking status			
Number of cigarettes smoked daily	NA	20 (20–30)	
Pack-years	NA	40 (24–49)	
Therapeutic interventions within 6 months after kidney biopsy			
ACE inhibitor or ARB therapy [n (%)]	65 (60.2)	48 (76.2)	0.044
Immunosuppressive treatment			0.413
No immunosuppressive agent	58 (53.7)	28 (44.4)	
Prednisolone [n (%)]	19 (17.6)	11 (17.5)	
Prednisolone + cyclosporine [n (%)]	31 (28.7)	24 (38.1)	
Outcomes			
30% reduction in eGFR [n (%)]	16 (14.8)	21 (33.3)	0.007
50% reduction in eGFR [n (%)]	6 (5.6)	11 (17.5)	0.017
Decline in eGFR (mL/min per 1.73 m^2 per year)	2.42 (−1.44 to 6.91)	4.01 (0.51–8.78)	0.046
ESRD [n (%)]	1 (0.9)	1 (1.6)	1.000
Death [n (%)]	8 (7.4)	3 (4.8)	0.748
Remission			
Complete remission [n (%)]	63 (58.3)	40 (63.5)	0.522
Partial remission [n (%)]	96 (88.9)	54 (85.7)	0.631
Relapse [n (%)]	14 (16.1)	12 (26.7)	0.170
Observation period (months)	36 (15–71)	39 (18–74)	0.375

Median (interquartile range), Conversion factors for units: SCr in mg/dL to μmol/L, ×88.4; eGFR (mL/min/1.73 m^2) = $194 \times Scr^{-1.094} \times Age^{-0.287} \times 0.739$ (if female), total cholesterol in mg/dL to mmol/L, ×0.02586.

Abbreviations: IMN, idiopathic membranous nephropathy; eGFR, estimated glomerular filtration rate; ACE inhibitor/ARB, angiotensin-converting enzyme inhibitor/angiotensin receptor blocker; SCr, serum creatinine; ESRD, end-stage renal disease; NA, not applicable.

Treatment during the observation period

An ACE inhibitor or ARB was newly prescribed within 6 months of kidney biopsy in 113 (66.1%) patients and was used by 156 (91.2%) by the end of follow-up. The enrolled patients were divided according to the treatment within 6 months of kidney biopsy into three groups: (1) the prednisolone group, comprising 30 patients (17.5%) who received prednisolone alone; (2) the cyclosporine group, comprising 55 patients (32.1%) who received prednisolone and cyclosporine; and (3) the supportive therapy group, comprising 86 patients (50.3%) who received neither prednisolone nor other immunosuppressive drugs. One patient in the cyclosporine group (0.6%) also received mizoribine. Most of the patients in the prednisolone group were prescribed prednisolone starting at 0.8–1.0 mg/kg/day orally and tapered according to the response to therapy, whereas most in the cyclosporine group started with cyclosporine at 1 to 2 mg/kg and prednisolone at 0.4–0.6 mg/kg. The cyclosporine dosage was adjusted to achieve the target whole-blood trough level, and the prednisolone dose was tapered according to the response to therapy. The time from renal biopsy to the initiation of immunosuppressive therapy was 0.7 months (interquartile range, 0.3–3.3 months). The duration of prednisolone use was 11 months (interquartile range, 8–25 months) in the prednisolone group and 14 months (interquartile range, 9–17 months) in the cyclosporine group.

Outcome data

The median observation time for the entire cohort was 37 months (interquartile range, 15–72 months). In total, 37 (21.6%) patients developed a 30% decline in eGFR before ESRD, 17 (9.9%) developed a 50% decline in eGFR before ESRD, and 2 (1.2%) progressed to ESRD.

The rates of avoiding a 30% decline in eGFR for 1, 5, and 10 years were 0.82 (95% confidence interval [CI], 0.71–0.90), 0.61 (95% CI, 0.46–0.74), and 0.56 (95% CI, 0.40–0.71), respectively, in current-/ex-smokers and 0.93 (95% CI, 0.86–0.97), 0.80 (95% CI, 0.69–0.88), and 0.74 (95% CI, 0.57–0.86) in those who had never smoked; therefore, current/ex-smokers were at higher risk for developing a 30% decline in eGFR ($P=0.012$; Fig. 1).

The eGFR decreased significantly faster in current/ex-smokers than in those who had never smoked (4.01 mL/min per 1.73 m^2 per year [interquartile range, 0.51–8.78 mL/min per 1.73 m^2 per year] versus 2.42 mL/min per 1.73 m^2 per year [interquartile range, −1.44 to 6.91 mL/min per 1.73 m^2 per year]).

The eGFR did not improve by the last follow-up visit in any of the 37 patients who experienced a 30% decline in eGFR.

Meanwhile, 103 (60.2%) patients achieved CR of proteinuria after a median follow-up of 14 months (interquartile range, 6–25 months). The cumulative probabilities of achieving CR within 1, 5, and 10 years were 0.31 (95% CI, 0.20–0.44), 0.77 (95% CI, 0.62–0.87), and 0.81 (95% CI, 0.65–0.90) in current-/ex-smokers and 0.43 (95% CI, 0.33–0.54), 0.80 (95% CI, 0.67–0.88), and 0.81 (95% CI, 0.65–0.92) in those who had never smoked. Therefore, smoking was not associated with the achievement of CR ($P=0.570$).

Among the patients who achieved a first remission, 26 (25.2%) relapsed at least once.

No patient progressed to ESRD before developing a 30% decline in eGFR.

Eleven (6.4%) patients died during follow-up, one due to infection, and one each to acute subdural hematoma, traffic accident, sudden death, and intestinal bleeding. Malignancy occurred in 5 (2.9%) patients; the diagnoses were esophageal cancer, stomach cancer, colon cancer, prostate cancer, and malignant lymphoma in one patient each.

Predictors of a 30% decline in eGFR

Univariate Cox proportional hazards models revealed that older age, female sex, initial use of cyclosporine combination therapy, and current smoking were significantly associated with the primary outcome (Table 2). Adjustment for clinically relevant factors revealed current smoking (adjusted hazard ratio [HR], 7.81 [95% CI, 3.17–19.7], $P<0.001$), female sex (adjusted HR, 3.58 [95% CI, 1.87–8.00], $P=0.002$), older age (adjusted HR, 1.71 [95% CI, 1.13–2.62], per 10 years, $P=0.010$), and use of cyclosporine in combination with prednisolone (adjusted HR, 2.67 [95% CI, 1.08–6.59], $P=0.034$) to be significant predictors of the primary outcome.

No interactive effect on the primary outcome was detected between use of cyclosporine and smoking (adjusted HR, 1.16 [95% CI, 0.61–2.24], $P=0.644$).

To confirm the robustness of our results, we similarly assessed predictors of a 50% decline in eGFR and found that current smoking (adjusted HR, 9.85 [95% CI, 2.68–41.0], $P<0.001$) and female sex (adjusted HR, 4.20 [95% CI, 1.19–15.3], $P=0.027$) were also significant predictors of this outcome (Table S1).

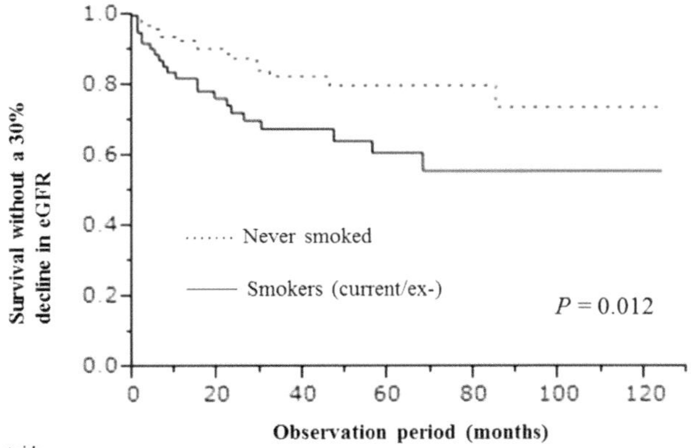

Number at risk							
Current/ex-smokers	63	40	24	17	10	6	2
Never smoked	108	67	41	29	16	8	3

Figure 1. Time to 30% decline in eGFR in current/ex-smokers and those who never smoked.

Table 2. Predictors of a 30% decline in eGFR.

	Univariate model		Multivariate model	
	HR (95% CI)	***P* value**	**HR (95% CI)**	***P* value**
Age (per 10 years)	1.47 (1.07–2.07)	0.018	1.71 (1.13–2.62)	0.010
Male (versus female)	0.43 (0.22–0.83)	0.012	0.28 (0.13–0.63)	0.002
Systolic blood pressure (per 10 mmHg)	1.06 (0.90–1.23)	0.455	1.07 (0.86–1.32)	0.546
Diastolic blood pressure (per 10 mmHg)	1.20 (0.94–1.53)	0.142	1.08 (0.77–1.52)	0.660
Serum albumin (per 1.0 g/dL)	0.80 (0.51–1.24)	0.317	1.32 (0.73–2.36)	0.359
Serum creatinine (per 1.0 mg/dL)	0.67 (0.18–1.98)	0.501	0.90 (0.19–3.13)	0.885
Urinary protein excretion (per 1.0 g/day)	1.03 (0.94–1.12)	0.519	1.02 (0.91–1.13)	0.673
Therapeutic interventions within 6 months after kidney biopsy				
ACE inhibitor or ARB therapy	0.72 (0.26–2.99)	0.598	0.90 (0.29–3.96)	0.874
Immunosuppressive treatment				
No immunosuppressive agent	Reference		Reference	
Prednisolone	0.84 (0.24–2.33)	0.758	1.30 (0.33–4.21)	0.687
Prednisolone + cyclosporine	2.18 (1.09–4.42)	0.027	2.67 (1.08–6.59)	0.034
Smokers (Current/Ex-)	2.24 (1.17–4.35)	0.015	4.00 (1.87–8.79)	<0.001
Ex-smokers	1.68 (0.64–3.93)	0.273	2.23 (0.79–5.79)	0.127
Current smokers	2.68 (1.29–5.52)	0.009	7.81 (3.17–19.7)	<0.001

HR, hazard ratio; CI, confidence interval.
Data are the HR, 95% CI, and *P* value from Cox proportional hazard regression analyses.
"Never smoked" was used as the reference category.
Adjusted for baseline characteristics (age, sex, systolic/diastolic pressure, serum creatinine level, urinary protein, use of ACE inhibitor or ARB within 6 months after kidney biopsy, and immunosuppressive therapy within 6 months after kidney biopsy).
Abbreviations: IMN, idiopathic membranous nephropathy; ACE, angiotensin-converting enzyme; ARB, angiotensin receptor blocker.

Dose-dependent association between smoking and a 30% decline in eGFR

Table 3 shows that the total smoking dose had a strong independent effect on the risk of renal progression. Both univariate and multivariate Cox proportional hazards models showed a significant association between the number of cigarettes per day and the primary outcome (adjusted HR, 1.61 [95% CI, 1.23–2.09], $P<0.001$, multivariate model 1). Cumulative smoking of ≥ 40 pack-years was also significantly associated with the primary outcome (adjusted HR, 5.56 [95% CI, 2.17–14.6], $P<0.001$, multivariate model 2). These results suggested that the risk of renal progression increased almost linearly with the number of cigarettes smoked.

Predictors of first complete remission

Univariate Cox proportional hazards models revealed a lower serum creatinine level, initial use of prednisolone monotherapy, and initial use of cyclosporine in combination with prednisolone to be significantly associated with first CR of proteinuria (Table S2). After adjustment for clinically relevant factors, the initial use of prednisolone monotherapy (adjusted HR, 2.15 [95% CI, 1.17–3.84], $P=0.015$) and cyclosporine in combination with prednisolone (adjusted HR, 2.90 [95% CI, 1.68–5.00], $P<0.001$) remained significant predictors of first CR of proteinuria. Neither a history of smoking (Table S2) nor the total smoking dose (Table S3) was associated with CR.

Discussion

We found that smoking increased the risk of renal dysfunction in Japanese patients with IMN in a dose-dependent manner, although former smoking did not appear to be a risk factor. These results highlight the clinical importance of smoking cessation in the treatment of patients with IMN.

Several cohort studies in the general population have suggested a dose-dependent association between smoking and CKD. The Cardiovascular Health Study identified smoking as a risk factor related to CKD progression in 4142 U.S. participants aged >65 years but did not include proteinuria as an independent variable [12]. The NHANRS II study followed 9082 middle-aged (49.3±13.3 years) U.S. participants for 13.2 years and showed a higher adjusted risk of end-stage kidney disease among those smoking >20 cigarettes per day. Baggio et al. studied 2981 elderly subjects from Italy and found smoking ≥21 cigarettes per day to be a very strong risk factor for pathological loss of kidney function [17]. Furthermore, the HUNT II study of 65,589 Norwegian participants revealed that the risk increased significantly as the cumulative amount of smoking (pack-years) increased; however, the risk significantly decreased as the years elapsed since smoking cessation increased among male ex-smokers aged <70 years [27]. Yamagata reported in a 10-year follow-up study of 123,764 Japanese participants aged ≥40 years who received community-based annual examinations that current smoking increased the risk of developing proteinuria, but that study did not evaluate the dose-dependency of the relationship between smoking and CKD [21]. These reports collectively identify smoking as a risk factor for the progression of CKD in the general population. Our present results were consistent with this literature, particularly the HUNT II study, in which current/ex-smokers reporting larger cumulative numbers of cigarettes smoked were at significantly higher risk of renal progression than were those who had never smoked.

Table 3. Influence of smoking dose on the risk of a 30% decline in eGFR.

	Univariate model		Multivariate model	
	HR (95% CI)	***P* value**	**HR (95% CI)**	***P* value**
Model 1				
No. of cigarettes (/10/d)	1.32 (1.05–1.63)	0.021	1.61 (1.23–2.09)	<0.001
Model 2				
1–20 pack-years	1.07 (0.17–3.75)	0.933	1.36 (0.20–5.94)	0.715
21–39 pack-years	1.64 (0.47–4.49)	0.399	3.51 (0.87–12.5)	0.076
≥40 pack-years	2.61 (1.21–5.48)	0.016	5.56 (2.17–14.6)	<0.001
Test for trend		0.015		<0.001

HR, hazard ratio; CI, confidence interval.
Data are the HR, 95% CI, and *P* value from Cox proportional hazard regression analyses.
"Never smoked" was used as the reference category. Models 1 and 2 are based on data from 168 patients because the number of cigarettes was missing for 1 current and 2 ex-smokers. Adjusted for baseline characteristics (age, sex, systolic/diastolic pressure, serum creatinine level, urinary protein, use of angiotensin-converting enzyme inhibitor or angiotensin receptor blocker within 6 months after kidney biopsy, and immunosuppressive therapy within 6 months after kidney biopsy).

Only a few studies of primary kidney disease have found a dose-dependent association between cigarette smoking and progression of primary glomerulonephritis. Yamamoto et al. identified cigarette smoking as a key dose-dependent prognostic factor for IgA nephropathy in a multivariate model. There has been only one case-control study addressing the relationship between smoking and nephrotic syndrome, which revealed no relationship between smoking and kidney progression in patients with MN [24]. However, that study failed to include baseline proteinuria and kidney function at study entry as independent variables. In contrast, we included those variables and identified smoking as an important dose-dependent prognostic factor in patients with IMN after adjustment for relevant confounders.

The present study identified immunosuppressive therapy as both a risk factor for renal progression (although urinary protein excretion was greater in such patients than in those who initially received supportive therapy) and the most significant independent predictor of achievement of CR. These results may, however, reflect indication bias, for which the present retrospective cohort study did not control. Furthermore, we should consider that unmeasured factors associated with treatment may not be included in the model.

Combination therapy with cyclosporine and prednisolone was frequently used for treatment of IMN in our cohort. Cattran et al. demonstrated that cyclosporine significantly decreased the rate of renal progression and reduced proteinuria in patients with IMN at high risk for progression and persistent nephrotic-range proteinuria [28,29]. Alexopoulos et al. also found that cyclosporine with or without corticosteroids effectively induced remission in the majority of nephrotic patients with IMN and well-preserved renal function [30]. Based on these findings, we often use cyclosporine in combination with corticosteroids for first-line treatment of patients with IMN. Although the 2012 Kidney Disease Improving Global Outcomes (KDIGO) clinical practice guideline for IMN recommends a cytotoxic agent (cyclophosphamide) for patients at high risk of progression [31], no patient in our study was treated with cyclophosphamide. This should be considered when interpreting our results.

Interestingly, our study identified female sex as an independent risk factor after adjustment for relevant clinical factors. Previous studies had shown male sex to be associated with a higher risk of developing ESRD [5–9]. In contrast, female sex has generally been associated with a relatively benign course [32]. However, these studies did not include smoking status as an independent variable, which may have caused overestimation of the relationship between male sex and risk of renal progression. Furthermore, Mina Yu reported in a cross-sectional study that menopause was an independent risk factor for CKD because of the accompanying loss of possibly cardioprotective estradiol production [33]. Previous studies of membranous nephropathy have generally enrolled younger patients than our study, suggesting that our study may have included a relatively large number of postmenopausal patients. Therefore, membranous nephropathy may lead to more rapid decline in GFR in postmenopausal women, who are already in an unfavorable hormonal state (i.e., estrogen deficient) with respect to the kidney. The generalizability of our results should be confirmed in another cohort study.

Although the exact mechanisms of the nephrotoxic effects of smoking are poorly understood, we can present some potential explanations of the relationship between smoking and CKD onset and progression. First, nephrotic syndrome increases oxidative stress by impairing antioxidant pathways [34]. The addition of smoking-induced oxidative stress to nephrotic syndrome-associated oxidative stress may accelerate renal progression [35–38]. Second, ex vivo studies have suggested that nicotine could promote mesangial cell proliferation and increase production of critical molecules involved in extracellular matrix production [39,40]. Third, smoking (or nicotine) could increase the plasma endothelin level [41], which has been shown to correlate with effective renal plasma flow in smokers [42]. Furthermore, Alves et al. reported that smoking aggravates the cyclosporine-induced impairment of GFR and that smoking in combination with cyclosporine induced periglomerular structural lesions and oxidative stress in a rat model of cyclosporine nephrotoxicity [43]. However, our results showed no interactive effect on renal function between use of cyclosporine and smoking. The external validity of the result should be confirmed in another study.

It is also possible that smoking might relate to medication adherence in some other way. A cross-sectional study showed that current smokers were less compliant with medication use than nonsmokers [44]. Therefore, we should consider the possibility of medication adherence in smokers. Moreover, we are aware that MN can itself have extra-renal associations and these should be considered for their possible relationship with smoking.

Our study has some limitations that must be discussed. First, underreporting of smoking and changes in smoking habits during the follow-up period can cause misclassification and tend to overestimate the effect of smoking on renal progression. Second, we did not address the relationship between smoking cessation and renal progression because our sample size was insufficient to evaluate it. Third, the patients in this study may not be representative of patients with IMN in other countries: different consequences of smoking have been reported in different populations [45]. We therefore advise caution when interpreting and generalizing our results.

Allowing for these methodological issues, our study has several advantages: it is one of the largest multicenter adult MN cohorts in Japan ever reported and is also, to the best of our knowledge, the first description of a relationship between smoking and renal dysfunction in patients with IMN.

In conclusion, our retrospective cohort study in patients with IMN showed cigarette smoking to be a key, dose-dependent predictor of IMN progression. All patients with IMN who smoke should be encouraged to quit.

Supporting Information

Table S1 Predictors of a 50% decline in eGFR.

Table S2 Predictors of first CR.

Table S3 Influence of smoking dose on first CR.

Table S4 The anonymous data set of 171 patients with IMN.

Acknowledgments

We are grateful for the time and efforts of the nephrologists who supported the present study: Dr. Shizunori Ichida, Dr. Hideaki Shimizu, Dr. Junichiro Yamamoto, Dr. Tomohiko Naruse, Dr. Hirofumi Tamai, Dr. Kei Kurata, Dr. Hirotake Kasuga, Dr. Arimasa Shirasaki, and Dr. Makoto Mizutani.

Author Contributions

Conceived and designed the experiments: MY MA SK S. Maruyama. Performed the experiments: MY MA RY SA SK T. Katsuno T. Kosugi WS NT YY MM YI S. Matsuo S. Maruyama. Analyzed the data: MY MA RY. Contributed reagents/materials/analysis tools: MY MA RY SK S. Maruyama. Contributed to the writing of the manuscript: MY MA S. Maruyama. Critically revised manuscript: MY MA S. Maruyama.

References

1. Fervenza FC, Sethi S, Specks U (2008) Idiopathic membranous nephropathy: diagnosis and treatment. Clin J Am Soc Nephrol 3: 905–919.
2. Cattran DC (2001) Idiopathic membranous nephropathy. Kidney Int 59: 1983–1994.
3. van den Brand JAJG, Hofstra JM, Wetzels JFM (2011) Low-molecular-weight proteins as prognostic markers in idiopathic membranous nephropathy. Clin J Am Soc Nephrol 6: 2846–2853.
4. du Buf-Vereijken PW, Branten AJ, Wetzels JF (2005) Idiopathic membranous nephropathy: outline and rationale of a treatment strategy. Am J Kidney Dis 46: 1012–1029.
5. Shiiki H, Saito T, Nishitani Y, Mitarai T, Research Group on Progressive Renal Diseases in Japan, et al. (2004) Prognosis and risk factors for idiopathic membranous nephropathy with nephrotic syndrome in Japan. Kidney Int 65: 1400–1407.
6. Marx BE, Marx M (1999) Prediction in idiopathic membranous nephropathy. Kidney Int 56: 666–673.
7. Troyanov S, Wall CA, Miller JA, Scholey JW, Cattran DC (2004) Idiopathic membranous nephropathy: definition and relevance of a partial remission. Kidney Int 66: 1199–1205.
8. Cattran DC, Pei Y, Greenwood CM, Ponticelli C, Passerini P, et al. (1997) Validation of a predictive model of idiopathic membranous nephropathy: its clinical and research implications. Kidney Int 51: 901–907.
9. Pei Y, Cattran D, Greenwood C (1992) Predicting chronic renal insufficiency in idiopathic membranous glomerulonephritis. Kidney Int 42: 960–966.
10. Noel LH, Zanetti M, Droz D, Barbanel C (1979) Long-term prognosis of idiopathic membranous glomerulonephritis. Study of 116 untreated patients. Am J Med 66: 82–90.
11. Zucchelli P, Ponticelli C, Cagnoli L, Passerini P (1987) Long-term outcome of idiopathic membranous nephropathy with nephrotic syndrome. Nephrol Dial Transplant 2: 73–78.
12. Bleyer AJ, Shemanski LR, Burke GL, Hansen KJ, Appel RG (2000) Tobacco, hypertension, and vascular disease: risk factors for renal functional decline in an older population. Kidney Int 57(5): 2072–2079.
13. Tozawa M, Iseki K, Iseki C, Oshiro S, Ikemiya Y, et al. (2002) Influence of smoking and obesity on the development of proteinuria. Kidney Int 62: 956–962.
14. Haroun MK, Jaar BG, Hoffman SC, Comstock GW, Klag MJ, et al. (2003) Risk factors for chronic kidney disease: a prospective study of 23,534 men and women in Washington County, Maryland. J Am Soc Nephrol 14(11): 2934–2941.
15. Stengel B, Tarver-Carr ME, Powe NR, Eberhardt MS, Brancati FL (2003) Lifestyle factors, obesity and the risk of chronic kidney disease. Epidemiology 14(4): 479–487.
16. Fox CS, Larson MG, Leip EP, Culleton B, Wilson PW, et al. (2004) Predictors of new-onset kidney disease in a community-based population. JAMA 29(7): 844–850.
17. Baggio B, Budakovic A, Perissinotto E, Maggi S, Cantaro S, et al (2005) Atherosclerotic risk factors and renal function in the elderly: the role of hyperfibrinogenaemia and smoking. Results from the Italian Longitudinal Study on Ageing (ILSA). Nephrol Dial Transplant 20(1): 114–123.
18. Hallan S, de Mutsert R, Carlsen S, Dekker FW, Aasarod K, et al. (2006) Obesity, smoking, and physical inactivity as risk factors for CKD: are men more vulnerable? Am J Kidney Dis 47(3): 396–405.
19. Ishani A, Grandits GA, Grimm RH, Svendsen KH, Collins AJ, et al. (2006) Association of single measurements of dipstick proteinuria, estimated glomerular filtration rate, and hematocrit with 25-year incidence of end-stage renal disease in the multiple risk factor intervention trial. J Am Soc Nephrol 17(5): 1444–1452.
20. Shankar A, Klein R, Klein BE (2006) The association among smoking, heavy drinking, and chronic kidney disease. Am J Epidemiol 164(3): 263–271.
21. Yamagata K, Ishida K, Sairenchi T, Takahashi H, Ohba S, et al. (2007) Risk factors for chronic kidney disease in a community-based population: a 10-year follow-up study. Kidney Int 71(2): 159–166.
22. Ejerblad E, Fored CM, Lindblad P, Fryzek J, Dickman PW, et al. (2004) Association between smoking and chronic renal failure in a nationwide population-based case-control study. J Am Soc Nephrol 15(8): 2178–2185.
23. Yamamoto R, Nagasawa Y, Shoji T, Iwatani H, Hamano T, et al. (2010) Cigarette smoking and progression of IgA nephropathy. Am J Kidney Dis 56(2): 313–324.
24. Stengel B, Couchoud C, Cénée S, Hémon D (2000) Age, blood pressure and smoking effects on chronic renal failure in primary glomerular nephropathies. Kidney Int 57(6): 2519–2526.
25. Hofstra JM, Wetzels JF (2012) Management of patients with membranous nephropathy. Nephrol Dial Transplant 27: 6–9.
26. Matsuo S, Imai E, Horio M, Yasuda Y, Tomita K, et al. (2009) Collaborators developing the Japanese equation for estimated GFR. Revised equations for estimated GFR from serum creatinine in Japan. Am J Kidney Dis 53: 982–992.
27. Hallan SI, Orth SR (2011) Smoking is a risk factor in the progression to kidney failure. Kidney Int 80: 516–523.
28. Cattran DC, Appel GB, Hebert LA, Hunsicker LG, Pohl MA, et al; North America Nephrotic Syndrome Study Group (2001) Cyclosporine in patients with steroid-resistant membranous nephropathy: a randomized trial. Kidney Int 59: 1484–1490.
29. Cattran DC, Greenwood C, Ritchie S, Bernstein K, Churchill DN, et al. (1995) A controlled trial of cyclosporine in patients with progressive membranous nephropathy. Canadian Glomerulonephritis Study Group. Kidney Int 47: 1130–1135.
30. Alexopoulos E, Papagianni A, Tsamelashvili M, Leontsini M, Memmos D (2006) Induction and long-term treatment with cyclosporine in membranous nephropathy with the nephrotic syndrome. Nephrol Dial Transplant 21: 3127–3132.
31. KDIGO Working Group (2012) KDIGO clinical practice guideline for glomerulonephritis. Kidney Int Suppl 2: 186–197.
32. Reichert LJ, Koene RA, Wetzels JF (1998) Prognostic factors in idiopathic membranous nephropathy. Am J Kidney Dis 31(1): 1–11.
33. Yu M, Ryu D-R, Kim S-J, Choi K-B, Kang D-H (2010) Clinical implication of metabolic syndrome on chronic kidney disease depends on gender and

menopausal status: results from the Korean National Health and Nutrition Examination Survey. Nephrol Dial Transplant 25: 469–477.
34. Soyoral YU, Aslan M, Emre H, Begenik H, Erdur FM, et al. (2011) Serum paraoxonase activity and oxidative stress in patients with adult nephrotic syndrome. Atherosclerosis 218(1): 243–246.
35. Nagasawa Y, Yamamoto R, Rakugi H, Isaka Y (2012) Cigarette smoking and chronic kidney diseases. Hypertens Res 35(3): 261–265.
36. Amaral S, Oliveira PJ, Ramalho-Santos J (2008) Diabetes and the impairment of reproductive function: possible role of mitochondria and reactive oxygen species. Curr Diabetes Rev 4(1): 46–54.
37. Maiese K, Chong ZZ, Shang YC (2007) Mechanistic insights into diabetes mellitus and oxidative stress. Curr Med Chem 14(16): 1729–1738.
38. Fatehi-Hassanabad Z, Chan CB, Furman BL (2010) Reactive oxygen species and endothelial function in diabetes. Eur J Pharmacol 636(1–3): 8–17.
39. Hua P, Feng W, Ji S, Raij L, Jaimes EA (2010) Nicotine worsens the severity of nephropathy in diabetic mice: implications for the progression of kidney disease in smokers. Am J Physiol Renal Physiol 299: F732–F739.
40. Jaimes EA, Tian RX, Raij L (2007) Nicotine: the link between cigarette smoking and the progression of renal injury? Am J Physiol Heart Circ Physiol 292: H76–H82.
41. Haak T, Jungmann E, Raab C, Usadel KH (1994) Elevated endothelin-1 levels after cigarette smoking. Metabolism 43(3): 267–269.
42. Gambaro G, Verlato F, Budakovic A (1998) Renal impairment in chronic cigarette smokers. J Am Soc Nephrol 9(4): 562–567.
43. Alves SA, Carlos CP, Mendes GEF, Oliveira SM, Luz MAM, et al. (2012) Previous exposure to cigarette smoke aggravates experimental cyclosporine-induced nephrotoxicity. Am J Nephrol 36: 334–341.
44. Sherman BW, Lynch WD (2014) The association of smoking with medical treatment adherence in the workforce of a large employer. Patient Prefer Adherence.8:477–486.
45. Sellers EM (1998) Pharmacogenetics and ethnoracial differences in smoking. JAMA 280: 179–180.

25

Mesangial Cell-Binding Activity of Serum Immunoglobulin G in Patients with Lupus Nephritis

Desmond Y. H. Yap, Susan Yung, Qing Zhang, Colin Tang, Tak Mao Chan*

Division of Nephrology, Department of Medicine, Queen Mary Hospital, The University of Hong Kong, Hong Kong

Abstract

In vitro data showed that immunoglobulin G (IgG) from patients with lupus nephritis (LN) could bind to cultured human mesangial cells (HMC). The clinical relevance of such binding was unknown. Binding of IgG and subclasses was measured in 189 serial serum samples from 23 patients with Class III/IV±V LN (48 during renal flares, 141 during low level disease activity (LLDA)). 64 patients with non-lupus glomerular diseases (NLGD) and 23 healthy individuals were used as controls. HMC-binding was measured with cellular ELISA and expressed as OD index. HMC-binding index of total IgG was 0.12±0.09, 0.36±0.25, 0.59±0.37 and 0.74±0.42 in healthy subjects, NLGD, LN patients during LLDA, and LN flares respectively ($P=0.046$, LN flare vs. LLDA; $P<0.001$, for healthy controls or NLGD vs. LN during flare or LLDA). Binding of serum IgG_1 to HMC was 0.05±0.05, 0.15±0.11, 0.41±0.38 and 0.55±0.40 for the corresponding groups respectively ($P=0.007$, LN flare vs. remission; $P<0.001$, for healthy controls or NLGD vs. LN during flare or remission). IgG_2, IgG_3 and IgG_4 from patients and controls did not show significant binding to HMC. Total IgG and IgG_1 HMC-binding index correlated with anti-dsDNA level ($r=0.26$ and 0.39 respectively, $P<0.001$ for both), and inversely with C3 ($r=-0.17$ and -0.45, $P<0.05$ for both). Sensitivity/specificity of total IgG or IgG_1 binding to HMC in predicting renal flares were 81.3%/39.7% (ROC AUC 0.61, $P=0.03$) and 83.8%/41.8% (AUC 0.63, $P=0.009$) respectively. HMC-binding by IgG_1, but not total IgG, correlated with mesangial immune deposition in LN renal biopsies under electron microscopy. Our results showed that binding of serum total IgG and IgG_1 in LN patients correlates with disease activity. The correlation between IgG_1 HMC-binding and mesangial immune deposition suggests a potential pathogenic significance.

Editor: Irun R. Cohen, Weizmann Institute of Science, Israel

Funding: This project was supported by the Hong Kong Society of Nephrology Research Grant 2009 awarded to Desmond Y. H. YAP and the endowment fund of the Yu Chiu Kwong Professorship in Medicine at University of Hong Kong awarded to T. M. Chan. S. Yung is supported by the Wai Hung Charitable Foundation. The funders had no role in study design, data collection and analysis, decision to publish, or preparation of the manuscript.

* Email: dtmchan@hku.hk

Introduction

Lupus nephritis (LN) is a severe manifestation in patients with systemic lupus erythematosus (SLE), and is an important cause of renal failure in some racial groups such as Asians [1,2]. The treatments to date are based on non-selective immunosuppression. The pathogenic mechanisms are multifactorial and complex, but increased understanding of the pathogenic mechanisms could lead to improvements in disease activity monitoring and treatment. SLE is a prototype autoimmune disease and is characterized by the production of different autoantibodies, resulting in immune-mediated injury to various organs including the kidneys [3,4]. The pathogenic importance of anti-dsDNA antibodies is exemplified by in vitro studies demonstrating their presence in renal eluates obtained from patients and mice with LN [5–7], and by clinical observations demonstrating a correlation between anti-dsDNA antibody titre and disease activity [8].

Mesangial cells have a central location in the glomerulus. Not only do mesangial cells provide structural support to adjacent capillary loops but it is well established that they also participate actively in disease mechanisms through the production of inflammatory and fibrotic growth factors [9,10]. Immunoglobulin deposition in the mesangial area, mesangial cell proliferation, and increase in mesangial matrix are constant features in renal biopsies of active LN [3,11]. Our group has previously reported that anti-dsDNA isolated from patients with LN can bind to human mesangial cells (HMC) and such binding correlates with clinical activity in selected LN patients and could contribute to intra-renal disease pathogenesis [12,13]. We also observed a correlation between anti-dsDNA and total IgG levels. In this study, we investigated whether the binding activity of total serum IgG and its subclasses to HMC might have clinical correlations in patients with LN, which have implications on the use of such binding as a biomarker for disease monitoring and further exploration into its pathogenic importance.

Materials and Methods

Patients

This study and the consent procedures were approved by the Institutional Review Board of the University of Hong Kong/ Hospital Authority Hong Kong West Cluster (HKU/HA HKW IRB). All included subjects have signed consent for the use of the serum samples in this study and the consent forms are kept in patients' case records. Patients attending follow-up at the SLE Clinic of Queen Mary Hospital, Hong Kong, with biopsy-proven Class III/IV±V LN and two or more episodes of renal flare during the period 2001 to 2013 were included. Histological

Table 1. Characteristics of 23 patients with Class III/IV±V lupus nephritis who had two or more episodes of renal flare during follow-up and included in the present study.

Age (year)	39.4±11.2
Female/Male	14/9
Duration of follow up (month)	138.2±80.5
Previous immunosuppressive exposure	
Prednisolone	23 (100%)
Cyclophosphamide	17 (73.9%)
Mycophenolate mofetil	18 (78.3%)
Azathioprine	19 (82.6%)
Calcineurin inhibitors	8 (34.8%)
Laboratory parameters at first renal flare	
Serum creatinine level (μmol/L)	111.8±56.4
Urine protein (g/D)	3.1±3.4
Anti-dsDNA level (iu/mL)	238.7±249.3
C3 level (mg/dL)	64.4±38.1

findings of LN were reported in accordance with the International Society of Nephrology/Renal Pathology Society (ISN/RPS) 2003 classification [14,15]. Standard treatment for active LN included corticosteroids combined with either cyclophosphamide or mycophenolate mofetil (MMF) as induction immunosuppression, followed by low-dose corticosteroids with either azathioprine or MMF as long-term maintenance immunosuppression. Disease activity was categorized as "active" or "low level disease activity" (LLDA) on the basis of both clinical and serologic parameters. "Active" disease had SLE Disease Activity Index (SLEDAI) score >10 with ≥4 points in the renal domain, and "low level disease activity" status was defined by SLEDAI score <4 with no points in the renal domain [16]. Patients with non-lupus glomerular diseases (NLGD) and healthy subjects (age- and sex-matched) were included as controls. The NLGD group included patients with IgA nephropathy, minimal change nephropathy, membranous nephropathy and ANCA-associated glomerulonephritis, and serum samples were obtained at presentation when the diagnoses were established by renal biopsy.

Laboratory methods

Archived serum samples from LN patients collected at baseline (i.e. at initiation of induction therapy) then serially at 3-month intervals with informed consent were retrieved. Single serum samples were obtained from patients with non-lupus glomerular diseases and healthy subjects.

HMC-binding activity of IgG in serum samples was measured using a cellular ELISA as previously described [12]. Briefly, HMC were seeded into 96-well microtitre plates at a density of 10,000 cells/cm^2. Cells were cultured in RPMI 1640 medium supplemented with 15% FCS and medium changed every 3 days. At 90% confluence HMC were growth arrested for 72 h, washed with PBS then fixed with 1% paraformaldehyde in PBS for 15 min. Cells were washed thrice with PBS in between steps, and all incubations were for 1 h at 37°C. HMC were blocked with 3% BSA followed by normal IgG (100 μg/ml) to block Fc receptor-mediated binding. HMC were incubated with serum samples (diluted 1:100, 100 μl) in triplicate, then incubated with anti-human IgG F(ab) conjugated with alkaline phosphatase. Degree of IgG binding to HMC was detected by incubation with para-nitrophenol phosphate at room temperature and with optical density measurement at $A_{405/420}$ when pre-established positive control sample showed an optical density of 1.5. The positive control was pooled serum from a patient with high HMC-binding activity. Seropositivity for HMC binding was denoted by results that exceed mean+3SD of results from healthy subjects. Circulating anti-dsDNA antibody titre was measured using a commercial ELISA (Microplate autoimmune anti-DNA quantitative ELISA) according to the manufacturer's instructions (BioRad, Hong Kong). Samples giving a value >60 IU/ml were considered positive. Kidney biopsies were performed within one week when renal flares were suspected clinically, and were reviewed by the same pathologist. The amount of mesangial deposits was semi-quantitated by electron microscopy (EM) in the following scale: 0 = no deposit; 1 = scanty deposits; 2 = moderate deposits; 3 = numerous deposits.

Data analysis and statistics

Continuous variables were expressed as mean±SD and analyzed by student's t-test, unless otherwise specified. Categorical variable were expressed as frequencies and percentages, and analyzed with Chi-square test where appropriate. Correlation of HMC-binding activity with clinical parameters was assessed by the Spearman's method. The sensitivity/specificity, positive and negative predictive value (PPV and NPV) of HMC-binding activity in predicting renal flares was calculated, and the Area Under Curve (AUC) of the Receiver Operator Characteristics (ROC) curves was determined. Statistical analysis was performed by Graphpad Prism 5 (La Jolla, California, USA) and two-tailed *P values*<0.05 was considered statistically significant.

Results

Patient characteristics

Twenty-three Chinese patients with biopsy-proven Class III/IV±V LN and who had experienced at least two episodes of renal flares during follow-up of 138.2±80.5 months were included (Table 1). A total of 276 serum samples were analyzed, with 189 samples from LN patients (48 during active renal flare and 141 during LLDA, 64 samples from patients with non-lupus glomer-

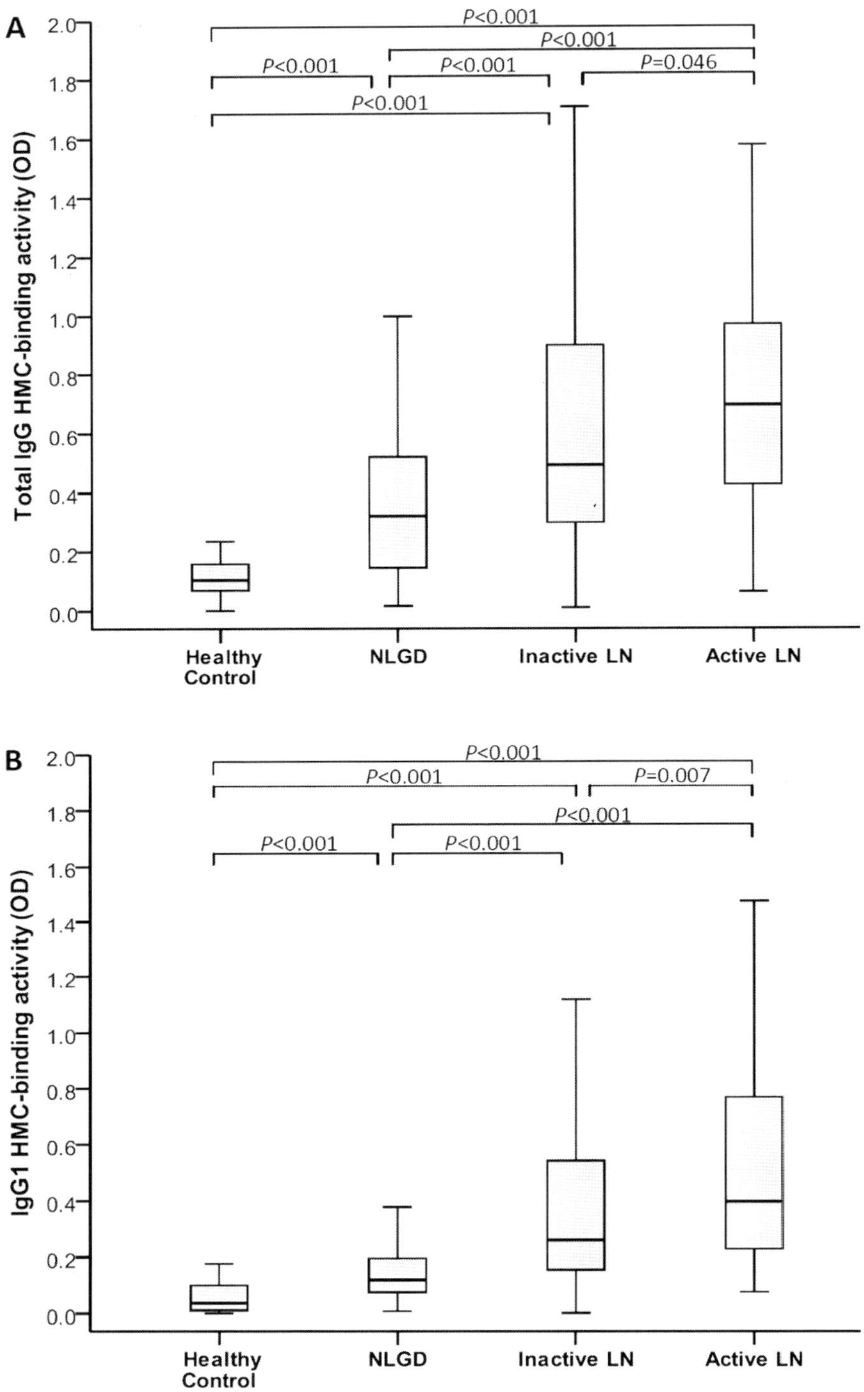

Figure 1. Mesangial cell-binding by (A) total IgG and (B) IgG_1 in serum samples of patients with inactive or active lupus nephritis, non-lupus glomerular diseases, and patients with inactive or active lupus nephritis, non-lupus glomerular diseases, and healthy controls.

ular diseases (NLGD), and 23 samples from healthy subjects respectively.

HMC-binding activity of serum total IgG and its subclasses in LN patients

Binding index of serum total IgG to HMC was 0.12±0.09, 0.36±0.25, 0.59±0.37 and 0.74±0.42 for healthy controls, NLGD, LN patients during LLDA, and active LN respectively (P=0.046, LN flare vs. LLDA; P<0.001, healthy controls or NLGD vs. active or inactive LN; P<0.001, NLGD vs. active or inactive LN) (Figure 1, A). Binding index of serum IgG_1 to HMC was 0.05±0.05, 0.15±0.11, 0.41±0.38 and 0.55±0.40 for healthy controls, NLGD, LN patients in LLDA, and active LN respectively (P= 0.007, LN flare vs. LLDA; P<0.001, healthy controls or

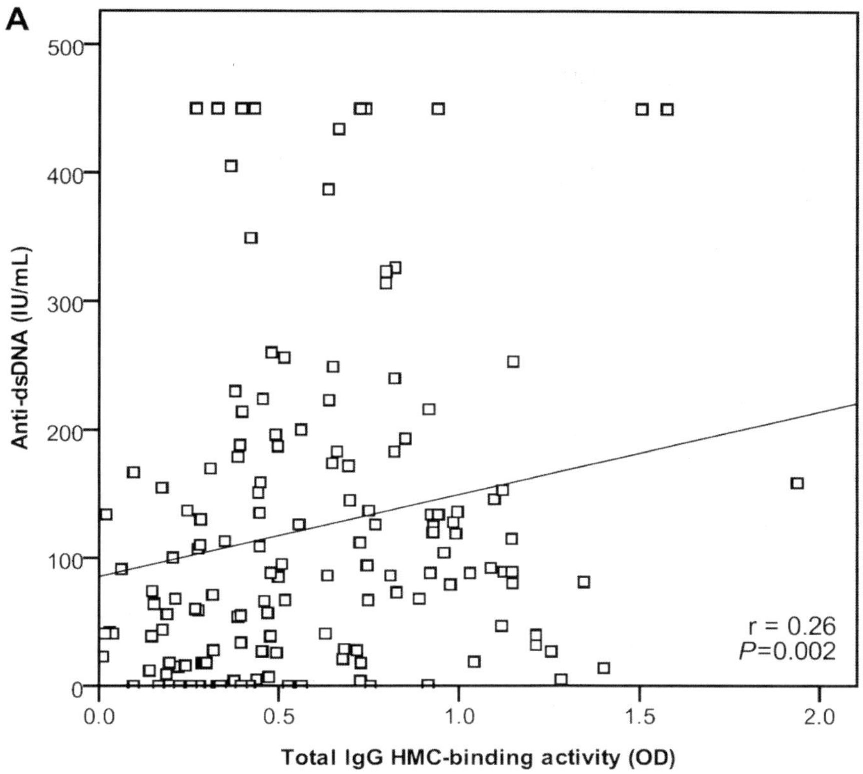

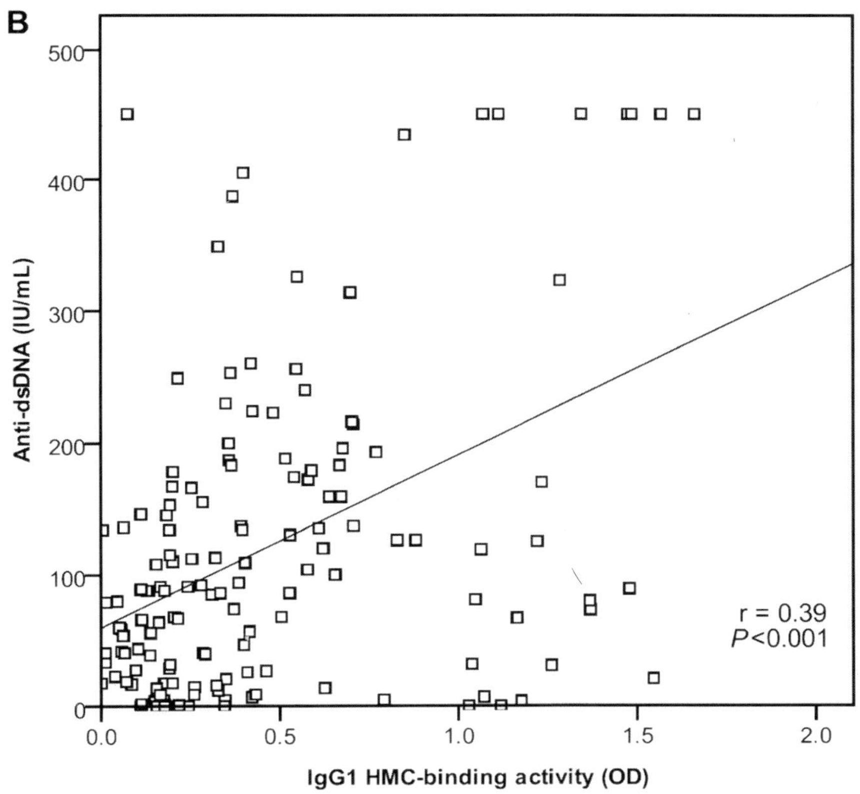

Figure 2. Correlation between mesangial cell-binding by (A) total IgG and (B) IgG_1 with anti-dsDNA level in 23 patients with Class III/IV±V lupus nephritis.

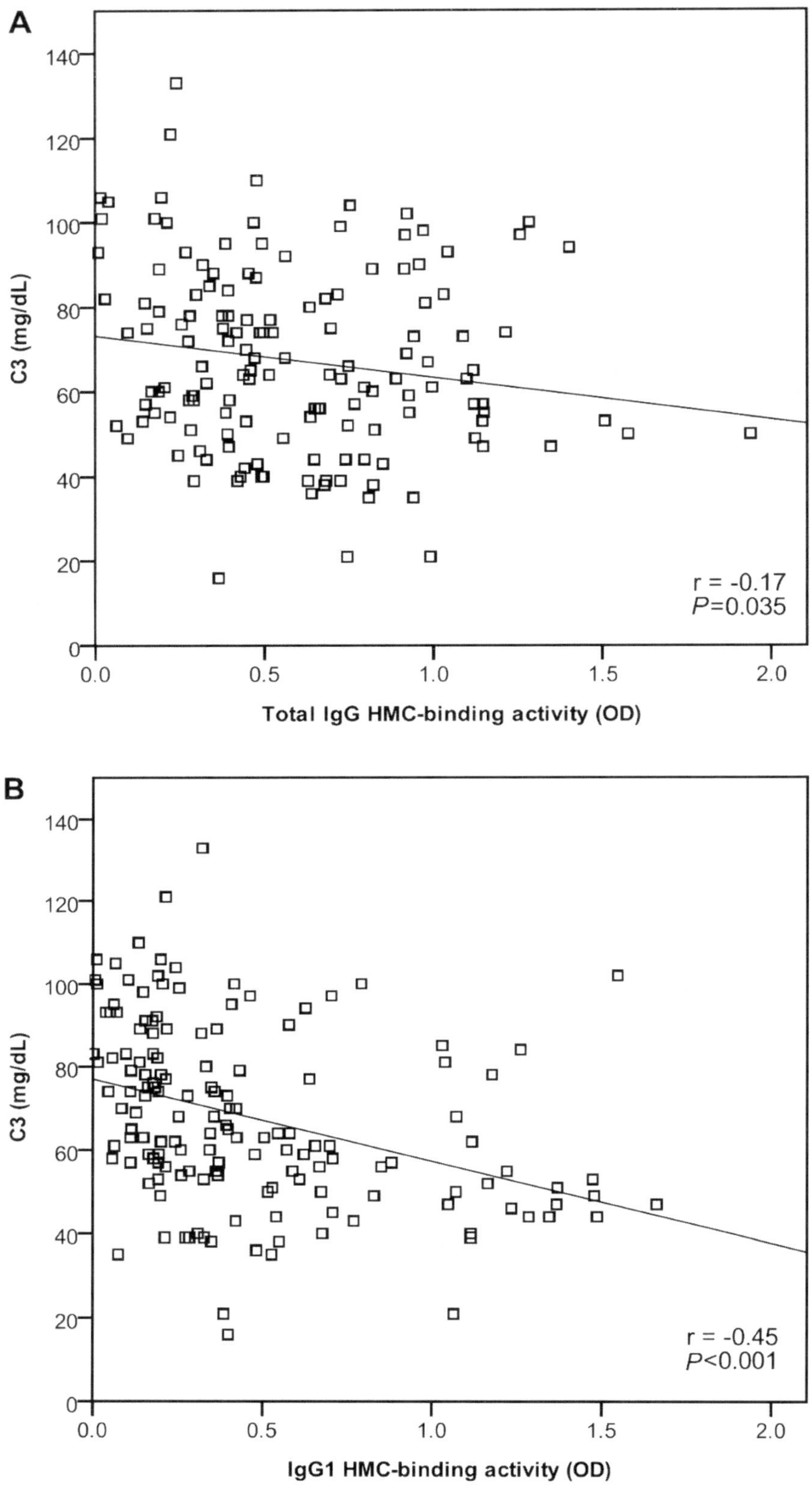

Figure 3. Negative correlation between mesangial cell-binding by (A) total IgG and (B) IgG_1 with C3 level in 23 patients with Class III/IV±V lupus nephritis.

A

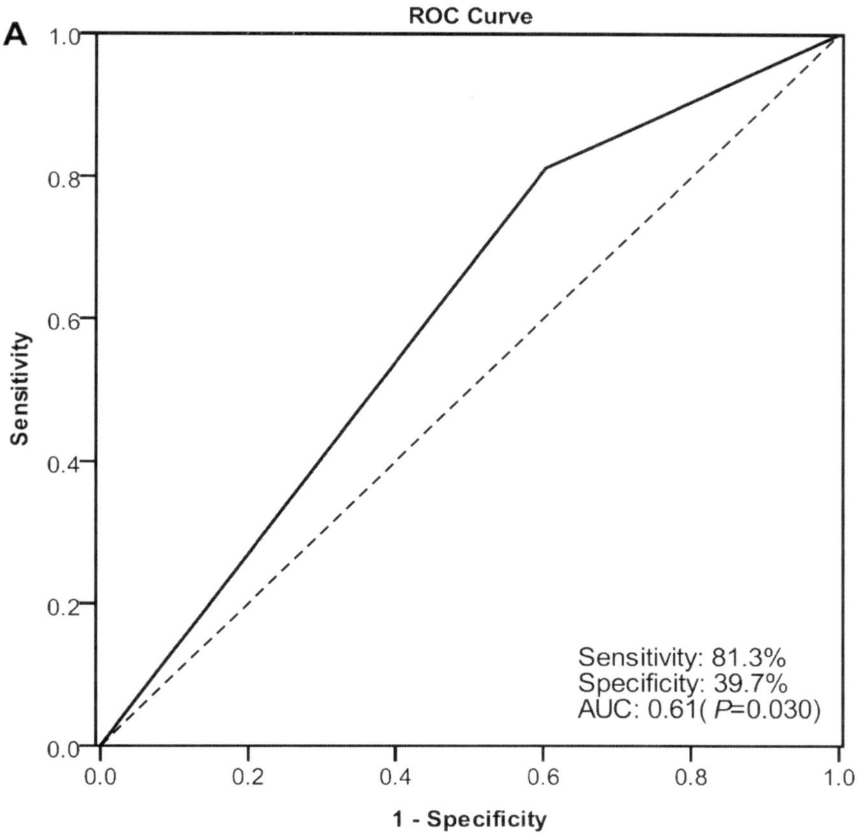
ROC Curve
Sensitivity
1 - Specificity
1.0
0.8
0.6
0.4
0.2
0.0
0.0
0.2
0.4
0.6
0.8
1.0
Sensitivity: 81.3%
Specificity: 39.7%
AUC: 0.61(P=0.030)

B

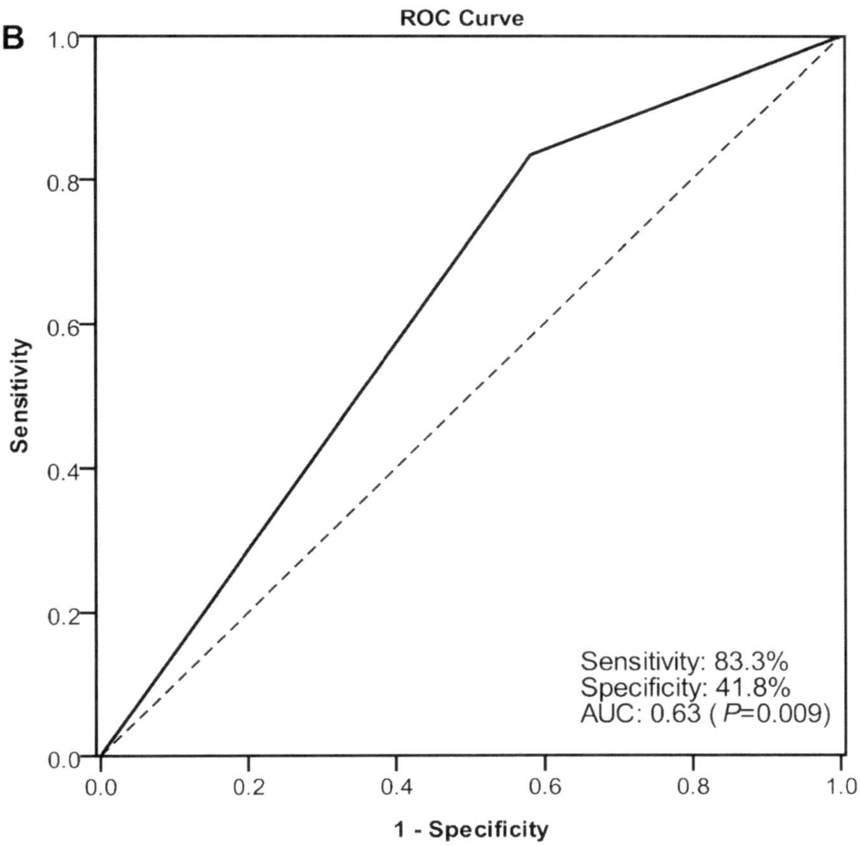
ROC Curve
Sensitivity
1 - Specificity
1.0
0.8
0.6
0.4
0.2
0.0
0.0
0.2
0.4
0.6
0.8
1.0
Sensitivity: 83.3%
Specificity: 41.8%
AUC: 0.63 (P=0.009)

Figure 4. Receiver Operator Characteristics (ROC) curve for sensitivity/specificity in renal flare prediction using the level of mesangial cell-binding by (A) total IgG and (B) IgG_1 in serum samples of 23 patients with Class III/IV±V lupus nephritis.

NLGD vs. active or inactive LN; $P<0.001$, NLGD vs. active or inactive LN) (Figure 1, B). There was no significant binding of serum IgG_2, IgG_3 or IgG_4 to HMC, which also did not vary between healthy controls, NLGD patients, and LN patients during flare or LLDA.

HMC binding by serum IgG and IgG_1 and clinical parameters

Total serum IgG and serum IgG_1 HMC-binding index both correlated positively with anti-dsDNA levels ($r = 0.26$ and 0.39 respectively, $P<0.001$ for both) (Figure 2, A&B). In contrast, both showed a negative correlation with C3 levels ($r = -0.17$ and -0.45 respectively, $P<0.05$ for both) (Figure 3, A&B). HMC-binding by IgG and IgG_1 was not related to the level of serum creatinine, serum albumin, or proteinuria at the time of blood sample collection ($P = 0.735$, 0.546 and 0.700 respectively for total IgG HMC-binding; $P = 0.628$, 0.443 and 0.170 for IgG_1 HMC-binding).

Overall sensitivity/specificity of total IgG or IgG_1 HMC-binding index in the prediction of renal flares (with or without systemic flares) was 81.3%/39.7% (AUC 0.61, $P = 0.030$) and 83.8%/41.8% (AUC 0.63, $P = 0.009$) respectively (Figure 4, A&B). The overall PPV and NPV of total IgG or IgG1 HMC-binding index in prediction of renal flares (with or without systemic flares) were 31.5%/86.2% and 32.8%/88.1% respectively. The sensitivity/specificity of total IgG or IgG_1 HMC-binding index to predict renal flares with concomitant systemic flares were 80.0%/35.1% (PPV: 12.1%; NPV: 94.1%) and 83.3%/36.1% (PPV: 12.7%; NPV: 95.1%), and 79.6%/38.6% (PPV: 28.2%; NPV: 86.2%) and 83.3%/40.8% (PPV: 28.7%; NPV: 89.6%) for renal flares without systemic flares. Two patients (8.7%) showed positive total IgG and IgG_1 binding to HMC during active renal flare when their anti-dsDNA and C3 levels remained within normal limits. Seropositivity of HMC-binding IgG_1 precedes renal flares by 43.8±62.9 days.

HMC binding by serum IgG and IgG_1 and mesangial immune deposition assessed by electron microscopy

Total IgG HMC-binding seropositivity was not related to the degree of mesangial immune deposition ($P = 0.733$). In contrast, patients seropositive for IgG_1 HMC-binding were more likely to show increased mesangial immune deposition at grades 2 or 3 (i.e. moderate to numerous) ($P = 0.016$). HMC-binding index of IgG_1, but not total IgG, also correlated positively with the mesangial deposition score ($r = 0.776$ and $P<0.001$ for IgG_1; $r = 0.263$ and $P = 0.363$ for total IgG).

Discussion

SLE is characterized by the production of various autoantibodies [4]. Previous studies have reported that different autoantibodies can bind to different renal components including podocytes, mesangial cells, endothelial cells, and renal tubular epithelial cells, and it has been speculated that such binding could have a pathogenic role in immune-mediated kidney injury [10,12,13,17–19]. Mesangial cells are located strategically at the centre of glomeruli and are juxtaposed to the capillary loops [9]. Mesangial immunoglobulin deposition and mesangial cell proliferation are cardinal histological features in LN [3,11]. Our previous investigations showed that anti-dsDNA antibodies from patients with LN could bind to HMC and trigger cellular responses involved in inflammation and fibrosis, and that such binding correlated with total serum IgG level (10,12). The present study sought to investigate the potential clinical correlations of the in vitro findings.

Our results showed a clear relationship between disease activity and HMC-binding by total serum IgG and IgG_1 in LN, and the degree of binding was significantly increased in LN compared with healthy subjects and patients with non-lupus glomerular diseases. Also, the positive correlation of IgG HMC-binding with anti-dsDNA level, and negative relationship with C3 level, prompted us to investigate whether HMC-binding index might serve as a biomarker for disease activity monitoring. In this context, previous studies have also found that active LN patients had significantly stronger IgG binding to isolated rat glomeruli in an *in vitro* assay when compared to SLE patients without nephritis [20]. That HMC-binding index of total IgG or IgG_1 was not related to serum creatinine, serum albumin, or proteinuria was not a disadvantage since these clinical parameters represent a summative outcome of both active disease and prior chronic damage and are also subject to modulating factors distinct from the lupus disease process such as hypertensive renal damage. Conventional serological parameters C3 and anti-dsDNA levels have been reported to show sensitivity and specificity of 49–79% and 51–74% respectively in the detection of disease flares [21–27]. The present results from samples collected serially in LN patients showed that in the majority of cases increased HMC-binding by IgG and IgG_1 was associated with increased disease activity, so that these parameters had sensitivities of over 80% in the predication of renal flares. However, seropositivity for HMC-binding by itself could be present in patients during remission and thus was non-specific for active disease. Notwithstanding its lack of specificity, assessment of HMC-binding index may be of value in the small proportion of patients in whom conventional serological parameters such as anti-DNA and C3 levels do not correlate with disease activity, as was demonstrated in two of the 23 patients studied, when both anti-DNA and C3 were still within the normal range at disease flare but serum HMC-binding IgG was positive.

The present results also have implications on pathogenic mechanisms in LN. Among the different IgG subclasses from LN patients tested, only IgG_1 showed significant binding to HMC. Furthermore, HMC-binding by IgG_1 correlated with clinical disease activity and also the degree of mesangial immune deposition as assessed by electron microscopy. In this context, previous studies have suggested that IgG_1 might be more pathogenic compared with other IgG subclasses in LN, attributed to its ability to fix complements [28,29]. Further studies are required to investigate the downstream cellular processes that follow the binding of HMC by IgG_1, and whether intervention or interruption of such binding could present a novel therapeutic approach.

Conclusions

The degree of mesangial cell binding by circulating IgG and IgG_1 in serum samples of patients with LN correlates with disease activity, and thus may complement anti-dsDNA and C3 as biomarkers for disease monitoring. Its relationship with mesangial immunoglobulin deposition in LN kidney tissue also suggests a pathogenic role.

Author Contributions

Conceived and designed the experiments: DY SY TMC. Performed the experiments: QZ. Analyzed the data: CT. Contributed reagents/materials/analysis tools: SY. Wrote the paper: DY TMC.

References

1. Bomback AS, Appel GB (2010) Updates on the treatment of lupus nephritis. J Am Soc Nephrol 21: 2028–2035.
2. Saxena R, Mahajan T, Mohan C (2011) Lupus nephritis: current update. Arthritis Res Ther 13: 240.
3. Golbus J, McCune WJ (1994) Lupus nephritis. Classification, prognosis, immunopathogenesis, and treatment. Rheum Dis Clin North Am 20: 213–242.
4. Tan EM, Schur PH, Carr RI, Kunkel HG (1966) Deoxybonucleic acid (DNA) and antibodies to DNA in the serum of patients with systemic lupus erythematosus. J Clin Invest 45: 1732–1740.
5. Winfield JB, Faiferman I, Koffler D (1977) Avidity of anti-DNA antibodies in serum and IgG glomerular eluates from patients with systemic lupus erythematosus. Association of high avidity antinative DNA antibody with glomerulonephritis. J Clin Invest 59: 90–96.
6. Kalunian KC, Panosian-Sahakian N, Ebling FM, Cohen AH, Louie JS, et al. (1989) Idiotypic characteristics of immunoglobulins associated with systemic lupus erythematosus. Studies of antibodies deposited in glomeruli of humans. Arthritis Rheum 32: 513–522.
7. Termaat RM, Assmann KJ, van Son JP, Dijkman HB, Koene RA, et al. (1993) Antigen-specificity of antibodies bound to glomeruli of mice with systemic lupus erythematosus-like syndromes. Lab Invest 68: 164–173.
8. Rovin BH, Zhang X (2009) Biomarkers for lupus nephritis: the quest continues. Clin J Am Soc Nephrol 4: 1858–1865.
9. Schlondorff D, Banas B (2009) The mesangial cell revisited: no cell is an island. J Am Soc Nephrol 20: 1179–1187.
10. Yung S, Chan TM (2012) Autoantibodies and resident renal cells in the pathogenesis of lupus nephritis: getting to know the unknown. Clin Dev Immunol 2012: 139365.
11. Mery JP, Morel-Maroger L, Boelaert J (1975) Immunoglobulin and complement deposits in lupus glomerulonephritis. Proc Eur Dial Transplant Assoc 11: 506–511.
12. Chan TM, Leung JK, Ho SK, Yung S (2002) Mesangial cell-binding anti-DNA antibodies in patients with systemic lupus erythematosus. J Am Soc Nephrol 13: 1219–1229.
13. Yung S, Cheung KF, Zhang Q, Chan TM (2010) Anti-dsDNA antibodies bind to mesangial annexin II in lupus nephritis. J Am Soc Nephrol 21: 1912–1927.
14. Tan EM, Cohen AS, Fries JF, Masi AT, McShane DJ, et al. (1982) The 1982 revised criteria for the classification of systemic lupus erythematosus. Arthritis Rheum 25: 1271–1277.
15. Weening JJ, D'Agati VD, Schwartz MM, Seshan SV, Alpers CE, et al. (2004) The classification of glomerulonephritis in systemic lupus erythematosus revisited. J Am Soc Nephrol 15: 241–250.
16. Bombardier C, Gladman DD, Urowitz MB, Caron D, Chang CH (1992) Derivation of the SLEDAI. A disease activity index for lupus patients. The Committee on Prognosis Studies in SLE. Arthritis Rheum 35: 630–640.
17. Chan TM, Cheng IK (1997) Identification of endothelial cell membrane proteins that bind anti-DNA antibodies from patients with systemic lupus erythematosus by direct or indirect mechanisms. J Autoimmun 10: 433–439.
18. Yung S, Tsang RC, Sun Y, Leung JK, Chan TM (2005) Effect of human anti-DNA antibodies on proximal renal tubular epithelial cell cytokine expression: implications on tubulointerstitial inflammation in lupus nephritis. J Am Soc Nephrol 16: 3281–3294.
19. Yung S, Cheung KF, Zhang Q, Chan TM (2013) Mediators of inflammation and their effect on resident renal cells: implications in lupus nephritis. Clin Dev Immunol 2013: 317682.
20. Budhai L, Oh K, Davidson A (1996) An in vitro assay for detection of glomerular binding IgG autoantibodies in patients with systemic lupus erythematosus. J Clin Invest 98: 1585–1593.
21. Rovin BH, Birmingham DJ, Nagaraja HN, Yu CY, Hebert LA (2007) Biomarker discovery in human SLE nephritis. Bull NYU Hosp Jt Dis 65: 187–193.
22. Moroni G, Radice A, Giammarresi G, Quaglini S, Gallelli B, et al. (2009) Are laboratory tests useful for monitoring the activity of lupus nephritis? A 6-year prospective study in a cohort of 228 patients with lupus nephritis. Ann Rheum Dis 68: 234–237.
23. Esdaile JM, Abrahamowicz M, Joseph L, MacKenzie T, Li Y, et al. (1996) Laboratory tests as predictors of disease exacerbations in systemic lupus erythematosus. Why some tests fail. Arthritis Rheum 39: 370–378.
24. Esdaile JM, Joseph L, Abrahamowicz M, Li Y, Danoff D, et al. (1996) Routine immunologic tests in systemic lupus erythematosus: is there a need for more studies? J Rheumatol 23: 1891–1896.
25. Coremans IE, Spronk PE, Bootsma H, Daha MR, van der Voort EA, et al. (1995) Changes in antibodies to C1q predict renal relapses in systemic lupus erythematosus. Am J Kidney Dis 26: 595–601.
26. Ho A, Barr SG, Magder LS, Petri M (2001) A decrease in complement is associated with increased renal and hematologic activity in patients with systemic lupus erythematosus. Arthritis Rheum 44: 2350–2357.
27. Ho A, Magder LS, Barr SG, Petri M (2001) Decreases in anti-double-stranded DNA levels are associated with concurrent flares in patients with systemic lupus erythematosus. Arthritis Rheum 44: 2342–2349.
28. Rothfield NF, Stollar BD (1967) The relation of immunoglobulin class, pattern of anti-nuclear antibody, and complement-fixing antibodies to DNA in sera from patients with systemic lupus erythematosus. J Clin Invest 46: 1785–1794.
29. Imai H, Hamai K, Komatsuda A, Ohtani H, Miura AB (1997) IgG subclasses in patients with membranoproliferative glomerulonephritis, membranous nephropathy, and lupus nephritis. Kidney Int 51: 270–276.

26

TRPC6 Single Nucleotide Polymorphisms and Progression of Idiopathic Membranous Nephropathy

Julia M. Hofstra[1], Marieke J. H. Coenen[2], Mascha M. V. A. P. Schijvenaars[2], Jo H. M. Berden[1], Johan van der Vlag[1], Lies H. Hoefsloot[2¤a], Nine V. A. M. Knoers[2¤b], Jack F. M. Wetzels[1], Tom Nijenhuis[1]*

1 Department of Nephrology, Radboud university medical center, Nijmegen, the Netherlands, **2** Department of Human Genetics, Radboud university medical center, Nijmegen, the Netherlands

Abstract

Background: Activating mutations in the Transient Receptor Potential channel C6 (TRPC6) cause autosomal dominant focal segmental glomerular sclerosis (FSGS). TRPC6 expression is upregulated in renal biopsies of patients with idiopathic membranous glomerulopathy (iMN) and animal models thereof. In iMN, disease progression is characterized by glomerulosclerosis. In addition, a context-dependent TRPC6 overexpression was recently suggested in complement-mediated podocyte injury in e.g. iMN. Hence, we hypothesized that genetic variants in TRPC6 might affect susceptibility to development or progression of iMN.

Methods & Results: Genomic DNA was isolated from blood samples of 101 iMN patients and 292 controls. By direct sequencing of the entire TRPC6 gene, 13 single nucleotide polymorphisms (SNPs) were identified in the iMN cohort, two of which were causing an amino acid substitution (rs3802829; Pro15Ser and rs36111323, Ala404Val). No statistically significant differences in genotypes or allele frequencies between patients and controls were observed. Clinical outcome in patients was determined (remission n = 26, renal failure n = 46, persistent proteinuria n = 29, follow-up median 80 months {range 51–166}). The 13 identified SNPs showed no association with remission or renal failure. There were no differences in genotypes or allele frequencies between patients in remission and progressors.

Conclusions: Our data suggest that TRPC6 polymorphisms do not affect susceptibility to iMN, or clinical outcome in iMN.

Editor: Michael Edward Zwick, Emory University School Of Medicine, United States of America

Funding: Financial support was provided by a Dutch Kidney Foundation grant (OW08) for J. M. H and J. F. M. W., a Kolff Career Stimulation Grant from the Dutch Kidney Foundation (KJPB 07.0001), a grant from the Genzyme Renal Innovations Program (GRIP) and a Ruby Diabetes Research Grant from the Dutch Diabetes Fund (2009.80.118) for T. N. http://www.nierstichting.nl http://www.genzyme.com/Responsibility/Grants-and-Giving.aspx http://www.diabetesfonds.nl The funders had no role in study design, data collection and analysis, decision to publish, or preparation of the manuscript.

* Email: Tom.Nijenhuis@Radboudumc.nl

¤a Current address: Department of Clinical Genetics, Erasmus Medical Centre, Rotterdam, the Netherlands
¤b Current address: Department of Medical Genetics, Utrecht Medical Centre, Utrecht, the Netherlands

Introduction

Membranous nephropathy (MN) is the leading cause of nephrotic syndrome in the adult Caucasian population and is characterized by immune complex deposition in the subepithelial layer of the glomerular basement membrane. In one third of patients, MN is caused by an underlying disease such as a malignancy, infection or a systemic disease. Until recently, no underlying cause could be identified in two thirds of patients and, therefore, the disease was considered to be idiopathic (iMN) in these patients. [1] In 2009 Beck *et al.* discovered antibodies against the M-type phospholipase A_2 receptor (PLA_2R), a membrane glycoprotein located on the podocyte, in patients with iMN. [2] Further studies showed that antibodies against PLA_2R are present in approximately 70% of Caucasian patients with active disease. [3,4] This finding thus provided evidence that iMN is an autoimmune disease.

A recent genome-wide association study showed that genetic variants in *HLA-DQA1* and *phospholipase A2 receptor* (*PLA2R1*) were most significantly associated with biopsy-proven iMN. [5] Association with *HLA* regions has been identified in many autoimmune diseases, the association with the *PLA2R1* gene supports the key role of the anti-PLA2R antibodies in the pathogenesis of the disease. In an additional study we assessed if rare genetic variants within the coding region of the *PLA2R1* gene could explain antibody formation. Although sequencing of the complete coding sequence of *PLA2R1* in 95 patients with iMN confirmed associations of common single nucleotide polymorphisms (SNPs) with iMN, rare variants were present in only a minority of patients (9%). [6] This data questions why iMN is rare, as these SNPs occur frequently in the general population. It could be hypothesized that a rare combination of (relatively) common events (genetic variants and/or environmental factors) might

constitute the pathogenetic trigger. In addition to *HLA* and *PLA2R1*, variants in other genes might be involved.

One of the biggest unresolved issues in patients with iMN is the highly variable disease course. Spontaneous remission occurs in about 40–50% of patients, but another 30–50% of patients progresses to end stage renal disease within 10 years. [7] Although several predictive strategies have been proposed, it remains difficult to identify patients with a high risk of disease progression. [8,9] Progression of disease is accompanied by glomerulsclerosis in renal biopsies. [10]

The Transient Receptor Potential channel C6 (TRPC6) is an ion channel that is expressed in podocytes at the slit diaphragm {Figure 1}. [11] This complex of interconnected proteins provides both physical linkage as well as a signaling platform that regulates podocyte behavior and architecture, and thereby affects glomerular permeability. TRPC6 was recognized as an important slit diaphragm component after *TRPC6* gain-of-function mutations were shown to be responsible for autosomal dominant focal segmental glomerulosclerosis (FSGS), a leading cause of steroid-resistant nephrotic syndrome that can rapidly progress to end-stage renal disease (ESRD). [11–15] Animal studies show that podocyte-specific transgenic TRPC6 overexpression leads to albuminuria and histological findings similar to human FSGS. [14,16] However, glomerular *TRPC6* expression is also increased in acquired human proteinuric diseases. Importantly, this occurs in human MN, as well as in the passive Heymann nephritis animal model for MN. [13,17] Furthermore, angiotensin II (AngII) activates specific TRPC6-mediated intracellular pathways in the podocyte. [17–20] Angiotensin receptor blockers, angiotensin converting enzyme inhibitors and calcineurin inhibitors, all three utilized to treat proteinuria in MN, were shown to inhibit these TRPC6-mediated cascades. [17,19] Thus, TRPC6 is not only primarily involved in the pathogenesis of FSGS, but could also mediate podocyte damage and/or progression to ESRD in other proteinuric diseases like MN. Therefore, we hypothesized that sequence variations in the *TRPC6* gene could affect susceptibility to development and/or progression of iMN.

In the present study, we screened a cohort of 101 biopsy-proven iMN patients for *TRPC6* sequence variations by direct sequencing of all 13 exons of the *TRPC6* gene. Furthermore, we assessed whether genetic variants were associated with disease progression and outcome in patients with iMN.

Subjects and Methods

Patients

The present study included iMN patients referred to our centre between 1995 and 2007. In all patients, the diagnosis of iMN was established by renal biopsy and secondary causes were excluded according to local routine clinical work up. [21] Baseline data on age, sex and ethnicity were present for all patients. To allow subgroup analysis of anti-PLA_2R positive patients, the presence of anti-PLA2R antibodies in the serum was evaluated. Serum samples at diagnosis were available for most patients. The assay for measuring anti-PLA_2R antibodies has been previously described. [22]

iMN patients were evaluated using a standardized protocol as previously described. [23] Patients were prospectively followed, and data on treatment and outcome (e.g. remission and renal survival) are obtained. For the current study we evaluated the occurrence of spontaneous remissions and/or renal failure. Spontaneous remission was defined as proteinuria <2.0 g/day with stable renal function in a patient not treated with immunosuppressive agents. Renal failure/progression was defined as an increase in serum creatinine >25% from baseline with a serum creatinine >135 μmol/l or an increase >50% from baseline.

Ethics statement

The study was approved by the ethics committee of the Radboud university medical center (Commissie Mensgebonden Onderzoek (CMO) Regio Arnhem Nijmegen, nr.9701-0016). All patients gave written informed consent prior to participation in the study.

Sequencing

DNA was purified from blood samples using salt extraction according to a previously described protocol. [24] All exons including splice sites in the *TRPC6* gene were sequenced. Sense and antisense primers were designed using Primer3. [25] PCR primers and conditions are given in Table 1. PCR products were purified using Multiscreen filter plates (Millipore Carrigtwohill, Cork, Ireland). Purified products were used for Sanger sequence analysis (bidirectional) with dye-termination chemistry (BigDye Terminator, version 3) on a 3730 DNA analyzer (Applied Biosystems, Inc., Foster City, CA, USA).

Analysis

TRPC6 sequences were analyzed for the presence of genetic variants in comparison with the published reference sequence for human *TRPC6* (mRNA NM_004621.5). Ethnically matched population allele frequencies of the identified variants were obtained from the 1000 Genomes project (1000 Genomes release 10 - March 2012). [26] Variants were considered to be common (previously reported with allele frequency >1%), rare (previously reported with allele frequency <1%), or novel (not previously reported in the 1000 Genome project nor in dbSNP 136).

SNP genotyping. SNPs that lead to amino acid substitutions, and/or that were rare (previously with allele frequency <1%), completed with SNPs that had a the minor allele frequency in the patient cohort of >10%, were selected for genotyping in 292 healthy individuals from the same geographical region (Table 2). Genotyping was performed using Taqman allelic discrimination assays (Invitrogen, Bleiswijk, The Netherlands) according to the instructions of the manufacturer. The fluorescent signal for allelic discrimination was determined after amplification using an end-point reading on the 7500 Fast Real-time System (Applied Biosystems). Automated allele calling was performed by allelic discrimination plots using SDS 1.4 software (Applied Biosystems). We included 5% duplicate samples in each plate as quality control.

Association analysis. Frequencies of SNPs identified in iMN patients were compared with genotype data of 379 Caucasian controls that were downloaded from the 1000 Genomes project (release 10). In an attempt to increase power, data of 292 healthy controls were added for variants in 5 SNPs, as detected with Taqman assay. Association analyses were performed using the whole genome analysis toolset PLINK (version 1.07). [27] Significance was set a $p<0.05$. SNPs with an allele frequency of 0.1 and higher were used to construct haplotypes. Haplotype analysis was also performed using PLINK. Next, frequencies of SNPs identified in patients with progressive disease (renal failure) were compared with frequencies observed in patients with a spontaneous remission of proteinuria as described above.

Power calculations. In order to be able to estimate the effect size of the genetic variants, we performed a genetic power calculation using the online Harvard Genetic Power Calculator (http://pngu.mgh.harvard.edu/~purcell/gpc/). ' We calculated the effect size that could be excluded with 80% power and a

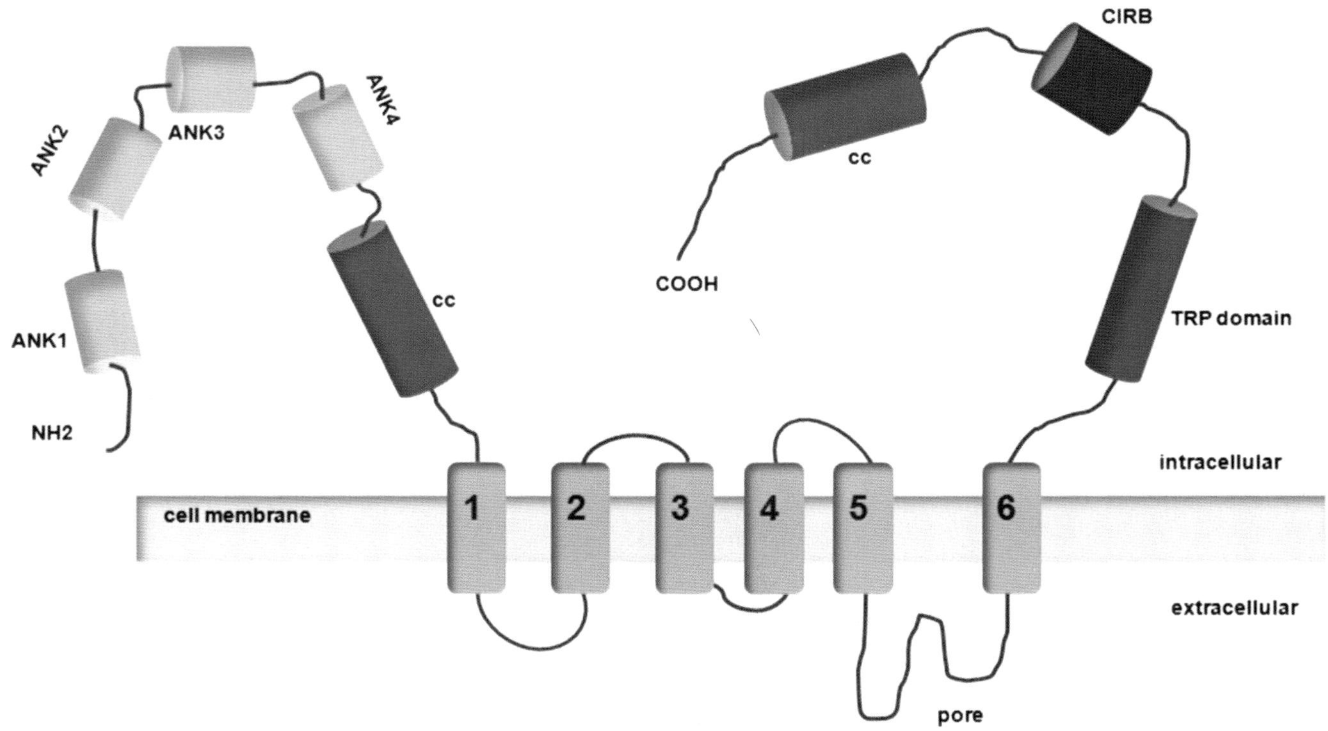

Figure 1. TRPC6 topology. Structure of the TRPC6 monomer. TRPC6 belongs to the large family of TRP channels, which contain six transmembrane domains, one pore-forming region and large intracellular N- and C-tails. Four subunits are required to assemble a functional channel. In the pococyte, TRPC6 is part of the slit diaphragm multiprotein complex. TRP: transient receptor potential, ANK: Ankyrin repeat, cc: coiled–coiled domain, CIRB: CaM/IP3R-binding domain.

two-sided p-value of 0.05, for various frequencies of the high-risk allele (ranging from 0.200 to 0.008).

Results

Patient characteristics

A total of 101 patients with biopsy proven iMN were included in the present study. Patients were mostly male (77%) and mean age at diagnosis was 51±15 years. All patients were of self-reported Caucasian ancestry. Serum samples at onset of disease were available for 92 patients, anti-PLA_2R antibodies were present in 62 samples (67%).

Sequencing

In 101 patients with iMN we identified eight sequence variants in the coding region of the *TRPC6* gene (Table 2). Of the eight coding variants observed, six were common SNPs and two were rare (See Methods for definitions). These rare variants (c.888G>A and c.2142G>T) were both encountered once in two different patients in a heterozygous state, but did not result in amino acid changes (synonymous mutations). Only two of the common SNPs resulted in an amino acid substitution (rs3802829; Pro15Ser and rs36111323, Ala404Val). Four additional common SNPs were observed in the intron regions, as well as one rare variant in the 5′-UTR (c1-10 C>A). The latter was present in 5 patients, all in a heterozygous state.

Association between *TRPC6* variants and occurrence of iMN

Control data were obtained from the 1000 Genomes project as described. To increase power to detect possible genotype frequency differences between our iMN cohort and the general population, 292 healthy Caucasian controls from the same geographical area were included as an additional control group for the frequency of five SNPs. These five SNPs were selected by previously specified criteria. Association analysis showed that there were no significant differences in the allele frequencies of both the coding and non-coding SNPs between the 101 iMN patients and ethnically matched controls (Table 2). Based on our power calculations, the effect sizes that could be excluded for the various frequencies of the high-risk allele were above 1.6 to 4. For the two SNPs leading to amino acid substitutions in exons, these were 1.7 and 1.8, respectively.

When analyzing associations for the subgroup of PLA_2R positive patients ($n = 62$), the synonymous SNP rs12366144 was more frequently present in patients than in controls ($p = 0.02$) (Table 2). However, when correcting for the multiple testing of 12 SNPs, (p-value should be less than $0.05/12 = 0.00417$), this significant association disappeared. Haplotype analysis was performed including all available SNPs, but no significant associations were determined.

Association between *TRPC6* variants and clinical outcome

After a median follow-up of 80 months (range 15–166) spontaneous remission had occurred in 26 patients, and 46 patients had progressed to renal failure. Of the remaining patients, six had persistent proteinuria >2.0 gram/day with stable renal

Table 1. Primers used to sequence the 13 exons of *TRPC6*.

Exon	F/R primer	Primer sequence 5′—3′
1	F primer	GTCTGCCCAGGTCCAGTTC
1	R primer	GTACACACGCGGGTTCAG
2_01	F primer	GATGAATGGCAAGTCATTTGG
2_01	R primer	AACCTCTTGCCTTCAGCAAA
2_02	F primer	GCCAATGAGCATCTGGAAAT
2_02	R primer	AGCCGTCATGACTGGATCTT
2_03	F primer	GATTGAACGGCCTCATGATT
2_03	R primer	GGTAGCGATCACAACTTTTGC
3	F primer	AACGTGGTATTCTCCATTATTGC
3	R primer	AGCACCAACAAGAACCAAAA
4	F primer	GCCATTTGTTTGTTGCCTGT
4	R primer	TGGAGATAAGATTTTTCCCCACT
5	F primer	GGAGATCATTGGAATGTGCAG
5	R primer	AATGAACCCAAGGCAACTGT
6	F primer	TTGGGACCAAATTTTGAAGG
6	R primer	GAGAATTGTGCAGTAACCGAACT
7	F primer	GGAGACTTCCATTCGAAAACC
7	R primer	CCAAAACATTATCCCATGGAC
8	F primer	TCACTAATTTGCAGACACTAAACAA
8	R primer	CGAAGAGCAGTCCATGCTT
9	F primer	CGATCACTGGGGTCTGAGAG
9	R primer	AAAGGGATGTGGCATAGTGG
10	F primer	AGGGAAGAACCCCGTAAGAA
10	R primer	GCTTCTGAACATCTGTCCCTTT
11	F primer	TTGGCAGCCACAAAGTCTAA
11	R primer	AAGAATCACATAGTTCAAGAACCTAAA
12	F primer	GGCTCACTACAGGGAGGAAG
12	R primer	GCTCTCCAGGCACTCTGC
13	F primer	TTTCCTCCTGTCCCACAGTC
13	R primer	GGCTCCAGATGATAGGATGG

F, forward; R, reverse.

function, 19 patients were censored for outcome analysis because of treatment with immunosuppressive agents, and four patients were lost to follow-up. None of the 13 identified *TRPC6* sequence variations correlated with remission or renal failure (Table 3). An additional analysis comparing those patients in whom spontaneous remission occurred (n = 26) to all others (n = 75) also did not show differences between groups (data not shown).

Discussion

In this study, 13 SNPs in the gene encoding *TRPC6* were identified in our cohort of 101 biopsy-proven iMN patients. None of the identified SNPs was associated with the occurrence of iMN *per se*. In addition, the presence of *TRPC6* SNPs was not associated with clinical outcome in terms of remission rate, persistence of proteinuria or progression to renal failure. Thus, our data do not confirm the hypothesis that *TRPC6* SNPs could confer susceptibility to, or alter the clinical course in iMN.

Pathogenesis of iMN has been an unsolved mystery for decades. The histological features of MN were first described in 1957. [28] The characteristic finding in kidney biopsies of subepithelial deposits that consisted of IgG and complement pointed to an immunological disease ontology. In a rat model of MN, Heymann's nephritis, the disease is caused by IgG antibodies targeting megalin, a protein expressed by both rat tubular cells and podocytes. [29] Since megalin is not present on human podocytes, other pathophysiological mechanisms and other antigenic targets have been considered. A major breakthrough came with the discovery by Beck *et al.* of circulating auto-antibodies against the M-type Phospholipase A_2 receptor (PLA2R), a protein expressed by human podocytes, in the majority of patients with iMN. [2] Anti-PLA2R antibodies in iMN are mainly of the IgG4 subclass, both in serum and in biopsies. IgG4 is considered not to activate complement, but immune deposits in iMN contain large amount of complement C3. It has been suggested that anti-PLA2R antibodies might activate the lectin pathway of the complement cascade by binding to Mannose Binding Lectin. [30] However, the mechanism by which the antibodies finally lead to the membranous phenotype with severe podocyte damage is still unknown. Furthermore, the trigger for autoantibody formation remains unclear. A rare combination of (relatively) common events (genetic variants and/or environmental factors) might serve as a pathogenetic trigger in a multi-hit setting.

Next to these remaining questions on pathogenetic issues, the substantial interindividual variability in the course and prognosis of the iMN is also unexplained as yet. Why is the disease benign with a single episode and spontaneous remission in some patients, and do other patients progress to ESRD after several treatment resistant episodes? The genetic profile of the patient may be one of the aspects contributing to this interindividual variability. In another glomerulopathy, IgA nephropathy, common polymorphisms in several genes (*MYH*, *TLR9*) were associated with disease progression and development of ESRD. [31,32] Since *TRPC6* gain-of-function mutations cause podocyte injury leading to hereditary FSGS, glomerular TRPC6 expression is increased in MN, and glomerulosclerosis occurs in progressive MN, we hypothesized that polymorphisms in *TRPC6*, contribute to the susceptibility to develop iMN and/or progress to end-stage renal disease. Of note, Chen *et al.* previously showed that three *TRPC6* SNPs, which they selected on reasons that were not clearly defined, did not correlate with the occurrence of MN. [33] In our study, all exons were sequenced including splice sites in the *TRPC6* gene to identify polymorphisms in the coding regions of *TRPC6* in an unbiased manner. While we identified *TRPC6* SNPs in iMN patients, we found no association of these SNPs with disease occurrence or progression, although based on the number of patients in our cohort a limited effect size could have been missed. This means that the alleles we identified could still have functional effects on TRPC6 channel activity, of which the resulting clinical effect would fall under the effect size we can rule out. However, the majority of the identified SNPs [11] were either intronic or synonomous, minimizing the chance of any functional relevance. The two SNPs causing predicted amino acid substitutions, although of interest, clearly did not contribute to the development of MN in all patients.

In the PLA2R positive patients, one SNP showed an association, but the statistical significance of this association was lost after correction for multiple testing. In terms of genetic association studies, our cohort is quite small and we, therefore, cannot exclude that our study is underpowered to find existing associations, especially with regard to haplotypes. As only the coding regions of the *TRPC6* gene were sequenced, information on intronic polymorphisms and/or SNPs in the promoter region of the gene that might influence expression of the TRPC6 protein, is lacking.

Table 2. *TRPC6* variants in patients with iMN (n = 101).

Chr	position	name	ref	All	CEU AF	AF patients	p-value	AF PLA2R	p-value*	ref cDNA	cDNA	prot. level	effect	exon	observations
11	101454244	rs191383391	G	G/T	0.017**	0.025	0.44	0.024	0.56	C	c.-10C>A		5'-ÚTR	1	
11	101454192	rs3802829	G	G/A	0.093**	0.089	0.85	0.113	0.48	C	c.43C>T	p.Pro15Ser	missense	1	NH2-terminal region
11	101453995	rs17096918	C	C/T	0.083	0.069	0.52	0.081	0.93	G	c.170+70G>A		intron		
11	101375549	rs10501986	T	T/C	0.480	0.495	0.71	0.492	0.81	A	c.171-20A>G		intron		
11	101374812	rs144891994	C	C/T	0 ^	0.005	NA	0.008	NA	G	c.888G>A	p.Thr296Thr	synonymous	2	CCD
11	101374626	rs4542378	G	G/A	0.480	0.490	0.80	0.492	0.81	C	c.945+129C>T		intron		
11	101359750	rs36111323	G	G/A	0.135**	0.165	0.24	0.156	0.52	C	c.1211C>T	p.Ala404Val	missense	4	linker region between CCD & TMD1
11	101347093	rs12366144	A	A/G	0.250**	0.292	0.20	0.347	0.02	T	c.1683T>C	p.Asn561Asn	synonymous	6	linker region between TMD3 & TMD4
11	101342958	rs61743044	G	G/A	0.020	0.020	1.00	0.024	0.75	C	c.2115C>T	p.Tyr705Tyr	synonymous	8	linker region between TMD5 & TMD6
11	101342931	rs144891994	C	C/A	0.008	0.005	0.66	0	0.32	G	c.2142G>T	p.Thr714Thr	synonymous	8	TMD 6
11	101325970	rs7105083	G	G/A	0.263	0.238	0.47	0.266	0.93	C	c.2485-138C>T		intron		
11	101325788	rs72984209	G	G/A	0.077	0.054	0.28	0.081	0.87	C	c.2529C>T	p.Phe843Phe	synonymous	11	
11	101323770	rs12805398	C	C/T	0.140**	0.158	0.49	0.153	0.69	G	c.2712G>A	p.Gln904Gln	synonymous	13	

Chr = chromosome; position = basepair position based on UCSC genome browser version Human Feb. 2009 (GRCh37/hg19) assembly; name = rs identifier; ref = genomic reference allele; all = alleles; CEU AF = allele frequencies variant allele in control population. Control population consists of Caucasian population from 1000 Genomes project (release 10 - March 2012), complemented with data form 292 geographically matched controls for variants marked with **; ^ = not reported in 1000 Genomes project; AF patient = patient minor allele frequencies; p-value = comparison allele frequencies controls and patients; AF PLA2R = minor allele frequencies in PLA2R positive patients (n = 62); p-value* = comparison allele frequencies controls and PLA2R positive patients; genomic level = NC_000002.11; ref cDNA = reference allele cDNA (given that TRPC6 is on the negative strand); cDNA = NM_004621.5; prot. level = NP_004612.2; CCD = coiled-coiled domain; TMD = transmembrane domain.

Table 3. Genotypes in iMN patients with clinical remission versus patients with renal failure.

	Genotype	Remission n = 26 (%)		Renal Failure n = 46 (%)		p-value*
rs191383391	CC	25	(96.2)	43	(93.5)	0.64
	CA	1	(3.8)	3	(6.5)	
rs3802829	CC	22	(84.6)	37	(80.4)	0.68
	CT	4	(15.4)	9	(19.6)	
rs17096918	GG	23	(88.5)	37	(80.4)	0.40
	GA	3	(11.5)	9	(19.6)	
rs10501986	AA	9	(34.6)	10	(21.7)	0.09
	AG	15	(57.7)	25	(54.3)	
	GG	2	(7.7)	11	(23.9)	
rs144891994	GG	26	(100)	46	(100)	1.00
rs4542378	CC	9	(34.6)	9	(19.6)	0.09
	CT	15	(57.7)	27	(58.7)	
	TT	2	(7.7)	10	(21.7)	
rs36111323*	GG	19	(73.1)	31	(67.4)	0.74
	GA	7	(26.9)	14	(30.4)	
rs61743044	CC	26	(100)	43	(93.5)	1.00
	CT	0	(0)	3	(6.5)	
rs12366144	TT	16	(61.5)	20	(43.5)	0.18
	TC	9	(34.6)	23	(50.0)	
	CC	1	(3.8)	3	(6.5)	
rs145077205	GG	25	(96.2)	46	(100)	0.18
	GT	1	(3.8)	0	(0)	
rs7105083	CC	15	(57.7)	26	(56.5)	0.91
	CT	10	(38.5)	18	(39.1)	
	TT	1	(3.8)	2	(4.3)	
rs72984209	CC	23	(88.5)	41	(89.1)	0.93
	CT	3	(11.5)	5	(10.9)	
rs12805398	GG	18	(69.2)	32	(69.6)	0.88
	GA	8	(30.8)	14	(30.4)	

*N = 45 for renal failure.
*P-value for minor allele frequencies-comparison (Mann-Whitney U).

Since it is *TRPC6* gain-of-function that is associated with podocyte injury, transcriptionally-mediated increased or diminished *TRPC6* expression as a result of genetic variants in *TRPC6* regulatory regions, might influence susceptibility and prognosis.

However, assuming that *TRPC6* SNPs do not affect occurrence and progression in iMN, the question still remains why TRPC6 is overexpressed in iMN. Since TRPC6 is overexpressed in several human glomerular diseases and animal models of podocyte injury and glomerular disease, it could be a common effector in the resulting podocyte injury.[13,17] We have previously shown that AngII-mediated activation of the deleterious calcineurin/NFAT pathway, which includes Ca^{2+} influx through TRPC6 itself, leads to enhanced transcriptional expression of TRPC6 in the podocyte.[17] In addition, antiproteinuric agents like angiotensin receptor blockers, angiotensin converting enzyme inhibitors, calcineurin inhibitors and vitamin D normalize TRPC6 expression in podocyte injury and experimental glomerular disease. [17,34] Alternatively, an interesting hypothesis could be that e.g. anti-PLA2R antibodies actually activate PLA2R on the surface of the podocyte. In cell types other than podocytes, Ca^{2+} influx was demonstrated to be coupled to PLA2R activation. [35] Hypothetically, binding of anti-PLA2R antibodies to PLA2R on the podocyte could activate Ca^{2+} influx through TRPC6 and/or increase TRPC6 expression. A recent study from Kistler et al.,suggests that increasing TRPC6 expression might at first actually serve to protect the podocyte from complement-mediated injury, which seems crucial in MN. [36] Eventually, prolonged TRPC6 overexpression might then become deleterious. While *TRPC6* SNPs do not appear to alter susceptibility to iMN occurrence and progression, this new hypothesis suggests that TRPC6 indeed plays a pathophysiological role in iMN.

Author Contributions

Conceived and designed the experiments: JMH MJHC JFMW TN. Performed the experiments: JMH MJHC MMVAPS. Analyzed the data: JMH MJHC TN. Contributed reagents/materials/analysis tools: MJHC LHH NVAMK. Contributed to the writing of the manuscript: JMH MJHC TN JB JvdV JFMW TN.

References

1. Glassock RJ (1992) Secondary membranous glomerulonephritis. Nephrol Dial Transplant 7 Suppl 1: 64–71
2. Beck LH Jr, Bonegio RG, Lambeau G, Beck DM, Powell DW, Cummins TD, et al. (2009) M-type phospholipase A2 receptor as target antigen in idiopathic membranous nephropathy. N Engl J Med 361: 11–21
3. Ronco P, Debiec H (2012) Pathogenesis of membranous nephropathy: recent advances and future challenges. Nat Rev Nephrol 8: 203–213
4. Hofstra JM, Wetzels JF (2012) Anti-PLA(2)R antibodies in membranous nephropathy: ready for routine clinical practice? Neth J Med 70: 109–113
5. Stanescu HC, Arcos-Burgos M, Medlar A, Bockenhauer D, Kottgen A, Dragomirescu L, et al. (2011) Risk HLA-DQA1 and PLA(2)R1 alleles in idiopathic membranous nephropathy. The New England journal of medicine. 364: 616–626
6. Coenen MJ, Hofstra JM, Debiec H, Stanescu HC, Medlar AJ, Stengel B, et al. (2013) Phospholipase A2 Receptor (PLA2R1) Sequence Variants in Idiopathic Membranous Nephropathy. J Am Soc Nephrol. 24: 677–683
7. van den Brand JA, Hofstra JM, Wetzels JF (2011) Low-molecular-weight proteins as prognostic markers in idiopathic membranous nephropathy. Clin J Am Soc Nephrol 6: 2846–2853
8. Hofstra JM, Fervenza FC, Wetzels JF (2013) Treatment of idiopathic membranous nephropathy. Nature reviews Nephrology 9: 443–458
9. van den Brand JA, Hofstra JM, Wetzels JF (2012) Prognostic value of risk score and urinary markers in idiopathic membranous nephropathy. Clin J Am Soc Nephrol 7: 1242–1248
10. Heeringa SF, Branten AJ, Deegens JK, Steenbergen E, Wetzels JF (2007) Focal segmental glomerulosclerosis is not a sufficient predictor of renal outcome in patients with membranous nephropathy. Nephrol Dial Transplant 22: 2201–2207
11. Reiser J, Polu KR, Moller CC, Kenlan P, Altintas MM, Wei C, et al. (2005) TRPC6 is a glomerular slit diaphragm-associated channel required for normal renal function. Nat Genet 37: 739–744
12. Winn MP, Conlon PJ, Lynn KL, Farrington MK, Creazzo T, Hawkins AF, et al. (2005) A mutation in the TRPC6 cation channel causes familial focal segmental glomerulosclerosis. Science 308: 1801–1804
13. Moller CC, Wei C, Altintas MM, Li J, Greka A, Ohse T, et al. (2007) Induction of TRPC6 channel in acquired forms of proteinuric kidney disease. J Am Soc Nephrol 18: 29–36
14. Krall P, Canales CP, Kairath P, Carmona-Mora P, Molina J, Carpio JD, et al. (2010) Podocyte-specific overexpression of wild type or mutant trpc6 in mice is sufficient to cause glomerular disease. PLoS One 5: e12859.
15. Hofstra JM, Lainez S, van Kuijk WH, Schoots J, Baltissen MP, Hoefsloot LH, et al. (2013) New TRPC6 gain-of-function mutation in a non-consanguineous Dutch family with late-onset focal segmental glomerulosclerosis. Nephrol Dial Transplant 28: 1830–1838
16. Goel M, Sinkins WG, Zuo CD, Estacion M, Schilling WP (2006) Identification and localization of TRPC channels in the rat kidney. Am J Physiol Renal Physiol. 290(5):F1241–F52.
17. Nijenhuis T, Sloan AJ, Hoenderop JG, Flesche J, van GH, Kistler AD, et al. (2011) Angiotensin II contributes to podocyte injury by increasing TRPC6 expression via an NFAT-mediated positive feedback signaling pathway. Am J Pathol 179: 1719–1732
18. Zhang H, Ding J, Fan Q, Liu S (2009) TRPC6 up-regulation in Ang II-induced podocyte apoptosis might result from ERK activation and NF-kappaB translocation. Exp Biol Med 234: 1029–1036
19. Schlondorff J, Del CD, Carrasquillo R, Lacey V, Pollak MR (2009) TRPC6 mutations associated with focal segmental glomerulosclerosis cause constitutive activation of NFAT-dependent transcription. Am J Physiol Cell Physiol 296: C558–C569
20. Eckel J, Lavin PJ, Finch EA, Mukerji N, Burch J, Gbadegesin R, et al. (2011) TRPC6 enhances angiotensin II-induced albuminuria. J Am Soc Nephrol 22: 526–535
21. Hofstra JM, Wetzels JF (2012) Management of patients with membranous nephropathy. Nephrol Dial Transplant 27: 6–9
22. Debiec H, Ronco P (2011) PLA2R autoantibodies and PLA2R glomerular deposits in membranous nephropathy. N Engl J Med 364: 689–690
23. Branten AJ, du Buf-Vereijken PW, Klasen IS, Bosch FH, Feith GW, Hollander DA, et al. (2005) Urinary excretion of beta2-microglobulin and IgG predict prognosis in idiopathic membranous nephropathy: a validation study. J Am Soc Nephrol 16: 169–174
24. Miller SA, Dykes DD, Polesky HF (1988) A simple salting out procedure for extracting DNA from human nucleated cells. Nucleic Acids Res 16:1215
25. Rozen S, Skaletsky H (2000) Primer3 on the WWW for general users and for biologist programmers. Methods Mol Biol 132: 365–386
26. GenomesProject (2010) A map of human genome variation from population-scale sequencing. Nature 467: 1061–1073
27. Purcell S, Neale B, Todd-Brown K, Thomas L, Ferreira MA, Bender D, et al. (2007) PLINK: a tool set for whole-genome association and population-based linkage analyses. Am J Hum Genet 81: 559–575
28. Jones DB (1957) Nephrotic glomerulonephritis. Am J Pathol 33: 313–329
29. Kerjaschki D, Farquhar MG (1982) The pathogenic antigen of Heymann nephritis is a membrane glycoprotein of the renal proximal tubule brush border. Proc Natl Acad Sci USA 79: 5557–5561
30. Ma H, Sandor DG, Beck LH (2013) The role of complement in membranous nephropathy. Semin Nephrol 33: 531–542
31. Suzuki H, Suzuki Y, Narita I, Aizawa M, Kihara M, Yamanaka T, et al. (2008) Toll-like receptor 9 affects severity of IgA nephropathy. J Am Soc Nephrol 19: 2384–2395
32. Cheng W, Zhou X, Zhu L, Shi S, Lv J, Liu L, et al. (2011) Polymorphisms in the nonmuscle myosin heavy chain 9 gene (MYH9) are associated with the progression of IgA nephropathy in Chinese. Nephrol Dial Transplant 26: 2544–2549
33. Chen WC, Chen SY, Chen CH, Chen HY, Lin YW, Ho TJ, et al. (2010) Lack of association between transient receptor potential cation channel 6 polymorphisms and primary membranous glomerulonephritis. Renal failure 32: 666–672
34. Sonneveld R, Ferre S, Hoenderop JG, Dijkman HB, Berden JH, Bindels RJ, et al. (2013) Vitamin D down-regulates TRPC6 expression in podocyte injury and proteinuric glomerular disease. Am J Pathol 182: 1196–1204
35. Brooks RC, McCarthy KD, Lapetina EG, Morell P (1989) Receptor-stimulated phospholipase A2 activation is coupled to influx of external calcium and not to mobilization of intracellular calcium in C62B glioma cells. J Biol Chem 264: 20147–20153
36. Kistler AD, Singh G, Altintas MM, Yu H, Fernandez IC, Gu C, et al. (2013) Transient Receptor Potential Channel 6 (TRPC6) Protects Podocytes during Complement-mediated Glomerular Disease. J Biol Chem 288: 36598–36609

27

Molecular Pathogenesis of Post-Transplant Acute Kidney Injury: Assessment of Whole-Genome mRNA and MiRNA Profiles

Julia Wilflingseder[1,2], Judith Sunzenauer[2], Eva Toronyi[3], Andreas Heinzel[4], Alexander Kainz[1,2], Bernd Mayer[4], Paul Perco[4], Gábor Telkes[3], Robert M. Langer[3], Rainer Oberbauer[1,2]*

1 Department of Nephrology and Dialysis, Medical University Vienna, Vienna, Austria, **2** Department of Nephrology and Transplantation, KH Elisabethinen, Linz, Austria, **3** Department of Transplantation and Surgery, Semmelweis University, Budapest, Hungary, **4** emergentec biodevelopment GmbH, Vienna, Austria

Abstract

Acute kidney injury (AKI) affects roughly 25% of all recipients of deceased donor organs. The prevention of post-transplant AKI is still an unmet clinical need. We prospectively collected zero-hour, indication as well as protocol kidney biopsies from 166 allografts between 2011 and 2013. In this cohort eight cases with AKI and ten matched allografts without pathology serving as control group were identified with a follow-up biopsy within the first twelve days after engraftment. For this set the zero-hour and follow-up biopsies were subjected to genome wide microRNA and mRNA profiling and analysis, followed by validation in independent expression profiles of 42 AKI and 21 protocol biopsies for strictly controlling the false discovery rate. Follow-up biopsies of AKI allografts compared to time-matched protocol biopsies, further baseline adjustment for zero-hour biopsy expression level and validation in independent datasets, revealed a molecular AKI signature holding 20 mRNAs and two miRNAs (miR-182-5p and miR-21-3p). Next to several established biomarkers such as lipocalin-2 also novel candidates of interest were identified in the signature. In further experimental evaluation the elevated transcript expression level of the secretory leukocyte peptidase inhibitor (SLPI) in AKI allografts was confirmed in plasma and urine on the protein level ($p<0.001$ and $p=0.003$, respectively). miR-182-5p was identified as a molecular regulator of post-transplant AKI, strongly correlated with global gene expression changes during AKI. In summary, we identified an AKI-specific molecular signature providing the ground for novel biomarkers and target candidates such as SLPI and miR-182-5p in addressing AKI.

Editor: Giovanni Camussi, University of Torino, Italy

Funding: This study was supported by grants from the Austrian Science Fund (FWF P-21436 and P-25726) and the European Union, grant MC-IOF#328613. The funders had no role in study design, data collection and analysis, decision to publish, or preparation of the manuscript.

* Email: rainer.oberbauer@meduniwien.ac.at

Introduction

Post-transplant acute kidney injury (AKI) is a frequent complication after kidney transplantation and is associated with shortened graft survival [1,2,3]. In spite of a remarkable progress in the field of transplantation medicine, the incidence of AKI over the last 20 years remained constant. Rates between 15 and 25% have been reported, which mainly depend on the definition of AKI but also showing substantial differences between centers [4,5].

Several risk factors contributing to the development of AKI after kidney transplantation have been identified, including donor age, prolonged cold and warm ischemic times, and the use of organs procured from non-heart beating donors [5,6]. Molecular mechanisms determining the fate of kidney allografts via triggering the development of AKI remain unclear as ischemia and reperfusion injury (IRI) occur at a varying degree in all transplanted organs.

Molecular and cellular alterations associated with IRI mainly include tissue damage caused by reactive oxygen species (ROS), nitric oxide or peroxynitrite [7], but also a decreased adenylate cyclase activity and consecutive low intracellular cAMP levels. Consequences are impaired endothelial cell barrier functions (vascular permeability and leakage) [8,9]. Furthermore, significant alterations at the transcriptional level in control of gene expression occur, such as upregulation of the hypoxia inducible factor 1A (HIF1A) or the nuclear factor kappa B (NF-kB), the central regulator of inflammatory response [10]. Later on in the response cascade of IRI, cell death via apoptosis and necrosis is triggered [11]. Additionally, the activation of innate and adaptive immune response is provoked and contributes to tissue damage and injury, comprising pattern recognition receptors (PRRs) such as Toll-like receptors (TLRs) and/or infiltration of macrophages and/or T-cells [12].

Furthermore, microRNAs (miRNAs) were identified to be involved in the molecular cascade following IRI. miRNAs are post-transcriptional modulators that regulate target genes by perfect- or semi-complementary base pairing, finally resulting in RNA degradation or inhibition of translation, respectively [13].

Godwin et al. and Shapiro et al. reported miRNA signatures after warm ischemia followed by reperfusion in mice kidneys [14,15], and our group recently showed a deregulation of miRNAs in human post-transplantation (TX) AKI biopsies [16]. However, our knowledge on how miRNAs regulate gene expression in injured kidney tissue and impact transcript and protein levels is fairly understood.

This study was designed to specifically elucidate molecular regulation patterns on the combined level of mRNA and microRNA expression of transplant kidneys diagnosed with AKI versus grafts showing prompt organ function.

Materials and Methods

Renal transplant biopsy specimen

The study protocol was approved by the Institutional Review Board (IRB) (Ethical Committee of the Semmelweis University Budapest # 20303-0/2010-1018EKU (821/PI/01)), and all recipients provided written informed consent to follow-up allograft biopsy and blood and urine samples for research. There was no need for informed consent for zero-hour biopsies from deceased donor organs according to the IRB protocol, as allowance to perform autopsy existed. Living donors gave written informed consent to zero-hour donor biopsy for research.

We prospectively collected zero-hour biopsies from 166 renal allograft recipients from March 2011 to April 2013. From these 166 recipients, 34 had a follow-up kidney biopsy within 12 days after transplantation with the following clinical conditions: (i) 16 rejections (eight Banff 1, two Banff 2, one antibody-mediated rejection, two Banff 1 rejections with humoral rejection signs and three Banff Borderline rejections), (ii) eight with acute tubular necrosis without rejection defined as AKI and (iii) ten protocol biopsies without pathology acting as control group (primary graft function). AKI was defined as acute tubular necrosis in the absence of cellular and/or humoral signs of rejection according to the Banff 2012 criteria [17]. The indication for AKI kidney biopsy was more than one dialysis session within the first week after transplantation and a serum creatinine above 4 mg/dL after the first week. Together with the post-TX biopsies, EDTA-plasma and urine was collected from the recipients. The biopsy specimens were immediately submerged in RNAlater^{TM} (Ambion, Austin, Texas, USA) ensuring maximal RNA quality. For the present study we used (i) eight biopsy pairs with histological lesions of acute tubular necrosis in the post-TX biopsies (AKI group) and (ii) ten allografts with primary function and protocol biopsies without pathology (PGF group).

RNA Extraction and Microarray Hybridization

Total RNA was isolated and purified using chloroform and trizol reagent (Invitrogen, Carlsbad, California USA). RNA yield and quality were checked with the Agilent 2100 Bioanalyzer (Agilent, Palo Alto, California, USA). Kidney mRNA expression analysis was performed according to the NuGEN-recommended protocol using the Affymetrix GeneChip Human Gene 2.0 ST Array. Affymetrix GeneChip miRNA 3.0 Arrays were used for miRNA profiling. Total RNA (1 μg per sample) was labeled using the FlashTag^{TM} Biotin HSR RNA Labeling Kit (Affymetrix, Santa Clara, California, USA) and hybridized to the arrays as described by the manufacturer.

miRNA and mRNA microarray analysis

Affymetrix data were pre-processed, normalized, and summarized using the robust multi-average (RMA) method with quantile normalization, and annotated using the corresponding annotation file (.cdf) in Bioconductor. Microarray raw data files are available in the Gene Expression Omnibus (GEO) at NCBI with the accession number GSE53773. Interquartile range and intensity filtering were used to exclude features with low variance and signal intensity (log_2 level <4) over all profiles [18]. Significance Analysis of Microarrays (SAM) was used to determine differentially regulated mRNAs and miRNAs comparing AKI and control group samples [19]. The false discovery rate (FDR) was set to < 10% and the minimum fold change to 1.5 in order to detect significantly differentially regulated transcripts. Further, the derived mRNA and miRNA AKI signatures were verified in independent datasets [16,20]. Principal component analysis was performed based on the covariance matrix to visualize the variance in the gene expression signatures of the allografts. Spearman correlation was applied to evaluate association of differentially regulated miRNAs and mRNAs. Functional grouping of genes was based on Gene Ontology (GO) terms utilizing the DAVID Functional Annotation platform [21]. Three algorithms were used to predict miRNA targets, namely DIANAmT, miRanda and Targetscan [22,23,24]. Only miRNA targets identified by all three prediction algorithms were included in further analysis. Additionally, experimentally validated targets were extracted for identified miRNAs from miRTarBase [25].

To extract biomarker candidates discussed in the context of AKI the text mining tool FABLE (http://fable.chop.edu/overview.jsp) was used [26], taking into account all genes having at least two scientific references with the following search terms: 'Acute kidney injury' and 'Biomarker'.

Quantitation of SLPI protein concentration

We used a quantitative sandwich enzyme-linked immunoassay (ELISA) to determine the protein concentration of SLPI in plasma and urine as described by the manufacturer (R&D Systems, Minneapolis, MN, USA, article# DPI00).

Statistical analysis of clinical data

Continuous data were analyzed by non-parametric Wilcoxon Rank Sum Test. Categorical data were evaluated by Chi-square test or Fisher's exact test where appropriate. A p-value below 0.05 was considered statistically significant. Statistical assessment was performed with SAS for Windows 9.3 (The SAS Institute, Inc., Cary, North Carolina, USA).

Results

Patient characteristics

We first analyzed two sequential biopsies in 18 different kidney grafts (Basic mRNA and miRNA dataset). The first biopsy was carried out at implantation after cold storage (zero-hour biopsy) and the second biopsy was taken within 12 days after transplantation. Eight allografts fulfilled histological criteria for acute tubular injury in the post-TX biopsy (AKI group), and the other ten allografts had primary graft function (PGF) serving as control group with no pathology in the post-TX biopsy (protocol biopsy). Demographic data on the 18 transplant donors and recipients are provided in Table 1. None of the demographic variables of the recipient and donor pairs were significantly different between the two groups. Median donor age was numerically higher in the AKI group (53 years; interquartile range (IQR): [46.8; 56.8]) when compared to the PGF group (42.3 years; IQR: [40.3; 50], $p = 0.28$). All deceased donors received catecholamines before organ retrieval. Median serum creatinine level at time of post-TX biopsy was 9.81 mg/dL in the AKI group and 1.54 mg/dL in the PGF group ($p<0.001$). Independent publicly available mRNA and

Table 1. Kidney donor and recipient characteristics comparing AKI and control groups in the Basic and independent validation datasets.

	Basic mRNA and miRNA dataset			*Independent mRNA dataset Famulski et al. [20]*			*Independent miRNA dataset Wilflingseder et al. [16]*		
Variable	**PGF**	**AKI**	***p*-value**	**Protocol Biopsy Cohort**	**AKI**	***p*-value**	**Protocol Biopsy Cohort**	**AKI**	***p*-value**
Number of total biopsies	20	16	na	11	28	na	10	14	na
Number of 0 h biopsies	10	8	na	0	0	na	0	0	na
Number of donor organs	10	8	na	10	26	na	10	13	na
Donor age (years)	42.5 (40.3; 50)	53 (46.8; 56.5)	0.284	55 (20–82)[b]	53 (22–69)[b]	>0.05	59.5 (54.0; 67.0)	51.0 (46.0; 64.0)	0.42
Donor sex (m/f)	4/6	5/3	0.637[a]	n. st.	n. st.	n. st.	6/4	5/8	0.41
Donor source (living/deceased)	0/10	2/6	0.183[a]	2/9	11/15	>0.05	6/4	0/13	<0.01[a]
Donor last creatinine (mg/dl)	0.94 (0.85; 1.19)	0.92 (0.78; 1.06)	0.475	n. st.	n. st.	n. st.	0.82 (0.69; 0.92)	0.95 (0.7; 1.4)	0.17
Recipient sex (m/f)	8/2	6/2	1.000[a]	n. st.	n. st.	n. st.	3/7	2/11	0.62
Recipient age (years)	57.6 (47.9; 62.9)	55.3 (50.1; 58.7)	0.824	49 (29–70)[c]	52 (16–75)[c]	>0.05	50.8 (41.3; 59.1)	53.5 (47.2; 65.1)	0.34
Transplant number (1/2/3/4/5)	9/1/0/0/0	6/0/2/0/0	0.183[a]	n. st.	n. st.	n. st.	10/0/0/0/0	10/1/1/0/1	1.00[a]
Cold ischemic time (hours)	13.5 (11.9; 17.6)	12.8 (7.5; 15.5)	0.398	n. st.	n. st.	n. st.	1.0 (0.0; 8)	11.5 (10; 17.5)	<0.01
PRA latest (%)	0 (0; 4.5)	2 (0; 18)	0.363	n. st.	n. st.	n. st.	0.0 (0.0; 0.0)	0.0 (0.0; 5.0)	0.02
Sum of HLA mismatches (0/1/2/3/4/5)	2/0/2/4/1/1	0/1/0/2/1/4	0.231[a]	n. st.	n. st.	n. st.	0/1/2/4/2/1	3/3/1/4/1/1	0.57
Immunosuppression (CNI/else)	9/1	8/0	1.000[a]	n. st.	n. st.	n. st.	9/1	12/1	1.00[a]
Induction therapy (none/IL2/ATG)	8/1/1	6/1/1	1.000[a]	n. st.	n. st.	n. st.	6/3/1	11/1/1	0.26[a]
Time from TX to biopsy (days)	7.5 (6.3; 9.8)	7 (6; 9.5)	0.651	42	16 (6–42)[c]	<0.001	104.5 (102; 109.5)	7 (2; 8)	<0.001
Serum creatinine at post-TX biopsy	1.54 (1.32; 1.73)	9.81 (5.74; 10.14)	<0.001	n. st.	n. st.	n. st.	n. st.	n. st.	n. st.

Continuous data are provided as median and 1st and 3rd quartile; categorical data are shown as counts.
na … not applicable,
[a]Fisher's exact test,
[b]mean (range),
[c]median (range),
n. st. … not stated.
PGF … primary graft function, AKI … acute kidney injury.

Table 2. AKI mRNA signature as verified in the independent evaluation dataset.

		post-TX		baseline adjusted		
Probe Set ID	**Gene Symbol**	**raw p-value**	**Fold change**	**raw p-value**	**Fold change**	**Gene Description**
16919547	SLPI	1.55E-03	5.67	1.20E-03	15.17	secretory leukocyte peptidase inhibitor
16775083	OLFM4	6.15E-03	2.86	2.98E-03	7.88	olfactomedin 4
16787902	SERPINA3	1.08E-03	2.03	2.91E-03	7.03	serpin peptidase inhibitor, clade A (alpha-1 antiproteinase, antitrypsin), member 3
16743647	**MMP7**	**3.42E-02**	**2.88**	**1.54E-02**	**4.06**	**matrix metallopeptidase 7 (matrilysin, uterine)**
16760792	CD163	2.77E-02	1.94	1.69E-02	3.12	CD163 molecule
16693414	**S100A8**	**7.43E-04**	**2.40**	**1.66E-02**	**3.09**	**S100 calcium binding protein A8**
16735751	LYVE1	7.55E-04	1.53	2.09E-03	2.28	lymphatic vessel endothelial hyaluronan receptor 1
17089525	**LCN2**	**5.02E-03**	**1.95**	**8.81E-03**	**2.28**	**lipocalin 2**
16707503	EXOC6	8.75E-04	1.52	1.88E-03	1.78	exocyst complex component 6
17024144	IFNGR1	4.61E-03	1.51	7.64E-03	1.77	interferon gamma receptor 1
17087615	LPPR1	5.54E-04	0.51	3.00E-03	0.57	lipid phosphate phosphatase-related protein type 1
16991527	CYFIP2	2.00E-03	0.55	2.80E-03	0.52	cytoplasmic FMR1 interacting protein 2
16695262	KCNJ10	3.92E-04	0.55	3.00E-04	0.52	potassium inwardly-rectifying channel, subfamily J, member 10
17101262	ARSF	1.46E-03	0.57	3.30E-03	0.47	arylsulfatase F
17094946	TRPM6	1.89E-02	0.62	2.19E-03	0.45	transient receptor potential cation channel, subfamily M, member 6
17072059	SLC30A8	2.29E-02	0.53	4.78E-03	0.45	solute carrier family 30 (zinc transporter), member 8
16773086	FGF9	4.37E-04	0.55	8.50E-04	0.45	fibroblast growth factor 9 (glia-activating factor)
16934643	PVALB	2.02E-04	0.39	2.75E-03	0.42	parvalbumin
17007950	PNPLA1	1.15E-03	0.50	1.10E-03	0.36	patatin-like phospholipase domain containing 1
16962671	TMEM207	1.57E-04	0.32	9.31E-04	0.33	transmembrane protein 207

bold......molecular features discussed as biomarker candidates of acute kidney injury.
Raw p-values and fold changes of verified differentially regulated genes are provided.

miRNA datasets were used for validation of findings in the Basic mRNA and miRNA dataset. The independent mRNA dataset comprised renal post-TX biopsies from allografts diagnosed with AKI (n = 28) and six week protocol biopsies (n = 11) published by Famulski et al. in 2012 [20] and the independent miRNA dataset consisted of miRNA profiles of AKI post-TX biopsies (n = 14) and three-month protocol biopsies (n = 10) from one of our previous studies [16]. Patient characteristics from these published datasets were extracted from the original publications and are also provided in Table 1. A significant difference was found in biopsy collection time between the AKI and protocol biopsy groups and no zero-hour biopsies were collected in these studies. Variables not found in the original publications are indicated as 'not stated'.

Molecular phenotype of post-transplant AKI

Differentially regulated genes in the injured kidney. In a first analysis we compared mRNA profiles of post-TX biopsies between the AKI (n = 8) and PGF group (n = 10) using the SAM method setting the FDR to <10%. In total, 245 differentially regulated genes were identified showing fold changes >1.5 (Table

Table 3. AKI miRNA signature as verified in the evaluation dataset.

			post-TX		baseline adjusted	
Probe Set ID	**miRNA Name**	**miRBase Accession**	**raw *p*-value**	**Fold change**	**raw *p*-value**	**Fold change**
hsa-miR-21-star_st	hsa-miR-21-3p	MIMAT0004494	1.64E-02	2.22	2.41E-02	3.34
hsa-miR-182_st	hsa-miR-182-5p	MIMAT0000259	1.62E-02	1.56	2.46E-03	1.88

Raw p-values and fold changes of verified differentially regulated miRNAs are provided.

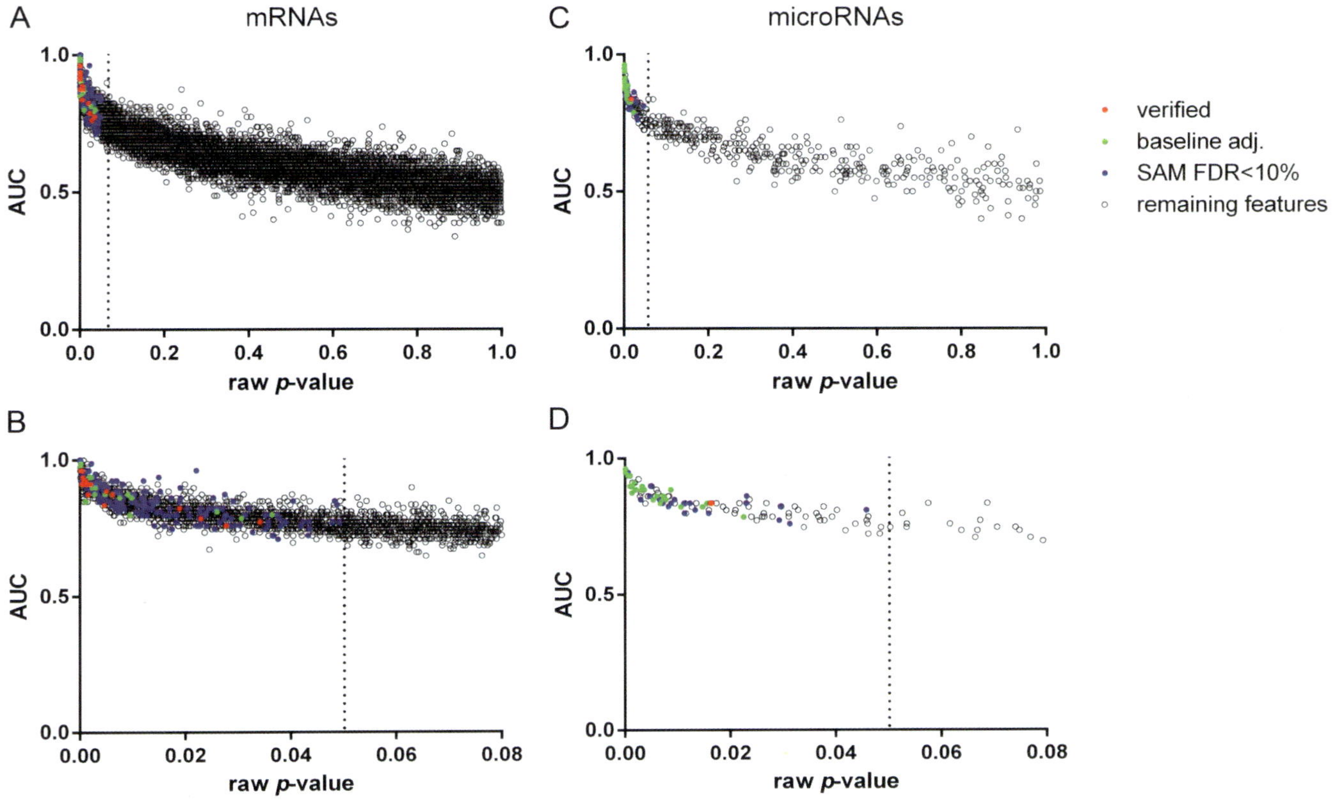

Figure 1. Raw p-values and area under the curve (AUC) of the investigated mRNAs and miRNAs comparing post-TX AKI and PGF allografts. (A) full p-value range of mRNAs (B) mRNAs with p-value<0.08 on the x-axis for specific visualization of features with a raw p-value<0.05 (C) full p-value range of microRNAs (D) microRNAs with raw p-value<0.08 on the x-axis; red: features verified in an independent dataset (20 mRNAs and two microRNAs), green: significant features after baseline adjustment (39 mRNAs and 29 miRNAs), blue: significant features identified by SAM (245 mRNAs and 49 microRNAs), black: remaining features (11,788 mRNAs and 393 microRNAs).

S1). Based on the 245 differentially regulated genes, principal component analysis (PCA) was performed. Samples were clustered utilizing the first three principal components that captured over 85% of the variance in the dataset (Figure S1).The 18 allografts separated into two distinct clusters in line with pathology stages, indicating that AKI allografts could be characterized based on the 245 differentially regulated genes. Functional annotation of the 245 genes revealed several significantly over-represented biological processes such as 'response to wounding', 'response to toxin', or 'response to metal ion and oxidation-reduction' (Table S2).

In a second step we also factored the mRNA expression levels of the zero-hour biopsies into the analysis by calculating the $\log_2$ expression difference between the two sequential biopsies of each allograft, and then again comparing AKI allografts vs. allografts with primary graft function (baseline adjustment). This analysis allowed us to identify the expression level trajectory in the development of AKI from implantation to the histological diagnosis of AKI in the recipient. 39 genes of the initial set of 245 genes still showed significant deregulation on the transcript level in the development of AKI (Table S3).

To assess the validity of the identified differentially regulated genes we evaluated our results in the mRNA dataset from Famulski et al., 2012 (GEO accession number: GSE30718) [20]. After re-analysis of this mRNA expression dataset utilizing the same statistical workflow as applied for our profiles, 932 genes were identified as significantly differentially regulated between the 28 AKI samples and 11 protocol biopsies without signs of AKI. A significant overlap was observed for our set of 39 baseline-adjusted AKI genes, with 20 also being present in the dataset from Famulski et al. (Chi-square test, $p<0.001$, using the total number of shared features on the Affymetrix arrays as reference, Table 2). The 20 shared genes could be categorized into the following biological processes: (i) 'response to wounding' (LYVE1, S100A8, SERPINA3, CD163; $p=0.02$), (ii) 'acute-phase response' (SERPINA3, CD163; $p=0.04$) and (iii) 'inflammatory response' (S100A8, SERPINA3, CD163; $p=0.04$).

Several of these deregulated genes were shown to be AKI biomarker candidates already discussed in the scientific literature according to FABLE analysis (highlighted bold in the gene lists, Table S1, S3 and Table 2), including MMP7, LCN2 and S100A8, supporting the validity of the identified AKI signature (Table 2).

Differentially regulated miRNAs in AKI. Deregulated miRNAs were identified following the same analysis workflow as used for deriving the mRNA profiles. 49 microRNAs were significantly upregulated in the AKI post-TX biopsies by more than 1.5 fold (SAM, FDR <10%, Table S4) compared to the PGF group. miRNAs with significant down-regulation were not detected. After expression baseline adjustment taking expression levels of the zero-hour biopsies into account, 29 miRNAs remained significantly differentially regulated (Table S5). For verification of the identified miRNAs a dataset recently published by our group was used (GEO accession number: GSE30282) [16]. We again re-analyzed this dataset by comparing miRNA profiles of AKI post-TX biopsies (n = 14) and three-month protocol

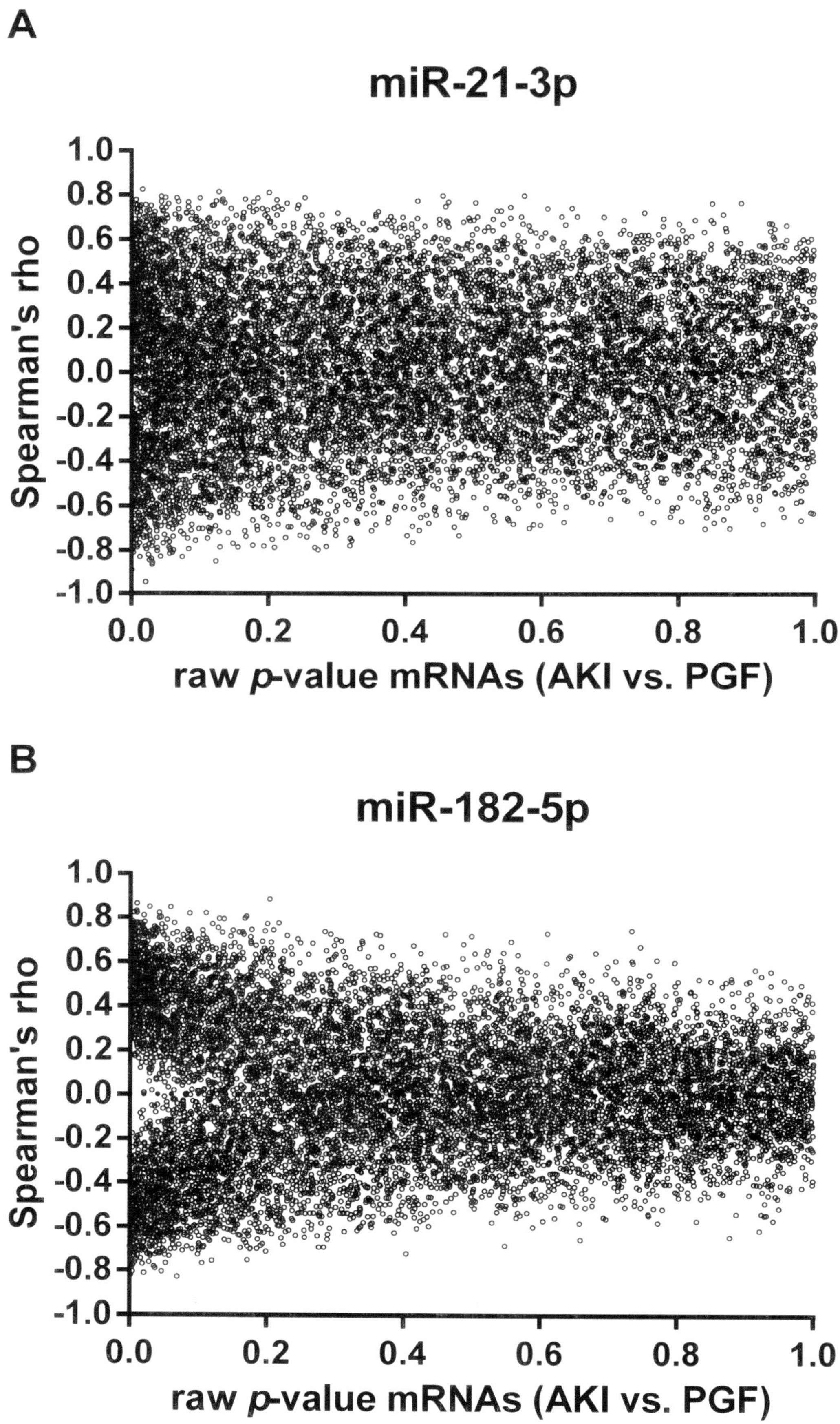
A
miR-21-3p
Spearman's rho
1.0
0.8
0.6
0.4
0.2
0.0
-0.2
-0.4
-0.6
-0.8
-1.0
0.0
0.2
0.4
0.6
0.8
1.0
raw p-value mRNAs (AKI vs. PGF)
B
miR-182-5p
Spearman's rho
1.0
0.8
0.6
0.4
0.2
0.0
-0.2
-0.4
-0.6
-0.8
-1.0
0.0
0.2
0.4
0.6
0.8
1.0
raw p-value mRNAs (AKI vs. PGF)

Figure 2. Correlation coefficients (Spearman's rho) of (A) miR-21-3p and (B) miR-182-5p and mRNAs plotted against the corresponding raw *p*-values of baseline adjusted mRNA levels comparing the AKI and PGF group.

biopsies (n = 10) of kidneys with no AKI history, and identified twelve miRNAs as significantly upregulated. Of these 12 miRNAs from our validation set, two miRNAs (miR-21-3p and miR-182-5p) were found in the baseline-adjusted list of 29 miRNAs (Table 3). Only five out of the 29 differentially regulated miRNAs were present as probes on the Affymetrix array that was used in our validation dataset. Therefore an overlap of two miRNAs was still statistically significant when taking into account the number of common and valid probes of mature miRNAs on the two different arrays (Fisher's exact test, p = 0.03).

Figure 1 shows the raw *p*-values of the investigated mRNAs and miRNAs resulting from the group comparisons of post-TX AKI and PGF allografts plotted against the area under the curve (AUC) of the receiver operating characteristic (ROC) curve computed for each individual transcript. Significantly differentially regulated mRNAs and miRNAs are highlighted in color. Indeed, baseline adjustment and verification in an independent dataset led to selection of features with a lower *p*-value and a higher AUC value, strengthening the utility of our analysis approach.

MicroRNA-182-5p expression is correlated with global gene expression response of post-transplant AKI

Spearman correlation was used to associate miRNA and mRNA expression levels. Correlation coefficients of the verified miRNAs, miR-21-3p and miR-182-5p, were calculated for the baseline-adjusted mRNA expression levels and plotted against the raw *p*-values of the mRNAs comparing AKI and PGF allografts (Figure 2). Apparently, the expression levels of miR-182-5p showed a more pronounced correlation with the differentially regulated mRNAs as indicated by the funnel at lower p-values in Figure 2B. Correlation with miR-21-3p expression levels did not exhibit this effect (Figure 2A) suggesting a central role of miR-182-5p in graft injury.

We identified three further miRNAs (miR-132-3p, miR-212-3p and miR-149-3p) not being covered in the verification data set with a similar correlation pattern as seen for miR-182-5p (Figure S2). Together these four miRNAs are highly correlated ($R<-0.7$ or >0.7) to 26 baseline adjusted differentially regulated mRNAs (Table S6), which can be categorized into the biological processes 'ECM-receptor interaction' ($p = 0.004$) and 'Focal adhesion' ($p = 0.02$). Further two genes with a negative correlation coefficient are potential direct targets of two miRNAs based on three miRNA target prediction algorithms (DIANAmT, miRanda and TargetScan). miR-182-5p is predicted to be a potential inhibitor of klotho (KL) and miR-149-3p of potassium inwardly-rectifying channel, subfamily J, member 10 (KCNJ10). None of the correlated genes were experimentally verified targets of the four miRNAs according to miRTarBase.

Validation of a potential novel biomarker of AKI in plasma and urine

To further assess the validity of our findings also on the protein level, we selected the protein product of the gene revealing the strongest association with AKI according to mRNA expression fold change, namely the secretory leukocyte peptidase inhibitor (SLPI). SLPI protein concentrations were determined in EDTA-plasma and urine of the 18 kidney allograft recipients. EDTA plasma and urine were collected at the same day as the post-TX biopsy. For three AKI patients only plasma was available due to lack of urine excretion. SLPI protein concentration was found to be significantly elevated in plasma as well as in urine of AKI patients when compared to the PGF group (Figure 3). Median SLPI concentration in plasma was 117 ng/ml (IQR: [96; 132]) in the AKI group and 71 ng/ml (IQR: [60; 72]) in the PGF group ($p<0.001$, Figure 3A). In urine the SLPI concentration was 73 ng/ml (IQR: [25; 156]) in the AKI group (n = 5) and 3.6 ng/ml (IQR: [2.5; 5.6]) in the PGF group ($p = 0.003$, Figure 3B). SLPI gene expression levels in the transplant kidneys were also highly correlated with SLPI protein concentrations in urine ($R = 0.77$) and plasma ($R = 0.57$), respectively. Relative gene expression of SLPI in post-TX biopsies is shown in Figure 3C.

Discussion

This study provides a comprehensive molecular picture of post-transplant AKI on the combined mRNA and miRNA level. As all transplant organs experienced IRI, the comparison between AKI and time-matched biopsies from allografts with primary function within the first days after transplantation allowed us to investigate the molecular profiles leading to poor initial graft function and acute tubular injury. Several known as well as novel molecules were identified.

The clinical consequences of post-transplant AKI leading to delayed graft function (DGF) were extensively investigated. A meta-analysis of 33 studies showed that recipients with DGF had an increase of relative risk (RR) by 41% to lose their graft in a median follow-up time of 3.2 years [2]. Further, DGF was associated with an augmented rate of acute rejection episodes (RR 18%–66%) and higher serum creatinine levels at the end of the follow-up period [2,27,28]. Therefore, prevention of DGF is of significant medical relevance, especially regarding limited donor pools and the acceptance of further marginal donor kidneys [29,30,31,32].

Our current understanding of the molecular mechanisms underlying post-transplant AKI is mainly based on investigations of IRI [33] and of zero-hour kidney transplant biopsies [34,35,36]. To our knowledge only one study so far analyzed the transcriptome of human renal allograft biopsies during AKI [20] which was also used as independent validation set for findings of the current study. Six-week protocol biopsies of allografts with no history of AKI and stable kidney function (n = 11) served as the control group in this study. The validation study for our miRNA findings was based on protocol biopsies procured after three months [16]. Aside these differences in follow-up time a significant overlap of deregulated mRNAs and miRNAs was found, providing us with a stable molecular AKI signature on mRNA and miRNA level. Several biomarker candidates were found in the list of differentially regulated genes, with some of them discussed as prognostic markers regarding future graft function such as lipocalin-2 (LCN2) and Kidney Injury Molecule 1 (HAVCR1) [37,38,39], allowing to deduce an association with intrinsic injury in the kidney linked to outcome. Hence, the consensus mRNA and miRNA AKI signature may be utilized to establish biomarkers providing a better approximation of the injury status in the organ. We evaluated one of these candidates, SLPI, on the protein level in plasma and urine of the transplant recipients. We could confirm the significantly elevated SLPI mRNA expression in injured allografts both in plasma and urine of AKI patients also on the protein level. Furthermore SLPI urine concentration was highly

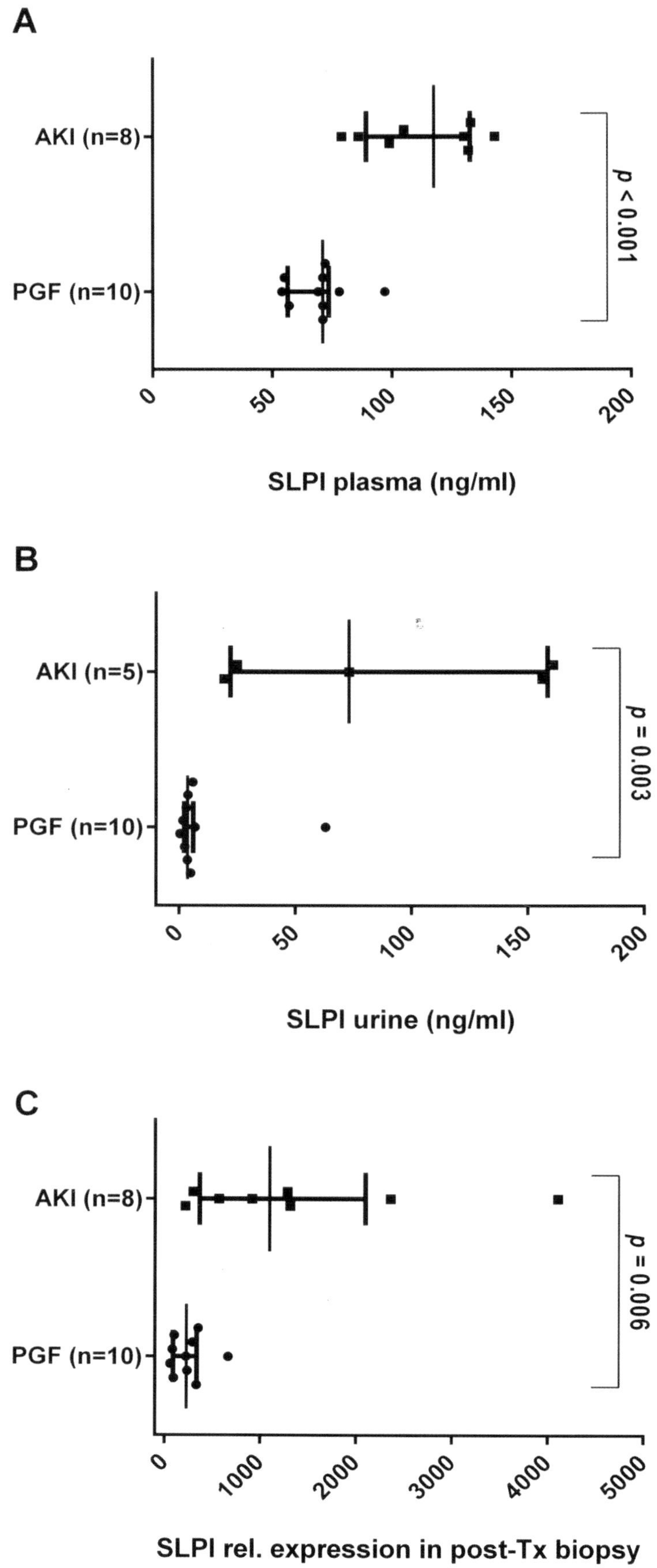
A
AKI (n=8)
PGF (n=10)
p < 0.001
0
50
100
150
200
SLPI plasma (ng/ml)
B
AKI (n=5)
PGF (n=10)
p = 0.003
0
50
100
150
200
SLPI urine (ng/ml)
C
AKI (n=8)
PGF (n=10)
p = 0.006
0
1000
2000
3000
4000
5000
SLPI rel. expression in post-Tx biopsy

Figure 3. SLPI protein concentration (ng/ml) measured by sandwich ELISA in (A) EDTA-plasma and (B) urine of AKI and PGF patients. Three AKI patients were anuric at the time of post-TX biopsy. (C) Relative gene expression levels of SLPI in post-TX biopsies. Individual data points as well as median, 1st and 3rd quartile are provided.

correlated with SLPI gene expression in the organ, indicating a link of elevated SLPI concentration in urine to the status of kidney damage in the organ itself. Tubule epithelial cells have already been identified by immunohistochemistry as the source of SLPI protein expression in the kidney [40]. However, further evaluation in larger patient cohorts is needed to assess the applicability of SLPI as a novel biomarker for AKI.

On the molecular level the most challenging part is to distinguish repair response from mechanisms causing devastating injury in the donor organ and subsequent detrimental effects on graft and patient survival. Final proof can only be accomplished in functional studies of the involved molecules. However, unbiased explorative analyses such as the present study are important for discovery, hypothesis generation and refinement. Therapeutic targets currently under investigation for DGF and IRI are summarized in two recently published reviews [5,41]. Inhibition of the Toll-like receptor 2 (TLR2) is one of the experimental strategies (clinicaltrials.gov: NCT01794663). TLR signaling leads to an accelerated immune response and can be activated by so called 'danger signals' (i.e. from damaged tissue) [42]. We found a higher expression of TLR2 in AKI allografts (Table S1).

miRNAs are currently under intense investigation as therapeutic agents and potent modifiers of immune response and tolerance [43]. miRNAs are shown to regulate entire molecular networks via simultaneous targeting of several hundred genes [44]. This makes miRNAs, in contrast to compounds targeting a single molecule, interesting for clinical phenotypes such as AKI where entire cellular processes are deregulated.

miR-182-5p expression is profoundly correlated with genes identified to be strongly associated with kidney tissue injury. miR-182-5p can be activated by IL2 and STAT5 and inhibits FOXO1 expression [45]. FOXO1 acts as a master cellular regulator of a variety of cellular processes including cell survival, apoptosis, proliferation and metabolism, and also plays a critical role in the homeostasis of cells of the immune system including T-cells, B-cells and neutrophils [46]. Further, the absence of FOXO1 was shown to severely curtail the development of FOXP3+ regulatory T-cells (Tregs). Those Tregs that nevertheless developed were found to be non-functional *in vivo* and down-regulation of FOXO1 in T-cells resulted in lymphocyte infiltration [47]. Further, BCL2 is a direct target of miR-182-5p and inhibition of miR-182-5p resulted in a higher protein expression of BCL2, suggesting potent anti-apoptotic effects [48,49].

Certainly there are limitations in the interpretation of the given kidney biopsy mRNA and miRNA profiles such as the limited sample size, which we aimed to compensate by controlling the FDR, and importantly via validation in independent sample cohorts. Additionally we confirmed differentially regulation of three mRNAs in the Basic dataset and two miRNAs in the independent miRNA dataset by qRT-PCR (Figure S3). Further, as microRNAs are post-transcriptional regulators which mainly inhibit translation of mRNAs into proteins [44], we based the identification of miRNA regulators on correlation analysis with the corresponding mRNA profiles of each allograft. This allowed us to capture the global impact on gene expression of the microRNA regulators [50].

Taken together, an AKI-specific molecular signature on the mRNA and miRNA level was identified. The identified molecules and processes set the stage for subsequent injury specific biomarker validation and functional studies uncovering the relation to immune-associated damage and repair response. This will lead to further improvement in understanding and potential clinical management of AKI.

Supporting Information

Figure S1 Principal component analysis based on the 245 differentially regulated genes comparing post-TX AKI and PGF allografts. The first three principal components (PC) were plotted, capturing 85% of the variance in the dataset. Acute kidney injury allografts (grey spheres) and allografts with primary kidney function (black spheres) form two distinct clusters.

Figure S2 Correlation coefficients (Spearman's rho) of (A) miR-132-3p and (B) miR-212-3p (C) miR-149-3p calculated for all mRNAs against the raw p-values of baseline adjusted mRNA levels between the AKI and PGF group.

Figure S3 qRT-PCR validation of significantly differentially regulated (A) mRNAs (SLPI, MMP7 and LCN2) and (B) miRNAs (miR-182-5p and miR-21-3p) between AKI and control group (PGF). Log_2 (relative expression) values are shown for the qRT-PCR and the array experiment. Individual data points as well as median, 1st and 3rd quartile are provided.

Table S1 245 significantly differentially regulated mRNAs comparing post-TX AKI and protocol biopsies from allografts with primary graft function.

Table S2 Significantly over-represented biological processes embedded in the post-TX mRNA signature (245 mRNAs).

Table S3 39 significantly differentially regulated mRNAs comparing AKI and PGF allografts after baseline adjustment.

Table S4 Significantly differentially regulated miRNAs comparing post-TX AKI and protocol biopsies from allografts with primary graft function.

Table S5 Significantly differentially regulated microRNAs comparing AKI and PGF allografts after baseline adjustment.

Table S6 Highly correlated genes (Spearman's rho >0.7 or <−0.7) to miR-182-5p, miR-132-3p, miR-212-3p and miR-149-3p out of the baseline adjusted differentially regulated gene list.

Author Contributions

Conceived and designed the experiments: JW RO. Performed the experiments: JW JS. Analyzed the data: JW AH PP. Contributed to the writing of the manuscript: JW RO BM. Collected clinical samples: ET GT RL. Prepared the figures: JW AK. Reviewed the manuscript: AH BM PP ET GT RL RO.

References

1. Hariharan S, McBride MA, Cherikh WS, Tolleris CB, Bresnahan BA, et al. (2002) Post-transplant renal function in the first year predicts long-term kidney transplant survival. Kidney Int 62: 311–318.
2. Yarlagadda SG, Coca SG, Formica RN Jr, Poggio ED, Parikh CR (2009) Association between delayed graft function and allograft and patient survival: a systematic review and meta-analysis. Nephrol Dial Transplant 24: 1039–1047.
3. Legendre C, Canaud G, Martinez F (2013) Factors influencing long-term outcome after kidney transplantation. Transpl Int.
4. Perico N, Cattaneo D, Sayegh MH, Remuzzi G (2004) Delayed graft function in kidney transplantation. Lancet 364: 1814–1827.
5. Siedlecki A, Irish W, Brennan DC (2011) Delayed graft function in the kidney transplant. Am J Transplant 11: 2279–2296.
6. Irish WD, Ilsley JN, Schnitzler MA, Feng S, Brennan DC (2010) A risk prediction model for delayed graft function in the current era of deceased donor renal transplantation. Am J Transplant 10: 2279–2286.
7. Chatterjee PK (2007) Novel pharmacological approaches to the treatment of renal ischemia-reperfusion injury: a comprehensive review. Naunyn Schmiedebergs Arch Pharmacol 376: 1–43.
8. Ogawa S, Gerlach H, Esposito C, Pasagian-Macaulay A, Brett J, et al. (1990) Hypoxia modulates the barrier and coagulant function of cultured bovine endothelium. Increased monolayer permeability and induction of procoagulant properties. J Clin Invest 85: 1090–1098.
9. Ogawa S, Koga S, Kuwabara K, Brett J, Morrow B, et al. (1992) Hypoxia-induced increased permeability of endothelial monolayers occurs through lowering of cellular cAMP levels. Am J Physiol 262: C546–554.
10. Eltzschig HK, Carmeliet P (2011) Hypoxia and inflammation. N Engl J Med 364: 656–665.
11. Hotchkiss RS, Strasser A, McDunn JE, Swanson PE (2009) Cell death. N Engl J Med 361: 1570–1583.
12. Chen GY, Nunez G (2010) Sterile inflammation: sensing and reacting to damage. Nat Rev Immunol 10: 826–837.
13. Fabian MR, Sonenberg N, Filipowicz W (2010) Regulation of mRNA translation and stability by microRNAs. Annu Rev Biochem 79: 351–379.
14. Godwin JG, Ge X, Stephan K, Jurisch A, Tullius SG, et al. (2010) Identification of a microRNA signature of renal ischemia reperfusion injury. Proc Natl Acad Sci U S A 107: 14339–14344.
15. Shapiro MD, Bagley J, Latz J, Godwin JG, Ge X, et al. (2011) MicroRNA expression data reveals a signature of kidney damage following ischemia reperfusion injury. PLoS One 6: e23011.
16. Wilflingseder J, Regele H, Perco P, Kainz A, Soleiman A, et al. (2013) miRNA profiling discriminates types of rejection and injury in human renal allografts. Transplantation 95: 835–841.
17. Solez K, Colvin RB, Racusen LC, Haas M, Sis B, et al. (2008) Banff 07 classification of renal allograft pathology: updates and future directions. Am J Transplant 8: 753–760.
18. Gentleman RC, Carey V, Huber W, Irizarry R, Dudoit S (2005) Bioinformatics and Computational Biology Solutions Using R and Bioconductor: Springer Publications
19. Tusher VG, Tibshirani R, Chu G (2001) Significance analysis of microarrays applied to the ionizing radiation response. Proc Natl Acad Sci U S A 98: 5116–5121.
20. Famulski KS, de Freitas DG, Kreepala C, Chang J, Sellares J, et al. (2012) Molecular phenotypes of acute kidney injury in kidney transplants. J Am Soc Nephrol 23: 948–958.
21. Huang da W, Sherman BT, Lempicki RA (2009) Systematic and integrative analysis of large gene lists using DAVID bioinformatics resources. Nat Protoc 4: 44–57.
22. Grimson A, Farh KK, Johnston WK, Garrett-Engele P, Lim LP, et al. (2007) MicroRNA targeting specificity in mammals: determinants beyond seed pairing. Mol Cell 27: 91–105.
23. Maragkakis M, Alexiou P, Papadopoulos GL, Reczko M, Dalamagas T, et al. (2009) Accurate microRNA target prediction correlates with protein repression levels. BMC Bioinformatics 10: 295.
24. Miranda KC, Huynh T, Tay Y, Ang YS, Tam WL, et al. (2006) A pattern-based method for the identification of MicroRNA binding sites and their corresponding heteroduplexes. Cell 126: 1203–1217.
25. Hsu SD, Lin FM, Wu WY, Liang C, Huang WC, et al. (2011) miRTarBase: a database curates experimentally validated microRNA-target interactions. Nucleic Acids Res 39: D163–169.
26. McDonald R, Pereira F (2005) Identifying gene and protein mentions in text using conditional random fields. BMC Bioinformatics 6 Suppl 1: S6.
27. Jayaram D, Kommareddi M, Sung RS, Luan FL (2012) Delayed graft function requiring more than one-time dialysis treatment is associated with inferior clinical outcomes. Clin Transplant 26: E536–543.
28. Quiroga I, McShane P, Koo DD, Gray D, Friend PJ, et al. (2006) Major effects of delayed graft function and cold ischaemia time on renal allograft survival. Nephrol Dial Transplant 21: 1689–1696.
29. Abecassis M, Bridges ND, Clancy CJ, Dew MA, Eldadah B, et al. (2012) Solid-organ transplantation in older adults: current status and future research. Am J Transplant 12: 2608–2622.
30. Cohen B, Smits JM, Haase B, Persijn G, Vanrenterghem Y, et al. (2005) Expanding the donor pool to increase renal transplantation. Nephrol Dial Transplant 20: 34–41.
31. Tso PL, Dar WA, Henry ML (2012) With respect to elderly patients: finding kidneys in the context of new allocation concepts. Am J Transplant 12: 1091–1098.
32. SRTR Annual report 2011.
33. Cavaille-Coll M, Bala S, Velidedeoglu E, Hernandez A, Archdeacon P, et al. (2013) Summary of FDA workshop on ischemia reperfusion injury in kidney transplantation. Am J Transplant 13: 1134–1148.
34. Hauser P, Schwarz C, Mitterbauer C, Regele HM, Muhlbacher F, et al. (2004) Genome-wide gene-expression patterns of donor kidney biopsies distinguish primary allograft function. Lab Invest 84: 353–361.
35. Perco P, Kainz A, Wilflingseder J, Soleiman A, Mayer B, et al. (2009) Histogenomics: association of gene expression patterns with histological parameters in kidney biopsies. Transplantation 87: 290–295.
36. Mueller TF, Reeve J, Jhangri GS, Mengel M, Jacaj Z, et al. (2008) The transcriptome of the implant biopsy identifies donor kidneys at increased risk of delayed graft function. Am J Transplant 8: 78–85.
37. Hall IE, Yarlagadda SG, Coca SG, Wang Z, Doshi M, et al. (2010) IL-18 and urinary NGAL predict dialysis and graft recovery after kidney transplantation. J Am Soc Nephrol 21: 189–197.
38. Szeto CC, Kwan BC, Lai KB, Lai FM, Chow KM, et al. (2010) Urinary expression of kidney injury markers in renal transplant recipients. Clin J Am Soc Nephrol 5: 2329–2337.
39. Shao X, Tian L, Xu W, Zhang Z, Wang C, et al. (2014) Diagnostic value of urinary kidney injury molecule 1 for acute kidney injury: a meta-analysis. PLoS One 9: e84131.
40. Ohlsson S, Ljungkrantz I, Ohlsson K, Segelmark M, Wieslander J (2001) Novel distribution of the secretory leucocyte proteinase inhibitor in kidney. Mediators Inflamm 10: 347–350.
41. Sharif A, Borrows R (2013) Delayed graft function after kidney transplantation: the clinical perspective. Am J Kidney Dis 62: 150–158.
42. Rosin DL, Okusa MD (2011) Dangers within: DAMP responses to damage and cell death in kidney disease. J Am Soc Nephrol 22: 416–425.
43. Chen CZ, Schaffert S, Fragoso R, Loh C (2013) Regulation of immune responses and tolerance: the microRNA perspective. Immunol Rev 253: 112–128.
44. He L, Hannon GJ (2004) MicroRNAs: small RNAs with a big role in gene regulation. Nat Rev Genet 5: 522–531.
45. Stittrich AB, Haftmann C, Sgouroudis E, Kuhl AA, Hegazy AN, et al. (2010) The microRNA miR-182 is induced by IL-2 and promotes clonal expansion of activated helper T lymphocytes. Nat Immunol 11: 1057–1062.
46. Peng SL (2008) Foxo in the immune system. Oncogene 27: 2337–2344.
47. Kerdiles YM, Stone EL, Beisner DR, McGargill MA, Ch'en IL, et al. (2010) Foxo transcription factors control regulatory T cell development and function. Immunity 33: 890–904.
48. Peng X, Li W, Yuan L, Mehta RG, Kopelovich L, et al. (2013) Inhibition of proliferation and induction of autophagy by atorvastatin in PC3 prostate cancer cells correlate with downregulation of Bcl2 and upregulation of miR-182 and p21. PLoS One 8: e70442.
49. Yan D, Dong XD, Chen X, Yao S, Wang L, et al. (2012) Role of microRNA-182 in posterior uveal melanoma: regulation of tumor development through MITF, BCL2 and cyclin D2. PLoS One 7: e40967.
50. van Rooij E (2011) The art of microRNA research. Circulation research 108: 219–234.

Permissions

All chapters in this book were first published in PLOS ONE, by The Public Library of Science; hereby published with permission under the Creative Commons Attribution License or equivalent. Every chapter published in this book has been scrutinized by our experts. Their significance has been extensively debated. The topics covered herein carry significant findings which will fuel the growth of the discipline. They may even be implemented as practical applications or may be referred to as a beginning point for another development.

The contributors of this book come from diverse backgrounds, making this book a truly international effort. This book will bring forth new frontiers with its revolutionizing research information and detailed analysis of the nascent developments around the world.

We would like to thank all the contributing authors for lending their expertise to make the book truly unique. They have played a crucial role in the development of this book. Without their invaluable contributions this book wouldn't have been possible. They have made vital efforts to compile up to date information on the varied aspects of this subject to make this book a valuable addition to the collection of many professionals and students.

This book was conceptualized with the vision of imparting up-to-date information and advanced data in this field. To ensure the same, a matchless editorial board was set up. Every individual on the board went through rigorous rounds of assessment to prove their worth. After which they invested a large part of their time researching and compiling the most relevant data for our readers.

The editorial board has been involved in producing this book since its inception. They have spent rigorous hours researching and exploring the diverse topics which have resulted in the successful publishing of this book. They have passed on their knowledge of decades through this book. To expedite this challenging task, the publisher supported the team at every step. A small team of assistant editors was also appointed to further simplify the editing procedure and attain best results for the readers.

Apart from the editorial board, the designing team has also invested a significant amount of their time in understanding the subject and creating the most relevant covers. They scrutinized every image to scout for the most suitable representation of the subject and create an appropriate cover for the book.

The publishing team has been an ardent support to the editorial, designing and production team. Their endless efforts to recruit the best for this project, has resulted in the accomplishment of this book. They are a veteran in the field of academics and their pool of knowledge is as vast as their experience in printing. Their expertise and guidance has proved useful at every step. Their uncompromising quality standards have made this book an exceptional effort. Their encouragement from time to time has been an inspiration for everyone.

The publisher and the editorial board hope that this book will prove to be a valuable piece of knowledge for researchers, students, practitioners and scholars across the globe.

List of Contributors

Norikazu Hinamoto, Daisuke Saito, Hiroko Yamasaki, Katsuyuki Tanabe, Tatsuyo Nasu, Hiroyuki Watatani, Haruyo Ujike, Masaru Kinomura and Hirofumi Makino
Department of Medicine and Clinical Science, Okayama University Graduate School of Medicine, Dentistry and Pharmaceutical Sciences, Okayama, Japan

Yohei Maeshima
Department of Medicine and Clinical Science, Okayama University Graduate School of Medicine, Dentistry and Pharmaceutical Sciences, Okayama, Japan
Department of Chronic Kidney Disease and cardiovascular disease, Okayama University Graduate School of Medicine, Dentistry and Pharmaceutical Sciences, Okayama, Japan

Hitoshi Sugiyama
Department of Medicine and Clinical Science, Okayama University Graduate School of Medicine, Dentistry and Pharmaceutical Sciences, Okayama, Japan
Center for Chronic Kidney Disease and Peritoneal Dialysis, Okayama University Graduate School of Medicine, Dentistry and Pharmaceutical Sciences, Okayama, Japan

Hikaru Sonoda
Discovery Research Laboratories, Shionogi, Osaka, Japan

Yasufumi Sato
Department of Vascular Biology, Institute of Development, Aging, and Cancer, Tohoku University, Sendai, Japan

Marc Vincent
INSERM U775, Centre Universitaire des Saints Pères, Paris, France

Nicolas Pallet
INSERM U775, Centre Universitaire des Saints Pères, Paris, France
Service de Biochimie, Hôpital Européen Georges Pompidou, Assistance Publique-Hôpitaux de Paris, Paris, France
Service de Néphrologie, Hôpital Européen Georges Pompidou, Assistance Publique-Hôpitaux de Paris, Paris, France
Université Paris Descartes, Paris, France

Jean-François Chassé
INSERM U775, Centre Universitaire des Saints Pères, Paris, France
Université Paris Descartes, Paris, France

Philippe Beaune
INSERM U775, Centre Universitaire des Saints Pères, Paris, France
Service de Biochimie, Hôpital Européen Georges Pompidou, Assistance Publique-Hôpitaux de Paris, Paris, France
Université Paris Descartes, Paris, France

Diane Nga-Matsogo and Alexandre Karras
Service de Néphrologie, Hôpital Européen Georges Pompidou, Assistance Publique-Hôpitaux de Paris, Paris, France

Sophie Chauvet, Charlene Levi and Eric Thervet
Service de Néphrologie, Hôpital Européen Georges Pompidou, Assistance Publique-Hôpitaux de Paris, Paris, France
Université Paris Descartes, Paris, France

Vannary Meas-Yedid and Jean-Christophe Olivo-Marin
Unitéd'Analyse d'image quantitative, Institut Pasteur, Paris, France

Paul Avillach
Departement d'informatique médicale, Hôpital Européen Georges Pompidou, Assistance Publique-Hôpitaux de Paris, Paris, France
Université Paris Descartes, Paris, France

Xiangju Wang, Andrew J. Kassianos, Steven Zuryn, Kathrein E. Roper, Andrew Osborne, Sandeep Sampangi and Helen Healy
Conjoint Kidney Research Laboratory, Pathology Queensland, Brisbane, Queensland, Australia
Department of Renal Medicine, Royal Brisbane and Women's Hospital, Brisbane, Queensland, Australia

Ray Wilkinson
Conjoint Kidney Research Laboratory, Pathology Queensland, Brisbane, Queensland, Australia
Department of Renal Medicine, Royal Brisbane and Women's Hospital, Brisbane, Queensland, Australia

Institute of Health and Biomedical Innovation, Queensland University of Technology, Brisbane, Queensland, Australia
Medical School, University of Queensland, Brisbane, Queensland, Australia

Vishwas Raghunath
Department of Renal Medicine, Royal Brisbane and Women's Hospital, Brisbane, Queensland, Australia

Leo Francis
Pathology Queensland, Brisbane, Queensland, Australia

Chin Lin
Graduate Institute of Life Sciences, National Defense Medical Center, Taipei, Taiwan, ROC

Hsin-Yi Yang, Chi-Ming Chu, Fu-Huang Lin, Sen-Yeong Kao and Sui-Lung Su
School of Public Health, National Defense Medical Center, Taipei, Taiwan, ROC

Chia-Chao Wu
Division of Nephrology, Department of Medicine, Tri-Service General Hospital, National Defense Medical Center, Taipei, Taiwan, ROC

Yuh-Feng Lin
Division of Nephrology, Department of Medicine, Tri-Service General Hospital, National Defense Medical Center, Taipei, Taiwan, ROC
Division of Nephrology, Department of Medicine, Shuang Ho Hospital, Graduate Institute of Clinical Medicine, Taipei Medical University, New Taipei City, Taiwan, ROC

Herng-Sheng Lee
Division of Pathology, Tri-Service General Hospital, National Defense Medical Center, Taipei, Taiwan, ROC

Kuo-Cheng Lu
Division of Nephrology, Department of Medicine, Cardinal Tien Hospital, School of Medicine, Fu Jen Catholic University, New Taipei City, Taiwan, ROC

Takashige Kuwabara, Hideki Yokoi, Hirotaka Imamaki, Akira Ishii, Kenichi Koga and Masashi Mukoyama
Department of Medicine and Clinical Science, Kyoto University Graduate School of Medicine, Kyoto, Japan

Kiyoshi Mori and Kazuwa Nakao
Department of Medicine and Clinical Science, Kyoto University Graduate School of Medicine, Kyoto, Japan
Medical Innovation Center, Kyoto University Graduate School of Medicine, Kyoto, Japan

Masato Kasahara
Department of Medicine and Clinical Science, Kyoto University Graduate School of Medicine, Kyoto, Japan
Department of EBM Research, Institute for Advancement of Clinical and Translational Science, Kyoto University Hospital, Kyoto, Japan

Shinji Yasuno and Kenji Ueshima
Department of EBM Research, Institute for Advancement of Clinical and Translational Science, Kyoto University Hospital, Kyoto, Japan

Akira Sugawara
Department of Nephrology, Osaka Red Cross Hospital, Osaka, Japan

Takashi Morikawa, Yoshio Konishi and Masahito Imanishi
Division of Nephrology and Hypertension, Osaka City General Hospital, Osaka, Japan

Akira Nishiyama
Department of Pharmacology, Kagawa University Medical School, Kagawa, Japan

Ya-Ling Zhai, Li Zhu, Su-Fang Shi, Li-Jun Liu, Ji-Cheng Lv and Hong Zhang
Renal Division, Department of Medicine, Peking University First Hospital, Beijing, China
Peking University Institute of Nephrology, Beijing, China
Key Laboratory of Renal Disease, Ministry of Health of China, Beijing, China
Key Laboratory of Chronic Kidney Disease Prevention and Treatment (Peking University), Ministry of Education, Beijing, China

Beatriz Santamaria and Luis Miguel Blanco-Colio
Laboratory of Nephrology, IIS-Fundacion Jimenez Diaz, Madrid, Spain

Ana Belen Sanz
Laboratory of Nephrology, IIS-Fundacion Jimenez Diaz, Madrid, Spain
REDinREN, Madrid, Spain

Marta Ruiz-Ortega
Laboratory of Nephrology, IIS-Fundacion Jimenez Diaz, Madrid, Spain
REDinREN, Madrid, Spain
Universidad Autonoma de Madrid, Madrid, Spain

Jesus Egido
Laboratory of Nephrology, IIS-Fundacion Jimenez Diaz, Madrid, Spain
Universidad Autonoma de Madrid, Madrid, Spain
IRSIN, Madrid, Spain

Alberto Ortiz
Laboratory of Nephrology, IIS-Fundacion Jimenez Diaz, Madrid, Spain
REDinREN, Madrid, Spain
Universidad Autonoma de Madrid, Madrid, Spain
IRSIN, Madrid, Spain

Luiz Stark Aroeira
Department of Immunology, Instituto de Investigación Biomédica de Vigo (IBIV), Vigo, Pontevedra, Spain

Teresa Bellon
Department of Nephrology, IDIPAZ, Madrid, Spain

Gloria del Peso and Maria Dolores Sanchez-Niño
Department of Nephrology, IDIPAZ, Madrid, Spain
REDinREN, Madrid, Spain

Jose Jimenez-Heffernan
Hospital Universitario de la Princesa, Madrid, Spain

Manuel Lopez-Cabrera
REDinREN, Madrid, Spain
Centro Biologia Molecular Severo Ochoa, Madrid, Spain

Rafael Selgas
Department of Nephrology, IDIPAZ, Madrid, Spain
REDinREN, Madrid, Spain

Zhao Cui, Shui-Yi Hu, Xiao-Yu Jia, Rui Yang, Xin Zheng, Jie Ao and Gang Liu
Renal Division, Department of Medicine, Peking University First Hospital, Peking University Institute of Nephrology, Key Laboratory of Renal Disease, Ministry of Health of China, Key Laboratory of Chronic Kidney Disease Prevention and Treatment (Peking University), Ministry of Education of China, Beijing, China

Rui Ma
Renal Division, Department of Medicine, Peking University First Hospital, Peking University Institute of Nephrology, Key Laboratory of Renal Disease, Ministry of Health of China, Key Laboratory of Chronic Kidney Disease Prevention and Treatment (Peking University), Ministry of Education of China, Beijing, China
Renal Division, Department of Medicine, First Affiliated Hospital of Guangxi Medical University, Nanning, Guangxi Zhuang Autonomous Region, China

Ming-Hui Zhao
Renal Division, Department of Medicine, Peking University First Hospital, Peking University Institute of Nephrology, Key Laboratory of Renal Disease, Ministry of Health of China, Key Laboratory of Chronic Kidney Disease Prevention and Treatment (Peking University), Ministry of Education of China, Beijing, China
Peking-Tsinghua Center for Life Sciences, Beijing, China

Yun-Hua Liao
Renal Division, Department of Medicine, First Affiliated Hospital of Guangxi Medical University, Nanning, Guangxi Zhuang Autonomous Region, China

Takahito Moriyama, Kayu Tanaka, Chihiro Iwasaki, Yasuko Oshima, Ayami Ochi, Hiroshi Kataoka, Mitsuyo Itabashi, Takashi Takei, Keiko Uchida and Kosaku Nitta
Department of Medicine, Kidney Center, Tokyo Women's Medical University, Tokyo, Japan

Michio Nagata
Department of Kidney and Vascular Pathology, University of Tsukuba, Tsukuba, Japan

Satoshi Hara
Department of Kidney and Vascular Pathology, University of Tsukuba, Tsukuba, Japan
Division of Rheumatology, Department of Internal Medicine, Kanazawa University of Graduate School of Medicine, Kanazawa, Japan

Kazuhiro Umeyama and Hiroshi Nagashima
Meiji University International Institute for Bio-Resource Research, Kawasaki, Japan

Takashi Yokoo
Division of Nephrology and Hypertension, Department of Internal Medicine, The Jikei University School of Medicine, Tokyo, Japan

Yu Du, Junhua Li, Fan He, Yongman Lv, Wei Liu and Hongyu Gao
Department of Nephrology, Tongji hospital affiliated to Tongji medical college, Huazhong University of Science and Technology, Wuhan, Hubei, China

Ping Wu
Department of Pathophysiology, Tongji Medical College, Huazhong University of Science and Technology, Wuhan, Hubei, China

Jiao Huang and Sheng Wei
Department of Epidemiology and Biostatistics, School of Public Health, Tongji Medical College, Huazhong University of Science and Technology, Wuhan, Hubei, China

Lotta Tengroth, Julia Arebro, Susanna Kumlien Georén and Lars-Olaf Cardell
Division of Ear, Nose and Throat Diseases, Department of Clinical Sciences, Intervention and Technology, Karolinska Institutet, Stockholm, Sweden

Ola Winqvist
Department of Medicine, Unit of Translational Immunology, Karolinska Institute, Stockholm, Sweden

Christine A. Murakami, Derek M. Fine, Mohamed G. Atta, Gregory M. Lucas and Michelle M. Estrella
Department of Medicine, Johns Hopkins University School of Medicine, Baltimore, Maryland, United States of America

Doaa Attia
Faculty of Medicine, Alexandria, Egypt

Naima Carter-Monroe
Department of Pathology, Johns Hopkins University School of Medicine, Baltimore, Maryland, United States of America

Phong T. Le, Meghan M. Pearce, Shubin Zhang, Edward M. Campbell and Alan J. Wolfe
Department of Microbiology and Immunology, Stritch School of Medicine, Loyola University Chicago, Maywood, Illinois, United States of America

Elizabeth R. Mueller, Cynthia A. Brincat and Linda Brubaker
Department of Obstetrics and Gynecology, Stritch School of Medicine, Loyola University Chicago, Maywood, Illinois, United States of America

Cynthia S. Fok
University of Minnesota, Department of Urology, Minneapolis, Minnesota, United States of America

Tao Zhang, Shaoshan Liang, Dacheng Chen, Chunxia Zheng, Caihong Zeng, Haitao Zhang and Zhihong Liu
National Clinical Research Center of Kidney Diseases, Jinling Hospital, Nanjing University School of Medicine, Nanjing 210002, P. R. China

Huimei Chen
National Clinical Research Center of Kidney Diseases, Jinling Hospital, Nanjing University School of Medicine, Nanjing 210002 P. R. China
Jiangsu Key Laboratory of Molecular Medicine, Nanjing University School of Medicine, Nanjing, 2100093, P. R. China

Chester Whitley
Department of Pediatrics, University of Minnesota, Minneapolis, United States of America

Michael Mauer
Department of Pediatrics, University of Minnesota, Minneapolis, United States of America
Department of Medicine, University of Minnesota, Minneapolis, United States of America

Emily Glynn, Alexey Sokolovskiy and Behzad Najafian
Department of Pathology, University of Washington, Seattle, United States of America,

Einar Svarstad
Department of Medicine, Haukeland University Hospital, Bergen, Norway
Department of Clinical Medicine, University of Bergen, Bergen, Norway

Camilla Tøndel
Department of Clinical Medicine, University of Bergen, Bergen, Norway
Department of Pediatrics, Haukeland University Hospital, Bergen, Norway

Marie-Claire Gubler
U983, Université René Descartes, Hôpital Necker-Enfants Malades AP-HP, Paris, France

Michael West
Division of Nephrology, Department of Medicine, Dalhousie University, Halifax, Nova Scotia, Canada

Martin Tepel, Christoffer Borst and Claus Bistrup
Department of Nephrology, Odense University Hospital, and University of Southern Denmark, Institute of Molecular Medicine, Cardiovascular and Renal Research, Institute of Clinical Research, Odense, Denmark

Niels Marcussen
Department of Pathology, Odense University Hospital, and University of Southern Denmark, Odense, Denmark

Nikolaos Pagonas, Timm H. Westhoff and Felix S. Seibert
Department of Nephrology, Charité, Campus Benjamin Franklin, Berlin, Germany
Medizinische Klinik I, Univ.-Klinik Marienhospital Herne, Ruhr-University Bochum, Bochum, Germany

Robert Arndt and Walter Zidek
Department of Nephrology, Charité, Campus Benjamin Franklin, Berlin, Germany

Ikechi G. Okpechi, Thandiwe A. L. Dlamini, Brian L. Rayner and Charles R. Swanepoel
Division of Nephrology and Hypertension, Groote Schuur Hospital and University of Cape Town, South Africa

Maureen Duffield
Division of Anatomical Pathology, National Health and Laboratory Services (NHLS), University of Cape Town, South Africa

George Moturi
Department of Medicine, Aga Khan University Hospital, Nairobi, Kenya

Noriaki Kitamura, Takahiro Yamaguchi and Yoshiko Iwai
Department of Molecular Biology, School of Medicine, University of Occupational and Environmental Health, Kitakyushu, Japan

Akihiro Kuma
Department of Molecular Biology, School of Medicine, University of Occupational and Environmental Health, Kitakyushu, Japan
Second Department of Internal Medicine, Cardiology and Nephrology, School of Medicine, University of Occupational and Environmental Health, Kitakyushu, Japan

Masahito Tamura and Yutaka Otsuji
Second Department of Internal Medicine, Cardiology and Nephrology, School of Medicine, University of Occupational and Environmental Health, Kitakyushu, Japan

Sohsuke Yamada
Department of Pathology and Cell Biology, School of Medicine, University of Occupational and Environmental Health, Kitakyushu, Japan

Ke-Yong Wang
Bio-information Research Center, University of Occupational and Environmental Health, Kitakyushu, Japan

Hiroto Izumi
Department of Occupational Pneumology, Institute of Industrial Ecological Science, University of Occupational and Environmental Health, Kitakyushu, Japan

Kimitoshi Kohno
The President Laboratory, University of Occupational and Environmental Health, Kitakyushu, Japan

Shi-Jun Li, Hui-Ping Chen, Ying-Hua Chen, Li-hua Zhang, Yuan-Mao Tu and Zhi-hong Liu
National Clinical Research Center of Kidney Diseases, Jinling Hospital, Nanjing University of Medcine, Nanjing, China

Li-Hao Chen, Suzanne L. Advani, Kerri Thai, M. Golam Kabir, Darren A. Yuen, Kim A. Connelly, Philip A. Marsden, Richard E. Gilbert and Andrew Advani
Keenan Research Centre for Biomedical Science and Li Ka Shing Knowledge Institute of St. Michael's Hospital, Toronto, Ontario, Canada

Manish M. Sood
Ottawa Hospital Research Institute, University of Ottawa, Ottawa, Ontario, Canada

Ian W. Gibson
Health Sciences Centre, University of Manitoba, Winnipeg, Manitoba, Canada

Darren J. Kelly
Department of Medicine, St. Vincent's Hospital, Melbourne, Victoria, Australia

Ying Fan, Wenzhen Xiao and Niansong Wang
Department of Nephrology, Shanghai Jiao Tong University Affiliated Sixth People's Hospital, Shanghai, China

John Cijiang He, Chengguo Wei, Weijia Zhang and Peter Y. Chuang
Division of Nephrology, Department of Medicine, Icahn School of Medicine at Mount Sinai, New York, New York, United States of America

Hans M. Larsson and Jeffrey A. Hubbell
Laboratory for Regenerative Medicine and Pharmacobiology, Institute for Bioengineering, School of Life Sciences and School of Engineering, Ecole Polytechnique Fédérale de Lausanne, Lausanne, Switzerland

Yann Barrandon and Francois Gorostidi
Laboratory of Experimental Surgery, Department of Experimental Surgery, Centre Hospitalier Universitaire Vaudois, Lausanne, Switzerland
Laboratory of Stem Cell Dynamics, Institute for Bioengineering, School of Life Sciences, Ecole Polytechnique Fédérale de Lausanne, Lausanne, Switzerland

Peter Frey
Laboratory for Regenerative Medicine and Pharmacobiology, Institute for Bioengineering, School of Life Sciences and School of Engineering, Ecole Polytechnique Fédérale de Lausanne, Lausanne, Switzerland
Laboratory of Experimental Pediatric Urology, Department of Pediatric Urology, Centre Hospitalier Universitaire Vaudois, Lausanne, Switzerland

Joerg Latus, Daniel Kitterer, M. Dominik Alscher and Niko Braun
Department of Internal Medicine, Division of Nephrology, Robert-Bosch Hospital, Auerbachstrasse 0, Stuttgart, Germany

Daniel Cadar, Klara Tenner-Racz and Paul Racz
Bernhard Nocht Institute for Tropical Medicine, WHO Collaborating Centre for Arbovirus and Haemmorrhagic Fever Reference and Research, Bernhard-Nocht-Strasse , Hamburg, Germany

German Ott
Department of Diagnostic Medicine, Division of Pathology, Robert-Bosch Hospital, Auerbachstrasse 110, Stuttgart, Germany

Jonas Schmidt-Chanasit
Bernhard Nocht Institute for Tropical Medicine, WHO Collaborating Centre for Arbovirus and Haemmorrhagic Fever Reference and Research, Bernhard-Nocht-Strasse , Hamburg, Germany
German Centre for Infection Research (DZIF), partner site Hamburg-Luebeck-Borstel, Hamburg, Germany

Makoto Yamaguchi, Shinichi Akiyama, Sawako Kato, Takayuki Katsuno, Tomoki Kosugi, Waichi Sato, Naotake Tsuboi, Yoshinari Yasuda, Masashi Mizuno, Yasuhiko Ito, Seiichi Matsuo and Shoichi Maruyama
Department of Nephrology, Nagoya University Graduate School of Medicine, Nagoya, Japan

Masahiko Ando
Center for Advanced Medicine and Clinical Research, Nagoya University Hospital, Nagoya, Japan

Ryohei Yamamoto
Department of Geriatric Medicine and Nephrology, Osaka University Graduate School of Medicine, Suita, Japan

Desmond Y. H. Yap, Susan Yung, Qing Zhang, Colin Tang and Tak Mao Chan
Division of Nephrology, Department of Medicine, Queen Mary Hospital, The University of Hong Kong, Hong Kong

Julia M. Hofstra, Jo H. M. Berden, Johan van der Vlag, Jack F. M. Wetzels and Tom Nijenhuis
Department of Nephrology, Radboud university medical center, Nijmegen, the Netherlands

Marieke J. H. Coenen, Mascha M. V. A. P. Schijvenaars, Lies H. Hoefsloot and Nine V. A. M. Knoers
Department of Human Genetics, Radboud university medical center, Nijmegen, the Netherlands

Julia Wil lingseder, Alexander Kainz and Rainer Oberbauer
Department of Nephrology and Dialysis, Medical University Vienna, Vienna, Austria
Department of Nephrology and Transplantation, KH Elisabethinen, Linz, Austria

Judith Sunzenauer
Department of Nephrology and Transplantation, KH Elisabethinen, Linz, Austria

Eva Toronyi, Gábor Telkes and Robert M. Langer
Department of Transplantation and Surgery, Semmelweis University, Budapest, Hungary

Andreas Heinzel, Bernd Mayer and Paul Perco
emergentec biodevelopment GmbH, Vienna, Austria

Index